INFLAMMATORY BOWEL DISEASE

Genetics, Barrier Function, Immunologic Mechanisms, and Microbial Pathways

T0339434

ANNALS OF THE NEW YORK ACADEMY OF SCIENCES
Volume 1072

INFLAMMATORY BOWEL DISEASE

Genetics, Barrier Function, Immunologic Mechanisms, and Microbial Pathways

Edited by
Wolfram W. Domschke, Martin F. Kagnoff, Torsten F. Kucharzik,
Lloyd F. Mayer, and Stephan R. Targan

Published by Blackwell Publishing on behalf of the New York Academy of Sciences
Boston, Massachusetts
2006

Library of Congress Cataloging-in-Publication Data

Inflammatory bowel disease : genetics, barrier function, immunologic
mechanisms, and microbial pathways / edited by Wolfram W.
Domschke ... [et al.].
   p. ; cm. – (Annals of the New York Academy of Sciences,
ISSN 0077-8923 ; v. 1072)
   ISBN-13: 978-1-57331-568-5 (alk. paper)
   ISBN-10: 1-57331-568-0 (alk. paper)
   1. Inflammatory bowel diseases–Congresses. I. Domschke,
Wolfram. II. New York Academy of Sciences. III. Series.
   [DNLM: 1. Inflammatory Bowel Diseases–genetics–Congresses.
2. Inflammatory Bowel Diseases–immunology–Congresses.
3. Inflammatory Bowel Diseases–microbiology–Congresses.
W1 AN626YL v.1072 2006 / WI 420 I4238 2006]

   RC862.I53I54 2006
   616.3'44–dc22

                  2006016183

The *Annals of the New York Academy of Sciences* (ISSN: 0077-8923 [print]; ISSN: 1749-6632 [online]) is published 28 times a year on behalf of the New York Academy of Sciences by Blackwell Publishing, with offices located at 350 Main Street, Malden, Massachusetts 02148 USA, PO Box 1354, Garsington Road, Oxford OX4 2DQ UK, and PO Box 378 Carlton South, 3053 Victoria Australia.

Information for subscribers: Subscription prices for 2006 are: Premium Institutional: $3850.00 (US) and £2139.00 (Europe and Rest of World).
Customers in the UK should add VAT at 5%. Customers in the EU should also add VAT at 5% or provide a VAT registration number or evidence of entitlement to exemption. Customers in Canada should add 7% GST or provide evidence of entitlement to exemption. The Premium Institutional price also includes online access to full-text articles from 1997 to present, where available. For other pricing options or more information about online access to Blackwell Publishing journals, including access information and terms and conditions, please visit www.blackwellpublishing.com/nyas.

Membership information: Members may order copies of the *Annals* volumes directly from the Academy by visiting www.nyas.org/annals, emailing membership@nyas.org, faxing 212-888-2894, or calling 800-843-6927 (US only), or +1 212 838 0230, ext. 345 (International). For more information on becoming a member of the New York Academy of Sciences, please visit www.nyas.org/membership.

Journal Customer Services: For ordering information, claims, and any inquiry concerning your institutional subscription, please contact your nearest office:
UK: Email: customerservices@blackwellpublishing.com; Tel: +44 (0) 1865 778315; Fax +44 (0) 1865 471775
US: Email: customerservices@blackwellpublishing.com; Tel: +1 781 388 8599 or 1 800 835 6770 (Toll free in the USA); Fax: +1 781 388 8232
Asia: Email: customerservices@blackwellpublishing.com; Tel: +65 6511 8000; Fax: +61 3 8359 1120
Members: Claims and inquiries on member orders should be directed to the Academy at email: membership@nyas.org or Tel: +1 212 838 0230 (International) or 800-843-6927 (US only).

Mailing: The *Annals of the New York Academy of Sciences* are mailed Standard Rate.
Postmaster: Send all address changes to *Annals of the New York Academy of Sciences*, Blackwell Publishing, Inc., Journals Subscription Department, 350 Main Street, Malden, MA 01248-5020. Mailing to rest of world by DHL Smart and Global Mail.

Disclaimer: The Publisher, the New York Academy of Sciences, and the Editors cannot be held responsible for errors or any consequences arising from the use of information contained in this publication; the views and opinions expressed do not necessarily reflect those of the Publisher, the New York Academy of Sciences, or the Editors.

Annals are available to subscribers online at the New York Academy of Sciences and also at Blackwell Synergy. Visit www.annalsnyas.org or www.blackwell-synergy.com to search the articles and register for table of contents e-mail alerts. Access to full text and PDF downloads of *Annals* articles are available to nonmembers and subscribers on a pay-per-view basis at www.annalsnyas.org.

The paper used in this publication meets the minimum requirements of the National Standard for Information Sciences Permanence of Paper for Printed Library Materials, ANSI Z39.48-1984.

ISSN: 0077-8923 (print); 1749-6632 (online)
ISBN-10: 1-57331-568-0 (paper); ISBN-13: 978-1-57331-568-5 (paper)

A catalogue record for this title is available from the British Library.

ANNALS OF THE NEW YORK ACADEMY OF SCIENCES

Volume 1072
August 2006

INFLAMMATORY BOWEL DISEASE
Genetics, Barrier Function, Immunologic Mechanisms, and Microbial Pathways

Editors
WOLFRAM W. DOMSCHKE, MARTIN F. KAGNOFF, TORSTEN F. KUCHARZIK,
LLOYD F. MAYER, AND STEPHAN R. TARGAN

This volume is the result of the international symposium **Inflammatory Bowel Disease: Research Drives Clinics—Genetics, Barrier Function, Immunological and Microbial Pathways**, held on September 1–3, 2005, in Münster, Germany.

CONTENTS

Part III. Barrier Function

The conference was supported by:

- Crohn's & Colitis Foundation of America (CCFA)
- Deutsche Forschungsgemeinschaft (DFG)

Major funding was received from:

- Baxter
- Braun
- Centocor
- Essex
- Falk

Financial assistance was received from:

- Abbott
- Altana
- Ardeypharm
- Ashai
- AstraZeneca
- Bayer Vital
- Eisai
- Ferring
- Förderkreis der Universität Münster
- Fresenius
- Fujinon GmbH
- Immundiagnostik
- Medinal Medizinprodukte GmbH
- Miltenyi Biotec
- MSD Sharp & Dohme
- New England Biolabs/Cell Signalling Technology
- Novartis
- Schering
- Sigma Tau
- UCB Celltech
- Wyeth Pharma

Preface

The International Symposium on Inflammatory Bowel Disease (IBD), on which this volume of the *Annals* is based, was held in Münster, Germany, September 2–3, 2005. At this meeting, about 450 participants from more than 30 countries gathered to translate recent advances in basic sciences into clinical IBD management and to explore potential future strategies for treatment. This translational effort informed and encompassed the orchestration of factors and processes that eventually lead to the manifest disease: these include genetic and immunologic factors, an interaction of the enteric microflora with the underlying mucosa, and a disrupted barrier function. Our vision was to have a symposium that might build bridges between basic scientists and clinicians as well as provide a discussion platform for both internationally renowned senior investigators and young researchers dedicated to unraveling the intricacies of the diseased intestinal mucosa. The present volume represents the symposium's plenary lectures as well as those poster presentations that were awarded poster prizes.

For enabling us to hold this IBD symposium and produce this volume, the organizers gratefully acknowledge the contributions of the German Research Council (DFG) and the Crohn's & Colitis Foundation of America (CCFA), which provided funding for travel scholarships, as well as the many industry contributors listed in the Table of Contents.

Finally, we wish to particularly acknowledge and express our appreciation to the scientific secretaries of the Münster symposium, Dr. Andreas Lügering and Dr. Christian Maaser, for their invaluable help in making both the meeting and the publication a success.

—WOLFRAM W. DOMSCHKE
Münster, Germany

—MARTIN F. KAGNOFF
La Jolla, California

—TORSTEN F. KUCHARZIK
Münster, Germany

—LLOYD F. MAYER
New York, New York

—STEPHAN R. TARGAN
Los Angeles, California

Ann. N.Y. Acad. Sci. 1372: xi (2006). © 2006 New York Academy of Sciences.
doi: 10.1196/annals.1326.040

Current Limitations of IBD Treatment

Where Do We Go from Here?

STEPHAN R. TARGAN

Inflammatory Bowel Disease Center and Immunobiology Research Institute, Celare-Sinai Medical Center, Los Angeles California 90048, USA

ABSTRACT: Great progress has been made over the last decade in the development of targeted specific therapies for inflammatory bowel disease. Nevertheless, accumulating experience with these modalities and results from ongoing investigations of agents currently on the market and those in development have demonstrated that efficacy may be limited to certain patient phenotypes. Recently, great interest has been applied to studies of the interplay between the adaptive and innate immune responses to achieve a better understanding of the immunopathogeneses of inflammatory bowel diseases as well as to identify targets for even more potent intervention.

KEYWORDS: inflammatory bowel disease; biologic therapy; anti-tumor necrosis factor (TNF); mucosal inflammation

Accelerated research over the last five years has led to great advances in scientific discovery and has expanded our understanding of the inflammatory bowel diseases and their underlying pathophysiologic mechanisms. Studies have provided evidence for the hypothesis that inflammatory bowel diseases are result of a genetic predisposition that leads to a mucosal immune regulatory cell defect and susceptibility to environmental triggers, particularly luminal bacteria, including specific antigens and pathogen-associated molecular patterns (PAMPs). Most recently it has become apparent that this dysfunction occurs from an abnormal relationship between innate immune responses to bacterial structures mediated via toll and other receptors and the adaptive immune response.

An imbalance between several effector cell types, including T cells and NK-T cells, and a vast array of T regulatory cells is the likely cause of inflammation. In addition to these findings, there have been several novel pathways and specific targets upon which to focus new therapeutics. The "holy grail" of IBD treatment is to avoid chronic steroid usage in an attempt to prevent disease progression

Address for correspondence: Dr. Stephan R. Targan, M.D., Cedars-Sinai Medical Center, 8700 Beverly Blvd., Suite D4063, Los Angeles CA 90048 USA. Voice: 310-423-0540; fax: 310-423-0224. e-mail: Stephan.Targan@cshs.org

Ann. N.Y. Acad. Sci. 1072: 1–8 (2006). © 2006 New York Academy of Sciences.
doi: 10.1196/annals.1326.032

TABLE 1. Initial efficacy of biologics for Crohn's Disease—anti-TNF

Drug	Absolute benefit (%)	Relative benefit (%)
Infliximab (Ref. 28)	$48^a/29^a$	282/725
Adalimumab (Ref. 29)	18^a	150
Certolizumab (Ref. 30)	$NS^a/32^b$	NS/178

[a] Primary
[n] Post hoc

and to eliminate the need for surgery, and, of course, to identify markers of disease susceptibility to prevent its expression. In 1993, when the effort began to identify specific interventions in the underlying disease process, there were very few products and only a single target being developed. In 2005, there are greater than 30 products, consisting of monoclonal antibodies, small-molecule molecular techniques including antisense mRNA, peptides, and vaccines. More than 10 targets are being pursued and multiple pathways are being explored, ranging from the bacterial host interaction and dendritic cell biology all the way to preventing cell recirculation into the mucosa by blocking integrin-adhesion molecules, globally and selectively, including the prevention of CCR9+ T cells from homing to the small bowel.

Therefore, two questions arise: (1) With several novel therapies already available, what are the limitations and (2) is there any need for further development? The first question addresses the efficacy of our current therapeutics, particularly immediate induction of remission, sustained maintenance of remission, and the value of subgroup analysis. Among the important considerations is initial efficacy of tribiologic therapies (TABLE 1), which at this point are predominantly inhibitors of TNF. The "absolute benefit" in therapeutic trials refers to the percentage difference between effectiveness of treatment among patients receiving active compound versus placebo. The absolute benefit of anti-TNF therapies, whether looking at response and/or remission, even with infliximab, ranges from 20–29%. Studies of the new anti-TNF compounds, adalimumab and certolizumab (under development) resulted in an absolute benefit of 32%. Among other biologics under development (TABLE 2), from

TABLE 2. Initial efficacy of biologics for Crohn's Disease—other

Drug	Absolute benefit (%)	Relative benefit (%)
Anti-α4 (Ref. 1)	$NS/15^a$	NS/107
Anti-IL-12 (Ref. 31)	50^b	200
Anti-IFN-γ (Ref. 2)	$61\ddagger/54^c$	436/∞
GMCSF (Ref. 32)	$10\S/22^a$	23/61

NOTE: $P = NS$.
[a] Secondary
[b] Primary
[c] Post hoc

TABLE 3. Initial efficacy of biologics for ulcerative colitis

Drug	Absolute benefit (%)	Relative benefit (%)
α4β7 (Ref. 33)	19[a]	136
Infliximab (Ref. 4)	31*/24	84/160
Anti-CD3 (Ref. 20)	~60%	?

[a] Primary

antiα4 to the administration of GMCSF, the absolute benefit is anywhere from 15 to 60%.

As can be assumed from the statistics shown, most of the biologics are effective in only a subpopulation of patients. The efficacy of induction of remission among biologics for ulcerative colitis treated with antiα4β7 and infliximab is 25–30%, and effectiveness decreases over the long term (TABLE 3). In general, there is less than 40% benefit over a placebo. Infliximab (anti-TNF), the most studied biologic, only induces sustained clinical remission at 54 weeks in fever than 25% of Crohn's disease patients, and factoring in steroid withdrawal at week 54, the number drops to below 20%. Thus, even with the best biologic long term, only 25% of patients can be maintained at 1 year. For nataluzimab (antiα4) the best absolute difference is 24% at 15 months with 50% able to get steroids. In ulcerative colitis, the Active Ulcerative Colitis I and II trials of infliximab have shown an absolute difference of 34% of patients in remission at week 30, and for those who have been able to discontinue steroids at week 30, the absolute difference is around 20%. In considering the overall population, even the most novel therapeutics that are either approved for treatment or are in late-phase development, the efficacy is limited.

The approach that considers disease subgroup analysis includes the supposition that subpopulations exist within the larger groups of patients with Crohn's disease and ulcerative colitis among which the efficacy rate and absolute response rates would be greater. Such has been demonstrated by the ENACT I trial[1] that initially appeared to be negative. Post-trial analysis demonstrated that where the initial intent to treat was negative, when the study population was separated into three groups, those patients who were C-reactive protein (CRP)-positive, those who were on immunomodulators, and those who were both CRP+ and on immunomodulators, the placebo rate decreased, the efficacy rate remained the same and thus a significant difference was shown between the treatment and placebo groups. Another case in which further analysis revealed a significant result is the trial of anti-interferon-γ for Crohn's disease.[2] Patients with elevated C-reactive protein levels greater than 4 mg/L had significant and somewhat durable responses to treatment, with up to 50% achieving remission and a marked decrease in the placebo effect.

Another issue that arises in the use of biologics, particularly monoclonal antibodies, is attenuation or loss of efficacy over time, secondary to the induction of antibodies to the therapeutic monoclonal. In infliximab treatment, several trials demonstrated 9–17% induction of these anti-antibodies.[3,4] When infliximab levels are correlated with anti-antibody development, treatment response following an infusion is shown to be affected by levels of anti-antibodies. The key result of these analyses is the finding that those patients who are on immunosuppressants prior to getting antibody infusions have the lowest level of anti-antibody development.

With such profound manipulations of the immune system come infectious complications. These infections will occur both early and late in treatment. A small percentage of patients after several infusions with anti-TNF modalities develop reactivation of latent tuberculosis and/or other intercellular pathogens, such as histoplasmosis or coccidioidomycosis.[5,6] Initially thought to induce very few infectious complications, in ongoing observation of patients receiving nataluzimab, it became clear that a very small percentage of patients (approximately 0.1%) developed multifocal leukoencephalopathy (PML) 1 to 2 years after infusion.[7–11] Therefore we have a long way to go in our peach for the Holy Grail of IBD treatment, despite the recent development of more potent biologics.

Where will we find the novel targets for therapeutic development and how are we going to investigate their optimal efficacy? Several genetic loci on various chromosomes have been shown to be linked with inflammatory bowel disease. The vast majority of these are related to Crohn's disease, but recently some associated with ulcerative colitis have been reported. The two associations that have been substantiated are functional variants within genes that are critically important for the host sampling of commensal bacterial populations. NOD2[12,13] variants are critically important for sampling muramyl dipeptide (a structure on gram-negative bacteria) and, most recently, a lack of bacterial signaling in the promoter was shown in IBD5-associated organic transporter gene (OCTN)[14] that alters the bacterial induction of host responses. It is likely that gene abnormalities occur in both innate immune pathways as well as adaptive immune pathways. It is quite possible that patients who have mild, nonprogressive disease may have a single gene defect with no defects in the adaptive immune response. On the other hand, those patients that have greater than one defect in innate immunity coupled with one or more gene defects in T cell or cytokine expression would have a markedly increased adaptive immune response that leads to severe disease.

As for the question of where and how we are going to come upon these targets, one approach would be to discover the specific genes within chromosomal regions and define which pathways are affected. Finally, a diligent awareness of general scientific accomplishments that will lead to novel findings may relate to aberrant functions in mucosal inflammation. An example of the latter is found by studying the biology of some TNF superfamily molecules. Specifically, transgenic mice expressing LIGHT[a]1 on T cells develop a mucosal

---

[a]Lymphotoxin-like inducible protein that competes with glycoprotein D for binding herpesvirus entry mediator in T cells.

inflammatory process, demonstrating that light can play a role in induction and perpetuation of mucosal inflammation.[15] In a second example, we and others have determined that there is increased expression of TL1A mRNA in biopsy of inflamed areas from Crohn's disease patients compared to normal specimens subjects, and others have demonstrated increased expression within monocytes and T cells within the mucosa of Crohn's disease patients (TL1A).[16,17] To substantiate the relevance of TL1A, in the first human genome-wide association study in both Japanese and European populations, it was found that genetic variants in the TL1A gene (TNF superfamily member 15) was associated with Crohn's disease.[18] Finally, determining which genetic manipulations in animal models are relevant to subpopulations of inflammatory bowel disease patients will allow us to more rapidly discover similarities between mouse and man that will accelerate target identification and potential drug development.

No matter what targets are discovered, novel delivery systems, including oral delivery of small molecules, rapidly acting short-term delivery drugs with residual efficacy, and genetically engineered bacteria must be a focus of consideration. One small molecule under investigation is an inhibitor of CCR9, which is expressed on lymphocytes and is important for selective trafficking to the small bowel. [19] Also under development, a short-term delivered drug with residual efficiency, is an antibody to CD3, a marker of T cells, which after two infusions has shown residual effects in some ulcerative colitis patients up to 2 years post infusion; this suggests that early limited exposure to this antibody may "reset" immune responses.[20] A similar approach recently has been used in new-onset type 1 diabetes where six infusions over 6 weeks prevented progression of loss of beta cells, persisting 1.5–2 years and suggesting that one can reset immune effector mechanisms by targeted and selected time frames.[21] Finally, genetic engineering of commensal bacteria for delivery of cytokines is being assessed for its potential benefit in therapeutics.[22] Bacteria producing the regulatory molecule IL-10 are currently being tested in pilot trials of patients with Crohn's disease.

Finally, to enhance target therapeutic efficacy, investigators should forego are the assumption that ulcerative colitis and Crohn's disease independent diseases. Instead the inflammatory bowel diseases should be regarded as a whole, with subclassifications based on overlapping and well-defined pathophysiologic destinctions. This approach was first suggested in 1989, in establishing a goal of defining "reagent-grade patients." This concept has evolved into the hypothesis that the clinical variability we see may be based upon a specific, genetically determined, immune imbalance that, when these individuals are exposed to specific types of bacterial products and their antigens, manifest in different clinical phenotypes. Recent findings from mouse studies have demonstrated that animals raised in bacteria-free environments do not develop colitis.[23] On the contrary, when exposed to multiple bacteria, the animals develop extensive colitis. However, if you expose the animal to only a single type of bacteria, such as *E. fecalis*, left-sided colitis develops, although, with a very slow onset. When the animal is repopulated with *E. coli*, a right-sided more rapidly aggressive disease ensues, with even more proximal stricturing. In human Crohn's disease, similar results were shown by assessing antibody responses to specific bacterial antigens that have been associated with Crohn's disease in comparison to healthy subjects and other inflammatory controls, suggesting a loss of tolerance to mucosa-associated bacteria.[24] However, loss of tolerance is not global; rather it is selective and the patient responses cluster into particular groups. So some patients have reactivity to a single bacterial antigen, others may react to two, and yet others may react to all three. Whether they have the number, of antibody responses from 0–3 relates to the aggressiveness of the disease in terms of disease progression and ultimate need for surgery.[25,26] Further association is noted when taking into consideration the magnitude of the reactivity. The greater the number, as well as the higher the response to these antibodies, the more aggressive the disease course.[25-27] A recent prospective study has shown that patients who express antibodies will have more rapid complications, such as internal penetrating disease or will more likely require surgery (M.C. Dubinsky, personal communication). Such findings suggest the potential benefits of intervention early on rather than after complications and possibly the prevention of progression of disease. In addition, continued investigation may well indicate selective pathways in individual patients based upon genetic underpinnings that lead to specific immunologic responses and the links to clinical phenotypes. Thus in 2006, there are too many targets and not enough patients to test each. It may well be more prudent to approach novel discovery in a much more select way. A goal is to define further these "reagent-grade patients" and by incorporating these definitions into study design or by substratifying patient groups afterward to fully appreciate effectiveness and to help identify novel target disease mechanisms.

REFERENCES

1. SANDBORN, W.J., J.F. COLOMBEL, R. ENNS, *et al.* 2005. Natalizumab induction and maintenance therapy for Crohn's disease. N. Engl. J. Med. **353:** 1912–1925.
2. HOMMES, D., T. MIKHAJLOVA, S. STOINOV, *et al.* 2004. Fontolizumab (Huzaf), a humanized anti-IFN-gamma antibody, has clinical activity and excellent tolerability in moderate to severe Crohn's disease. Gastroenterology **127:** 332.
3. BREEDVELD, F.C., P. EMERY, E. KEYSTONE, *et al.* 2004. Infliximab in active early rheumatoid arthritis. Ann. Rheum. Dis. **63:** 149–155.
4. RUTGEERTS, P., W.J. SANDBORN, B.G. FEAGAN, *et al.* 2005. Infliximab for induction and maintenance therapy for ulcerative colitis. N. Engl. J. Med. **353:** 2462–2476.
5. BERGSTROM, L., D.E. YOCUM, N.M. AMPEL, *et al.* 2004. Increased risk of coccidioidomycosis in patients treated with tumor necrosis factor alpha antagonists. Arthritis Rheum. **50:** 1959–1966.
6. RYCHLY, D.J. & J.T. DIPIRO. 2005. Infections associated with tumor necrosis factor-alpha antagonists. Pharmacotherapy **25:** 1181–1192.

7. ADELMAN, B., A. SANDROCK & M.A. PANZARA. 2005. Natalizumab and progressive multifocal leukoencephalopathy. N. Engl. J. Med. **353:** 432–433.
8. ALVAREZ-CERMENO, J.C., J. MASJUAN & L.M. VILLAR. 2005. Progressive multifocal leukoencephalopathy, natalizumab, and multiple sclerosis. N. Engl. J. Med. **353:** 1744–1746.
9. BERGER, J.R. & I.J. KORALNIK. 2005. Progressive multifocal leukoencephalopathy and natalizumab–unforeseen consequences. N. Engl. J. Med. **353:** 414–416.
10. KLEINSCHMIDT-DEMASTERS, B.K. & K.L. TYLER. 2005. Progressive multifocal leukoencephalopathy complicating treatment with natalizumab and interferon beta-1a for multiple sclerosis. N. Engl. J. Med. **353:** 369–374.
11. VAN ASSCHE, G., M. VAN RANST, R. SCIOT, et al. 2005. Progressive multifocal leukoencephalopathy after natalizumab therapy for Crohn's disease. N. Engl. J. Med. **353:** 362–368.
12. HUGOT, J.P., M. CHAMAILLARD, H. ZOUALI, et al. 2001. Association of NOD2 leucine-rich repeat variants with susceptibility to Crohn's disease. Nature **411:** 599–603.
13. OGURA, Y., D.K. BONEN, N. INOHARA, et al. 2001. A frameshift mutation in NOD2 associated with susceptibility to Crohn's disease. Nature **411:** 603–606.
14. PELTEKOVA, V.D., R.F. WINTLE, L.A. RUBIN, et al. 2004. Functional variants of OCTN cation transporter genes are associated with Crohn disease. Nat. Genet. **36:** 471–475.
15. KINJO, Y., & M. KRONENBERG. 2005. Valpha14i NKT cells are innate lymphocytes that participate in the immune response to diverse microbes. J. Clin. Immunol. **25:** 522–533.
16. BAMIAS, G., C. MARTIN, III, M. MARINI, et al. 2003. Expression, localization, and functional activity of TL1A, a novel Th1-polarizing cytokine in inflammatory bowel disease. J. Immunol. **171:** 4868–4874.
17. PREHN, J.L., S. MEHDIZADEH, C.J. LANDERS, et al. 2004. Potential role for TL1A, the new TNF-family member and potent costimulator of IFN-gamma, in mucosal inflammation. Clin. Immunol. **112:** 66–77.
18. YAMAZAKI, K., D. MCGOVERN, J. RAGOUSSIS, et al. 2005. Single nucleotide polymorphisms in TNFSF15 confer susceptibility to Crohn's disease. Hum. Mol. Genet. **14:** 3499–3506.
19. PAPADAKIS, K.A., C. LANDERS, J. PREHN, et al. 2003. CC chemokine receptor 9 expression defines a subset of peripheral blood lymphocytes with mucosal T cell phenotype and Th1 or T-regulatory 1 cytokine profile. J. Immunol. **171:** 159–165.
20. TARGAN, S., B.A. SALZBERG, L. MAYER, et al. 2005. A phase I-II study: multiple dose levels of visilizumab are well tolerated and produce rapid and sustained improvement in ulcerative colitis patients refractory to treatment with Iv steroids (ivsr-Uc). Gastroenterology **128:** A-75.
21. KILLESTEIN, J. 2002. Anti-CD3 monoclonal antibody in new-onset type 1 diabetes mellitus. N. Engl. J. Med. **347:** 1116–1117.
22. MACPHERSON, A.J., D. GATTO, E. SAINSBURY, et al. 2000. A primitive T cell-independent mechanism of intestinal mucosal IgA responses to commensal bacteria. Science **288:** 2222–2226.
23. KIM, S.C., S.L. TONKONOGY, C.A. ALBRIGHT, et al. 2005. Variable phenotypes of enterocolitis in interleukin 10-deficient mice monoassociated with two different commensal bacteria. Gastroenterology **128:** 891–906.

24. LANDERS, C.J., O. COHAVY, R. MISRA, *et al.* 2002. Selected loss of tolerance evidenced by Crohn's disease-associated immune responses to auto- and microbial antigens. Gastroenterology **123:** 689–699.
25. ARNOTT, I.D., C.J. LANDERS, E.J. NIMMO, *et al.* 2004. Sero-reactivity to microbial components in Crohn's disease is associated with disease severity and progression, but not NOD2/CARD15 genotype. Am. J. Gastroenterol. **99:** 2376–2384.
26. MOW, W.S., E.A. VASILIAUSKAS, Y.C. LIN, *et al.* 2004. Association of antibody responses to microbial antigens and complications of small bowel Crohn's disease. Gastroenterology **126:** 414–424.
27. TARGAN, S.R., C.J. LANDERS, H. YANG, *et al.* 2005. Antibodies to CBir1 flagellin define a unique response that is associated independently with complicated Crohn's disease. Gastroenterology **128:** 2020–2028.
28. HANAUER, S.B., B.G. FEAGAN, G.R. LICHTENSTEIN, *et al.* 2002. Maintenance infliximab for Crohn's disease: the ACCENT I randomised trial. Lancet **359:** 1541–1549.
29. SANDBORN, W.J., S.B. HANAUER, M. LUKAS, *et al.* 2005. Induction and maintenance of clinical remission and response in subjects with Crohn's disease treated during a 6-month open-label period with fully human anti-tnf-α monoclonal antibody adalimumab (humira). Gastroenterology **128:** A-111.
30. SCHREIBER, S., P. RUTGEERTS, R.N. FEDORAK, *et al.* 2005. A randomized, placebo-controlled trial of certolizumab pegol (CDP870) for treatment of Crohn's disease. Gastroenterology **129:** 807–818.
31. MANNON, P.J., I.J. FUSS, L. MAYER, *et al.* 2004. Anti-interleukin-12 antibody for active Crohn's disease. N. Engl. J. Med. **351:** 2069–2079.
32. KORZENIK, J.R., B.K. DIECKGRAEFE, J.F. VALENTINE, *et al.* 2005. Sargramostim for active Crohn's disease. N. Engl. J. Med. **352:** 2193–2201.
33. FEAGAN, B.G., G.R. GREENBERG, G. WILD, *et al.* 2005. Treatment of ulcerative colitis with a humanized antibody to the alpha4beta7 integrin. N. Engl. J. Med. **352:** 2499–2507.

CARD15/NOD2 Mutations in Crohn's Disease

JEAN-PIERRE HUGOT

Department of Paediatric Gastroenterology, INSERM Avenir U458,
Hôpital Robert Debré, 48 Bd. Sérurier, 75019 Paris, France

ABSTRACT: Inflammatory bowel diseases (IBDs) are complex genetic disorders characterized by a complex interplay between genetic and environmental risk factors. At least ten genes or anonymous loci have been proposed to play a role in IBD. Among them, the best studied is CARD15/NOD2, a gene coding for a protein involved in bacterial recognition by cells involved in innate immunity. Despite a large amount of work, a consensus model explaining the effect of Card 15/NoD2 mutations did not emerge, and the disease mechanisms are still subject to debate.

KEYWORDS: inflammatory bowel disease; Crohn's disease; NOD2; CARD15; complex genetic disorders; innate immunity

INTRODUCTION

Crohn's disease (CD) was until recently a disease of unknown etiology. This lack of knowledge limits not only the diagnostic procedures, but also the development of specific treatments. The main goal of geneticists is to try to fill this gap and to provide etiological data to the scientific community. From this point of view, important results have been recently obtained that can be considered as a breakthrough toward a better understanding of CD mechanisms. These advances allowed the formulation of physiopathological hypotheses, which are now under investigation using functional models.

CROHN'S DISEASE SUSCEPTIBILITY GENES

As early as 1934, CD was recognized as a familial disorder and this observation was further confirmed by many groups in the middle of the 20th century. The proportion of familial aggregations was on average 8% to 10%, with large fluctuations between studies. Familial aggregations argue for genetic factors

Address for correspondence: J-P. Hugot, M.D., Ph.D., INSERM Avenir U458, Hôpital Robert Debré, 48 Bd. Sérurier, 75019 Paris, France. Voice: 33-1-40-03-57-12; fax: 33-1-40-03-57-66.
e-mail: jean-pierre.hugot@rdb.aphp.fr

Ann. N.Y. Acad. Sci. 1072: 9–18 (2006). © 2006 New York Academy of Sciences.
doi: 10.1196/annals.1326.011

playing a role in the disease and the recent discovery of inflammatory bowel disease (IBD) susceptibility genes confirms this interpretation. However, environmental risk factors shared by family members seem also to contribute to the familial aggregations. Indeed, looking at the sibships with multiple-affected siblings, we observed that the birth order of affected sibs is significantly different from a random distribution.[1] This observation that affected sibs form clusters strongly suggests that environmental factors also play a role in familial aggregations of the disease.

In the 1990s, analysis of the disease segregation in the pedigrees suggested that a major recessive gene could explain the predisposition to CD. This point of view was definitively ruled out by the results of the genome screens. In fact, among the many genome scans published today, none of them was able to identify a gene with an attributable relative risk in siblings (λs) of IBD patients higher than 2. This observation indicates that there is no major gene, with a large effect on the phenotype variance for IBD. Thus, the model of inheritance derived from the genome-wide scans is a complex interplay between many genetic risk factors with a modest individual contribution for each one. In other words, a given IBD susceptibility gene is neither necessary nor sufficient for disease development. However, it is interesting to note that the initial conclusions of the segregation analyses are partially true, at least for caspase recruitment domains (CARD)15/ nucleotide-binding oligomerization domain (NOD)2, for which a dose–effect is observed (see below).

Considering the CD phenotype, researchers studied genes involved in the immune system, such as HLA genes, TNFα or its receptors, interleukins, ICAM1, toll-like receptors (TLRs), vitamin D receptor, and interferon. Alternatively, genes playing a role in epithelial functions (e.g., mucins), drug resistance (MDR1), or cancer predisposition (e.g., hMLH1) were also proposed as candidate genes. Several authors found iteratively an association between IBD and HLADRB1, TNFα, TLRs, and MDR1, which are among the most studied candidate genes today. Unfortunately, for most of the other investigated candidate genes, conflicting data are often observed and discrepancies between studies are sometimes difficult to resolve.

Using an alternative approach, some geneticists screened the whole genome in order to get IBD genes. This strategy does not require any hypothesis on gene function and lets geneticists discover unexpected or even unknown genes. Using this positional cloning approach, several groups in the world delineated regions of significant linkage on chromosomes 1, 5, 6p, 10, 12, 14, 16p, 16q, and 19 that certainly contain IBD loci.[2–8](FIG. 1). In most cases, the relevant genes are still unknown and the above-mentioned regions of linkage have to be investigated further. However, on chromosomes 5, 10, and 16, searchers were lucky enough to find, after several years of effort, an association between CD and genetic polymorphisms.

On chromosome 5q, polymorphisms within the SLC22A4/5 genes coding for the organic cationic transporters (OCTN) 1 and 2 were reported by a Canadian

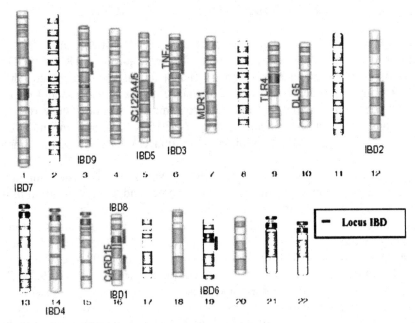

FIGURE 1. Loci and genes proposed to be involved in the genetic predisposition to inflammatory bowel diseases.

group to be associated with CD.[9] These CD-associated polymorphisms are in strong linkage disequilibrium (i.e., they are usually carried together on the same chromosome). It is thus difficult to understand which one is the most important. One polymorphism alters the properties (K_m and V_{max}) of the protein, while the other one modifies the expression level of the other gene. As a result, a defect in both OCTN1 and OCTN2 transporters seems to be associated with CD. OCTN1 and OCTN2 are transporters for a wide variety of small molecules including xenobiotics and carnitine. However, we do not know which transported molecule may be relevant for CD.

At the same time, polymorphisms within DLG5, located on chromosome 10, were reported by a German group to be associated with CD.[10] The associated polymorphisms induce nonconservative changes in the protein sequence but their functional effect has not yet been tested. The encoded protein is a scaffolding protein containing several PDZ domains. Its function is not yet clearly defined.

On chromosome 16, genetic variations on NOD2 gene were initially reported by two independent groups to be associated with CD.[11,12] Thereafter, this observation was widely reproduced by many investigators.[13–17] Altogether, these data allow concluding that NOD2 (later named CARD15 by the HUGO International Gene Nomenclature Committee) is one of the CD genes.

CARD15/NOD2 IN CLINICAL PRACTICE

CARD15/NOD2 is mutated in about 50% of CD patients and 20% of healthy controls in Caucasian populations.[18] In consequence, CARD15/NOD2 mutations are neither necessary nor sufficient for disease occurrence. This observation is in accordance with the retained complex genetic model for CD, where genetic risk factors contribute only to a small proportion of the variance. For example, it has been calculated that CARD15/NOD2 represents no more than 20% of CD genetic susceptibility. In addition, CARD15/NOD2 mutations are very rare in Asian or African populations.

The disease risk associated with CARD15/NOD2 mutations was initially estimated in the range of 2 to 3 for heterozygotes and from 20 to 40 in mutated homozygotes or compound heterozygotes.[11,12,18] A recent meta-analysis has refined these values and the odds ratio of the disease in mutation carriers is estimated to be 2.20 (95% CI: 1.84–2.62), 2.99 (95% CI: 2.38–3.74), and 4.09 (95% CI: 3.23–5.18) for the three main mutations R702W, G908R, and 1007fs, while the odds ratio for double mutants is estimated to be 17.1 (95% CI: 10.7–27.2).[19] The risk of disease may appear relatively high in this last population of people with mutations on two of the two chromosomes. However, considering the prevalence of the disease in the general population (usually estimated in the range of 1/1,000), the disease risk is no higher than 1 or few percents. As a result, and in the absence of preventive actions available to date, the information derived from CARD15/NOD2 genotyping is limited for clinical practice.

CARD15/NOD2 has no role in the genetic predisposition to ulcerative colitis (UC). However, a recent report indicates that the development of pouchitis after colectomy and ileo-anal anastomosis may be associated with CARD15/NOD2 mutations.[20]

The main CARD15/NOD2 mutations (R702W, G908R, and 1007fs) are associated with some phenotypic subgroups of patients.[18] The age of onset is lower in patients with mutations. A pure colonic inflammation is also less often encountered. Finally, strictures and/or fistulas are more common in patients with mutations. All these associations are even more significant for patients with two mutations than in patients with a single-dose mutation.[18] Unfortunately, here too, these findings have a limited impact in clinical practice. Finally, no relationship was observed between the genotype and the response or the adverse reactions under anti-TNF antibody therapy.

CARD15/NOD2 AND DISEASE MECHANISMS

CARD15/NOD2 is a protein with three functional portions.[21] The C terminal part of the protein contains a leucine-rich repeat (LRR) domain that is known to play a role in protein–protein interactions. The middle part of the protein is characterized by a NOD involved in protein self-oligomerization. At last, the

N terminal part of the protein contains two CARDs known to play a role in apoptosis and NF-κB activation pathways.

Such a structure is reminiscent of very old proteins involved in host–pathogen interactions. For example, CARD15/NOD2 has resemblance to the N gene involved in the resistance to mosaic virus in plants. In case of virus infection in plants without the resistance gene, the mosaic virus is able to disseminate and to infect the whole organism. On the other hand, in the presence of the N resistance gene, the leaves in contact with the virus develop a strong local reaction associated with a limited diffusion of the virus.

This early observation indicated that CARD15/NOD2 is involved in innate immunity. The expression profile of the gene given by Northern blot analyses confirmed this point of view. CARD15/NOD2 is mainly expressed in phagocytes including monocytes, macrophages, dendritic cells, and polymorphonuclear cells.[22,23] CARD15 was further detected in epithelial cells *in vitro* and *in vivo* after activation by proinflammatory cytokines.[23–25] More recently, the Nunez group found that in the mouse and human intestine, CARD15/NOD2 is mainly expressed by Paneth cells.[26,27] These cells specialize in host defense, producing antibacterial peptides and lysozyme at the bottom of the crypts, and CARD15/NOD2 seems to be involved in defensin production.[28] As a result, CARD15/NOD2 is thought to have a pivotal role in the innate immune defense of the crypts, limiting the invasion by bacteria present in the gut lumen.

Innate immunity is driven by a few pathogen-associated molecular patterns (PAMPs), which are present in most of the noneukaryotic cells. The host molecules involved in PAMP recognition are known as pattern recognition receptors (PPRs). Two main families of PPRs have been discovered in human beings: the toll-like receptors (TLRs) and the NODs. TLRs are transmembranous molecules able to recognize lipopeptides (TLR1 and 6), lipoteichoic acid (TLR2 and 6), DNA from viruses (TLR3, 7, and 8), lipopolysaccharide (TLR4), flagellin (TLR5), bacterial DNA (TLR9), and still unknown other molecules (for review see Ref. 29). NODs are seen as the intracellular counterpart of the TLRs. NOD1 (also known as CARD4) and NOD2 are activated by some fractions of peptidoglycan, a major component of the bacterial wall.[30–33]

The poorly purified PAMPs used in initial experiments might have led to erroneous conclusions. For example, NOD2 was initially considered as a lipopolysaccharide receptor, while it is now known that it recognizes muramyldipeptide (MDP), a peptidoglycan fraction.[34] More recently, Travassos *et al.* showed that TLR2 is a receptor for lipoteichoic acid but not for peptidoglycan.[35] As a result, NOD1 and NOD2 now appear with the peptidoglycan recognition proteins as the only known proteins involved in the host response induced by peptidoglycan. Peptidogycan recognition proteins are considered as lytic enzymes (secreted or stored in vesicles) while the NODs are seen as intracellular sensors of peptidogycan even whether we do not yet know whether peptidogycan products directly interact with the NODs.

Lesage *et al.* analyzed the mutational spectrum of the gene. They found at least 60 genetic polymorphisms within the gene, including 30 with a putative functional effect.[18] The mutations are localized all along the gene, excepting the CARD domains, where no mutation was observed in the first domain and only three in the second domain. Considering that the CARDs are certainly the effectors of the protein, this first observation suggests that mutated proteins are deregulated rather than structurally inactive. The observation of many mutations in the regulatory parts of the protein confirms this point of view and suggests that CD results in a lack of CARD15 regulation.

An excess of CD patients carrying two mutations on two chromosomes is widely recognized and it has been calculated that the risk of developing the disease in double-dose mutation carriers is 5- to 10-fold higher than the risk for people carrying only one mutation.[11,12,18,19] This dosage effect is consistent with a loss-of-function model, where the molecular defect of the gene lowers its efficiency. This loss-of-function model was confirmed by many data from several groups using *in vitro* models of transiently transfected cell lines.[12,30–32] *Ex vivo* analyses performed on circulating monocytes from CD patients confirmed that CD-associated mutations are characterized by a loss of response to MDP.[36] However, there is no demonstration today that MDP response is linked to the CD phenotype. Finally, the loss-of-function model were disputed very recently after the observation that mice carrying the 1007fs human homologue mutation were characterized by an excess of IL1β production.[37]

Under MDP activation, CARD15 is able to activate the NF-κB pathway via a Rick/Rip2 interaction.[38] Because NF-κB is a key pathway in inflammatory response, CARD15 is considered as a proinflammatory molecule. The recent report by Madea *et al.* that CARD15/NOD2 is able to activate IL1β via the caspase 1 pathway confirms the proinflammatory properties of CARD15/NOD2.[37] However, by its CARDs, CARD15 may also play a role in apoptosis pathways, but little is known about the proapoptotic function of the protein and this lack of data makes it difficult to come to definite conclusions about the exact functions of the gene.

One of the most pressing questions is to understand how a loss-of-function model (suggested by genetic and functional data) may induce an inflammatory condition as CD. Most authors suggest that a defect of the innate immunity induces a proliferation of bacteria and a consequent inflammation in the host tissues driven by the adaptive immune system. Unfortunately, this point of view remains speculative. As a result, others have tried to find alternative explanations. Watanabe *et al.* showed that NOD2 limits the proinflammatory effects driven by TLR2 stimulation.[39] Chen *et al.* also considered NOD2 as an anti-inflammatory molecule under certain circumstances.[40] Netea *et al.* recently suggested that CD results from defective production of anti-inflammatory (interleukin-10 and tumor growth factor β) cytokines.[41] Finally, Madea *et al.* proposed a gain-of-function model for CARD15/NOD2 mutations in mice.[37] As a result, many conflicting data are available today and additional experiments are now required in order to reconcile them.

CARD15/NOD2 AS A TOOL FOR FURTHER RESEARCH

CARD15/NOD2 is not only associated with CD, but it is also associated with two other disorders: Blau syndrome (BS) and graft-versus-host disease (GVHD).[42,43] BS is a rare autosomal dominant disorder characterized by skin rashes, arthritis, and uveitis, but no gut lesions. Like CD, the inflammatory lesions contain granulomas. BS mutations are located in the middle of the NBD domain and they induce a basal activation of the NF-κB pathway without MDP stimulation.[30] The clinical and histological resemblance between BS and CD argue for a common unified mechanism for these two inflammatory disorders. In consequence, one could be tempted by a common gain-of-function model for CD and BS.[37] However, this concept is certainly too simple, considering that there is no gut lesion in BS patients.

In the case of bone marrow graft, the mortality and the morbidity related to the graft, especially GHVD, are associated with the three main CD mutations (R702W, G908R, and 1007fs).[43] The risk is low in case of no mutation in both donor and recipient of the graft. It is intermediate in case of mutation in the donor or in the recipient, and it is high in case of mutation in donor and recipient. This observation suggests that mutations in both epithelial and circulating cells are important in the disease.

Even if difficult to interpret, the connection between BS and GVHD through CARD15/NOD2, provides a unique opportunity to understand the function of the protein and to make joint progress on these three conditions.

Because CD is a complex genetic disorder, the final understanding of disease mechanisms will require integrating genetic and environmental risk factors in a unified system. The discovery of CD susceptibility genes provides a unique opportunity to identify new environmental factors. In fact, little is known about the environmental causes of the disease. Cigarette-smoking is the best studied, but it does not appear as the unique risk factor, and additional epidemiological studies are required.

CARD15/NOD2 identification allowed confirming that bacteria likely have a crucial role in the occurrence of CD lesions. Even if it may appear as a paradox that a genetic risk factor allows focusing on an environmental risk factor, this conclusion may be one of the most important results of the genetic approach. It is a nice illustration of the interdependence between genetic and environmental risk factors in complex genetic disorders.

The gut flora as a whole is usually proposed to be an etiological factor for CD. This opinion is mainly supported by the presence of MDP in nearly all bacteria species. However, the gut flora hypothesis does not explain the long-term trend in incidence of the disease. Gut flora has always been genetically at risk present in persons. Thus if gut flora as a whole is a risk factor, a constant incidence of CD over time should be observed. It can be postulated that external environmental factors (e.g., diet changes or antibiotic use) have altered the gut flora composition during the 20th century. However, in that case, the entire gut flora can no longer be considered as a risk factor and the question moves toward more specific components of the flora. In addition, it is not easy to explain why CD lesions may occur in segments of the digestive tract as different as the stomach, jejunum, or colon in terms of gut flora colonization. Finally, the intracytoplasmic location of CARD15 suggests that the infectious agents involved in CD are able to interact with the cytoplasm of the cell. Such bacteria can be intracytoplasmic or have a secretory apparatus. In both cases, they exhibit some invasive properties that are not observed in the common saprophytes of the gut.

As an alternative to the gut flora hypothesis, several specific viruses and bacteria have been proposed as etiologic agents for CD including *Mycobacteriu paratuberculosis, Listeria monocytogenes, Yersini enterolitica, Escherichia coli,* and measles virus, but none of them can be definitively pinpointed as a causal agent at the present time.[44–48] Studying their interaction with CARD15/NOD2 could allow progress in understanding their putative role in CD.

REFERENCES

1. HUGOT, J.P., J.P. CÉZARD, C JF, *et al.* 2003. Clustering of Crohn's disease within affected sibships. Eur. J. Hum. Genet. **11:** 179–184.
2. HUGOT, J.P., P. LAURENT-PUIG, C. GOWER-ROUSSEAU, *et al.* 1996. Mapping of a susceptibility locus for Crohn's disease on chromosome 16. Nature **379:** 821–823.
3. SATSANGI, J., M. PARKES, E. LOUIS, *et al.* 1996. Two stage genome-wide search in inflammatory bowel disease provides evidence for susceptibility loci on chromosomes 3, 7 and 12. Nat. Genet. **14:** 199–202.
4. HAMPE, J., S. SCHREIBER, S.H. SHAW, *et al.* 1999. A genomewide analysis provides evidence for novel linkages in inflammatory bowel disease in a large European cohort. Am. J. Hum. Genet. **64:** 808–816.
5. RIOUX, J.D., M.S. SILVERBERG, M.J. DALY, *et al.* 2000. Genomewide search in Canadian families with inflammatory bowel disease reveals two novel susceptibility loci. Am. J. Hum. Genet. **66:** 1863–1870.
6. CHO, J.H., D.L. NICOLAE, L.H. GOLD, *et al.* 1998. Identification of novel susceptibility loci for inflammatory bowel disease on chromosomes 1p, 3q, and 4q: evidence for epistasis between 1p and IBD1. Proc. Natl. Acad. Sci. USA **95:** 7502–7507.
7. DUERR, R.H., M.M. BARMADA, L. ZHANG, *et al.* 2000. High-density genome scan in Crohn disease shows confirmed linkage to chromosome 14q11-12. Am. J. Hum. Genet. **66:** 1857–1862.
8. HAMPE, J., S.H. SHAW, R. SAIZ, *et al.* 1999. Linkage of inflammatory bowel disease to human chromosome 6p. Am. J. Hum. Genet. **65:** 1647–1655.
9. PELTEKOVA, V.D., R.F. WINTLE, L.A. RUBIN, *et al.* 2004. Functional variants of OCTN cation transporter genes are associated with Crohn disease. Nat. Genet. **36:** 471–475.
10. STOLL, M., B. CORNELIUSSEN, C.M. COSTELLO, *et al.* 2004. Genetic variation in DLG5 is associated with inflammatory bowel disease. Nat. Genet. **36:** 476–480.
11. HUGOT, J.P., M. CHAMAILLARD, H. ZOUALI, *et al.* 2001. Association of NOD2 leucine-rich repeat variants with susceptibility to Crohn's disease. Nature **411:** 599–603.

12. OGURA, Y., D.K. BONEN, N. INOHARA, *et al.* 2001. A frameshift mutation in NOD2 associated with susceptibility to Crohn's disease. Nature **411:** 537–539.

13. HAMPE, J., A. CUTHBERT, P.J. CROUCHER, *et al.* 2001. Association between insertion mutation in NOD2 gene and Crohn's disease in German and British populations. Lancet **357:** 1925–1928.

14. AHMAD, T., A. ARMUZZI, M. BUNCE, *et al.* 2002. The molecular classification of the clinical manifestations of Crohn's disease. Gastroenterology **122:** 854–866.

15. CUTHBERT, A.P., S.A. FISHER, M.M. MIRZA, *et al.* 2002. The contribution of NOD2 gene mutations to the risk and site of disease in inflammatory bowel disease. Gastroenterology **122:** 867–874.

16. VERMEIRE, S., G. WILD, K. KOCHER, *et al.* 2002. CARD15 genetic variation in a Quebec population: prevalence, genotype-phenotype relationship, and haplotype structure. Am. J. Hum. Genet. **71:** 74–83.

17. MURILLO, L., J.B. VAN CRUSIUS, A.A. BODEGRAVEN, *et al.* 2002. CARD15 gene and the classification of Crohn's disease. Immunogenetics **54:** 59–61.

18. LESAGE, S., H. ZOUALI, J.P. CÉZARD, *et al.* 2002. CARD15/NOD2 mutational analysis and genotype-phenotype correlation in 612 patients with inflammatory bowel disease. Am. J. Hum. Genet. **70:** 845–857.

19. ECONOMOU, M., T.A. TRIKALINOS, K.T. LOIZOU, *et al.* 2004. Differential effects of NOD2 variants on Crohn's disease risk and phenotype in diverse populations: a metaanalysis. Am. J. Gastroenterol. **99:** 2393–2404.

20. MEIER, C.B., R.A. HEGAZI, J. AISENBERG, *et al.* 2005. Innate immune receptor genetic polymorphisms in pouchitis: is CARD15 a susceptibility factor? Inflamm. Bowel Dis. **11:** 965–971.

21. OGURA, Y., N. INOHARA, A. BENITO, *et al.* 2001. Nod2, a Nod1/Apaf-1 family member that is restricted to monocytes and activates NF-kB. J. Biol. Chem. **276:** 4812–4818.

22. GUTIERREZ, O., C. PIPAON, N. INOHARA, *et al.* 2002. Induction of Nod2 in myelomonocytic and intestinal epithelial cells via nuclear factor-kB activation. J. Biol. Chem. **277:** 41701–41705.

23. BERREBI, D., R. MAUDINAS, J.P. HUGOT, *et al.* 2003. CARD15 overexpression in inflamed Crohn's disease colons by mononuclear and epithelial cells. Gut **52:** 840–846.

24. ROSENSTIEL, P., M. FANTINI, K. BRAUTIGAM, *et al.* 2003. TNF-alpha and IFN-gamma regulate the expression of the NOD2 (CARD15) gene in human intestinal epithelial cells. Gastroenterology **124:** 1001–1009.

25. HISAMATSU, T., M. SUZUKI, H.C. REINECKER, *et al.* 2003. CARD15/NOD2 functions as an antibacterial factor in human intestinal epithelial cells. Gastroenterology **124:** 993–1000.

26. LALA, S., Y. OGURA, C. OSBORNE, *et al.* 2003. Crohn's disease and the NOD2 gene: a role for Paneth cells. Gastroenterology **125:** 47–57.

27. OGURA, Y., S. LALA, W. XIN, *et al.* 2003. Expression of NOD2 in Paneth cells: a possible link to Crohn's ileitis. Gut **52:** 1591–1597.

28. KOBAYASHI, K.S., M. CHAMAILLARD, Y. OGURA, *et al.* 2005. Nod2-dependent regulation of innate and adaptive immunity in the intestinal tract. Science **307:** 731–734.

29. AKIRA, S. & K. TAKEDA. 2004. Toll-like receptor signalling. Nat. Rev. Immunol. **4:** 499–511.

30. CHAMAILLARD, M., D. PHILPOTT, S.E. GIRARDIN, *et al.* 2003. Gene-environment interaction modulated by allelic heterogeneity in inflammatory diseases. Proc. Natl. Acad. Sci. USA **100:** 3455–3460.

31. GIRARDIN, S.E. *et al*. 2003. Nod2 is a general sensor of peptidoglycan through muramyl dipeptide (MDP) detection. J. Biol. Chem. **278:** 8869–8872.
32. INOHARA, N. *et al*. 2003. Host recognition of bacterial muramyl dipeptide mediated through NOD2. implications for Crohn's disease. J. Biol. Chem. **278:** 5509–5512.
33. GIRARDIN, S.E., L.H. TRAVASSOS, M. HERVE, *et al*. 2003. Peptidoglycan molecular requirements allowing detection by Nod1 and Nod2. J. Biol. Chem. **278:** 41702–41708.
34. INOHARA, N., Y. OGURA, FF. CHEN, *et al*. 2001. Human Nod1 confers responsiveness to bacterial lipopolysaccharides. J. Biol. Chem. **276:** 2551–2554.
35. TRAVASSOS, L.H., S.E. GIRARDIN, D.J. PHILPOTT, *et al*. 2004. Toll-like receptor 2-dependent bacterial sensing does not occur via peptidoglycan recognition. EMBO Rep. **5:** 1000–1006.
36. LI, J., T. MORAN, E. SWANSON, *et al*. 2004. Regulation of IL-8 and IL-1beta expression in Crohn's disease associated NOD2/CARD15 mutations. Hum. Mol. Genet. **13:** 1715–1725.
37. MAEDA, S., L.C. HSU, H. LIU, *et al*. 2005. Nod2 mutation in Crohn's disease potentiates NF-kappaB activity and IL-1beta processing. Science **307:** 734–738.
38. INOHARA, N. *et al*. 2000. An induced proximity model for NF-kappa B activation in the Nod1/RICK and RIP signaling pathways. J. Biol. Chem. **275:** 27823–27831.
39. WATANABE, T., A. KITANI, P.J. MURRAY & W. STROBER. 2004. NOD2 is a negative regulator of toll like receptor 2-medated T helper type 1 responses. Nat. Immunol. **5:** 800–808.
40. CHEN, C.M., Y. GONG, M. ZHANG & J.J. CHEN. 2004. Reciprocal cross-talk between Nod2 and TAK1 signaling pathways. J. Biol. Chem. **279:** 25876–25882.
41. NETEA, M.G., B.J. KULLBERG, D.J. DE JONG, *et al*. 2004. NOD2 mediates anti-inflammatory signals induced by TLR2 ligands : implications for Crohn's disease. Eur. J. Immunol. **34:** 2052–2059.
42. MICELI-RICHARD, C., S. LESAGE, M. RYBOJAD, *et al*. 2001. CARD15 mutations in Blau syndrome. Nat. Genet. **29:** 19–20.
43. HOLLER, E., G. ROGLER, H. HERFARTH, *et al*. 2004. Both donor and recipient NOD2/CARD15 mutations associate with transplant-related mortality and GvHD following allogeneic stem cell transplantation. Blood **104:** 889–894.
44. GREENSTEIN, R.J. 2003. Is Crohn's disease caused by a mycobacterium? Comparisons with leprosy, tuberculosis, and Johne's disease. Lancet Infect. Dis. **3:** 507–514.
45. BULL, T.J., E.J. MCMINN, K. SIDI-BOUMEDINE, *et al*. 2003. Detection and verification of *Mycobacterium avium* subsp. Paratuberculosis in fresh ileocolonic mucosal biopsy specimens from individuals with and without Crohn's disease. J. Clin. Microbiol. **41:** 2915–2923.
46. KALINOWSKI, F., A. WASSMER, M.A. HOFMANN, *et al*. 1998. Prevalence of enteropathogenic bacteria in surgically treated chronic inflammatory bowel disease. Hepato-Gastroenterology **45:** 1552–1558.
47. LAMPS, L.W., K.T. MADHUSUDHAN, J.M. HAVENS, *et al*. 2003. Pathogenic Yersinia DNA is detected in bowel and mesenteric lymph nodes from patients with Crohn's disease. Am. J. Surg. Pathol. **27:** 220–227.
48. DARFEUILLE-MICHAUD, A., C. NEUT, N. BARNICH, *et al*. 1998. Presence of adherent *Escherichia coli* strains in ileal mucosa of patients with Crohn's disease. Gastroenterology **115:** 1405–1413.

Innate Immune Sensing of Microbes by Nod Proteins

THOMAS A. KUFER, DIANA J. BANKS, AND DANA J. PHILPOTT

Immunité Innée et Signalisation, Institut Pasteur, 28, Rue du Docteur Roux, 75724 Paris, Cedex 15, France

ABSTRACT: Nod1 and Nod2 are proteins involved in innate immune defense. These intracellular surveillance proteins detect bacterial peptidoglycan, although requiring distinct motifs to achieve sensing. Detection through Nod1 and Nod2 initiates proinflammatory signaling via NF-κB activation, which is necessary for clearance of infecting pathogens from the host. The peptidoglycan product sensed by Nod1 is a motif characteristic of Gram-negative bacteria plus some Gram-positive bacteria, such as *Bacillus* and *Listeria* spp. The specificity of Nod1 to detect this subset of bacteria might represent a selective advantage for the host in certain cases when Gram-negative bacteria represent the main threat, such as in the epithelial cells lining the intestinal mucosa. In contrast, Nod2 has been implicated as a general sensor for both Gram-positive and Gram-negative bacteria since muramyl dipeptide (MDP), which is the minimal motif in all peptidoglycans, is the structure recognized by Nod2. Mutations in Nod2 have been associated with autoinflammatory disease in humans, including Crohn's disease. Interestingly, the most common mutation in Nod2 associated with Crohn's disease results in protein product that no longer detects MDP. Although the implications of these findings are still not fully understood, it appears that lack of bacterial sensing through a loss of interaction between mutant Nod2 and MDP contributes to the pathology of disease. A loss of surveillance activity by Nod2 may result in the inability of local responses in the intestinal mucosa to control bacterial infection, thereby initiating systemic responses and leading to aberrant inflammation.

KEYWORDS: Nod1; Nod2; toll-like receptor; peptidoglycan; innate immunity; bacterial infection; NF-κB

INTRODUCTION

Eukaryotes use the innate and adaptive immune systems to detect and eliminate pathogens. Immediately following infection, the innate immune system is

Present address and address for correspondence: D. J. Philpott, Department of Immunology, University of Toronto, King's College Circle, Toronto, Ontario, Canada MS5 IA8. Voice: 416-978-7527; fax: 416-978-1938.

e-mail: dana.philpott@utoronto.ca

Ann. N.Y. Acad. Sci. 1072: 19–27 (2006). © 2006 New York Academy of Sciences.
doi: 10.1196/annals.1326.020

activated, providing a first line of defense against microbes.[1] Through the sensing of pathogen-associated molecular patterns (PAMPs) by specific pattern-recognition molecules (PRMs), the innate immune system detects the presence of pathogens.[1] This sensing of microbial PAMPs by host PRMs leads to the activation of signaling pathways, which initiate a defense response designed to destroy the microbe.

Both plants and animals rely on this system of sensing PAMPs by PRMs. PAMPs include essential cell wall components of bacteria, such as peptidoglycan and lipopolysaccharide (LPS), as well as flagella and bacterial nucleic acid motifs.[2] It has been shown that PAMPs can be recognized by either extracellular or intracellular PRMs. For instance, toll-like receptors (TLRs), which are expressed on the surface of various mammalian cells and in distinct subcellular structures, are instrumental in sensing extracellular PAMPs or those that are internalized into specialized compartments. Recently, members of the NAIP [neuronal apoptosis inhibitory protein], CIITA [MHC class II transcription activator], HET-E [incompatibility locus protein from *Podospora anserine*] and TP1 [telomerase-associated protein]) NACHT–leucine-rich repeat (LRR) protein family (NLRs), including Nod1 and Nod2, have been shown to detect cytosolic pathogen-associated molecular patterns (PAMPs) and are critical for defense against intracellular bacteria.[2] Recent findings suggest that both "outside-in" signaling, via TLRs, as well as "inside-in" signaling, through NLRs, are important in eukaryote defense mechanisms against microbial infection.[2]

NOD1 AND NOD2—INTRACELLULAR PEPTIDOGLYCAN SENSORS

Studies with the invasive Gram-negative bacteria, *Shigella flexneri*, first showed that a sensing system was likely present within epithelial cells.[3] Only invasive bacteria were shown to be able to induce the activation of proinflammatory signaling. Indeed, the presentation of bacterial products to the cytosol of epithelial cells through microinjection is sufficient to activate the NF-κB pathway and drive the induction of proinflammatory gene expression.[3] It was later shown that Nod1, a protein of the NLR family and surprisingly similar in domain organization to plant resistance proteins, is implicated in this sensing system.[4] Other invasive Gram-negative bacteria, including enteroinvasive *Escherichia coli*[5] and *Pseudomonas aeruginosa*,[6] are capable of interacting with Nod1. Finally, it was demonstrated that not only invasive bacteria can be detected by Nod1. Indeed, *Helicobacter pylori (H. pylori)*, a Gram-negative extracellular pathogen that interacts intimately with its host cell, also activates NF-κB through a Nod1-dependent pathway.[7] In this case, *H. pylori* likely "contaminates" the target cell with Nod1 elicitors transferred via a type IV secretion apparatus, which can be likened to a molecular syringe that the bacteria uses

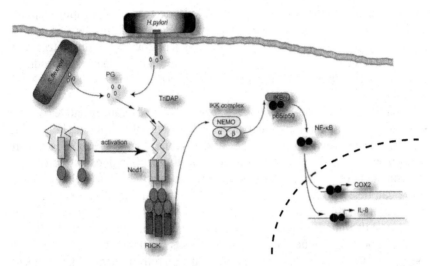

FIGURE 1. Nod1 activation pathway stimulated by bacterial infection. Peptidoglycan is transferred into epithelial cells by invasive bacteria, such as *S. flexneri* or by specialized transporters from extracellular bacteria, such as *H. pylori*. Once inside the cell, peptidoglycan may be converted into the active ligand, TriDAP, in order to specifically stimulate Nod1. TriDAP sensing leads to Nod1 oligomerization and subsequent recruitment of the serine/threonine kinase, RICK (also known as Rip2). RICK can then directly activate the NF-κB pathway through activation of the IKK complex, leading to degradation of IκBα and release of NF-κB. This transcription factor can then translocate to the nucleus where it targets the promoters of many genes involved in the inflammatory response, leading to expression of factors, such as IL-8 and Cox-2.

to transfer key virulence factors into the host cell (see FIGURE 1 for scheme of Nod1 activation by infection).

One focus of our group and others in the field was to identify the bacterial ligand that stimulated the Nod proteins. For Nod1, it appeared clear early in our studies that the activating component was from Gram-negative bacteria. Our original studies had shown that Gram-positive extracts were either incapable of activating Nod1 or did so very poorly. Using a candidate approach, we tested a number of potential Nod1 agonists isolated from Gram-negative bacteria, including LPS and lipoproteins. However, it was finally discovered that Gram-negative type peptidoglycan could stimulate the Nod1 pathway very efficiently.[8] Peptidoglycan is a complex structure of carbohydrate chains of β (1–4)-linked, alternating N-acetylglucosamine (G) and N-acetylmuramic acid (M) sugars cross-linked by short peptide bridges between the sugar backbone. What is more or less distinct about peptidoglycan from Gram-negative bacteria is the presence of diaminopimelic acid (DAP) in the third position of the peptide chain; in most Gram-positive bacteria, this amino acid is a lysine.

Since PG is a complex molecule, we then focused on identifying the minimal motifs active toward the Nod proteins. Through HPLC fractionation followed by mass spectrometry we showed that Nod1 detects a single muropeptide, GM-Tri$_{DAP}$, produced as a peptidoglycan degradation product in Gram-negative bacterial metabolism.[8] The minimal peptidoglycan motif detected by Nod1 has revealed that, out of the GM-Tri$_{DAP}$ muropeptide naturally produced by bacteria, the dipeptide moiety D-Glu-mesoDAP is sufficient to trigger Nod1 activation.[9,10]

Nod2 is a general sensor for both Gram-positive and Gram-negative bacteria since biochemical and functional analyses have identified muramyl dipeptide (MDP), the minimal motif in all peptidoglycans, as the essential structure recognized by Nod2.[11,12] Further analysis of the peptidoglycan structural requirements allowing sensing by Nod2 have shown that, in addition to MDP, Nod2 can detect Muramyl-Tri$_{Lys}$ but not Muramyl-Tri$_{DAP}$.[9] Interestingly, the most common mutation in Nod2 associated with Crohn's disease, which is a frame-shift mutation resulting in the truncation of the terminal LRR,[13,14] results in protein product that no longer detects peptidoglycan.[11,12] Although the implications of these findings are still not fully understood, it appears that lack of bacterial sensing may contribute to the pathology of this disease, at least in some cases. A loss of surveillance activity by Nod2 may result in the inability of local responses in the intestinal mucosa to control bacterial infection, thereby initiating systemic responses and leading to aberrant inflammation.

SENSING SPECIFICITIES BETWEEN HUMAN AND MURINE NOD1

Our interests were then to examine whether additional NLR proteins were involved in detecting fragments of peptidoglycan. One peptidoglycan fragment in particular, called tracheal cytotoxin or TCT, has been known for years to have proinflammatory potential,[15,16] and our studies clearly showed that this fragment was detected by neither Nod1 nor Nod2.[9] In general, it was demonstrated that TCT has a limited potential of inducing the secretion of proinflammatory products from human monocyte-derived macrophages.[17] In contrast, TCT is highly active toward murine macrophages, where picomolar amounts induce robust cytokine secretion. Interestingly, the Nod1 ligand, Muramyl-Tri$_{DAP}$, is a very poor agonist of cytokine secretion in murine cells. Using cells derived from mice deficient in Nod1, we showed that TCT was in fact dependent on Nod1, begging the question that perhaps murine and human Nod1 have distinct ligand specificities. This was shown to be indeed the case since transfection of a murine Nod1 into human cells switched their specificity from Muramyl-Tri$_{DAP}$ to TCT.[17] This difference of peptide specificity likely relies on punctual differences between the primary amino acid sequences of LRR from human and mouse Nod1.[18] Our characterization of distinct muropeptide requirements to achieve peptidoglycan sensing by human Nod1 and murine Nod1 likely has important implications in the study of human pathogens that use mouse models of infection to understand the pathogenesis of disease. Indeed, specific peptidoglycan signatures may render a certain pathogen unable to colonize alternative hosts on account of differences in sensing specificities of the machinery of the host's innate immune system.

BIOLOGICAL EFFECTS OF NOD LIGANDS

As mentioned above, Nod ligands can induce cytokine secretion from human and murine cells. We have recently examined in detail the specific effects of Nod ligands on primary human cells, specifically monocytes and dendritic cells (DCs). The Nod2 ligands, MDP and Muramyl-Tri$_{Lys}$, are potent inducers of cytokine secretion, including IL-6, TNF, and IL-1β, but in particular IL-8, in both monocytes and DCs, whereas the Nod1 ligand appears to be less potent.[19] Strikingly, neither Nod ligand can induce the maturation of DCs, as measured by increased expression of CD80, CD86, and MHCII. However, both Nod ligands can synergize with low and ineffective doses of LPS to allow for a robust production of cytokines as well as costimulatory molecules in the case of DCs.[19] These findings suggest that during a bacterial insult, multiple ligands, acting through cell surface TLRs and cytoplasmic Nod proteins, act in synergy to potentiate the innate response and influence the nature and direction of the adaptive immune response.

NOD2 FRAME-SHIFT MUTATION IN CROHN'S DISEASE: A LOSS-OF-FUNCTION MUTATION

As discussed above, the most common mutation in Nod2 associated with Crohn's disease is a frame-shift mutation that results in a truncated molecule lacking the last LRR. *In vitro* studies have used ectopic expression of this mutant protein to show that it no longer functions to sense the Nod2 ligand, MDP.[11,12] Importantly, the molecule can still activate the NF-κB pathway when overexpressed, demonstrating that the mutated protein nevertheless retains some function. Studies using human cells derived from patients with this mutation corroborate these findings; cells from patients with the frame-shift mutation in Nod2 can no longer respond to MDP.[12,20,21] What is important to stress, however, is that cells derived from these patients can still respond to other stimulants; LPS, for example, induces similar levels of IL-1β from cells isolated from Nod2 frame-shift mutation patients compared to cells isolated from either healthy controls or Crohn's patients with distinct Nod2 or other mutations.[20,22] Surprisingly, a recent study from our group in collaboration with Mihai Neata and colleagues showed that cells derived from Nod2 frame-shift mutation patients no longer detect Nod2- or Nod1-activating agonists.[22] These findings therefore suggest that Crohn's disease patients carrying this mutation in Nod2 have overall defects in peptidoglycan sensing. How this influences disease development is the important part of the puzzle that remains to be solved.

NOD2 FUNCTION IN THE MOUSE

As discussed above, there seems to be evidence from human data that supports the idea for a loss-of-function scenario during Crohn's disease. Moreover, studies using Nod2-deficient mice also report a general lack of responsiveness to MDP.[17,23,24] Although these animals have normal intestinal physiology, and antigen-presenting cells respond normally to various TLR agonists, higher susceptibility to oral infection with *L. monocytogenes* is observed.[24] Similar to reduced levels of defensins in the gut of Crohn's patients,[25,26] Nod2-deficient mice show altered antimicrobial peptide expression.

These data, however, contrast with the clinical picture of Crohn's disease. The disease is associated with high levels of proinflammatory cytokines, which are products of NF-κB target genes, and thereby argue against a loss-of-function phenotype.[27] Antibodies against TNF-α, IL-6, and IL-12 and direct inhibition of NF-κB are, at least in part, effective therapies for Crohn's disease, indicating that a dampened NF-κB response to bacterial products seems contrary to Crohn's disease susceptibility.[28]

To look at this problem in more detail, a recent study described the phenotype of a knockout–knockin mouse with a mutation in Nod2 homologous to the major frame-shift mutation in human Crohn's disease.[29] Although these animals did not show abnormalities of the gastrointestinal tract, and isolated macrophages respond normally to TLR agonists, the release of IL-1 upon MDP or peptidoglycan stimulation was markedly elevated. Furthermore, increased intestinal inflammation in a dextran sodium sulfate model was observed, which was paralleled by enhanced IL-1, IL-6, and Cox-2 expression, and apoptosis of lamina propria macrophages.[29] These surprising gain-of-function findings would give an explanation for the phenotype observed in Crohn's disease, but are in stark contrast to reports discussed above using cells derived from human patients. Thus, future research on the species-specific role of Nod2 is needed to clarify these discrepancies.

CONCLUSIONS

Nod1 and Nod2 have now been defined as representatives of a new family of cytoplasmic pathogen-recognition molecules. These two proteins recognize distinct motifs found in the peptidoglycan of bacteria and initiate defensive responses in the host through the activation of NF-κB. What will be interesting in the future will be to define the responses downstream of Nod proteins and to compare these responses to those downstream of the TLRs. In this way, the specificity of responses emanating from these different PRRs can be characterized in order to better understand the individual role of these families of proteins in defense responses against microbial infection.

Why does the host require an intracellular means of pathogen detection in addition to the TLRs? The cytoplasmic detection system mediated by Nods likely plays a key role in host defense in those tissues where TLRs are absent or expressed at low levels.[30,31] This occurs in epithelial cells that line mucosal surfaces, as, for example, in colonic epithelial cells. Since these cells live in constant contact with the microbial flora, expression of TLRs and/or their cofactors is downregulated, especially on the surface epithelium, in order to avoid stimulation of the cells by PAMPs and aberrant inflammation of these tissues. However, when these cells are infected with invasive pathogens or pathogens that interact intimately with the plasma membrane, PAMPs can be transferred to the intracellular compartment, where they interact with Nod proteins and this then initiates the defense response. Thus, Nod proteins likely function as key sentinel molecules to alter host defenses to microbial aggression and maintain intestinal homeostasis.

ACKNOWLEDGMENTS

The authors would like to thank members of the "Immunité Innée et Signalisation" group and Stephen Girardin for helpful discussions. T.A.K. is supported by a fellowship from the Federation of European Biochemical Societies (FEBS) and D.J.B. by a summer student fellowship from the Samuel Lunenfeld Research Institute, Toronto, Canada.

Note Added in Proof

Our group[32] and that of Gabriel Nunez[33] recently described a novel interacting partner of Nod2, called Erbin, which appears to alter Nod2 function. Erbin is a member of the LRR and PDZ domain–containing family of proteins (LAPs) and is important for targeting certain proteins to the basolateral membrane of epithelial cells. The specific interaction of Nod2 with Erbin also appears important for its membrane targeting[33] as well as to regulate NFκB activity.[32,33] Furthermore, infection with *S. flexneri* altered the interaction of Erbin and Nod2, allowing the transient release of Nod2, which is likely important for its activation.[33] Finally, since the frame-shift mutant of Nod2 that is associated with Crohn's disease could not interact with Erbin,[32,33] one can speculate that disrupted interaction between these two proteins may contribute to the disregulation of mutant Nod2 and have an impact on disease development.

REFERENCES

1. JANEWAY, C.A., JR. & R. MEDZHITOV. 2002. Innate immune recognition. Annu. Rev. Immunol. **20**: 197–216.
2. KUFER, T.A., J.H. FRITZ & D.J. PHILPOTT. 2005. NACHT-LRR proteins (NLRs) in bacterial infection and immunity. Trends Microbiol. **13**: 381–388.
3. PHILPOTT, D.J. *et al.* 2000. Invasive *Shigella flexneri* activates NF-kappa B through a lipopolysaccharide-dependent innate intracellular response and leads to IL-8 expression in epithelial cells. J. Immunol. **165**: 903–914.
4. GIRARDIN, S.E. *et al.* 2001. CARD4/Nod1 mediates NF-kappaB and JNK activation by invasive *Shigella flexneri*. EMBO Rep. **2**: 736–742.
5. KIM, J.G., S.J. LEE & M.F. KAGNOFF. 2004. Nod1 is an essential signal transducer in intestinal epithelial cells infected with bacteria that avoid recognition by toll-like receptors. Infect. Immun. **72**: 1487–1495.
6. TRAVASSOS, L.H. *et al.* 2005. Nod1 participates in the innate immune response to *Pseudomonas aeruginosa*. J. Biol. Chem. **280**: 36714–36718.
7. VIALA, J. *et al.* 2004. Nod1 responds to peptidoglycan delivered by the *Helicobacter pylori* cag pathogenicity island. Nat. Immunol. **5**: 1166–1174.
8. GIRARDIN, S.E. *et al.* 2003. Nod1 detects a unique muropeptide from gram-negative bacterial peptidoglycan. Science **300**: 1584–1587.
9. GIRARDIN, S.E. *et al.* 2003. Peptidoglycan molecular requirements allowing detection by Nod1 and Nod2. J. Biol. Chem. **278**: 41702–41708.
10. CHAMAILLARD, M. *et al.* 2003. An essential role for NOD1 in host recognition of bacterial peptidoglycan containing diaminopimelic acid. Nat. Immunol. **4**: 702–707.
11. GIRARDIN, S.E. *et al.* 2003. Nod2 is a general sensor of peptidoglycan through muramyl dipeptide (MDP) detection. J. Biol. Chem. **278**: 8869–8872.
12. INOHARA, N. *et al.* 2003. Host recognition of bacterial muramyl dipeptide mediated through NOD2: implications for Crohn's disease. J. Biol. Chem. **278**: 5509–5512.
13. HUGOT, J.P. *et al.* 2001. Association of NOD2 leucine-rich repeat variants with susceptibility to Crohn's disease. Nature **411**: 599–603.
14. OGURA, Y. *et al.* 2001. A frameshift mutation in NOD2 associated with susceptibility to Crohn's disease. Nature **411**: 603–606.
15. FLAK, T.A. & W.E. GOLDMAN. 1999. Signalling and cellular specificity of airway nitric oxide production in pertussis. Cell. Microbiol. **1**: 51–60.
16. FLAK, T.A. *et al.* 2000. Synergistic epithelial responses to endotoxin and a naturally occurring muramyl peptide. Infect. Immun. **68**: 1235–1242.
17. MAGALHAES, J.G. *et al.* 2005. Murine Nod1 but not its human orthologue mediates innate immune detection of tracheal cytotoxin. EMBO Rep. **6**: 1201–1207.
18. GIRARDIN, S.E. *et al.* 2005. Identification of the critical residues involved in peptidoglycan detection by Nod1. J. Biol. Chem. **280**: 38648–38656.
19. FRITZ, J.H. *et al.* 2005. Synergistic stimulation of human monocytes and by toll-like receptor 4 and NOD1- and NOD2-activating agonists. Eur. J. Immunol. **35**: 2459–2470.
20. LI, J. *et al.* 2004. Regulation of IL-8 and IL-1beta expression in Crohn's disease associated NOD2/CARD15 mutations. Hum. Mol. Genet. **13**: 1715–1725.
21. NETEA, M.G. *et al.* 2004. NOD2 mediates anti-inflammatory signals induced by TLR2 ligands: implications for Crohn's disease. Eur. J. Immunol. **34**: 2052–2059.

22. NETEA, M.G. *et al.* 2005. The frameshift mutation in Nod2 results in unresponsiveness not only to Nod2– but also Nod1-activating peptidoglycan agonists. J. Biol. Chem. **280**: 35859–35867.
23. PAULEAU, A.L. & P.J. MURRAY. 2003. Role of Nod2 in the response of macrophages to toll-like receptor agonists. Mol. Cell. Biol. **23**: 7531–7539.
24. KOBAYASHI, K.S. *et al.* 2005. Nod2-dependent regulation of innate and adaptive immunity in the intestinal tract. Science **307**: 731–734.
25. WEHKAMP, J. *et al.* 2004. NOD2 (CARD15) mutations in Crohn's disease are associated with diminished mucosal alpha-defensin expression. Gut **53**: 1658–1664.
26. WEHKAMP, J. *et al.* 2005. Reduced Paneth cell {alpha}-defensins in ileal Crohn's disease. Proc. Natl. Acad. Sci. USA **102**: 18129–18134.
27. BOUMA, G. & W. STROBER. 2003. The immunological and genetic basis of inflammatory bowel disease. Nat. Rev. Immunol. **3**: 521–533.
28. PHILPOTT, D.J. & J. VIALA. 2004. Towards an understanding of the role of NOD2/CARD15 in the pathogenesis of Crohn's disease. Best Pract. Res. Clin. Gastroenterol. **18**: 555–568.
29. MAEDA, S. *et al.* 2005. Nod2 mutation in Crohn's disease potentiates NF-kappaB activity and IL-1beta processing. Science **307**: 734–738.
30. BACKHED, F. & M. HORNEF. 2003. Toll-like receptor 4-mediated signaling by epithelial surfaces: necessity or threat? Microbes Infect. **5**: 951–959.
31. PHILPOTT, D.J., S.E. GIRARDIN & P.J. SANSONETTI. 2001. Innate immune responses of epithelial cells following infection with bacterial pathogens. Curr. Opin. Immunol. **13**: 410–416.
32. KUFER, T.A. *et al.* 2006. Role for erbin in bacterial activation of Nod2. Infect. Immun. **74**: 3115–3124.
33. MCDONALD, C. *et al.* 2005. A role for Erbin in the regulation of Nod2-dependent NF-kappaB signaling. J. Biol. Chem. **280**: 40301–40309.

Animal Models of Inflammatory Bowel Disease

Lessons from Enteric Infections

LARS ECKMANN

University of California, San Diego, Department of Medicine, La Jolla, California 92093, USA

ABSTRACT: Mouse models of intestinal inflammation have played a key role in understanding the mechanisms that govern the inflammatory response in the intestine, and in designing new therapeutic strategies in the treatment of patients with inflammatory bowel disease (IBD). Most of these models use chemical challenges, whereas relatively few robust models of intestinal inflammation caused by microbial infection are known. Two common models of infectious murine colitis and typhlitis are infection with the murine epithelial-adherent pathogen, *Citrobacter rodentium*, and infection of streptomycin-pretreated mice with *Salmonella typhimurium*. Studies in these models have helped to define the interactions between bacterial pathogens and host immune defenses, thus broadening the understanding of host–microbial interactions in the intestinal tract. Furthermore, such models help to determine the physiologic consequences of neutralizing specific mediators and signaling pathways implicated in inflammation on antimicrobial host defense.

KEYWORDS: mucosal immunology; inflammation; microbial pathogenesis; intestinal microbiota; animal models

INTRODUCTION

Inflammatory bowel disease (IBD) is characterized by chronic relapsing inflammation of the intestine leading to diarrhea, abdominal pain, and weight loss. Patients with long-standing disease have an increased risk of developing colorectal cancer. Ulcerative colitis (UC) and Crohn's disease (CD) are the two major manifestations of IBD, yet it has become increasingly clear over recent years that these are not homogeneous disease conditions. Rather,

Address for correspondence: Lars Eckmann, University of California, San Diego, Department of Medicine 0665, 9500 Gilman Drive, La Jolla, California 92093-0665. Voice: 858-534-0683; fax: 858-822-6454.
e-mail: leckmann@ucsd.edu

Ann. N.Y. Acad. Sci. 1072: 28–38 (2006). © 2006 New York Academy of Sciences.
doi: 10.1196/annals.1326.008

genetic linkage studies and immunological phenotyping indicate that multiple subgroups of IBD exist, which are likely to have different etiologies and exhibit differential responses to therapy.[1,2]

The notion that intestinal inflammation represents a common phenotypic pathway of several diseases with different etiologies arose initially from studies in murine models of immune dysregulation, in which disruption of each of several genes encoding proteins with distinct immunological functions caused intestinal inflammation.[3–5] Subsequent studies have considerably expanded the list of genes whose loss in mice is associated with the development of spontaneous colitis or enteritis or increased susceptibility to experimental challenges causing these conditions.[6] Furthermore, investigation of the mechanisms that govern immune responses to varying microbes and defined antigens in murine models have led to important insights into basic features of immune regulation. Most notably, mouse models were critical in developing the "Th1/Th2" paradigm that CD4 T cells can differentiate in a polarized manner into cells that express distinct cytokine profiles and stimulate specific immune effector mechanisms.[7] These immunological concepts provided the intellectual framework to explore the mechanisms of immune dysregulation in IBD and gave rise to new treatment hypotheses for the disease. To give a recent example, based on the importance of IL-12 and/or IL-23 in mouse models of immune-driven intestinal inflammation,[8] pilot studies in humans with IBD revealed that blockade of IL-12p40 may be efficacious in treating CD.[9] Together, these considerations illustrate the critical importance of mouse models for understanding the pathogenesis of human IBD, and for developing new therapeutic strategies in preclinical trials.

Although intestinal inflammation is the central disease-causing feature of IBD, and hence the process targeted by therapeutic interventions, this physiological host response normally serves a beneficial purpose in the defense against enteric microbes. Absence of immune and inflammatory responses renders the host unable to defend itself against infection with food- and water-borne microbial pathogens. In contrast, these responses are not needed for normal health and fertility in animals not exposed to microbial pathogens. Thus, investigation of the physiological functions of intestinal immunity and inflammation is important for understanding host defense against enteric pathogens and for designing effective vaccination strategies. Insights in this area are also important for developing novel treatment approaches in IBD, as they might help to minimize the risk that a therapeutic intervention compromises critical host defenses against commonly encountered enteric pathogens. Furthermore, commensal enteric bacteria are involved in the development of intestinal inflammation in many animal models, and are likely to contribute to the development of IBD in humans.[10] Insights into the host responses to enteric bacteria, both pathogenic and commensal, are therefore likely to enhance the mechanistic understanding of IBD pathogenesis, which in turn is key for developing effective preventive and therapeutic measures.

MOUSE MODELS OF INFECTIOUS COLITIS

For several biological and practical reasons mice are the most commonly used animal models for research in immunology and infectious diseases. Mice and humans are placental mammals with closely related genomes, since 99% of mouse genes have a homolog in the human genome and 80% of mouse genes have an ortholog in conserved syntenic intervals in the human genome (1:1 orthologs).[11–13] Fewer than 1% of mouse genes (~100 genes) have no apparent human homolog, although they could have functionally active, yet extremely diverged and thus unrecognizable, human counterparts. Furthermore, many immunologic processes are similar in humans and mice, although some differences exist in selected areas, such as the repertoire of antimicrobial peptides of the α-defensin family.[14] Mice can be engineered genetically to harbor defined knockout or knockin mutations, and a plethora of research reagents is available. Finally, mice are relatively small and have a short generation time, facilitating effective breeding and experimental schemes.

Murine infection models are widely employed for a range of infectious agents, particularly those causing systemic infections. Somewhat surprisingly, very few good mouse models are available for investigating host defenses and inflammatory responses in the intestinal tract. Although intestinal infection through oral gavage is effective for infecting the host with many enteric pathogens, this route often does not lead to significant microbial colonization or inflammation in the intestine. For example, oral infection of normal adult mice with the invasive gram-negative bacteria, *Salmonella*, leads to systemic infection of spleen and liver, but causes only modest infection of the intestinal tract and very little intestinal inflammation.[15] However, two intestinal infection models, employing *Citrobacter rodentium* in normal mice and *Salmonella typhimurium* in antibiotic-pretreated mice, have gained prominence over the last few years, because infections are robust and cause significant intestinal inflammatory disease.

Citrobacter rodentium–Induced Colitis

C. rodentium (initially termed *Citrobacter freundii* biotype 4280) is a gram-negative murine pathogen that was first identified in veterinary medicine as the microbial agent responsible for causing transmissible murine colonic hyperplasia in mouse breeding colonies.[16,17] Subsequent studies revealed that the bacteria attach intimately to the colonic and cecal epithelium and form characteristic subcellular lesions termed *attaching and effacing* (A/E) *lesions*.[18] Similar lesions are formed by two important human enteric pathogens, enteropathogenic *Escherichia coli* (EPEC) and enterohemorrhagic *E. coli* (EHEC).[19,20] EPEC causes watery diarrhea worldwide, particularly in young children in developing countries, while EHEC infection can lead to hemorrhagic colitis upon consumption of undercooked meat in developed countries.[19,20] A/E lesions are characterized by localized destruction (effacement) of brush border microvilli, intimate attachment of the bacterium to the apical host cell membrane, and formation of an underlying pedestal-like structure in the host cell. The A/E lesion-forming pathogens generally do not invade deeper layers of the mucosa or spread systemically, making them predominantly mucosal pathogens. EHEC, but not EPEC or *C. rodentium*, elaborates specific enterotoxins, Shiga-like toxins, important in pathogenesis.[20] *C. rodentium* shares other important functional and structural similarities with clinical EPEC isolates. The bacterial gene coding for the outer membrane protein responsible for intimate attachment, intimin, is functionally homologous in *C. rodentium* and clinical EPEC strains.[21] Furthermore, the murine and human infections with these pathogens are characterized by similar antibody responses to the bacteria. Taken together, these results suggest that *C. rodentium* is functionally similar to EPEC, thus making murine *C. rodentium* infection a model for human infections with EPEC.

Oral *C. rodentium* infection of normal adult mice causes transient colonization of cecum and colon, which peaks after 1 week, and is cleared over the ensuing 2–3 weeks (FIG. 1). Bacterial colonization is limited to the intestinal mucosa, with only a few bacteria reaching systemic sites or the bloodstream.[22] After bacterial eradication, mice are resistant to a secondary bacterial challenge.[23] Infection is normally accompanied by only modest morbidity (weight loss, diarrhea) and minimal mortality in adult mice, although significant morbidity, such as retarded growth, and high mortality can occur in suck-

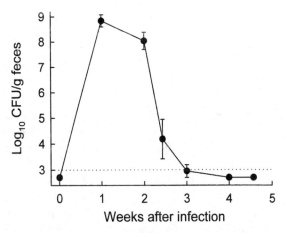

FIGURE 1. Time course of *C. rodentium* infection in normal mice. Adult C57BL/6 mice were infected orally with 5×10^8 *C. rodentium*. At the indicated times after infection, fecal pellets were collected, weighed, and homogenized. Homogenates were plated in serial dilutions on selective agar plates (MacConkey) and incubated overnight, after which colonies were counted. The *dotted line* indicates the sensitivity of the assay.

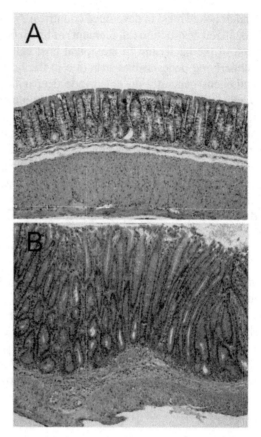

FIGURE 2. *C. rodentium*-induced colitis in normal mice. Paraffin sections of the colon of adult C57BL/6 mice, either uninfected (**A**) or 2 weeks after oral *C. rodentium* infection (**B**), were prepared and stained with hematoxylin/eosin. Infected mice show marked crypt hyperplasia and mixed inflammatory cell infiltration of mucosa and submucosa.

ling mice.[24] Infection leads to crypt hyperplasia, loss of goblet cells, and mucosal infiltration with lymphocytes, macrophages, neutrophils, and mast cells in colon and cecum[16,17,23] (FIG. 2). The lymphocytic host response to *C. rodentium* is characterized by mucosal infiltration with CD3+ T cells, particularly the CD4+ subset.[25] In addition, the cytokines interleukin-12 (IL-12) and gamma-interferon (IFN-γ) are upregulated in the colon of infected mice, indicating a bias toward a T helper cell-type 1 immune response.[26] T cells are important for clearance of *C. rodentium*, since mice with deficient $\alpha\beta$ T cells or CD4 T cells cannot control infection and exhibit high morbidity and mortality.[22,27] Moreover, mice develop IgG and IgA antibody responses to several bacterial proteins involved in virulence, including intimin, EspA, EspB, and Tir,[28] and B cells are absolutely required for bacterial clearance.[23,27] Despite the mucosal localization of the bacteria, secretory IgA or IgM antibodies, which are the dominant isotypes in mucosal secretions, play no role in host defense against *C. rodentium*, whereas IgG antibodies confer modest passive immune protection against oral challenge.[23] These data suggest that IgG acts as an immune effector against the bacteria, although it is not clear how circulating IgG can fulfill this function against luminal bacteria. B cells may also act as immune sensor cells during infection, perhaps in antigen presentation, as suggested by the marked delay in normal mucosal responses in B cell–deficient mice compared to normal mice after infection.[23]

Besides T and B lymphocytes, cells and mediators of innate immunity play a role in host defense against *C. rodentium*. The acute inflammatory cytokine, tumor necrosis factor (TNF)-α, is induced upon infection, and is required for effective clearance.[29] We found recently that IL-6, a multifunctional cytokine involved in B cell functions and the acute-phase response, is upregulated in the colon of infected mice. IL-6 deficiency leads to markedly delayed bacterial eradication, and greater infection-associated mucosal inflammation, suggesting that IL-6 exerts mucosa-protective functions in this model. This is in contrast to the findings in T cell–dependent models of experimental colitis, where IL-6 ablation was shown to attenuate inflammation.[30,31] Furthermore, signaling through the lymphotoxin β receptor is required for effective host defense against *C. rodentium*.[32] In its absence, mice fail to eradicate infection normally and exhibit more severe colitis, findings which caution that treatment of IBD with agents directed against the lymphotoxin β receptor signaling pathway is likely to render patients more susceptible to infection with certain enteric pathogens.[32] Among innate immune cells, a role for mast cells has been demonstrated in host defense against *C. rodentium*. Thus, mast cell–deficient mice show more severe colonic inflammation and increased bacterial dissemination into systemic sites, leading to higher mortality after *C. rodentium* infection than that in wild-type animals.[33] Neutrophil numbers also increase in the colon after infection, but their involvement in host defense is not clear at present.

Salmonella-induced Colitis in Streptomycin-Treated Mice

Salmonella are gram-negative food-borne enteric bacterial pathogens that can cause diarrheal disease or severe systemic infection in humans. Many different species exist, which fall into two major groups: *Salmonella typhi*, the cause of systemic typhoid fever, and nontyphoid *Salmonella* (e.g., *S. typhimurium*, *S. dublin*) that cause mostly intestinal disease, although the latter can also cause systemic disease.[34] Human intestinal disease induced by nontyphoid *Salmonella* is characterized by acute neutrophilic mucosal inflammation. In contrast, oral infection of mice with these bacteria causes no major intestinal disease, but rather systemic infection resembling typhoid fever in humans. Only in the end stages of disseminated *Salmonella* infection in mice can significant mucosal inflammation and destruction be observed in small intestine and colon. This lack of mucosal disease upon *Salmonella* infection can be partly overcome by treating mice with an oral antibiotic, such as strepto-mycin or kanamycin, before oral infection with *Salmonella*.[35,36] The antibiotics diminish the normal intestinal microbiota, allowing the inoculated *Salmonella* to colonize the lumen of cecum and colon more effectively than without an-tibiotic conditioning. Consequently, *Salmonella* grow to high density in the intestine within a day, which is accompanied by marked mucosal inflamma-tion over the same time period.[36] Thus, conditioning by oral antibiotics breaks the colonization resistance normally conferred by the microbiota[35] and allows orally inoculated *Salmonella* to establish intestinal infection rapidly and cause infection-associated colitis and typhlitis in normal mice. Similar results have been obtained after infection of germ-free mice with *S. typhimurium*, underlin-ing the importance of the normal microbiota in limiting *Salmonella*-induced intestinal inflammation in mice.[37]

Intestinal inflammation in the model is characterized by rapid crypt loss, epithelial erosions and goblet cell loss, mucosal and submucosal infiltration with acute inflammatory cells, particularly neutrophils, and marked edema, in the cecum and, to a lesser degree, in the colon.[36,38](FIG. 3). The model is especially useful for examining the early (4–72 h) intestinal events that occur after oral *Salmonella* infection, while the overwhelming intestinal infection probably causes severe, presumably lethal systemic disease at later stages (5–7 days), although this has not reported in detail. The *Salmonella* infectious colitis/typhlitis model has been used to examine the role of specific bacterial virulence factors in causing intestinal disease, and the importance of host factors in intestinal defense against *Salmonella*. For example, studies in this model have shown that flagella, appendages of the outer bacterial membrane required for motility, are required for effective colonization and induction of intestinal inflammation.[39] This effect appears to be mostly related to bacterial chemotaxis, since nonflagellated bacteria failed to get close to the epithelium.[39] Furthermore, the adaptor molecule MyD88, which is required for signaling through most toll-like receptors, was shown to be important for inducing colitis after infection with bacterial mutants lacking the *Salmonella* pathogenicity island (SPI)-2 secretion system, but not those lacking the SPI-1 system.[40] Virulence factors of the SPI-2 locus are important for bacterial survival in macrophages, while those of the SPI-1 locus are primarily involved in invasion of the intestinal epithelium.[38] Thus, SPI-2-dependent intracellular proliferation of the bacteria triggers MyD88-dependent innate immune responses in the intestinal tract.[40]

CONCLUSIONS

Mouse models of infectious colitis can help to determine the interactions between bacterial pathogens and host immune defenses, thus broadening the

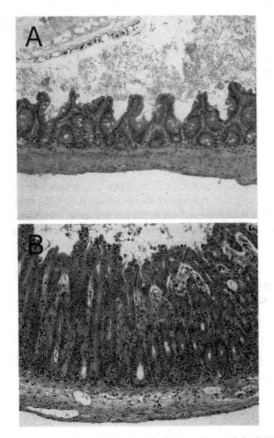

FIGURE 3. *Salmonella*-induced intestinal inflammation. Adult C57BL/6 mice were given 20 mg streptomycin orally, and infected 24 h later with *S. typhimurium* 14028 by oral gavage. Paraffin sections of the cecum 48 h after infection (**B**), or from uninfected control mice (**A**), were prepared and stained with hematoxylin/eosin. Infected mice exhibit extensive crypt hyperplasia, epithelial erosions at the surface, and edema and mixed inflammatory cell infiltration of mucosa and submucosa.

understanding of host–microbial interactions in the intestinal tract. Furthermore, such models help to define the physiologic consequences of neutralizing specific mediators and signaling pathways on antimicrobial host defense. These insights are important for assessing potential untoward side effects that novel pharmacological interventions might have in patients with IBD. In this regard, it is important to realize that microbial infection as the proximal cause of mucosal inflammation is a dynamic stimulus that changes in response to host defenses (FIG. 4). Interventions designed to inhibit a particular proinflammatory pathway in the host may, paradoxically, exacerbate mucosal inflammation, because the pathway might be required for effective host defense against infection, so that its loss results in a greater microbial load and thus a stronger stimulus for mucosal inflammation. Such considerations may also apply to

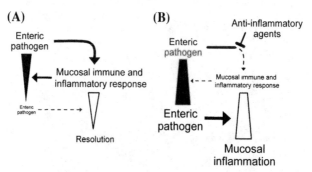

FIGURE 4. Potential paradoxical effects of anti-inflammatory agents in infectious colitis. (**A**) Physiologic response. Infection of the intestinal tract with an enteric pathogen causes induction of a mucosal immune and inflammatory response, which leads to destruction of the pathogen. As a consequence, reduction of the pathogen load attenuates the stimulus for a mucosal response, thus ultimately leading to resolution. (**B**) Potential effects of anti-inflammatory agents. Blockade of the mucosal immune and inflammatory response to infection prevents eradication of the pathogen. The ensuing increased pathogen burden provides an enhanced stimulus for a mucosal inflammatory response. Thus, anti-inflammatory agents may paradoxically lead to increased mucosal inflammation in response to a microbial challenge.

understanding the pathogenesis of IBD, and the consequence of specific therapeutic interventions, where enteric bacteria are likely to play a role in the initiation and maintenance of mucosal inflammation.

ACKNOWLEDGMENTS

This work was supported by NIH Grants RR17030, AI56075, DK35108, and a grant from the Crohn's and Colitis Foundation of America.

REFERENCES

1. VERMEIRE, S. & P. RUTGEERTS. 2005. Current status of genetics research in inflammatory bowel disease. Genes Immun. **6:** 637–645.
2. AHMAD, T., S. MARSHALL & D. JEWELL. 2003. Genotype-based phenotyping heralds a new taxonomy for inflammatory bowel disease. Curr. Opin. Gastroenterol. **19:** 327–335.
3. KUHN, R., J. LOHLER, D. RENNICK, *et al.* 1993. Interleukin-10-deficient mice develop chronic enterocolitis. Cell **75:** 263–274.
4. MOMBAERTS, P., E. MIZOGUCHI, M.J. GRUSBY, *et al.* 1993. Spontaneous development of inflammatory bowel disease in T cell receptor mutant mice. Cell **75:** 274–282.
5. SADLACK, B., H. MERZ, H. SCHORLE, *et al.* 1993. Ulcerative colitis-like disease in mice with a disrupted interleukin-2 gene. Cell **75:** 253–261.
6. STROBER, W., I.J. FUSS & R.S. BLUMBERG. 2002. The immunology of mucosal models of inflammation. Annu. Rev. Immunol. **20:** 495–549.

7. ELSON, C.O., Y. CONG, V.J. McCRACKEN, et al. 2005. Experimental models of inflammatory bowel disease reveal innate, adaptive, and regulatory mechanisms of host dialogue with the microbiota. Immunol. Rev. **206:** 260–276.

8. NEURATH, M.F., I. FUSS, B.L. KELSALL, et al. 1995. Antibodies to interleukin 12 abrogate established experimental colitis in mice. J. Exp. Med. **182:** 1281–1290.

9. MANNON, P. J., I.J. FUSS, L. MAYER, et al. 2004. Anti-interleukin-12 antibody for active Crohn's disease. N. Engl. J. Med. **351:** 2069–2079.

10. SARTOR, R.B. 2004. Therapeutic manipulation of the enteric microflora in inflammatory bowel diseases: antibiotics, probiotics, and prebiotics. Gastroenterology **126:** 1620–1633.

11. LANDER, E.S., L.M. LINTON, B. BIRREN, et al. 2001. Initial sequencing and analysis of the human genome. Nature **409:** 860–921.

12. VENTER, J.C., M.D. ADAMS, E.W. MYERS, et al. 2001. The sequence of the human genome. Science **291:** 1304–1351.

13. WATERSTON, R.H., K. LINDBLAD-TOH, E. BIRNEY, et al. 2002. Initial sequencing and comparative analysis of the mouse genome. Nature **420:** 520–562.

14. PATIL, A., A.L. HUGHES & G. ZHANG. 2004. Rapid evolution and diversification of mammalian alpha-defensins as revealed by comparative analysis of rodent and primate genes. Physiol. Genomics **20:** 1–11.

15. HEFFERNAN, E.J., J. FIERER, G. CHIKAMI, et al. 1987. Natural history of oral *Salmonella dublin* infection in BALB/c mice: effect of an 80-kilobase-pair plasmid on virulence. J. Infect. Dis. **155:** 1254–1259.

16. BARTHOLD, S.W., G.L. COLEMAN, P.N. BHATT, et al. 1976. The etiology of transmissible murine colonic hyperplasia. Lab. Anim. Sci. **26:** 889–894.

17. LUPERCHIO, S.A. & D.B. SCHAUER. 2001. Molecular pathogenesis of *Citrobacter rodentium* and transmissible murine colonic hyperplasia. Microbes Infect. **3:** 333–340.

18. SCHAUER, D.B. & S. FALKOW. 1993. Attaching and effacing locus of a *Citrobacter freundii* biotype that causes transmissible murine colonic hyperplasia. Infect. Immun. **61:** 2486–2492.

19. KAPER, J.B., J.P. NATARO & H.L. MOBLEY. 2004. Pathogenic *Escherichia coli*. Nat. Rev. Microbiol. **2:** 123–140.

20. WELINDER-OLSSON, C. & B. KAIJSER. 2005. Enterohemorrhagic *Escherichia coli* (EHEC). Scand. J. Infect. Dis. **37:** 405–416.

21. FRANKEL, G., A.D. PHILLIPS, M. NOVAKOVA, et al. 1996. Intimin from enteropathogenic *Escherichia coli* restores murine virulence to a *Citrobacter rodentium* eaeA mutant: induction of an immunoglobulin A response to intimin and EspB. Infect. Immun. **64:** 5315–5325.

22. BRY, L. & M.B. BRENNER. 2004. Critical role of T cell-dependent serum antibody, but not the gut-associated lymphoid tissue, for surviving acute mucosal infection with *Citrobacter rodentium*, an attaching and effacing pathogen. J. Immunol. **172:** 433–441.

23. MAASER, C., M.P. HOUSLEY, M. IIMURA, et al. 2004. Clearance of *Citrobacter rodentium* requires B cells but not secretory immunoglobulin A (IgA) or IgM antibodies. Infect. Immun. **72:** 3315–3324.

24. BARTHOLD, S.W., G.L. COLEMAN, R.O. JACOBY, et al. 1978. Transmissible murine colonic hyperplasia. Vet. Pathol. **15:** 223–236.

25. HIGGINS, L.M., G. FRANKEL, G. DOUCE, et al. 1999. Citrobacter rodentium infection in mice elicits a mucosal Th1 cytokine response and lesions similar to those in murine inflammatory bowel disease. Infect. Immun. **67:** 3031–3039.

26. SIMMONS, C.P., N.S. GONCALVES, M. GHAEM-MAGHAMI, et al. 2002. Impaired resistance and enhanced pathology during infection with a noninvasive, attaching-effacing enteric bacterial pathogen, Citrobacter rodentium, in mice lacking IL-12 or IFN-gamma. J. Immunol. **168:** 1804–1812.
27. SIMMONS, C.P., S. CLARE, M. GHAEM-MAGHAMI, et al. 2003. Central role for B lymphocytes and CD4+ T cells in immunity to infection by the attaching and effacing pathogen Citrobacter rodentium. Infect. Immun. **71:** 5077–5086.
28. GHAEM-MAGHAMI, M., C.P. SIMMONS, S. DANIELL, et al. 2001. Intimin-specific immune responses prevent bacterial colonization by the attaching-effacing pathogen Citrobacter rodentium. Infect. Immun. **69:** 5597–5605.
29. GONCALVES, N.S., M. GHAEM-MAGHAMI, G. MONTELEONE, et al. 2001. Critical role for tumor necrosis factor alpha in controlling the number of luminal pathogenic bacteria and immunopathology in infectious colitis. Infect. Immun. **69:** 6651–6659.
30. YAMAMOTO, M., K. YOSHIZAKI, T. KISHIMOTO, et al. 2000. IL-6 is required for the development of Th1 cell-mediated murine colitis. J. Immunol. **164:** 4878–4882.
31. KITAMURA, K., Y. NAKAMOTO, S. KANEKO, et al. 2004. Pivotal roles of interleukin-6 in transmural inflammation in murine T cell transfer colitis. J. Leukoc. Biol. **76:** 1111–1117.
32. SPAHN, T.W., C. MAASER, L. ECKMANN, et al. 2004. The lymphotoxin-beta receptor is critical for control of murine Citrobacter rodentium-induced colitis. Gastroenterology **127:** 1463–1473.
33. WEI, O.L., A. HILLIARD, D. KALMAN, et al. 2005. Mast cells limit systemic bacterial dissemination but not colitis in response to Citrobacter rodentium. Infect. Immun. **73:** 1978–1985.
34. FIERER, J. & M. SWANCUTT. 2000. Non-typhoid Salmonella: a review. Curr. Clin. Top. Infect. Dis. **20:** 134–157.
35. QUE, J.U. & D.J. HENTGES. 1985. Effect of streptomycin administration on colonization resistance to Salmonella typhimurium in mice. Infect. Immun. **48:** 169–174.
36. BARTHEL, M., S. HAPFELMEIER, L. QUINTANILLA-MARTINEZ, et al. 2003. Pretreatment of mice with streptomycin provides a Salmonella enterica serovar Typhimurium colitis model that allows analysis of both pathogen and host. Infect. Immun. **71:** 2839–2858.
37. STECHER, B., A.J. MACPHERSON, S. HAPFELMEIER, et al. 2005. Comparison of Salmonella enterica serovar Typhimurium colitis in germfree mice and mice pretreated with streptomycin. Infect. Immun. **73:** 3228–3241.
38. COOMBES, B.K., B.A. COBURN, A.A. POTTER, et al. 2005. Analysis of the contribution of Salmonella pathogenicity islands 1 and 2 to enteric disease progression using a novel bovine ileal loop model and a murine model of infectious enterocolitis. Infect. Immun. **73:** 7161–7169.
39. STECHER, B., S. HAPFELMEIER, C. MULLER, et al. 2004. Flagella and chemotaxis are required for efficient induction of Salmonella enterica serovar Typhimurium colitis in streptomycin-pretreated mice. Infect. Immun. **72:** 4138–4150.
40. HAPFELMEIER, S., B. STECHER, M. BARTHEL, et al. 2005. The Salmonella pathogenicity island (SPI)-2 and SPI-1 type III secretion systems allow Salmonella serovar typhimurium to trigger colitis via MyD88-dependent and MyD88-independent mechanisms. J. Immunol. **174:** 1675–1685.

Molecular Approaches to the Role of the Microbiota in Inflammatory Bowel Disease

CHARLES O. ELSON,[a] YINGZI CONG,[a] FENGXIA QI,[b]
ROBERT M. HERSHBERG,[c] AND STEPHAN R. TARGAN[d]

[a] University of Alabama at Birmingham, Birmingham,
Alabama 35294-0007, USA

[b] Division of Oral Biology and Medicine, School of Dentistry,
University of California at Los Angeles, Los Angeles, California, USA

[c] Dendrion Inc., Seattle, Washington, USA

[d] Cedars-Sinai Medical Center, Los Angeles, California, USA

ABSTRACT: The microbiota plays a crucial role in experimental models of inflammatory bowel disease, but the exact mechanisms of its effects are unknown. These studies took two molecular approaches to this question. The first used amplification of the 16s ribosomal DNA to define microbial diversity in the colon. Although there were differences in colitic and non-colitic mice, we could not determine whether this was primary or secondary to the disease. The second approach used serologic expression cloning to identify the microbial proteins stimulating the pathogenic immune response. Previously unknown microbial flagellins were the dominant cluster of antigens identified. About half of the sera from patients with Crohn's disease have IgG antibodies to these flagellins.

KEYWORDS: microbiota; colitis; antibodies; flagellin; ribosomal DNA

INTRODUCTION

In recent years many novel models of inflammatory bowel disease have been identified in rodents. In most instances, disease is abolished under germ-free conditions or ameliorated by antibiotics or by limited bacterial colonization.[1] These data establish that the microbiota is crucial for the development of experimental IBD. However, the microbiota is extremely complex and exactly

Address for correspondence: Charles O. Elson, M.D., Division of Gastroenterology and Hepatology, The University of Alabama, Birmingham, 633 Zeigler Research Building, 703 S. 19th Street, Birmingham, AL 35294-0007. Voice: 205-934-6060; fax: 205-934-8493.
e-mail: coelson@uab.edu

Ann. N.Y. Acad. Sci. 1072: 39–51 (2006). © 2006 New York Academy of Sciences.
doi: 10.1196/annals.1326.010

how these commensal bacteria contribute to chronic intestinal inflammation remains unclear.

In this report we took two approaches to address this issue. The first approach was to ask whether there is a qualitative and/or quantitative difference in the bacterial biota between colitic and healthy mice, either during neonatal development or later in life. In addition, we asked whether the composition of the colon microbiota shifts in colitis, a change that may contribute to perpetuation of disease. Because most members of the microbiota have not been cultured, we have used a culture-independent technique to identify them on the basis of PCR amplification of the ribosomal RNA gene.[2] Ribosomal RNA is universal to all bacteria (and eukaryotics), thus all living forms of life can now be related to each other via sequence variation at the ribosomal RNA coding region (rDNA). The amplicons of such PCR reactions were separated and the pattern characterized by denaturing gradient gel electrophoresis (DGGE).[3,4] The microbial profile of the healthy animal, as represented by distinct rDNA amplicons, was compared to that of mice with intestinal inflammation or of mice highly susceptible to colitis. Amplicons unique to either healthy or colitic mice were sequenced and compared to the RNA database to determine their affiliation with known bacterial entities.

The second approach to the issue of how the microbiota contributes to IBD was to use the host immune response as a reporter to identify the key antigens recognized in colitis. This approach used sera from a colitis-susceptible strain, C3H/HeJBir mice, that can develop colitis spontaneously under certain housing conditions.[5] We had previously found that C3H/HeJBir mice develop strong B cell and T cell responses to enteric bacterial antigens.[6] Transfer of enteric bacterial antigen–activated T cells from C3H/HeJBir mice into histocompatible C3H SCID/SCID recipients induces colitis, whereas transfer of similarly treated T cells from noncolitic parent strain C3H/HeJ does not.[7] Western analysis has shown that serum IgG from colitic C3H/HeJBir mice binds to a limited set of proteins from the microbiota, indicating that the immune-response microbiota is highly selective.[6] We used serologic expression cloning with sera from C3H/HeJBir mice to probe a DNA expression library of the cecal microbiota to identify the immunodominant microbial antigens stimulating pathogenic B cell and T cell immune responses in experimental colitis. Interestingly, previously unknown bacterial flagellins represented the largest group of antigens involved in experimental IBD, and about half of patients with Crohn's disease have seroreactivity to these same flagellins.[8]

MATERIALS AND METHODS

DNA Isolation

Bacteria from the murine cecum were suspended in 1 mL of TE (10 mM Tris-HCl, pH 8.0, 0.1 mM EDTA) with 150 μL of phenol (TE buffered), and

0.2 g of silicon/zirconium beads (0.1 mm diameter) were added. The sample was disrupted at 5,000 rpm for 30 sec in a mini-bead beater (Biospec Products, Bartlesville, OK, USA), put on ice for 30 sec to dissipate the heat generated during the process, then treated for another 30 sec. The same process was repeated four times to achieve a total beating time of 2 min. After adding another 150 μL of phenol to the mixture, the tube was vortexed briefly, then centrifuged for 5 min at 14,000 rpm. The supernatant (800 μL) was transferred to a new tube, and 400 μL of phenol:chloroform/isoamylalcohol (50:50 [24:1]) was added. The mixture was vortexed and centrifuged for another 5 min. The supernatant (750 μL) was extracted again with 500 μL phenol:chloroform/isoamyl alcohol. After centrifugation, 600 μL of the supernatant was mixed with 60 μL of 3M Na-acetate, pH 5.2, and 420 μL of isopropanol. The mixture was centrifuged for 5 min at 14,000 rpm at room temperature. The DNA pellet was washed with 70% ethanol and air-dried. The pellet was resuspended in 0.5 mL TE containing 10 μg RNase A and incubated at 37°C for 30 min. The suspension was extracted with 400 μL phenol:chloroform/isoamylalcohol, and precipitated with 0.7 volume of isopropanol in the presence of 0.3 M Na-acetate as described above. Then the DNA pellet was suspended in 200 μL TE, and quantified by spectrophotometry at 260 nm as well as by agarose gel electrophoresis.

Primers for PCR Amplification of the 16S rDNA from Mice Cecal Microbiota

To design primers appropriate for amplification of mice intestinal microbiota, we compared 16S rDNA sequences from diverse bacteria, such as enterobacteria, *Helicobacter* from humans and animals and streptococci, etc., by ClustalW sequence analysis. Based on the conserved regions, three sets of primers as listed in TABLE 1 were designed. A set of primers, bac1 and bac2, as described by Rupf *et al.* was used as a control.[9]

TABLE 1. Primers used in 16S rDNA analysis

Primer	Sequence
F46	5′-GCCTAAYACATGCAAGT-3′
GC-F46	5′-GC*-GCCTAAYACATGCAAGT
R335	5′-CTCCCGTAGGAGTCTGG-3′
F319	5′-CCAGACTCCTACGGGAG-3′
R517	5′-ACCGCGGCTGCTGGCAC-3′
F504	5′-CAGCAGCCGCGGTAATAC-3′
R886	5′-TTGCGRYCGTACTCCCC-3′
BAC1	5′-GC*-ACTACGTGCCAGCAGCC-3′
BAC2	5′-GGACTACCAGGGTATCTAATCC-3′

GC*: sequence the GC-clamp is 5′-CGCCGGGCCGCGGCCCGCCCGCCCGCGGGGGCACGGG GG-3′.

PCR Conditions

PCR was performed under the following conditions: 20 mM Tris-HCl, pH 8.4, 50 mM KCl, 2.5 mM $MgCl_2$, 100 mM each dNTPs, 250 nM primers, 200 ng total cecal DNA and 2 U Taq DNA polymerase in 100 μL reaction. The reaction was conducted in a Perkin–Elmer thermocycler under conditions that differ for each set of primer. For bac1/bac2 and F507/R886 primers, the parameters were 94°C for 3 min, 62°C for 30 sec, 72°C for 30 sec, 1 cycle; 94°C for 1 min, 62°C for 30 sec, 72°C for 30 sec, 30 cycles; followed by 94°C for 1 min, 62°C for 30 sec, and 72°C for 5 min for 1 cycle. For primer sets F46/R335, and F319/R517, the annealing temperature was 56°C, and the other parameters remained the same as for the bac1/bac2 primer set.

Denaturing Gradient Gol Electrophoresis

DGGE was performed by using the Bio-Rad DCode apparatus designed specifically for TGGE and DGGE. The denaturing gel consists of either 6% (for PCR products generated with bac1/bac2 or bac1/R886 primer sets) or 8% (for PCR products generated with GCF46/R335 and GCF319/R517 primer sets) acrylamide:bis (37.5 :1), 8 M urea, 20% deionized formamide, 2% glycerol, 1 × TAE, 0.1% ammonium persulfate (APS) and 0.05% TEMED. One hour after polymerization, the gel was assembled onto the apparatus. Twenty microliters of the PCR product was loaded and the gel was run at 100 V for 17 h with a denaturing gradient of 30% to 70% urea/formamide. After completion of electrophoresis, gels were stained with ethidium bromide (1 μg/mL) for 5 min.

Gel Elution, Cloning, and Sequencing

For ethidium bromide–stained gels, the band of interest was excised under a long-wavelength UV light, crushed and suspended in 50 μL TE. The suspension was incubated at 37°C for 1 h and centrifuged for 5 min at room temperature. One microliter of the supernatant was used for PCR amplification using the respective primers without the GC-clamp. The PCR products were cloned into TA-cloning vector pCRII (Invitrogen Carlsbad, CA). Positive clones were selected, and the plasmid isolated. DNA sequencing of the plasmid insert was performed by using an automated sequencing system in the UAB Cancer Research Center's core facility

Gel and Sequence Analyses

Digital images were saved to disk as TIFF files for subsequent comparisons and analyses. Bands (amplicons) cut out of gels representing unique genotypes were cloned and sequenced in both directions as described above. A BLAST

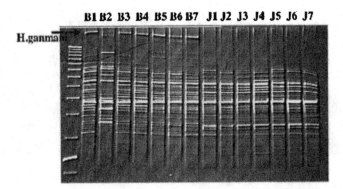

FIGURE 1. DGGE analysis of cecal bacterial 16s rDNA from C3H/HeJ and colitis-prone C3H/HeJBir mice. Both C3H/HeJ and colitis-prone C3H/HeJBir mice were born in the same room under the same conditions. After weaning at approximately 4 weeks, mice from each strain were ear-tagged and placed in the same cage for an additional 4 weeks. All were sacrificed at 8 weeks and their cecal bacteria collected for analysis using PCR amplification of the rDNA gene followed by DGGE. B1–B7, C3H/HeJBir mice; J1–J7, C3H/HeJ mice.

2.0^{10} search of Genbank sequences was done to with each sequence to identify an exactly matching sequence of a known bacteria or the "nearest neighbor" to it.

RESULTS

Cecal Microbial Profiles from Healthy and Colitic Adult C3H Mice

In the first set of experiments, cecal bacterial profiles were defined in control C3H/HeJ and colitis-prone C3H/HeJBir adult mice. Both sets of mice were born in the same room under the same conditions. After weaning at approximately 4 weeks, mice from each strain were ear-tagged and placed in the same cage for an additional 4 weeks. All were sacrificed at 8 weeks and their cecal bacteria collected for analysis using PCR amplification of the rDNA gene followed by DGGE. The patterns of amplicons seen on DGGE were similar, although there was a band that appeared in the C3H/HeJBir mice, but not in the C3H/HeJ mice. This was cloned and sequenced and identified as *Helicobacter ganmani (H. ganmani)* (FIG. 1), a recently identified mouse commensal.[11]

Neonatal Microbial Colonization in Colitis-Prone versus Healthy C3H Mice

During neonatal colonization of mice with enteric bacteria, there are large swings in culturable bacterial strains that occur in a sequential manner between

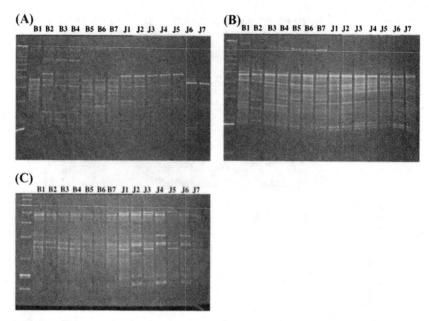

FIGURE 2. DGGE analysis of cecal bacterial 16s rDNA. Both C3H/HeJ and colitis-prone C3H/HeJBir mice were born in the same room and housed in the same cages. Groups of mice were sacrificed at age of 2 **(A)**, 4 **(B)**, or 6 **(C)** weeks and their cecal bacteria collected for analysis using PCR amplification of the rDNA gene followed by DGGE. B1–B7, C3H/HeJBir mice; J1–J7, C3H/HeJ mice.

the 10th and 14th days after birth.[12–14] These profound rearrangements of the bacterial populations in mice gradually stabilize, with the adult pattern being acquired by approximately 4 weeks. The microbiota is then thought to remain stable throughout adult life. Because the mice shown in FIGURE 1 were raised separately up to 4 weeks, we conducted a second experiment in which pregnant mice of the two strains were placed into the same large cage and the progeny ear-tagged so that they could be identified. In this experiment, the litters were raised in the same environment from birth. Interestingly, 2-week-old mice from each strain showed two different distinct patterns of bands. For instance, 4 of the 7 C3H/HeJBir mice shared the same pattern and the other 3 had a distinctive, different pattern that was shared (FIG. 2A). The C3H/HeJ mice had a similar dichotomy. By 6 weeks of age these differences were largely gone, with most of the C3H/HeJBir mice sharing the same pattern of bands (FIG. 2C). There was a bit more microbial diversity in the C3H/HeJ mice, but again many of the bands were similar to those seen in the C3H/HeJBir mice.

Alteration of the Enteric Microbiota by Chronic Colitis

An emerging body of data indicates that the enteric microbiota interacts with the epithelial layer and the mucosal immune system. Thus, alterations

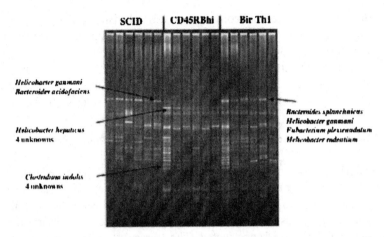

FIGURE 3. DGGE analysis of cecal bacteria in colitis. For C3H/HeJBir CD4$^+$ T cell transfer colitis, 2×10^6 CD4$^+$ Th1 cells reactive to cecal bacterial antigens were transferred into histocompatible C3H/HeSnJ SCID mice; the recipients developed colitis with focal lesions. For CD4$^+$ CD45RB^{hi}–induced colitis, 10^6 CD4$^+$ CD45RB^{hi} T cells from C3H/HeJBir mice were transferred into C3H/HeSnJ SCID mice; the recipients developed diffuse colitis. Control C3H/HeSnJ mice received no cells. All mice were kept in the same large cage and sacrificed 2 months later.

in the epithelium and mucosal lymphocytes that occur in colitis might cause, in turn, alterations of the bacterial microbiota. To address this question we used two different T cell transfer models of colitis. The first was the now well-established CD4$^+$CD45RB^{hi} T cell transfer model.[15] We have previously found that the transfers of CD4$^+$CD45RB^{hi} T cells from C3H/HeJBir mice into C3H-SCID mice induce a diffuse colitis throughout the colon and cecum, as is seen with other inbred strains. The second T cell adoptive transfer model involved the adoptive transfer into C3H/SCID mice of a memory CD4$^+$Th1 cell line from C3H/HeJBir mice that is reactive to enteric bacterial antigens.[7] SCID recipients of such transfers develop colitis that tends to be focal and more severe in the cecum than in the colon. C3H/SCID mice that received only saline solution instead of T cells served as the control. Again, the mice were ear-tagged and kept in the same cage. In both models the colitis tends to be maximal at approximately 8 weeks after transfer and that was the point at which the experiment was terminated. Cecal bacteria were collected from six mice from each group and analyzed as above. The results are shown in FIGURE 3. The DGGE patterns show that not only is the microbiota shifted in colitis, but also that it is shifted differently in the two T cell adoptive transfer models. A number of the bands that were distinctive in each model were cloned and sequenced and the bacteria identified are shown in FIGURE 3.

We conclude from these studies that this molecular approach to identification of the microbiota coupled with DGGE and sequencing is a valid and valuable methodology that will allow analysis of the microbiota in both health and diseased states. There were differences identified in the colonic microbiota between control C3H/HeJ and colitis-prone C3H/HeJBir mice. Whether these differences are a response to or a driver of colitis remains unclear from this microbe-centric approach. It is clear that induction of colitis alters the enteric microbiota, and the pattern of the shift depends on how the colitis is induced, that is, by a naïve or memory CD4 T cell. These results illustrate some of the complexity involved in dissecting the role of the enteric microbiota in IBD.

Which Microbiota Antigens Drive the Host Pathogenic Response?

The alternative approach to how the microbiota contribute to IBD is to use the host immune response as a reporter to identify the key microbial proteins stimulating pathogenic adaptive responses. To address this question serologic expression cloning was used. First a lambda phage expression library of total cecal bacterial DNA was constructed. The library was then screened using serum IgG from colitic C3H/HeJBir mice. Positive clones were collected and rescreened two more times. At the end of the process the remaining 60 clones were sequenced. There were no nucleotide matches for any of these clones in GenBank, but many had some homology to existing bacterial proteins. The most surprising result was that about a quarter of the total were previously unknown flagellins from enteric bacteria.[8] These flagellins appeared to cluster into the *C. coccoides* group, which are known to form a major part of the bacterial flora.

Two of these flagellins, CBir1 and FlaX, were expressed and studied in detail. Interestingly, reactivity to them was identified in multiple mouse colitis models, such as mdr1α knockout mice and IL-10-deficient mice on the C3H, C57BL6, and BALB/c genetic backgrounds. A CD4[+] T cell line from C3H/HeJBir mice was generated that reacted only with CBir1 flagellin but not other bacterial proteins. Adoptive transfer of this anti-flagellin T cell line resulted in a severe colitis in C3H/SCID recipients.[8]

The wide reactivity among multiple strains and models of colitis in mice prompted us to ask whether there might be reactivity to this flagellin in humans. Indeed, approximately half of patients with Crohn's disease had serum IgG antibodies to CBir1 flagellin. Such reactivity was significantly more frequent in patients with Crohn's disease than in sera from patients with ulcerative colitis, disease controls, or normal individuals.

DISCUSSION

These studies used the C3H/HeJBir mouse, a strain that was originally generated by a program of selective breeding at the Jackson Laboratory. It is derived from the common laboratory strain, C3H/HeJ, which is known to have a deletion mutation in TLR4.[16] The C3H/HeJ breeding stock at the Jackson Laboratory sporadically developed a self-limited juvenile right-sided colitis. The

C3H/HeJBir substrain was derived from such a colitic C3H/HeJ female. This new substrain developed spontaneous colitis when raised under certain housing conditions.[5] C3H/HeJBir mice are also very susceptible to colitis induction by chemical agents, and this susceptibility is genetically determined.[17,18] Analysis of C3H/HeJBir substrain demonstrated that these mice have strong B cell and Th1 cell responses to cecal bacterial antigens (CBA). Western analysis of their IgG seroreactivity to CBA revealed that their B cell/antibody response is highly selective, with a small number of bands identified out of the hundreds of thousands of proteins present. Transfer of cecal bacterial antigen-activated CD4[+] T cells into C3H SCID mice results in a focal colitis that is very similar to what is seen in the spontaneous disease. Because the host–microbiota interaction in C3H/HeJBir mice results in colitis, this experimental model is particularly well suited to studies on the interaction between the microbiota and the host that can lead to chronic intestinal inflammation.

The first question addressed was whether the colitis-prone C3H/HeJBir strain might have an alteration of the microbiota, compared to the closely related but noncolitic C3H/HeJ parental strain, which favors the development of colitis. The microbiota varies qualitatively and quantitatively along the length of intestine reaching 10^{12} organisms/gm of cecum content.[19] The microbiota is very complex and functions as a multicellular organ with metabolic activity equivalent to the liver. Current estimates are that there are as many as 800 species and > 7,000 strains in the microbiota.[20] These bacteria have a profound effect upon the host, inducing alterations in the epithelium, the vascular supply of the intestine, the intestinal nervous system, and the mucosal immune system.[20] The microbiota also plays an important role in the energy metabolism of the host.[21] The microbiota represents the greatest mass of antigen encountered by the host immune system and response to these antigens is continuous, as demonstrated by the 3–5 gm of IgA released into the intestine each day in normal humans. Thus, it is not unreasonable to postulate that a dysbiosis of the microbiota could alter the microbial–host dialogue sufficient to result in a chronic inflammatory disease of the intestine.

The sheer complexity of the microbiota is daunting, as is the failure of current culture techniques to grow most of these organisms. The development of ribosomal DNA gene analysis has been a technical breakthrough that allows definition of the microbiota without the need for culture. This technique was developed by microbial ecologists for application to the study of soil and marine microbes.[22] The application of this technique to human and mouse biota is revealing the major outlines of the microbiota composition in both mouse and man.[23,24,21] Although the major divisions and phyla seem to be similar between mouse and man, there is great diversity in species and strains.[20]

The examination of whether dysbiosis might exist in the colitis-prone C3H/HeJBir strain was addressed by using this 16S rDNA technique. When adult C3H/HeJBir mice were compared to the control C3H/HeJ mice, some differences were indeed found. For one, *H. ganmani* was identified in C3H/HeJBir mice, but not in C3H/HeJ.[11] This is of interest because *Helicobacter* has been implicated in intestinal inflammation. The best example of this is *Helicobacter pylori* induction of gastritis. There are a variety of *Helicobacter* present in the colon of normal mice, most of which are commensals, but some, such as *Helicobacter hepaticus*, have been implicated in the induction of gut inflammation in immunodeficient mice.[25]

Because neonates acquire their microbiota from their mother, we next asked whether litters of these two strains raised in the same cages would have differences in microbiota. Interestingly, there were significant differences identified in neonates of each strain at 2 weeks of age, when the flora are just being acquired and the mice are still suckling. As the mice aged in the same cage, most of these differences disappeared, but there did appear to be more diversity of microbial strains in the C3H/HeJ mice than in C3H/HeJBir mice, even though these mice were raised in the same cage and shared the same environment.

Because the microbiota interacts with the epithelial layer and with the innate and adaptive immune system of the host,[26] we next asked whether the microbiota is stable in colitis. We reasoned that changes that occur in colitis, including the inflammatory cell response, increased transudation of serum, increased oxygen tension, increased NO production, etc., could certainly have a substantial effect on the microbiota. To address this question we used two different T cell-induced colitis models. The first was the transfer of CD45RB[hi] naïve CD4 T cells from C3H/HeJBir mice into C3H SCID mice. The second was the transfer of bacteria-reactive, memory effector CD4 T cells from C3H/HeJBir mice into C3H SCID recipients. C3H SCID mice that were mock-injected with saline solution served as controls. All mice were again housed in the same cage. The results are quite clear that the microbiota shifted in colitis and changed its composition from the base line. Interestingly, the pattern of change was different depending on whether a memory or naïve T cell was transferred, even though both models are mediated through CD4[+] Th1 cell responses to the microbiota. These results support the idea that the microbiota is in dynamic equilibrium with the host and that the microbiota changes its composition in response to the microenvironmental changes that occur in colitis.

Taken together, these results indicate that there are some differences in the microbiota between the colitis-prone C3H/HeJBir mouse and its closely related, but phenotypically different, C3H/HeJ parental strain. However, the data do not tell us whether these differences are secondary to some mild inflammatory component present in the C3H/HeJBir mouse or whether they are a primary driver of disease. Given that dynamic changes in the microbiota were seen in the induced colitis models, we favor the former possibility, but this is a classic "chicken and egg" question. These studies do illustrate the complexity in the system and the inherent difficulty in trying to identify dysbiosis as a driver of inflammatory bowel disease.

Even if one or more bacteria in the microbiota were identified as being present only in colitic mice, the significance of this finding in relation to the development of colitis would be difficult to establish. Thus, a second approach was used, which was to use the host immune response to report which microbial antigens were stimulating the pathogenic response. This approach was based on observations mentioned earlier that C3H/HeJBir mice have high titer IgG antibodies to a limited set of proteins present in the cecal microbiota using Western analysis. Indeed, the same pattern of bands was identified using sera from C3H/HeJBir mice separated in time by more than a year and was quite reproducible among different groups of C3H/HeJBir mice. Other inbred strains with colitis also have limited reactivity to CBA, but not necessarily to the same bands as recognized by C3H/HeJBir mice (unpublished data).

The Western analysis data showing that the immune response was highly selective were confirmed by the serologic expression cloning that identified only 60 microbial genes. The dominance of previously unknown bacterial flagellins among these clones was unexpected. However, flagellins are able to activate the innate immune system through interaction with the toll-like receptor 5 and thus have inherent adjuvanticity that is not shared with most other bacterial proteins.[27,28] Secondly, these flagellins appear to derive from the *Clostridia coccioides* cluster, which are known to be highly represented in the bacterial flora. This cluster was not previously implicated in patients with Crohn's disease, and thus it is particularly interesting that half of patients with Crohn's disease have antibodies to flagellins from these bacteria. The reactivity of Crohn's sera to these flagellins demonstrates that this unbiased approach to identification of the host response to the microbiota has yielded unexpected dividends.

Subsequent work in Crohn's disease patients has shown that antibodies to CBir1 flagellin are associated with small bowel involvement, fibrostenosis, and internal perforating phenotypes, that is, with more complicated Crohn's disease.[29] This reactivity is independent of reactivity to ASCA, I2, or *E. coli* OmpC antigens. Interestingly, some 44% of patients with Crohn's disease who are pANCA-positive were positive for anti-CBir1 flagellin, but only 4% of pANCA-positive ulcerative colitis patients had similar reactivity. Thus, the antiflagellin response may well be able to distinguish pANCA-positive patients with Crohn's disease from pANCA patients with ulcerative colitis. The antiflagellin response thus might become a useful biomarker for the complicated Crohn's disease.

ACKNOWLEDGMENTS

This work was supported in part by grants from the Crohn's and Colitis Foundation of America, the Eli and Edythe Broad Foundation, and the National Institutes of Health (DK44240 and DK71176).

We acknowledge the expert technical assistance of Wayne Duck in these experiments.

REFERENCES

1. ELSON, C.O. & C.T. WEAVER. 2003. Experimental mouse models of inflammatory bowel disease: new insights into pathogenic mechanisms. *In* Inflammatory Bowel Disease: From Bench to Bedside. S.R. Targan, F. Shanahan & L.C. Karp, Eds.: 67–99. Kluwer Academic Publishers. Dordrecht.
2. LANE, D.J. *et al.* 1985. Rapid determination of 16S ribosomal RNA sequences for phylogenetic analysis. Proc. Natl. Acad. Sci. USA **82:** 6955–6959.
3. FELSKE, A., A.D.L. AKKERMANS & W.M. DE VOS. 1998. Quantification of 16S rRNA in complex bacterial communities by multiple competitive reverse transcription-PCR in temperature gradient gel electrophoresis fingerprints. Appl. Environ. Microbiol. **64:** 4581–4587.
4. KROES, I., P.W. LEPP & D.A. RELMAN. 1999. Bacterial diversity within the human subgingival crevice. Proc. Natl. Acad. Sci. USA **96:** 14547–14552.
5. SUNDBERG, J.P. *et al.* 1994. Spontaneous, heritable colitis in a new substrain of C3H/HeJ mice. Gastroenterology **107:** 1726–1735.
6. BRANDWEIN, S.L. *et al.* 1997. Spontaneously colitic C3H/HeJBir mice demonstrate selective antibody reactivity to antigens of the enteric bacterial flora. J. Immunol. **159:** 44–52.
7. CONG, Y. *et al.* 1998. CD4$^+$ T cells reactive to enteric bacterial antigens in spontaneously colitic C3H/HeJBir mice: increased T helper cell type 1 response and ability to transfer disease. J. Exp. Med. **187:** 855–864.
8. LODES, M.J. *et al.* 2004. Bacterial flagellin is a dominant antigen in Crohn's disease. J. Clin. Invest. **113:** 1296–1306.
9. RUPF, S., K. MERTE & K. ESCHRICH. 1999. Quantification of bacteria in oral samples by competitive polymerase chain reaction. J. Dent. Res. **78:** 850–856.
10. ALTSCHUL, S.F. *et al.* 1997. Gapped BLAST and PSI-BLAST: a new generation of protein database search programs. Nucleic Acids Res. **25:** 3389–3402.
11. ROBERTSON, B.R. *et al.* 2001. *Helicobacter ganmani* sp. nov., a urease-negative anaerobe isolated from the intestines of laboratory mice. Int. J. Syst. Evol. Microbiol. **51:** 1881–1889.
12. SCHAEDLER, R.W., R. DUBOS & R. COSTELLO. 1974. The development of the bacterial flora in the gastrointestinal tract of mice. J. Exp. Med. **122:** 59–70.
13. MUSHIN, R. & R. DUBOS. 1965. Colonization of the mouse intestine with *Escherichia coli*. J. Exp. Med. **122:** 745–757.
14. SAVAGE, D.C. & R. DUBOS. 1968. Alterations in the mouse cecum and its flora produced by antibacterial drugs. J. Exp. Med. **128:** 97–110.
15. POWRIE, F. *et al.* 1993. Phenotypically distinct subsets of CD4+ T cells induce or protect from chronic intestinal inflammation in C. B-17 scid mice. Int. Immunol. **5:** 1461–1471.
16. POLTORAK, A. *et al.* 1998. Defective LPS signaling in C3H/HeJ and C57BL/10ScCr mice: mutations in Tlr4 gene. Science **282:** 2085–2088.
17. MAHLER, M. *et al.* 1999. Genetic analysis of susceptibility to dextran sulfate sodium-induced colitis in mice. Genomics **55:** 147–156.
18. BRISTOL, I.J. *et al.* 2000. Heritable susceptibility for colitis in mice induced by IL-10 deficiency. Inflamm. Bowel Dis. **6:** 290–302.

19. MACFARLANE, G.T. & S. MACFARLANE. 1997. Human colonic microbiota: ecology, physiology and metabolic potential of intestinal bacteria. Scan. J. Gastroenterol. **222**(Suppl.): 3–9.
20. BACKHED, F. *et al.* 2005. Host-bacterial mutualism in the human intestine. Science. **307**: 1915–1920.
21. LEY, R.E. *et al.* 2005. Obesity alters gut microbial ecology. Proc. Natl. Acad. Sci. USA **102**: 11070–11075.
22. DELONG, E.F. & N.R. PACE. 2001. Environmental diversity of bacteria and archaea. Syst. Biol. **50**: 470–478.
23. WANG, X. *et al.* 2003. Molecular characterization of the microbial species that colonize human ileal and colonic mucosa by using 16S rDNA sequence analysis. J. Appl. Microbiol. **95**: 508–520.
24. ECKBURG, P.B. *et al.* 2005. Diversity of the human intestinal microbial flora. Science **308**: 1635–1638.
25. ZHANG, L. *et al.* 2005. Natural colonization with *Helicobacter* species and the development of inflammatory bowel disease in interleukin-10-deficient mice. Helicobacter **10**: 223–230.
26. LORENZ, R.G., V.J. MCCRACKEN & C.O. ELSON. 2005. Animal models of intestinal inflammation: ineffective communication between coalition members. Springer Semin. Immunopathol. **27**: 233–247.
27. HAYASHI, F. *et al.* 2001. The innate immune response to bacterial flagellin is mediated by toll-like receptor 5. Nature **410**: 1099–1103.
28. HONKO, A.N. & S.B. MIZEL. 2005. Effects of flagellin on innate and adaptive immunity. Immunol. Res. **33**: 83–102.
29. TARGAN, S.R. *et al.* 2005. Antibodies to CBir1 flagellin define a unique response that is associated independently with complicated Crohn's disease. Gastroenterology **128**: 2020–2028.

CCR6 and CCL20

Partners in Intestinal Immunity and Lymphorganogenesis

IFOR R. WILLIAMS

Department of Pathology, Emory University School of Medicine, Whitehead 105D, 615 Michael St., Atlanta, Georgia 30322, USA

ABSTRACT: The CCR6 chemokine receptor is expressed by most B cells and subsets of T cells and dendritic cells (DCs) found in the gut mucosal immune system. CCL20, the single chemokine ligand for CCR6, is selectively made by the follicle-associated epithelium (FAE) overlying Peyer's patches (PPs) and isolated lymphoid follicles (ILFs). CCL20 contributes to the recruitment of CCR6-expressing B cells to these structures. CCL20 expression by the intestinal epithelium is also highly inducible in response to inflammatory stimuli. Thus, CCL20 functions as both an inflammatory and homeostatic chemokine. Interactions between CCR6 and CCL20 play a role at several stages in the development of intestinal lymphoid structures. A subset of the c-kit$^+$ lymphoid precursors found in cryptopatches (CPs) expresses CCR6. Recruitment of B cells to CPs and the subsequent expansion and organization of these B cells allows differentiation of some of these structures into ILFs. In CCR6 knockout mice, PPs are smaller with fewer follicles and the development of ILFs is compromised. These defects in the development of mucosal inductive sites in CCR6-deficient mice are responsible for decreased IgA production to oral antigens. CCR6 can be included with CXCR5 and CCR7 in a list of chemokine receptors that participate in shaping the organized lymphoid structures that are part of the intestinal immune system.

KEYWORDS: CCR6; chemokines; lymphoid organogenesis; isolated lymphoid follicles

INTRODUCTION

Most cases of human inflammatory bowel disease are associated with a breakdown of normal immune tolerance to components of the commensal enteric flora. Evidence is accumulating that this loss of tolerance involves

Address for correspondence: Ifor R. Williams, Department of Pathology, Emory University School of Medicine, Whitehead 105D, 615 Michael St., Atlanta, GA 30322, USA. Voice: 404-727-8547; fax: 404-727-8538.

e-mail: irwilli@emory.edu

Ann. N.Y. Acad. Sci. 1072: 52–61 (2006). © 2006 New York Academy of Sciences.

doi: 10.1196/annals.1326.036

dysregulated responses of both the innate and adaptive immune responses. Inappropriate innate immune responses to components of the commensal enteric flora can lead to generation of effector responses under circumstances where regulatory responses are more appropriate. The initiation and sustenance of both effector and regulatory adaptive immune responses in the intestine is facilitated by the presence of organized intestinal lymphoid tissues. The compartmentalization characteristic of organized lymphoid tissues is largely the result of the concerted action of chemokines and chemokine receptors. Through the action of chemokines, B and T lymphocyte subsets are positioned in specific zones with access to the antigen-presenting cells (APC) and stromal cells that support the lymphocytes.[1] CCR6 is a CC chemokine receptor that contributes to both lymphorganogenesis and mucosal immunity in the intestine.

The organized lymphoid tissues of the intestine include cryptopatches (CPs), isolated lymphoid follicles (ILFs), Peyer's patches (PPs), and the mesenteric lymph node (MLN).[2] All of these structures except for the MLN arise in close proximity to a layer of epithelium. The epithelium actively participates in a chemokine dialogue that shapes these structures via selective production of chemokines by the follicle-associated epithelium (FAE), a specialized epithelium located above the lymphoid component of ILFs and PPs.[3,4] The FAE lacks several specialized types of epithelial cells that are normally present in the epithelium covering the surrounding villi and crypts, including goblet cells, enteroendocrine cells, and Paneth cells. The FAE also contains microfold (M) cells, specialized cells characterized morphologically by short, blunt-ended microvilli and functionally by high efficiency uptake of particulate antigens from the intestinal lumen. Immediately beneath the M cells are intraepithelial pockets that contain lymphocytes and dendritic cells (DCs). Antigenic material entering through M cells is delivered into the intraepithelial pocket and gains access to APC populations located in the subepithelial dome region (SED) beneath the FAE.

EXPRESSION PATTERN OF THE CCR6 LIGAND CCL20

Profiling of gene expression by the FAE in the intestine has revealed a set of transcripts that are expressed at significantly higher levels in the FAE than in intestinal epithelial cells that form the rest of the intestinal lining. Chemokines selectively expressed by the FAE include CCL20 (in mice and humans), CCL9 (in mice), and CCL23 (in humans).[4,5] The enhanced constitutive expression of CCL20 by the FAE has been demonstrated at both the mRNA level and the protein level. This article will critically examine the different proposed functions of CCL20 and CCR6 in the intestine, focusing on the role of CCR6 in controlling the positioning of DC subsets and how CCR6 is involved in the development of intestinal lymphoid structures. Insights into the specific role of CCR6 in these processes have been gained through identification of phenotypic abnormalities in CCR6 knockout mice.

The CCL20 gene was identified by several independent laboratories as a novel chemokine gene expressed by a variety of cell types. The original names for the gene product included macrophage inflammatory protein-3α (MIP-3α), liver activation-related chemokine (LARC), and Exodus-2.[6–8] CCL20 was demonstrated to be a ligand for an orphan G-protein-coupled receptor that was designated CCR6.[9,10] Expression studies have identified CCR6 on most B cells, effector memory T cells, and some subsets of DCs. While CCL20 remains the only known chemokine ligand for CCR6, human β-defensin 1 and 2 have been identified as additional ligands for CCR6.[11] These human β-defensin ligands have a significantly lower affinity for the CCR6 receptor. Whether the β-defensins can substitute for CCL20 in any physiological responses that require CCR6 is not yet known.

Most chemokines can be classified as either inflammatory or homeostatic chemokines on the basis of how their gene expression is regulated.[12] Inflammatory chemokines are involved in the recruitment of leukocytes to sites of injury and inflammation. Examples of inflammatory chemokines that are markedly induced above basal levels following an inflammatory insult include CXCL8, CCL2, and CXCL10. In contrast, homeostatic chemokines are usually constitutively expressed by the cells that make them. Examples include CXCL12, CXCL13, CCL19, CCL21, CCL25, and CCL28. A subset of these chemokines (CXCL12, CXCL13, CCL19, and CCL21) are known as lymphoid chemokines and provide chemotactic gradients that guide B cells and T cells into specific compartments within organized lymphoid tissues. Most of these lymphoid chemokines (CXCL13, CCL19, and CCL21) are also induced following stimulation of stromal cells through the lymphotoxin β receptor (LTβR), which is critical for development of all secondary lymphoid structures.

CCL20 is expressed by a variety of epithelial cell types including keratinocytes, pulmonary epithelial cells, and intestinal epithelial cells.[13–15] CCL20 is typically expressed at a low basal level, but can be strongly induced by proinflammatory signals including primary cytokines (e.g., TNF-α) and Toll-like receptor (TLR) agonists originating from microbes.[16] In microarray analyses of the epithelial transcriptome following specific proinflammatory stimuli, CCL20 is typically found to be one of the most highly induced genes. CCL20 is also expressed at higher levels in colonic biopsy tissue from patients with inflammatory bowel disease than in normal colonic tissue.[17] This pattern of CCL20 expression fits the general pattern expected of an inflammatory chemokine. CCL20 can play several different roles following its induction by inflammatory stimuli. In addition to the chemotaxis of CCR6-expressing cells, there is also evidence that CCL20 can act as an antimicrobial peptide.[15,18] When CCL20 expression is highly induced on epithelial cells in response to TLR agonists, the antimicrobial peptide action of CCL20 may contribute to protecting the local environment from microbes with the potential to cause invasive disease.

However, CCL20 exhibits a distinct pattern of regulation on epithelial tissues located adjacent to organized lymphoid structures. In the FAE that covers intestinal lymphoid aggregates, such as PPs and mature ILFs, the follicle-associate epithelial cells constitutively express significantly more CCL20 than do crypt and villous epithelial cells.[19] The same pattern occurs in the epithelial cells on the surface of human tonsils and in the mouse nasal-associated lymphoid tissue (NALT).[20,21] The increased basal expression of CCL20 by the enterocytes of the FAE is evidence that lymphoepithelial cross-talk is occurring, and the CCL20 synthesized by the FAE contributes to recruitment of CCR6-expressing cells to organized lymphoid aggregates in the intestine. Further support for this idea comes from the observation that CCL20 expression by epithelial cells is increased after stimulation of the LTβR by either its natural ligand LTα1β2 or agonist antibodies directed against the receptor.[19] CCL20 expression by the epithelial cells over mouse PPs can be detected at embryonic day 18.5, which is approximately 1 day after clusters of cells expressing LTβ are first detected.[19] These observations suggest that CCL20 and CCR6 participate in a positive amplification circuit that contributes to lymphoid organogenesis in the gut, with CCL20 recruiting cells (B cells and possibly also lymphoid tissue inducer cells) to the vicinity of the epithelium, which can further stimulate epithelial CCL20 expression by virtue of expression of surface LTα1β2. This prediction is supported by the morphological studies of gut-associated lymphoid tissue (GALT) structures including PPs and ILFs in CCR6-deficient mice, as described below. Considering the full spectrum of properties of CCL20, CCL20 is perhaps best regarded as both an inflammatory chemokine and a homeostatic chemokine involved in lymphorganogenesis.

PHENOTYPIC ABNORMALITIES IN CCR6-DEFICIENT MICE

Analysis of mice deficient in CCR6 has provided a series of new insights into how CCL20–CCR6 interactions function in tandem with the classic "homeostatic" chemokines to promote the assembly and maintenance of organized lymphoid structures located beneath epithelial surfaces. Four independently derived strains of CCR6 mice have been described.[22–25] This article will attempt to integrate the published findings from the groups studying CCR6-deficient mice, focusing specifically on the contributions of CCR6 to DC positioning in the PP and to the development of organized lymphoid structures in the intestine.

Before the first published report on the phenotype of CCR6-deficient mice, it was already known through the work of Iwasaki and Kelsall that the CD11c[+] DCs within PPs could be divided into subsets that were CD8α[+] (and CD11b[-]), CD11b[+] (and CD8α[-]), and negative for both CD8α and CD11b.[26] The CD11b[+] subset was shown to express mRNA for CCR6 and migrate to CCL20 in chemotaxis assays. Expression of CCR6 by most CD11b[+] DCs in PPs was established by analysis of CCR6–enhanced green fluorescent protein (EGFP) knockin mice.[24] Because of the selective expression of CCL20 by the FAE located above the SED of the PPs, it was proposed that recruitment of CD11b[+] DCs to the SED region was dependent on CCR6 and a chemotactic gradient of CCL20. Initial reports on two independent strains of CCR6-deficient mice suggested that CD11b[+] DC were absent from the vicinity of the SED in PPs.[22,23] However, a subsequent study examining PPs from all four reported strains of CCR6-deficient mice found that the number of CD11b[+] DC in the SED region was not significantly diminished.[5] The same study also showed that mouse CCL9, a chemokine that attracts CCR1[+] cells, was selectively expressed by the FAE and could chemoattract CD11b[+] DCs from PPs *in vitro*. FAE cells in human PPs were later shown to selectively express a CCL23, a homologue of mouse CCL9.[4] These findings and published studies showing that migration of new DCs into the lung is impaired in the absence of CCR6[27] suggest that the effects of CCR6 deficiency on the migration of DCs in PPs are more apparent in the course of an acute immunological response than under normal steady-state conditions, which permit other chemokines to attract CD11b[+] DC to the SED region. One of the mutant CCR6 alleles developed in mice includes an EGFP knockin allele that allows the EGFP to be used as a reporter to identify CCR6[+] cells and to identify the position and movements of CCR6[+] cells *in vivo* without using antibody staining.[24] Mice with a GFP knockin construct inserted into the CX3CR1 gene have been used, by means of *in situ* confocal microscopy, to visualize the extension of dendrites belonging to CXC3R1-expressing lamina propria DCs through the epithelial layer to reach the intestinal lumen.[28] Use of similar techniques to study mice that are heterozygous and homozygous for the CCR6–EGFP knockin allele may lead to a better understanding of the contribution of an intact CCR6 receptor to migration of CCR6[+] DC subsets within PPs. Recent studies have demonstrated that CCR6 = Expressing DCs are recruited into the subepithelial dome area of murine PPs in response to invasion by *Salmonella* of the FAE.[29]

Decreased size of small intestinal PPs has been described in two of the CCR6 knockout models, although the total number of PPs remained in the normal range.[23,29] The smaller PPs in CCR6 null mice have a decreased number of B cell–containing follicles and decreased cellularity. In addition, the percentage of M cells within the PPs FAE of CCR6-deficient mice is significantly decreased.[29] These observations indicate that CCR6 plays a significant role in the later stages of GALT development, in contrast to other chemokine receptors, such as CXCR5 and CCR7, which are also critical for earlier stages of lymphoid structure development.[31–33] CCR6 expression on B cells appears to be required for full recruitment of B cells to lymphoid follicles in structures such as PPs. Given that PPs are an important inductive site for the development of IgA responses to antigens encountered in the gut lumen, the impairment in mucosal IgA responses to oral antigens in CCR6-deficient[22] mice can be attributed, at least in part, to the compromised development of PPs.

CCR6 IN CPs AND ILFs

Because ILFs share multiple features with PPs including the presence of an FAE layer containing M cells and the ability to serve as an inductive site for mucosal IgA responses,[34] the effect of CCR6 deficiency on ILF development was also examined. Compared to C57BL/6 control mice, CCR6-deficient mice were found to have fewer immature ILFs.[35] Immature ILFs are thought to be precursors of mature ILFs that contain B cell aggregates, but are smaller and have not yet developed germinal centers.[36] In addition to comparing the number of ILFs in CCR6-deficient and wild-type mice, the effects of CCR6 deficiency have been examined in two mouse models that feature significantly increased ILF development compared to wild-type mice. In the first model, mice are treated *in utero* with LTβR-Ig on embryonic day 16 to block the development of PPs and peripheral lymph nodes. These mice cannot develop normal PPs after birth because the normal developmental window for PPs development has passed. In place of PPs, these mice develop a greater number of ILFs in a process stimulated by the presence of the commensal enteric flora. In the second model, transfer of T cell–depleted bone marrow is used to rescue the development of intestinal lymphoid structures including CPs and ILFs in mice that have a targeted mutation in CD132 or γ_c, the common γ chain of the IL-2 receptor, and consequently are profoundly lymphopenic and lack any endogenous CPs or ILFs. When *in utero* LTβR-Ig treatment was used to stimulate a greater extent of ILFs development, the number of immature and mature ILFs increased in CCR6-deficient mice compared to untreated controls.[35] However, the extent of ILFs development remained substantially compromised compared to the wild-type controls treated with LTβR-Ig in parallel. Consistent with these results, transfer of CCR6-deficient bone marrow to CD132 null mice also yields significantly fewer ILFs than does transfer of wild-type bone marrow. These findings indicate that CCR6 plays similar roles in both ILF and PP development, even though development of these structures begins at different points in time during development.

The origin of immature ILFs is still under investigation. CPs may function as precursor structures that can develop into immature ILFs when seeded with a sufficient number of B cells. The development of both CPs and ILFs is dependent on the presence of LTα and LTβR.[37] LTα1β2 interactions with the LTβR are required to initiate the development of other organized lymphoid aggregates (e.g., lymph nodes and PPs) that result from initial productive interactions between lymphoid tissue inducer cells and stromal organizer cells. Another common feature identified in both CPs and ILFs is the presence of a network of supporting stromal cells expressing LTβR-dependent markers including VCAM-1 and FDC-M1.[36] The original description of CPs in mice reported the presence of occasional B220$^+$ B cells in these structures.[38] Lymphoid aggregates with features somewhere between those of classic CP and fully developed ILFs have been described recently.[39] These structures may represent intermediates in a process through which some CPs can transition into ILFs.

Analysis of small intestinal tissue from CCR6-deficient mice also revealed the presence of CP that included the same major cell populations found in the CPs of wild-type mice (i.e., lymphoid precursor cells, DCs, and stromal cells).[40] However, an unexpected observation made as part of these studies was that a subset of the c-kit[+] lymphoid precursor cells in CPs express CCR6. This was demonstrated by finding EGFP fluorescence within CPs from CCR6–EGFP knockin mice and by direct staining of CPs in wild-type mice with monoclonal antibodies to mouse CCR6. The functional significance of CCR6 expression by lymphoid precursor cells in CPs has not yet been defined. Some of these CCR6[+] cells may be lymphoid tissue inducer cells. Clusters of presumed lymphoid tissue inducer cells expressing the RORγt isoform of the RORγ receptor have been identified within CPs using RORγt-EGFP knockin mice.[41]

SUMMARY

CCR6-deficient mice exhibit an interesting combination of mucosal immune defects, with some occurring as a result of altered lymphoid aggregate development in the intestine and others arising as a result of the absence of CCR6 in one or more of the cellular subsets known to normally express CCR6. Identification of CCR6 expression on lymphoid precursors in CPs and the demonstration of defects in ILF and PP development in CCR6-deficient mice have contributed to a better understanding of the role of CCL20–CCR6 interactions during the emergence and establishment of intestinal lymphoid structures.

ACKNOWLEDGMENTS

Research in the author's laboratory has been supported by grants from the NIH (DK 064730) and the Crohn's and Colitis Foundation of America. Core facilities used in this research are supported with the assistance of the Emory Digestive Disease Research Development Center (NIH DK 064399). I wish to thank the members of my laboratory who have contributed to the experimental findings discussed in this manuscript. In particular, I would like to thank Torsten Kucharzik and Andreas Lügering for their efforts in developing and characterizing the CCR6–EGFP knockin mice and Rebekah Taylor for her studies on lymphoid organogenesis in the intestine. I also thank my collaborator Rodney Newberry and members of his laboratory for their work on ILF development in CCR6-deficient mice.

REFERENCES

1. OHL, L., G. BERNHARDT, O. PABST, *et al.* 2003. Chemokines as organizers of primary and secondary lymphoid organs. Semin. Immunol. **15:** 249–255.
2. TAYLOR, R.T. & I.R. WILLIAMS. 2005. Lymphoid organogenesis in the intestine. Immunol. Res. **33:** 167–182.
3. OWEN, R.L. & A.L. JONES. 1974. Epithelial cell specialization within human Peyer's patches: an ultrastructural study of intestinal lymphoid follicles. Gastroenterology **66:** 189–203.
4. ANDERLE, P., M. RUMBO, F. SIERRO, *et al.* 2005. Novel markers of the human follicle-associated epithelium identified by genomic profiling and microdissection. Gastroenterology **129:** 321–327.
5. ZHAO, X., A. SATO, C.S. DELA CRUZ, *et al.* 2003. CCL9 is secreted by the follicle-associated epithelium and recruits dome region Peyer's patch $CD11b^+$ dendritic cells. J. Immunol. **171:** 2797–2803.
6. ROSSI, D.L., A.P. VICARI, K. FRANZ-BACON, *et al.* 1997. Identification through bioinformatics of two new macrophage proinflammatory human chemokines: MIP-3α and MIP-3β. J. Immunol. **158:** 1033–1036.
7. HIESHIMA, K., T. IMAI, G. OPDENAKKER, *et al.* 1997. Molecular cloning of a novel human CC chemokine liver and activation-regulated chemokine (LARC) expressed in liver: chemotactic activity for lymphocytes and gene localization on chromosome 2. J. Biol. Chem. **272:** 5846–5853.
8. HROMAS, R., C.H. KIM, M. KLEMSZ, *et al.* 1997. Isolation and characterization of Exodus-2, a novel C-C chemokine with a unique 37-amino acid carboxyl-terminal extension. J. Immunol. **159:** 2554–2558.
9. BABA, M., T. IMAI, M. NISHIMURA, *et al.* 1997. Identification of CCR6, the specific receptor for a novel lymphocyte-directed CC chemokine LARC. J. Biol. Chem. **272:** 14893–14898.
10. LIAO, F., R. ALDERSON, J. SU, *et al.* 1997. STRL22 is a receptor for the CC chemokine MIP-3α. Biochem. Biophys. Res. Commun. **236:** 212–217.
11. YANG, D., O. CHERTOV, S.N. BYKOVSKAIA, *et al.* 1999. β-defensins: linking innate and adaptive immunity through dendritic and T cell CCR6. Science **286:** 525–528.
12. VON ANDRIAN, U.H. 2003. Introduction: chemokines—regulation of immune cell trafficking and lymphoid organ architecture. Semin. Immunol. **15:** 239–241.
13. NAKAYAMA, T., R. FUJISAWA, H. YAMADA, *et al.* 2001. Inducible expression of a CC chemokine liver- and activation-regulated chemokine (LARC)/macrophage inflammatory protein (MIP)-3α/CCL20 by epidermal keratinocytes and its role in atopic dermatitis. Int. Immunol. **13:** 95–103.
14. IZADPANAH, A., M.B. DWINELL, L. ECKMANN, *et al.* 2001. Regulated MIP-3α/CCL20 production by human intestinal epithelium: mechanism for modulating mucosal immunity. Am. J. Physiol. Gastrointest. Liver Physiol. **280:** G710–G719.
15. STARNER, T.D., C.K. BARKER, H.P. JIA, *et al.* 2003. CCL20 is an inducible product of human airway epithelia with innate immune properties. Am. J. Respir. Cell Mol. Biol. **29:** 627–633.
16. FUJIIE, S., K. HIESHIMA, D. IZAWA, *et al.* 2001. Proinflammatory cytokines induce liver and activation-regulated chemokine/macrophage inflammatory protein-3α/CCL20 in mucosal epithelial cells through NF-κB. Int. Immunol. **13:** 1255–1263.

17. PULESTON, J., M. COOPER, S. MURCH, et al. 2005. A distinct subset of chemokines dominates the mucosal chemokine response in inflammatory bowel disease. Aliment. Pharmacol. Ther. **21:** 109–120.

18. YANG, D., Q. CHEN, D.M. HOOVER, et al. 2003. Many chemokines including CCL20/MIP-3α display antimicrobial activity. J. Leukoc. Biol. **74:** 448–455.

19. RUMBO, M., F. SIERRO, N. DEBARD, et al. 2004. Lymphotoxin β receptor signaling induces the chemokine CCL20 in intestinal epithelium. Gastroenterology **127:** 213–223.

20. RODIG, S.J., D. JONES, A. SHAHSAFAEI, et al. 2002. CCR6 is a functional chemokine receptor that serves to identify select B-cell non-Hodgkin's lymphomas. Hum. Pathol. **33:** 1227–1233.

21. RANGEL-MORENO, J., J. MOYRON-QUIROZ, K. KUSSER, et al. 2005. Role of CXC chemokine ligand 13, CC chemokine ligand (CCL) 19, and CCL21 in the organization and function of nasal-associated lymphoid tissue. J. Immunol. **175**.

22. COOK, D.N., D.M. PROSSER, R. FORSTER, et al. 2000. CCR6 mediates dendritic cell localization, lymphocyte homeostasis, and immune responses in mucosal tissue. Immunity **12:** 495–503.

23. VARONA, R., R. VILLARES, L. CARRAMOLINO, et al. 2001. CCR6-deficient mice have impaired leukocyte homeostasis and altered contact hypersensitivity and delayed-type hypersensitivity responses. J. Clin. Invest. **107:** R37–R45.

24. KUCHARZIK, T., J.T. HUDSON, III, R.L. WAIKEL, et al. 2002. CCR6 expression distinguishes mouse myeloid and lymphoid dendritic cell subsets: demonstration using a CCR6 EGFP knock-in mouse. Eur. J. Immunol. **32:** 104–112.

25. BIRAGYN, A., P.A. RUFFINI, C.A. LEIFER, et al. 2002. Toll-like receptor 4-dependent activation of dendritic cells by β-defensin 2. Science **298:** 1025–1029.

26. IWASAKI, A. & B.L. KELSALL. 2000. Localization of distinct Peyer's patch dendritic cell subsets and their recruitment by chemokines, macrophage inflammatory protein (MIP)-3α, MIP-3β, and secondary lymphoid organ chemokine. J. Exp. Med. **191:** 1381–1394.

27. OSTERHOLZER, J.J., T. AMES, T. POLAK, et al. 2005. CCR2 and CCR6, but not endothelial selectins, mediate the accumulation of immature dendritic cells within the lungs of mice in response to particulate antigen. J. Immunol. **175:** 874–883.

28. NIESS, J.H., S. BRAND, X. GU, et al. 2005. CX3CR1-mediated dendritic cell access to the intestinal lumen and bacterial clearance. Science **307:** 254–258.

29. SALAZAR-GONZALEZ, R.M., J.H. NIESS, D.J. ZAMMIT, et al. 2006. CCR6-mediated dendridic cell activation of pathogen-specific T cells in Peyer's patches. Immunity **24:** 623–632.

30. LÜGERING, A., M. FLOER, S. WESTPHAL, et al. 2005. Absence of CCR6 inhibits CD4+ regulatory T-cell development and M-cell formation inside Peyer's patches. Am. J. Pathol. **166:** 1647–1654.

31. FORSTER, R., A.E. MATTIS, E. KREMMER, et al. 1996. A putative chemokine receptor, BLR1, directs B cell migration to defined lymphoid organs and specific anatomic compartments of the spleen. Cell **87:** 1037–1047.

32. FORSTER, R., A. SCHUBEL, D. BREITFELD, et al. 1999. CCR7 coordinates the primary immune response by establishing functional microenvironments in secondary lymphoid organs. Cell **99:** 23–33.

33. OHL, L., G. HENNING, S. KRAUTWALD, et al. 2003. Cooperating mechanisms of CXCR5 and CCR7 in development and organization of secondary lymphoid organs. J. Exp. Med. **197:** 1199–1204.
34. LORENZ, R.G. & R.D. NEWBERRY. 2004. Isolated lymphoid follicles can function as sites for induction of mucosal immune responses. Ann. N.Y. Acad. Sci. **1029:** 44–57.
35. McDONALD, K.G., J.S. McDONOUGH, I. WILLIAMS, et al. 2005. CC chemokine receptor 6 is essential for isolated lymphoid follicle formation [abstract]. Gastroenterology **128:** Suppl. 2, A–21.
36. LORENZ, R.G., D.D. CHAPLIN, K.G. McDONALD, et al. 2003. Isolated lymphoid follicle formation is inducible and dependent upon lymphotoxin-sufficient B lymphocytes, lymphotoxin β receptor, and TNF receptor I function. J. Immunol. **170:** 5475–5482.
37. TAYLOR, R.T., A. LUGERING, K.A. NEWELL, et al. 2004. Intestinal cryptopatch formation in mice requires lymphotoxin α and the lymphotoxin β receptor. J. Immunol. **173:** 7183–7189.
38. KANAMORI, Y., K. ISHIMARU, M. NANNO, et al. 1996. Identification of novel lymphoid tissues in murine intestinal mucosa where clusters of c-kit$^+$ IL-7R$^+$ Thy1$^+$ lympho-hemopoietic progenitors develop. J. Exp. Med. **184:** 1449–1459.
39. PABST, O., H. HERBRAND, T. WORBS, et al. 2005. Cryptopatches and isolated lymphoid follicles: dynamic lymphoid tissues dispensable for the generation of intraepithelial lymphocytes. Eur. J. Immunol. **35:** 98–107.
40. LÜGERING, A., T. KUCHARZIK, D. SOLER, et al. 2003. Lymphoid precursors in intestinal cryptopatches express CCR6 and undergo dysregulated development in the absence of CCR6. J. Immunol. **171:** 2208–2215.
41. EBERL, G. & D.R. LITTMAN. 2004. Thymic origin of intestinal αβ T cells revealed by fate mapping of RORγt$^+$ cells. Science **305:** 248–251.

Apoptosis as a Therapeutic Tool in IBD?

ANDREAS LÜGERING, PIA LEBIEDZ, STEFAN KOCH,
AND TORSTEN KUCHARZIK

Department of Medicine B, University of Münster, Münster, Germany

ABSTRACT: Defective apoptosis of mucosal cell populations seems to be a relevant pathogenetic mechanism in inflammatory bowel disease (IBD). It has been suggested that the induction of apoptosis in various effector cells may be a relevant therapeutic mechanism in IBD. Indeed, it was shown that different drugs used for treatment of IBD have the capacity to induce apoptosis in T cells or monocytes *in vitro* and *in vivo*. However, it remains unclear whether these observations are related to clinical efficacy of these agents. TNF-α is one of the most relevant proinflammatory mediators in IBD and anti-TNF treatment has been shown to be of particular benefit for patients with IBD. It could subsequently be shown that various anti-TNF-α agents, such as infliximab and adalimumab, can induce apoptosis in activated monocytes and lymphocytes *in vitro* and *in vivo*. This mechanism requires reverse signaling via transmembranous TNF, thereby eliciting a signal transduction cascade that results in programmed cell death. Although other mechanisms might also contribute to the clinical effect of anti-TNF-α, current data suggest that apoptosis is a relevant mechanism that is associated with clinical efficacy of anti-TNF agents. Induction of apoptosis in activated monocytes or T cells may be regarded as therapeutic tool not only for anti-TNF agents, but also for other drugs used in IBD. Future strategies should focus on identification of mechanisms that prevent apoptosis in the mucosa of patients with IBD and in targeting apoptotic pathways as a therapeutic strategy in IBD.

KEYWORDS: apoptosis; mononuclear cells; anti-TNF; IBD; target

INTRODUCTION

Inflammatory bowel disease is characterized by a dense infiltrate of mucosal cells that mainly consist of activated T cells and macrophages.Extensive studies over the last decades have shown that activated T cells[1,2] as well as monocytes and macrophages[3,4] play an intriguing role in pathogenesis of IBD, whereas the mechanisms that lead to the persistence of chronic inflammation in

Address for correspondence: Torsten Kucharzik, M.D., Department of Medicine B, University of Münster, Albert-Schweitzer-Str. 33, D-48129 Münster, Germany. Voice: +49-251-8347574; fax: +49-251-8347576.
e-mail: kucharz@uni-muenster.de

Ann. N.Y. Acad. Sci. 1072: 62–77 (2006). © 2006 New York Academy of Sciences.
doi: 10.1196/annals.1326.013

IBD patients are not well characterized. Increased proliferation or insufficient apoptosis might contribute to increased numbers of inflammatory cells in IBD mucosa. Apoptosis is involved in the regulation and function of the immune system and also in the removal of potential harmful cells. Dysfunction or dysregulation of the apoptotic program has indeed been implicated in multiple immune disorders, such as rheumatoid arthritis. Similarly, there is increasing evidence that intrinsic defects in the control of programmed cell death in the mucosal cell department are implicated in the pathogenesis of inflammatory bowel disease.[5–9] Properties of apoptosis induction in lamina propria T cells of patients with Crohn's disease and ulcerative colitis have been determined and it could be shown that mucosal T cells are highly resistant to apoptosis.[8,10] As apoptosis of activated T cells is an important mechanism of peripheral immune tolerance, these findings may explain the perpetuation of inflammatory reactions in IBD mucosa. Recent observations suggest that the apoptotic defect of mucosal T cells in Crohn's disease occurs at the level of the mitochondria in the intrinsic pathway of apoptosis.[9] As defective apoptosis of mucosal cell populations appears to be important pathogenetic mechanisms for mucosal inflammation in IBD, it has been speculated that removal of potentially harmful cells by induction of apoptosis might be a therapeutic tool in inflammatory bowel disease.

Over the last few years various therapeutic agents have therefore been examined regarding their capacity to induce apoptosis in effector cell populations in IBD. It could be shown that most agents, such as steroids,[11,12] sulphasalazine,[10] infliximab,[13,14] azathioprine,[15] methotrexate,[16,17] cyclosporin,[18] tacrolimus,[19] or thalidomide[20] have the capacity to induce apopotosis in monocytes or lymphocytes. Different molecular apoptotic pathways seem to be used by different drugs, which may explain differential therapeutic effects of these agents.

Although extensive *in vitro* studies have been shown that apoptosis can be induced in lymphocytes and monocytes by a variety of drugs used in IBD, it remains unclear whether apoptosis also occurs *in vivo* and more importantly if induction of apoptosis is indeed the integral effect of these drugs.

TNF-α is one of the predominant proinflammatory mediators of inflammation in IBD and induction of apoptosis has been intensively investigated for different anti-TNF agents during the last couple of years. The following review will therefore focus on the role of anti-TNF agents and their capacity to induce apoptosis in lymphocytes and monocytes as well as the importance of anti-TNF-induced apoptosis as a relevant mechanism of action in IBD.

ROLE OF TNF-α IN INFLAMMATORY BOWEL DISEASE

Multiple studies over the last decades provided evidence that TNF is a crucial proinflammatory cytokine in various inflammatory disorders and, therefore, has been approached for therapy.[21-23] TNF is a member of ~20 related cytokines that act through members of the TNF receptor family, and its initial form is a 26-kDa transmembrane protein (mTNF). After cleavage from the cell surface by a metalloproteinase called TNF-α-converting enzyme (TACE) TNF is subsequently released as a 17-kDa protein (sTNF). After trimerization it binds to two different receptors: TNF receptor I (p55), the primary receptor for sTNF that is constitutively expressed by most cell types, and TNF receptor II (p75), the main receptor for mTNF expressed in a highly regulated manner.[24] TNF is predominantly expressed by tissue macrophages and T cells and stimulates inflammation by activating gene transcription through IKK/NFκB and JNK/AP-1 signaling, thereby inducing, for example, cytokine and chemokine expression. TNF is also capable of triggering apoptosis; however, the mechanisms involved in this process are not completely understood, but likely involve NFκB activation followed by activation of c-Flip expression and limitation of JNK activity.[25]

In Crohn's disease, the lamina propria of the gut contains abundant TNF-producing cells, and increased concentrations of TNF have also been found in the stool of children with Crohn's disease.[26,27] The *in vivo* action of TNF-α seems pleiotropic and includes an increase in the ability of neutrophil granulocytes to adhere to vascular endothelial cells,[28] promoting transmigration of neutrophils through the endothelium[29] and formation of vascular thrombin.[30] These mechanisms may also be relevant in the pathogenesis of IBD. Additional mechanisms of TNF-α have been suggested, such as stimulation of a Th1 T cell response[31] and activation of endogenous matrix metalloproteinases (MMPs), which result in mucosal damage and subsequent fibrosis[32] (FIG. 1). Different therapeutic strategies, such as the use of steroids, pentoxifylline, and thalidomide have been shown to reduce TNF expression in various models.[33-36]

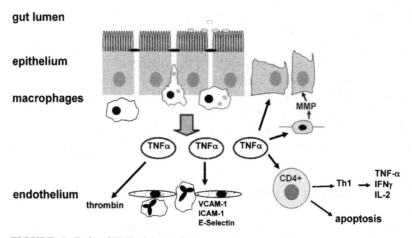

FIGURE 1. Role of TNF-alpha in the mucosal immune system.

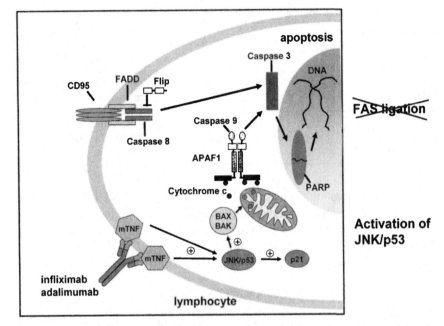

FIGURE 2. Apoptosis induced by anti-TNF agents is linked to the mitochondrial pathway of apoptosis but not to Fas ligation.

As an example for small molecules with TNF-inhibiting functions, thalidomide has proven effective in the therapy of refractory Crohn's disease, but is seldom used because of its severe side effects.[37–39] The exact mechanism of action of thalidomide is still not completely understood, but thalidomide has been proven to inhibit TNF-α production by enhanced mRNA degradation, for example, in human monocytes.[40] Furthermore, thalidomide reduces TNF-α and IL-12 production in CD patients[36,41] and modulates the density of adhesion molecules on the cell surface. The tetravalent guanylhydrazone CNI-1493, an inhibitor of MAP kinases, has also proven to have beneficial effects in the treatment of Crohn's disease by reduction of TNF production and inhibition of inflammatory tissue damage.[42] However, these therapeutic approaches do not specifically reduce TNF function but exert their therapeutic potential by various different mechanisms.

About 15 years ago a chimeric antibody specific for human TNF was generated by grafting a mouse Fab region into 75% human IgG1κ constant region, and initial phase I/II studies in RA could demonstrate a prompt onset of benefits within hours in patients with long-standing active disease[43]; and the first successfully treated CD patient was subsequently reported in 1993.[23] In 1998 the FDA approved infliximab for Crohn's disease after clinical efficacy and safety had been demonstrated in two trials for refractory luminal CD and fistulizing CD. Meanwhile, the indications for infliximab have been extended on

TABLE 1. Induction of apoptosis by different therapeutics used in IBD

Therapeutic Agent in IBD	Apoptotic Cell Population
Steroids	monocytes, T lymphocytes
Sulfasalazine	T lymphocytes
Infliximab	monocytes, T lymphocytes
Adalimumab	monocytes, T-lymphocytes
Methotrexate	T lymphocytes
Azathioprine	T lymphocytes
Cyclosporine	T lymphocytes
Thalidomide	monocytes

the basis of various multicentric prospective trials (ACCENT I/II), including induction and maintenance treatment as well as systemic manifestations of CD.[44,45] Recently, clinical efficacy of infliximab could also be demonstrated for patients with chronic active ulcerative colitis (ACT1/ACT2 trials).[46]

OTHER ANTI-TNF AGENTS

Because infliximab can also induce severe side effects, such as formation of human antichimeric antibodies (HACA) or allergic reactions, multiple TNF-neutralizing strategies have been constructed in order to reduce side effects and to improve the clinical efficacy of the treatment.

Adalimumab is a recombinant human monoclonal IgG1 antibody directed against human TNF that is already in clinical use for rheumatoid arthritis. Adalimumab is able to bind to soluble and transmembrane TNF-α and is under phase III clinical trials for therapeutic use in inflammatory bowel disease. First results suggest beneficial effects in severe-to-moderate Crohn's disease, particularly in cases of infliximab-associated infusion reactions.[47,48]

Etanercept is a fusion protein consisting of the p75-part of TNF receptor II and the Fc domain of a human IgG1. Etanercept has been shown to be effective in rheumatoid arthritis to a similar extent as adalimumab or infliximab.[49] However, in a small trial including 43 patients (20 patients completed the trial) designed for a large therapeutic effect, Sandborn *et al.* were not able to find a positive influence of etanercept on the course of Crohn's disease.[50] Therefore, etanercept is thought to be ineffective.

Onercept is a recombinant unmodified human TNF I receptor (p55). First results suggested a potential therapeutic effect in CD,[51] but these observation could not be confirmed in a larger trial, suggesting that both recombinant TNF receptors are not effective in the treatment of CD.

CDP571 is a humanized IgG4 monoclonal antibody consisting of 95% human and 5% mouse protein. CDP571 has been tested in clinical trials and shown to be effective in patients with moderate-to-severe Crohn's disease,[52,53] but seems to be less effective than infliximab.

CDP870 (certolizumab) is a humanized PEG (polyethyleneglycol)-conjugated anti-TNF Fab-fragment that can be applicated subcutaneously. Recently, it has been shown that CDP870 has clinical efficacy in Crohn's disease, at least in a subgroup of patients who have high CRP values.[54]

Although the current clinical data do not allow a final comparison regarding the efficacy of the different anti-TNF reagents, it can be concluded that (1) anti-TNF antibodies are efficient in the therapy of Crohn's disease, and that (2) in contrast to RA receptor-binding approaches are inefficient even though the receptor fusion protein constructs are capable of binding soluble TNF as well as membrane-bound TNF. These observations suggest that mere neutralization of TNF is not the only therapeutic effect and that different mechanisms might be involved in CD and RA.

INDUCTION OF APOPTOSIS BY ANTI-TNF ACTION *IN VITRO* AND *IN VIVO*

Multiple data, such as clinical inefficacy of receptor fusion constructs as well as long-lasting therapeutic effects, suggest that anti-TNF therapy is based on more than mere neutralization of sTNF and also exerts its function through different mechanisms. Indeed, multiple studies could show that anti-TNF antibodies are likely to directly interact with different cellular subsets of the immune system, such as monocytes and lymphocytes as well as epithelial cells, and various molecular mechanisms have been described recently.

Multiple observations over the last few decades have indicated that programmed cell death plays a central role during the development of organisms.[55] Apoptosis is a relevant mechanism for the function of the immune system and various data have shown that dysregulation of apoptotic cell death may be a relevant mechanism in inflammatory disorders, such as rheumatoid arthritis.[56] Similarly, several reports suggested that mucosal T cells found in the inflamed mucosa of Crohn's disease patients are resistant to apoptotic stimuli.[5,6,9] Therefore, proapoptotic stimulation seems to be an intriguing therapeutic mechanism. Indeed, early studies analyzing the lamina propria cellular infiltrate after infliximab challenge showed a significant loss of CD68+ monocytes as well as CD4+ and CD8+ T lymphocytes.[57] A later report by our group could show that infliximab induces apoptosis in freshly isolated monocytes;[14] corresponding observations were found by Waetzig *et al.*[58] The induction of apoptosis does not seem to require the Fas/FasL signal transduction pathway, but rather involves upregulation of Bax/Bak followed by mitochondrial release of cytochrome *c*. In a recent report, Shen *et al.* could extend these observations by showing that the humanized anti-TNF antibody adalimumab is also capable of inducing monocyte apoptosis, whereas the recombinant fusion protein etanercept is not.[59] Taken together, there is ample *in vitro* evidence that the anti-TNF antibody infliximab induces monocyte apoptosis. Because apoptosis is supposed to rapidly occur *in vivo*, this mechanism would explain the fast therapeutic effect of anti-TNF agents seen in Crohn's disease and also the observation that in some patients therapeutic effects extend far beyond the circulating half-life of the antibody; however, the nature of the process also makes it difficult to analyze it more carefully *in vivo* and to correlate it to therapeutic effects. Similarly, the induction of T cell apoptosis *in vitro* in peripheral blood lymphocytes as well as in lamina propria lymphocytes by infliximab was shown by Hove et al.[60] and confirmed later.[60–62] Corresponding to the observations found in monocytes, the effect was absent when cells were incubated with etanercept, suggesting that the lack of efficacy of this reagent in the therapy of Crohn's disease might be related to the induction of apoptosis. Further confirming these observations, a recent report could show that the reduced rate of apoptotic T cells found in the lamina propria of patients suffering from active CD is reverted after infliximab treatment,[63] although the results are potentially not only reflecting direct apoptotic effects, but also including other immunomodulatory mechanisms 10 weeks after drug administration. Another successful approach to detect *in vivo* apoptosis after anti-TNF therapy was recently demonstrated by van den Brande et al., who employed scintigraphic annexin V labeling.[64]

Reverse Signaling is Linked to Anti-TNF-Induced Apoptosis

There is ample evidence that the immunosuppressive efficacy of anti-TNF agents (infliximab, adalimumab) is not only mediated by binding of soluble TNF, but moreover involves a direct interference with intracellular signaling events, a process described as "reverse signaling." Initially, the conserved cytoplasmatic part of mTNF through various species suggested that the transmembrane ligand might transduce bidirectional signals,[65] and further observations could demonstrate that a dimeric form of the type I soluble TNF receptor is indeed able to dephosphorylate mTNF. Binding of sTNF-R to mTNF induced an increase in intracellular calcium levels,[66] further substantiating the presence of an associated signaling pathway in a macrophage cell line. More recent data could show that reverse signaling might serve as a silencing signal, as monocytes were found to be resistant toward LPS stimulation after incubation with TNF-binding agents.[67,68] In T cells, reverse signaling through mTNF could provide a costimulatory signal for IL-4 and IFN-γ transcription and induce adhesion molecule expression.[69] Recently, Mitoma et al. showed that stably transfected Jurkat T cells constitutively expressing mutant forms of mTNF undergo apoptosis after incubation with infliximab, suggesting that this effector mechanism described in earlier reports is linked to reverse signaling.[62] The induction of apoptosis was associated with induced interleukin-10 production and G0/G1 cycle arrest, and all events, were inhibited by substitution of intracytoplasmatic serine residues of mTNF. The detailed analysis of intracellular signaling pathways showed an upregulation of Bax, Bak, and p21[WAF/CIP1] and phosphorylation of c-JUN kinase. In contrast, etanercept was not capable of inducing similar events, whereas both TNF-binding reagents induced E-selectin expression, indicating that at least two different signal transduction pathways are involved. The data also confirm previous results obtained from peripheral and lamina propria T cells regarding the induction of apoptosis[60] and further extend these observations, as effects mediated by TNF-RI and TNF-RII can be excluded. In a different setting, Kirchner *et al.* could demonstrate that anti-TNF reagents potentially exert their effects on monocytes through two different mechanisms:[67] whereas the secretion of "death factor x" secreted by monocytes after LPS stimulation was dependent on protein kinase C (PKC), the secretion of LPS-induced cytokines was not. Interestingly, the latter was not observed after incubation with etanercept, whereas anti-TNF antibodies 195F and infliximab as well as etanercept both suppressed the release of endothelial apoptosis factors.

Influence of Anti-TNF Treatment on MAP Kinases

Mitogen-activated protein kinases (MAPKs) are conserved among eukaryotes and are key players in several signaling events, and their particular influence in inflammatory processes has been extensively shown.[70] Preliminary data on the MAPK inhibitor CNI-1493 showed that this agent might also be effective in Crohn's disease.[42] TNF is known to act as a regulator and effector of MAPK signaling, and inhibition of JNKs and/or p38 MAPK leads to reduced expression of TNF in CD patients.[42] To evaluate whether antagonizing TNF by antibody treatment influences MAPK activation in CD patients, Waetzig *et al.* characterized the activation of p38 subtypes (p38α-δ), c-Jun N-terminal kinases (JNKs), and the extracellular signal-regulated kinases (ERK)1/2 after infliximab treatment in the inflamed intestinal mucosa.[58] During the first 48 h after infusion, a significant transient increase of p38α was observed predominantly in macrophages, whereas no differences were described for JNK1/2. In this report, similar results were found in myelomonocytotic THP-1, but not in Jurkat T cells, whereas colonic CD4 T cells were found to activate p38 after infliximab challenge in a later report indicating the dependency on the particular system. Interestingly, the proapoptotic effect of infliximab did not seem to be related to p38 activation, as cotreatment with a p38 inhibitor abrogated p38-mediated TNF induction, but not monocyte apoptosis. In more recent updates, the authors found preliminary evidence for the hypothesis that p38 signaling contributes to the diversity of responses to infliximab treatment. Interestingly, while both infliximab and etanercept reduced STAT3 tyrosine phosphorylation of lamina propria T cells, only infliximab influenced p38 phosphorylation, indicating that different signaling pathways are involved.[71] However, although the authors hypothesize that the signal transduction might be mediated by reverse

TABLE 2. Clinical efficacy of various anti-TNF agents in IBD correlated with the capacity to induce apoptosis

Anti-TNF-α agent	Monocyte Apoptosis	Lymphocyte Apoptosis	Clinical Response in CD
Infliximab	yes	yes	yes
Adalimumab	yes	yes	yes
Etanercept	no	no	no
Onercept	yes	n.d.	no
CDP 571	n.d.	n.d.	yes
CDP 870	no	no	yes
Thalidomide	yes	n.d.	yes

n.d. = not defined.

signaling through mTNF, no direct evidence was described. In contrast, Mitoma *et al.* recently demonstrated that JNK activation might be crucial for cellular responses to infliximab. In their publication, MAPK-activation was shown in transfected Jurkat T cells and induction of apoptosis after infliximab challenge correlated to JNK phosphorylation, whereas both phenomena were absent after incubation with etanercept.[62] We could recently show that another anti-TNF agent, thalidomide, which is also capable of inducing monocyte apoptosis, is associated with activation of Act1, while JNK1/2, p38, and ERK1/2 remain unaffected.[20] It therefore appears likely that different proapoptotic anti-TNF agents use different signaling pathways, all of which result in programmed cell death.

ARE APOPTOSIS-RELATED MECHANISMS IMPORTANT IN ANTI-TNF TREATMENT?

Several groups have convincingly shown that anti-TNF agents, such as infliximab and adalimumab, can induce apoptosis in monocytes and lymphocytes *in vitro* and *in vivo*. However, the more important question is whether apoptotis-related mechanisms associated with these agents are important for the clinical efficacy of these drugs. This hypothesis is difficult to prove as there is no simple method to quantify apoptosis *in vivo* as dying cells are usually rapidly removed by macrophages.

Recently, Hlavaty *et al.* developed an apoptotic pharmacogenetic index (API) as a clinical predictor for a response to infliximab treatment. The apoptotic index was based on well-characterized polymorphisms in Fas, Fas-ligand, and caspase-9, which are known to be associated with low apoptotic activity. Applying this technique, the investigators were able to demonstrate that response to treatment positively correlates with apoptosis, while nonresponse is associated with a low apoptotic index.[72] These data suggest that apoptosis is indeed linked to the clinical response to anti-TNF agents.

Considering this observation there is a simple link between the capacity for induction of apoptosis in lymphocytes or monocytes and clinical efficacy in IBD: Anti-TNF agents, such as infliximab and adalimumab have clinical efficacy in IBD and exert strong proapoptotic effects. In contrast, etanercept, which has been reported not to induce apoptosis in monocytes and lymphocytes, has no clinical efficacy in IBD (TABLE 2). However, the situation seems to be more complex. Recently, Waetzig *et al.* could show that the TNF receptor fusion protein, soluble TNF-RI, also exerts proapoptotic effects in monocytes via reverse signaling.[73] These data raise the question of why receptor fusion proteins are not efficacious in Crohn's disease even though they have proapoptotic properties. In addition, recent data show that CDP870 (certolizumab), which exhibits clinical efficacy in Crohn's disease, does not induce apoptosis in immune cells even though it has even higher binding capacities to TNF compared to infliximab in these studies.[74] These data would suggest that apoptosis is not required for clinical efficacy.

Other preliminary data have shown that immune cell apoptosis after infliximab treatment can be detected in responders as well as nonresponders, whereas phosphorylation of p38 downstream effectors ATF-2 and Hsp27 differed between both groups.[75] These results suggest that differential signaling of the p38 MAPK pathway, but not necessarily induction of apoptosis, might contribute to the diversity of responses to infliximab treatment.

Even more confusing, and in contrast to data described earlier, are recent reports suggesting that etanercept as well as infliximab induce apoptosis in macrophages, but not lymphocytes in rheumatoid arthritis (RA) joints.[76] These data raise the question of whether macrophages and lymphocytes behave differently in RA compared to Crohn's disease.

Taken together, even though there are more and more data suggesting that induction of apoptosis by anti-TNF drugs is at least in part linked to clinical efficacy in IBD, there are still many open questions and it is conceivable that other mechanisms might also contribute to the clinical efficacy of anti-TNF agents.

OTHER POTENTIAL MECHANISMS OF ANTI-TNF EFFECTS BESIDES INDUCTION OF APOPTOSIS

Because induction of apoptosis cannot explain all of the observed clinical phenomena of anti-TNF treatment, it is likely that other mechanisms might also contribute to the anti-inflammatory capacity of anti-TNF reagents.

Ehrenstein *et al.* recently showed that regulatory T cells might constitute a target for anti-TNF therapies.[77] They found that the compromised function of regulatory T cells in RA was restored by anti-TNF therapy. These observations are quite intriguing, as the regulatory T cells have been implicated in the pathogenesis of gut inflammation.

TNF has also been suggested to play a role in the increased paracellular permeability that has been observed in IBD by influencing tight junction formation, while it also increases epithelial cell apoptosis and bacterial translocation across the epithelium.[78] Zeissig and colleagues[79] were able to show that anti-TNF therapy is able to restore the decreased epithelial cell permeability, and corresponding data were found by Suenaert *et al.* by using permeation of[51]Cr-EDTA through the small intestine.[80] The reduced barrier function in CD patients was found to be related to increased epithelial cell apoptosis, whereas expression of tight junction proteins was not affected. The normalization of epithelial resistance after anti-TNF therapy correlated to the reduction of epithelial cell apoptosis as measured by TUNEL. Similarly, Marini and colleagues found in a murine model of Crohn's-like ileitis spontaneously developing in SAMP/YitFc mice that TNF neutralization with an anti-mouse TNF antibody mitigates the severity of colitis by abrogation of intestinal epithelial cell apoptosis.[81]

Cell cycle arrest through reverse signaling induced by infliximab, which has recently been shown by Mitoma *et al.*,[62] may also contribute to the clinical effects of anti-TNF treatment.

CONCLUSIONS

Defects in the apoptosis of mucosal cell populations are an important factor in the pathogenesis of IBD. A variety of therapeutic agents that are used for treatment of IBD have the capacity to induce apoptosis in immune cells, such as monocytes/macrophages and lymphocytes *in vitro*. It has been shown that reverse signaling by transmembraneous TNF is required for inducing a signaling cascade, which results in programmed cell death. Because TNF fusion proteins such as etanercept do not induce reverse signaling, this may explain the missing clinical efficacy of this drug. It therefore appears likely that apoptosis is a relevant mechanisms in anti-TNF treatment and potentially also for other drugs used for IBD treatment. However, induction of apoptosis cannot explain every clinical feature of anti-TNF antibody treatment, and results from different anti-TNF drugs are inconclusive regarding their capacity to induce apoptosis in the immune cell population. It therefore appears likely that other mechanisms, for example, reduction of epithelial permeability or induction of regulatory T cells, might also play an important mechanistic role. It is also conceivable that different anti-TNF agents use different pathways.

The molecular apoptotic pathways that are affected by different drugs used in the treatment of IBD are likely to be different, which might explain their additional or even synergistic therapeutic effects. Therefore, these drugs may have additional or even synergistic therapeutic effects.

Future strategies might include identification of underlying apoptotic pathways to identify targets that may be used as a therapeutic tool. This will also help to further identify predictors of response. Because both monocytes/ macrophages and T lymphocytes contribute substantially to pathogenesis of mucosal inflammation in IBD, the therapeutic induction of apoptosis may affect both or all of these cell populations. Further analysis is needed to identify mechanisms that prevent adequate apoptosis in the mucosa of patients with refractory IBD to evaluate new strategies for the treatment of patients with IBD.

REFERENCES

1. NEURATH, M.F., S. FINOTTO & L.H. GLIMCHER. 2002. The role of Th1/Th2 polarization in mucosal immunity. Nat. Med. **8:** 567–573.
2. STROBER, W., I.J. FUSS & R.S. BLUMBERG. 2002. The immunology of mucosal models of inflammation. Annu. Rev. Immunol. **20:** 495–549.
3. RUGTVEIT, J. *et al.* 1997. Cytokine profiles differ in newly recruited and resident subsets of mucosal macrophages from inflammatory bowel disease. Gastroenterology **112:** 1493–1505.
4. ROGLER, G. 2004. Update in inflammatory bowel disease pathogenesis. Curr. Opin. Gastroenterol. **20:** 311–317.
5. BOIRIVANT, M. *et al.* 1999. Lamina propria T cells in Crohn's disease and other gastrointestinal inflammation show defective CD2 pathway-induced apoptosis. Gastroenterology **116:** 557–565.
6. INA, K. *et al.* 1999. Resistance of Crohn's disease T cells to multiple apoptotic signals is associated with a Bcl-2/Bax mucosal imbalance. J. Immunol. **163:** 1081–1090.
7. ATREYA, R. *et al.* 2000. Blockade of interleukin 6 trans signaling suppresses T-cell resistance against apoptosis in chronic intestinal inflammation: evidence in Crohn disease and experimental colitis in vivo. Nat. Med. **6:** 583–588.
8. ITOH, J. *et al.* 2001. Decreased Bax expression by mucosal T cells favours resistance to apoptosis in Crohn's disease. Gut **49:** 35–41.
9. STURM, A. *et al.* 2004. Divergent cell cycle kinetics underlie the distinct functional capacity of mucosal T cells in Crohn's disease and ulcerative colitis. Gut **53:** 1624–1631.
10. DOERING, J. *et al.* 2004. Induction of T lymphocyte apoptosis by sulphasalazine in patients with Crohn's disease. Gut **53:** 1632–1638.
11. SCHMIDT, M. *et al.* 1999. Glucocorticoids induce apoptosis in human monocytes: potential role of IL-1 beta. J. Immunol. **163:** 3484–3490.
12. SCHMIDT, M. *et al.* 2001. Role of the CD95/CD95 ligand system in glucocorticoid-induced monocyte apoptosis. J. Immunol. **166:** 1344–1351.
13. TEN HOVE, T. *et al.* 2002. Infliximab treatment induces apoptosis of lamina propria T lymphocytes in Crohn's disease. Gut **50:** 206–211.
14. LUGERING, A. *et al.* 2001. Infliximab induces apoptosis in monocytes from patients with chronic active Crohn's disease by using a caspase-dependent pathway. Gastroenterology **121:** 1145–1157.
15. TIEDE, I. *et al.* 2003. CD28-dependent Rac1 activation is the molecular target of azathioprine in primary human CD4+ T lymphocytes. J. Clin. Invest. **111:** 1133–1145.

16. GENESTIER, L. *et al.* 1998. Immunosuppressive properties of methotrexate: apoptosis and clonal deletion of activated peripheral T cells. J. Clin. Invest. **102:** 322–328.
17. CUTOLO, M. *et al.* 2000. Antiproliferative and antiinflammatory effects of methotrexate on cultured differentiating myeloid monocytic cells (THP-1) but not on synovial macrophages from patients with rheumatoid arthritis. J. Rheumatol. **27:** 2551–2557.
18. NAUJOKAT, C. *et al.* 2003. Cell cycle- and activation-dependent regulation of cyclosporin A-induced T cell apoptosis. Biochem. Biophys. Res. Commun. **310:** 347–354.
19. MIGITA, K. & K. EGUCHI. 2001. FK 506-mediated T-cell apoptosis induction. Transplant. Proc. **33:** 2292–2293.
20. GOCKEL, H.R. *et al.* 2004. Thalidomide induces apoptosis in human monocytes by using a cytochrome c-dependent pathway. J. Immunol. **172:** 5103–5109.
21. FELDMANN, M. & R.N. MAINI. 2001. Anti-TNF alpha therapy of rheumatoid arthritis: what have we learned? Annu. Rev. Immunol. **19:** 163–196.
22. RUTGEERTS, P., G. VAN ASSCHE & S. VERMEIRE. 2004. Optimizing anti-TNF treatment in inflammatory bowel disease. Gastroenterology **126:** 1593–1610.
23. DERKX, B. *et al.* 1993. Tumour-necrosis-factor antibody treatment in Crohn's disease. Lancet **342:** 173–174.
24. LOCKSLEY, R.M., N. KILLEEN & M.J. LENARDO. 2001. The TNF and TNF receptor superfamilies: integrating mammalian biology. Cell **104:** 487–501.
25. VARFOLOMEEV, E.E. & A. ASHKENAZI. 2004. Tumor necrosis factor: an apoptosis JuNKie? Cell **116:** 491–497.
26. BREESE, E.J. *et al.* 1994. Tumor necrosis factor alpha-producing cells in the intestinal mucosa of children with inflammatory bowel disease. Gastroenterology **106:** 1455–1466.
27. NICHOLLS, S. *et al.* 1993. Cytokines in stools of children with inflammatory bowel disease or infective diarrhea. J. Clin. Pathol. **46:** 757–760.
28. GAMBLE, J.R. *et al.* 1985. Stimulation of the adherence of neutrophils to umbilical vein endothelium by human recombinant tumor necrosis factor. Proc. Natl. Acad. Sci. USA **82:** 8667–8671.
29. CARLOS, T.M. & J.M. HARLAN. 1994. Leukocyte-endothelial adhesion molecules. Blood **84:** 2068–2101.
30. LEVI, M. *et al.* 1993. Pathogenesis of disseminated intravascular coagulation in sepsis. JAMA **270:** 975–979.
31. PLEVY, S.E. *et al.* 1997. A role for TNF-alpha and mucosal T helper-1 cytokines in the pathogenesis of Crohn's disease. J. Immunol. **159:** 6276–6282.
32. PENDER, S.L. *et al.* 1998. Suppression of T cell-mediated injury in human gut by interleukin 10: role of matrix metalloproteinases. Gastroenterology **115:** 573–583.
33. BARNES, P.J. 1998. Anti-inflammatory actions of glucocorticoids: molecular mechanisms. Clin. Sci. (Lond). **94:** 557–572.
34. DIAB-ASSEF, M. *et al.* 2002. The phosphodiesterase inhibitor, pentoxifylline, alters rat intestinal epithelial cell proliferation via changes in the expression of transforming growth factors. Scand. J. Gastroenterol. **37:** 206–214.
35. REIMUND, J.M. *et al.* 1997. In vitro effects of oxpentifylline on inflammatory cytokine release in patients with inflammatory bowel disease. Gut **40:** 475–480.

36. BAUDITZ, J., S. WEDEL & H. LOCHS. 2002. Thalidomide reduces tumour necrosis factor alpha and interleukin 12 production in patients with chronic active Crohn's disease. Gut **50:** 196–200.
37. GORDON, J.N. & P.M. GOGGIN. 2003. Thalidomide and its derivatives: emerging from the wilderness. Postgrad. Med. J. **79:** 127–132.
38. EHRENPREIS, E.D. *et al.* 1999. Thalidomide therapy for patients with refractory Crohn's disease: an open-label trial. Gastroenterology **117:** 1271–1277.
39. VASILIAUSKAS, E.A. *et al.* 1999. An open-label pilot study of low-dose thalidomide in chronically active, steroid-dependent Crohn's disease. Gastroenterology **117:** 1278–1287.
40. SAMPAIO, E.P. *et al.* 1991. Thalidomide selectively inhibits tumor necrosis factor alpha production by stimulated human monocytes. J. Exp. Med. **173:** 699–703.
41. SETTLES, B. *et al.* 2001. Down-regulation of cell adhesion molecules LFA-1 and ICAM-1 after in vitro treatment with the anti-TNF-alpha agent thalidomide. Cell. Mol. Biol. (Noisy-le-Grand) **47:** 1105–1114.
42. HOMMES, D. *et al.* 2002. Inhibition of stress-activated MAP kinases induces clinical improvement in moderate to severe Crohn's disease. Gastroenterology **122:** 7–14.
43. ELLIOTT, M.J. *et al.* 1993. Treatment of rheumatoid arthritis with chimeric monoclonal antibodies to tumor necrosis factor alpha. Arthritis Rheum. **36:** 1681–1690.
44. HANAUER, S.B. *et al.* 2002. Maintenance infliximab for Crohn's disease: the ACCENT I randomised trial. Lancet **359:** 1541–1549.
45. RUTGEERTS, P. *et al.* 2004. Comparison of scheduled and episodic treatment strategies of infliximab in Crohn's disease. Gastroenterology **126:** 402–413.
46. RUTGEERTS, P. *et al.* 2005. Infliximab for induction and maintenance therapy for ulcerative colitis. N. Engl. J. Med. **353:** 2462–2476.
47. YOUDIM, A. *et al.* 2004. A pilot study of adalimumab in infliximab–allergic patients. Inflamm. Bowel Dis. **10:** 333–338.
48. SANDBORN, W.J. *et al.* 2004. An open-label study of the human anti-TNF monoclonal antibody adalimumab in subjects with prior loss of response or intolerance to infliximab for Crohn's disease. Am. J. Gastroenterol. **99:** 1984–1989.
49. HOCHBERG, M.C. *et al.* 2003. Comparison of the efficacy of the tumour necrosis factor alpha blocking agents adalimumab, etanercept, and infliximab when added to methotrexate in patients with active rheumatoid arthritis. Ann. Rheum. Dis. **62 Suppl 2**: ii13–16.
50. SANDBORN, W.J. *et al.* 2001. Etanercept for active Crohn's disease: a randomized, double-blind, placebo-controlled trial. Gastroenterology **121:** 1088–1094.
51. RUTGEERTS, P. *et al.* 2003. Treatment of active Crohn's disease with onercept (recombinant human soluble p55 tumour necrosis factor receptor): results of a randomized, open-label, pilot study. Aliment. Pharmacol. Ther. **17:** 185–192.
52. SANDBORN, W.J. *et al.* 2004. CDP571, a humanised monoclonal antibody to tumour necrosis factor alpha, for moderate to severe Crohn's disease: a randomised, double blind, placebo controlled trial. Gut **53:** 1485–1493.
53. SANDBORN, W.J. *et al.* 2001. An engineered human antibody to TNF (CDP571) for active Crohn's disease: a randomized double-blind placebo-controlled trial. Gastroenterology **120:** 1330–1338.
54. SCHREIBER, S. *et al.* 2005. A randomized, placebo-controlled trial of certolizumab pegol (CDP870) for treatment of Crohn's disease. Gastroenterology **129:** 807–818.

55. DANIAL, N.N. & S.J. KORSMEYER. 2004. Cell death: critical control points. Cell **116:** 205–219.
56. POPE, R.M. 2002. Apoptosis as a therapeutic tool in rheumatoid arthritis. Nat. Rev. Immunol. **2:** 527–535.
57. BAERT, F.J. *et al.* 1999. Tumor necrosis factor alpha antibody (infliximab) therapy profoundly down-regulates the inflammation in Crohn's ileocolitis. Gastroenterology. **116:** 22–28.
58. WAETZIG, G.H. *et al.* 2002. p38 mitogen-activated protein kinase is activated and linked to TNF-alpha signaling in inflammatory bowel disease. J. Immunol. **168:** 5342–5351.
59. SHEN, C. *et al.* 2005. Adalimumab induces apoptosis of human monocytes: a comparative study with infliximab and etanercept. Aliment. Pharmacol. Ther. **21:** 251–258.
60. VAN DEN BRANDE, J.M. *et al.* 2003. Infliximab but not etanercept induces apoptosis in lamina propria T-lymphocytes from patients with Crohn's disease. Gastroenterology **124:** 1774–1785.
61. DI SABATINO, A. *et al.* 2004. Defective mucosal T cell death is sustainably reverted by infliximab in a caspase dependent pathway in Crohn's disease. Gut **53:** 70–77.
62. MITOMA, H. *et al.* 2005. Infliximab induces potent anti-inflammatory responses by outside-to-inside signals through transmembrane TNF-alpha. Gastroenterology **128:** 376–392.
63. DI SABATINO, A. *et al.* 2004. Infliximab downregulates basic fibroblast growth factor and vascular endothelial growth factor in Crohn's disease patients. Aliment. Pharmacol. Ther. **19:** 1019–1024.
64. VAN DEN BRANDE JMH, B.R., Z. DETKOVA, H. BRAAT, *et al.* 2004. In vivo imaging of infliximab induced apoptosis in Crohn's disease patients. Gastroenterology **126:** A205.
65. SMITH, C.A., T. FARRAH & R.G. GOODWIN. 1994. The TNF receptor superfamily of cellular and viral proteins: activation, costimulation, and death. Cell **76:** 959–962.
66. WATTS, A.D. *et al.* 1999. A casein kinase I motif present in the cytoplasmic domain of members of the tumour necrosis factor ligand family is implicated in 'reverse signalling.' EMBO J. **18:** 2119–2126.
67. KIRCHNER, S. *et al.* 2004. Effect of different tumor necrosis factor (TNF) reactive agents on reverse signaling of membrane integrated TNF in monocytes. Cytokine **28:** 67–74.
68. KIRCHNER, S. *et al.* 2004. LPS resistance in monocytic cells caused by reverse signaling through transmembrane TNF (mTNF) is mediated by the MAPK/ERK pathway. J. Leukoc. Biol. **75:** 324–331.
69. FERRAN, C. *et al.* 1994. Anti-tumor necrosis factor modulates anti-CD3-triggered T cell cytokine gene expression in vivo. J. Clin. Invest. **93:** 2189–2196.
70. DONG, C., R.J. DAVIS & R.A. FLAVELL. 2002. MAP kinases in the immune response. Annu. Rev. Immunol. **20:** 55–72.
71. ROSENSTIEL, P. *et al.* 2005. Differential modulation of p38 mitogen activated protein kinase and STAT3 signalling pathways by infliximab and etanercept in intestinal T cells from patients with Crohn's disease. Gut **54:** 314–315; author reply 316–6.
72. HLAVATY T.P.M., S. JOOSSENS, G. CLAESSENS, *et al.* 2005. Prediction of response to infliximab in luminal and fistulizing Crohn's disease based on a decision making model using an apoptotic pharmacogenetic index and clinical predictors. Gastroenterology **128:** A309.

73. WAETZIG, G.H. *et al.* 2005. Soluble tumor necrosis factor (TNF) receptor-1 induces apoptosis via reverse TNF signaling and autocrine transforming growth factor-beta1. FASEB J. **19:** 91–93.
74. FOSSATI, G. *et al.* 2004. Effect of the anti-TNF agents adalimumab, infliximab and certolizumab pegol on the induction of apoptosis in activated peripheral blood lymphocytes. Gastroenterology **128:** A512.
75. WAETZIG, G.H. *et al.* 2003. Differential p38 mitogen-activated protein kinase target phosphorylation in responders and nonresponders to infliximab. Gastroenterology **125:** 633–634; author reply 635–636.
76. CATRINA, A.I. *et al.* 2005. Evidence that anti-tumor necrosis factor therapy with both etanercept and infliximab induces apoptosis in macrophages, but not lymphocytes, in rheumatoid arthritis joints: extended report. Arthritis Rheum. **52:** 61–72.
77. EHRENSTEIN, M.R. *et al.* 2004. Compromised function of regulatory T cells in rheumatoid arthritis and reversal by anti-TNFalpha therapy. J. Exp. Med. **200:** 277–285.
78. BRUEWER, M. *et al.* 2003. Proinflammatory cytokines disrupt epithelial barrier function by apoptosis-independent mechanisms. J. Immunol. **171:** 6164–6172.
79. ZEISSIG, S. *et al.* 2004. Downregulation of epithelial apoptosis and barrier repair in active Crohn's disease by tumour necrosis factor alpha antibody treatment. Gut **53:** 1295–1302.
80. SUENAERT, P. *et al.* 2002. Anti-tumor necrosis factor treatment restores the gut barrier in Crohn's disease. Am. J. Gastroenterol. **97:** 2000–2004.
81. MARINI, M. *et al.* 2003. TNF-alpha neutralization ameliorates the severity of murine Crohn's-like ileitis by abrogation of intestinal epithelial cell apoptosis. Proc. Natl. Acad. Sci. USA **100:** 8366–8371.

The Intestinal Microvasculature as a Therapeutic Target in Inflammatory Bowel Disease

OSSAMA A. HATOUM,[a] JAN HEIDEMANN,[b] AND DAVID G. BINION[a]

[a]Department of Medicine, Medical College of Wisconsin, Milwaukee, Wisconsin 53226, USA

[b]Department of Medicine B, University of Munster, D-48129 Munster, Germany

ABSTRACT: Chronic inflammation is a complex biologic process which involves immune as well as non-immune cells including the microvasculature and its endothelial lining. Growing evidence suggests that the microvasculature plays an integral role in the pathophysiology of inflammatory bowel disease (IBD; Crohn's disease and ulcerative colitis). The microvasculature contributes to chronic inflammation through altered leukocyte recruitment, impaired perfusion, and angiogenesis leading to tissue remodeling. These diverse areas of IBD microvascular biology represent therapeutic targets that are currently undergoing investigation.

KEYWORDS: Crohn's disease; ulcerative colitis; IBD; endothelial dysfunction; microvessels; MAdCAM-1; ICAM-1; CCR9; natalizumab; alicaforsen; ridogrel; MLN02; traficet-EN; angiogenesis

INTRODUCTION

The microcirculation and its endothelial lining play a central role in the initiation and perpetuation of the inflammatory response as well as in tissue remodeling in chronic inflammation. Investigation into the cellular and molecular mechanisms in human inflammatory bowel disease (IBD; Crohn's disease, ulcerative colitis) has demonstrated a central role for the intestinal microvascular endothelium in both normal mucosal immunity as well as in the dysregulated chronic inflammation that characterizes IBD, prompting investigation of novel therapeutic strategies targeting the microvasculature. Chronically inflamed IBD gut microvessels demonstrate an enhanced capacity for leukocytes adherence following inflammatory activation and to have alterations in selective leukocyte recruitment compared to uninvolved areas of bowel. In

Address for correspondence: David G. Binion, M.D., Division of Gastroenterology and Hepatology, Department of Medicine, Medical College of Wisconsin, 9200 W. Wisconsin Ave., Milwaukee, WI 53226, USA. Voice: 414-456-6845; fax: 414-564-6214.

e-mail: dbinion@mcw.edu

Ann. N.Y. Acad. Sci. 1072: 78–97 (2006). © 2006 New York Academy of Sciences.

doi: 10.1196/annals.1326.003

addition to the role of the vasculature in leukocyte trafficking, both forms of IBD are characterized by refractory mucosal damage and ulceration with an impaired capacity to heal, which suggests decreased perfusion and chronic ischemia in the IBD gut. Recent investigation of submucosal microvessels from patients with Crohn's disease and ulcerative colitis as well as gut microvessels from rodent models of IBD has confirmed this hypothesis, demonstrating microvascular dysfunction with impaired vasodilatiory capacity in the chronically inflamed intestine. The tissue remodeling, which characterizes IBD, is also accompanied by angiogenesis, particularly in the bowel wall and the serosal surfaces of the gut, suggesting that antiangiogenic treatment regimens may play a role in the restoration of gut architecture. We review the role of the microvasculature in human chronic intestinal inflammation and IBD pathogenesis, as well as emerging strategies targeting the vasculature focusing on (1) cell adhesion molecules (CAM), (2) chemokines, (3) microvascular physiology, and (4) angiogenesis.

MICROVASCULAR CAM AND IBD

Contribution of Local Endothelial Cells to IBD Pathogenesis

Endothelial cells are now appreciated to play an early and rate-limiting step in the inflammatory process, where endothelial activation in response to cytokines, bacterial products, and inflammatory mediators leads to leukocyte recruitment from the circulation.[1] Endothelial activation results in a rapid pattern of gene expression, where CAM and chemokines expressed by endothelial cells will mediate enhanced leukocyte interaction, which progresses through the sequential process of transient adhesion (saltation), firm adhesion, and leukocyte transmigration. Local accumulation of leukocytes is a central feature of gut mucosal inflammatory reactions occurring at sites of a microbial infection or in the setting of a disrupted intestinal epithelial barrier, features commonly observed in IBD. The process of leukocyte accumulation is dependent on the active emigration of circulating leukocytes, which follows a multistep sequence of margination, leukocyte–endothelial cell adhesion, transendothelial migration, as well as chemotactic leukocyte locomotion to the site of inflammation. In recent years, the central role of the endothelial cells lining the postcapillary microvasculature in the process of leukocyte recruitment in inflammation has been defined. Indeed, some of the most potent activators of endothelial cells are the cytokines IL-1 and TNF-α, both of which are known to play a key role in IBD pathogenesis.[2,3] The recognition that leukocytes must firmly adhere to vascular endothelial cells in order for gut inflammation to proceed in IBD has resulted in an intensive effort to define the molecular mechanisms that mediate these cell–cell interactions.

Research performed using primary endothelial cells derived from human gut (human intestinal microvascular endothelial cells ([HIMECs]) has provided an *in vitro* system to define key aspects of microvascular physiology of the gut in IBD. Observations by Binion *et al.* have shown that HIMECs derived from actively inflamed IBD mucosa display a marked increase in leukocyte-binding capacity as compared to HIMECs derived from healthy areas of resected human bowel as well as uninvolved areas of IBD intestine, not exposed to chronic inflammation.[4,5] These acquired changes in the involved HIMECs in IBD are long-lived, and persist during the lifetime in which the endothelial cells can be cultured *in vitro.*[6] These findings strongly suggest that intestinal endothelial cells may play an important role in the pathophysiology of chronic, destructive inflammation in IBD. In addition, these data also suggest that intestinal endothelial cells exposed to the stress of chronic inflammation in IBD acquire a proinflammatory phenotype, which may further contribute to the perpetuation of the inflammatory process. Mechanisms underlying leukocyte hyperadhesion in IBD gut endothelial cells are discussed in further detail in the section Microvascular Dysfunction in IBD further in this review.

Altered Leukocyte Recruitment in IBD: Microvascular Expression of Peripheral Node Addressin

Studies investigating potential alterations in leukocyte homing patterns in IBD were carried out by Salmi *et al.*[7] Using an *ex vivo* leukocyte-binding assay on thin sections of resected control and IBD bowel, these investigators demonstrated that naïve lymphocytes were preferentially recruited to the IBD intestinal microvascular endothelium compared to control intestinal microvessels, which bound increased numbers of memory lymphocytes. These findings were confirmed by Burgio *et al.*,[8] who also demonstrated an altered pattern of leukocyte binding in Crohn's disease, where naïve monocytes and T cells were again preferentially recruited to the chronically inflamed intestine. These findings suggest that an inappropriate population of naïve immune cells is recruited to the chronically inflamed intestine, an antigenically rich environment.

A novel, yet well-characterized rodent model of spontaneous chronic intestinal inflammation is the SAMP/Yit mouse.[9] Using a selective adoptive transfer approach in recipient SCID animals, Rivera-Nieves and colleagues characterized the specific subsets of leukocytes that were responsible for the generation of chronic gut inflammation.[10] Similar to human IBD studies, a population of CD4+ T cells expressing the L-selectin molecule in combination with alpha4beta7 was found to play a key role in the development of chronic gut inflammation. These findings from both human IBD as well as an animal model of spontaneous gut chronic inflammation suggest that an inappropriate population of naïve immune cells is recruited to the chronically inflamed intestine, an antigenically rich environment. This pattern of inappropriate immune cell recruitment in chronic inflammation suggests a mechanism that may contribute to perpetuation of chronic inflammation.[11]

The SAMP/Yit mouse has also been recently used to develop a novel strategy for ultrasound diagnosis of chronic gut inflammation. Bachmann and co-workers successfully conjugated rat anti-mouse antibodies detecting mucosal addressin (MAd)CAM-1 to the external surface of lipid-shelled microbubbles to produce a targeted contrast agent for use with transabdominal ultrasound to detect experimental ileitis.[12] This novel imaging strategy has immediate potential as a research tool for monitoring *in vivo* mucosal inflammation in whole animals with colitis. The ability to more accurately assess inflammatory mechanisms integral to the disease process using a noninvasive ultrasound approach carries great potential for both diagnostic technique and a strategy to monitor disease activity and therapeutic efficacy.

Selective Adhesion Molecule Blockade in Animal Models of IBD

Rolling interactions of leukocytes on the endothelial intraluminal surface are mediated by selectins and their corresponding mucin-type ligands. The selectins, designated as L-, P-, and E-selectins, represent a family of adhesive receptors expressed on leukocytes (L-selectin), platelets, and endothelial cells (P-selectin) or endothelial cells alone (E-selectin).[13,14] In contrast to integrins and immunoglobulin superfamily members that mediate an array of cell–cell interactions throughout the body, selectin function is uniquely restricted to the vascular system. Recent development of an accurate method to quantify *in vivo* expression of molecules exposed on the endothelial surface, based on the injection of radio-labeled monoclonal antibodies,[15] has facilitated characterization of adhesion molecule expression in various animal models of colitis. Although a consistent increase in P- and E-selectin expression has been documented in experimental colitis, immunoneutralization of these adhesion molecules has little impact on the inflammatory process in the colon.[16] The lack of strong preclinical animal studies has limited researchers' enthusiasm for targeting these molecules in patients with IBD.

The importance of CAM in the pathogenesis of chronic gut inflammation has focused both on immunolocalization studies on histologic sections as well as functional experiments blocking specific CAM to define a contributing role in the disease process. Immunolocalization of CAM in human IBD has demonstrated marked increase in E-selectin and intercellular cell adhesion molecule 1 (ICAM-1) expression in gut microvascular endothelium, while vascular cell adhesion molecule-1 (VCAM-1) expression was less clearly demonstrated.[16,17] In contrast, rodent models of IBD have demonstrated increased levels of all three of these CAMs, including VCAM-1 in the intestinal microcirculation. Rodent models where VCAM-1 has been demonstrated to play a role in chronic gut inflammation include TNBS-colitis,[18] dextran sodium sulfate (DSS)-colitis,[19] and peptidoglycan/polysaccharide-induced colitis in rats,[20] as well as in colitis appearing in IL-10 knockout mice.[21] In using rodent models of colitis, immunoneutralization of adhesion molecules has shown a consistent benefit for VCAM-1 blockade,[18,19] whereas inconsistent results have been obtained following immunoneutralization of ICAM-1 or MAdCAM-1.[19] Furthermore, studies in the SAMP/Yit mouse have demonstrated significant benefit in animals who received anti-CAM blockade when two molecules were targeted simultaneously, while no clinical benefit was seen in animals treated with single agents.[9]

Selective Adhesion Molecule Blockade in Human IBD

Targeting endothelial–leukocyte interaction for therapeutic benefit in patients with IBD has received intense interest, as three experimental agents have been investigated in six placebo-controlled trials in IBD.[22] Initial investigation of antiadhesion molecule therapy in IBD targeted the ICAM-1. ICAM-1, a member of the immunoglobulin superfamily, is an inducible transmembrane glycoprotein that is constitutively expressed at low levels on vascular endothelial cells and a subset of leukocytes and will play a central role in the recruitment and retention of leukocytes in inflammatory foci.[23,24] In response to cytokines and other proinflammatory mediators, microvascular endothelial cells in the human intestine will upregulate their expression of ICAM-1, leading to increased leukocyte adhesion through interaction with their primary counterligands, the β_2-integrins, leukocyte function-associated antigen 1 (LFA-1), and Mac-1.[25,26]

Following experimental success in the use of humanized antibodies targeting ICAM-1 in patients with refractory rheumatoid arthritis,[27] investigators initiated trials targeting increased ICAM-1 expression in Crohn's disease patients. Alicaforsen (ISIS 2302; ISIS Pharmaceuticals, Carlsbad, CA, USA), a 20-base phosphorothioate oligodeoxynucleotide designed to specifically hybridize to a sequence in the 3'-untranslated region of the human ICAM-1 message, represented one of the earliest attempts to develop antisense treatment of human disease.[28,29] Following infusion and cellular uptake, the oligodeoxynucleotide-RNA heterodimer formed serves as a substrate for the ubiquitous nuclease RNase-H, with subsequent cleavage and reduction in cellular-specific message content and consequent reduction in ICAM-1 expression.[29,30] Phosphorothioate oligodeoxynucleotides achieve relative nuclease resistance over DNA by the substitution of a sulfur molecule for one of the nonbridging oxygen molecules in each phosphodiester linkage.[31,32] Initial clinical attempts to use alicaforsen in the treatment of Crohn's disease were made by Yacyshyn *et al.*,[33] who reported a steroid-sparing effect, as well as inducing remission in up to 40% of treated patients. Subsequent clinical trials of alicaforsen have not demonstrated success, but may have suffered from insufficient dosing as well as difficulties in trial design.[34] Trials of alicaforsen in enema formulation for ulcerative colitis are also being carried out at the present time.[35]

Podolsky *et al.* defined an important role for integrin–integrin ligand interaction in chronic colitis, which develops in the cotton-top tamarin, a New World primate that is susceptible to the development of a spontaneous form of IBD similar to human ulcerative colitis.[16] These authors demonstrated that leukocytes expressing the alpha4 integrin will interact with endothelial integrin ligands and play an essential role in the pathogenesis of chronic colitis. Animals treated with an anti-alpha4 antibody demonstrated clinical improvement,[36] and the success of these early observations provided the basis for the development of novel therapeutic strategies targeting interaction of leukocytes expressing the alpha4 integrin (alpha4beta1 VLA4 and alpha4beta7) with their endothelial ligands, including MAdCAM-1, in human trials.[37]

The most extensive investigation of antialpha4 integrin antibody therapy for the treatment of Crohn's disease involved studies with the humanized antibody natalizumab (Elan Pharmaceuticals, San Diego, CA, USA), which targets the alpha4 integrin on leukocytes expressing alpha4beta1 as well as alpha4beta7. Natalizumab has undergone extensive investigation in the treatment of chronic inflammation in multiple sclerosis as well as Crohn's disease.[38,39] In a pivotal phase II trial of natalizumab in Crohn's disease, natalizumab failed to who had significant benefit and meet primary end points. However, a subset of patients who had objective markers of inflammation (i.e., elevated C-reactive protein) demonstrated significant and sustained improvement during the induction and maintenance trial.

Although natalizumab showed benefit in a subset of patients with Crohn's disease with objective evidence of inflammation, the emergence of infections complications halted development of this reagent. However, the development of a severe, and life-threatening JC viral reactivation encephalitis prompted a voluntary withdrawal of this agent in early 2005, interrupting pivotal trials in the Crohn's disease population. The potential development of natalizumab in Crohn's disease treatment remains in question, dependent largely on these safety issues.

A second selective leukocyte adhesion receptor antagonist targeting interaction of alpha4-expressing leukocytes with MAdCAM-1 on the gut endothelium in patients with IBD has also undergone extensive evaluation. MLN02 (Millenium Pharmaceuticals, Cambridge, MA, USA) is a humanized antibody that specifically targets leukocytes expressing alpha4beta7 integrin, which is the specific ligand for the MAdCAM-1. MLN02 demonstrated success in a multicenter, double-blind, placebo-controlled phase II trial in ulcerative colitis patients treated only with mesalamine compounds.[40] Two infusions of MLN02 resulted in significant improvement in rates of remission and response. The results of this trial indicate that an antialpha4 integrin inhibition strategy will also be effective in the treatment of patients with ulcerative colitis, and Crohn's disease. More importantly, the severe infectious complications associated with the less-selective antialpha4 integrin blockade produced by natalizumab were not witnessed in these early trials with the more selective MLN02 reagent.

CHEMOKINES AND THE INTESTINAL
MICROVASCULATURE IN IBD

Chemokines are an expanding superfamily of chemoattractant cytokines, which play a central role in the initiation and promotion of inflammatory reactions, as well as additional functions in cellular homeostasis and repair in a variety of cell types, including vascular endothelial cells. Increased production of chemokines involved in leukocyte recruitment in response to inflammatory stimuli is well described in the setting of IBD.[41,42] Because chemokines are secreted from cells and engage specific cell surface receptors in order to exert biologic effect, there is strong potential that agents that specifically target select chemokine pathways may be developed for the treatment of specific immune and inflammatory disorders.

During inflammation, RANTES, MCP-1, MCP-3, and MIP-1 exhibit potent promigratory and activating potentials for eosinophils, basophils, and T cells. Recent evidence has shown that a restricted expression of chemokines in the mucosal surfaces of the gut may play a critical role in selective leukocyte trafficking to this highly specialized immune compartment. The chemokine TECK,[43–45] expressed on the vascular endothelium in the small intestine, has been shown to play a key role in selective leukocyte recruitment, with leukocytes expressing the chemokine receptor CCR9. This work implies that select leukocyte recruitment is regulated through restricted expression of various chemokine–chemokine receptor ligands in the intestine, and may play a role in the altered leukocyte recruitment found in IBD.

The potential for blocking CCR9 interaction with specific intestinal chemokine expression was explored by Wei et al. Using the C-C chemokine receptor 9 antagonist CCX282 (Traficet-EN, ChemoCentryx, Inc., Mountain View, CA, USA),[46,47] these investigators were able to demonstrate a clinical benefit in a rodent model of inflammation. In human FDA phase I trial results, the orally available compound was well tolerated and demonstrated sustained levels of the drug. Currently, phase II trials evaluating the efficacy of Traficet-EN are being initiated.

MICROVASCULAR DYSFUNCTION IN IBD

Diminished Mucosal Perfusion: Intraoperative and Endoscopic Studies

Intestinal vascular remodeling and damage are an early pathologic finding that may precede the development of overt mucosal ulceration in IBD. These areas of greatest microvascular alteration and damage correlated histologically with vascular penetration through the muscularis propria and in regions of dense angiogenesis seen in distal areas of the mucosal circulation. Funayama et al. investigated remodeling in the intestinal microcirculation from Crohn's disease–resected bowel using tissue histometry.[48] These authors suggested that circulatory disturbances occur in the early stages of Crohn's disease, which may then lead to increased vascular resistance in the area between the deep submucosal and the distal mesenteric arteries, possibly contributing to a local gut ischemia. The potential for an ischemic injury to the IBD bowel was furthered by Wakefield *et al.*, who identified occlusive fibrinoid lesions in the small arteries and arterioles supplying Crohn's disease–affected areas of intestine that were not demonstrated in uninvolved areas of bowel using scanning electron micrographs of corrosion microcasts of the gut microvasculature.[49] Morphologically, the chronically inflamed microvessels were tapered and stenosed compared to vessels from areas of uninvolved Crohn's disease and control bowel. Taken together, these studies suggest that the microvascular anatomy undergoes extensive remodeling and plays a role in the pathogenesis of chronic inflammatory lesions, with the degree of vascular damage correlating with the severity of intestinal injury.

Attempts to characterize physiologic alterations in intestinal blood flow in IBD have used both direct and indirect methods to quantify perfusion. Early studies by Hulten *et al.* demonstrated that chronically inflamed IBD tissues (in both chronically active and quiescent disease) showed diminished gut perfusion compared to controls, which correlated most closely with histologic evidence of persistent ulceration and intestinal fibrosis.[50] These studies were performed intraoperatively on IBD patients undergoing resection, using a radiotracer "washout" technique. Because these studies were performed on patients with refractory "end-stage" disease, which was being treated surgically, there is a possibility that the apparent ischemic injury was a late-stage alteration in the disease process. These early studies were complemented by more recent *in vivo* investigation with endoscopic approaches to quantify mucosal blood flow. Angerson *et al.* demonstrated similar findings using endoscopic Doppler laser flowmetry, where chronically inflamed Crohn's disease bowel demonstrated significantly decreased perfusion.[51] Further support for diminished mucosal perfusion in the chronically inflamed IBD intestine was demonstrated by Tateishi and colleagues using laser Doppler flowmetry intraoperatively in Crohn's disease patients undergoing resection.[52] These observations over the past two and a half decades have consistently demonstrated that the most severe decrease in vascular perfusion is found in association with fibrotic strictures in patients with long-standing Crohn's disease.[51]

Microvascular Dysfunction in IBD Arterioles: Microvascular Physiologic Studies

Refractory, poorly healing wounds, such as foot and leg ulcers in patients with peripheral vascular disease and long-standing diabetes mellitus, are associated with tissue ischemia and have been linked to microvascular dysfunction.[53-58] In IBD intestine, similar poorly healing and refractory mucosal ulcerations occur in the gut lining: these are suggestive of tissue hypoperfusion and an ischemic component to the pathologic picture. This question of whether there is an impaired vasodilation capacity in the chronically inflamed IBD intestinal arterioles was addressed directly by Hatoum et al.[59] These investigators directly examined the vasodilator responses in freshly isolated human intestinal arterioles by measuring in vitro vasodilator capacity in response to acetylcholine (Ach; an endothelial-dependent vasodilator). Gut arterioles, 50–150 microns in diameter, from IBD and control (non-IBD) intestinal specimens were suspended and perfused immediately following resection. Non-IBD intestinal arterioles dilated dose-dependently to Ach, while chronically inflamed IBD arterioles (in both Crohn's disease and ulcerative colitis) demonstrated a diminished vasodilatory capacity to Ach (non-IBD microvascular maximal dilation (MD): $82 \pm 2\%$, $n = 34$ compared to IBD microvascular MD: $15 \pm 2\%$, $n = 33$, respectively; $P = < 0.05$). This decreased vasodilator capacity was directly related to a loss of nitric oxide (NO)–dependent function in the IBD microvessels exposed to chronic inflammation in vivo. The chronically inflamed IBD vessels were found to be heavily dependent on cyclo-oxygenase (COX)–derived vasodilator compounds to maintain vascular tone and dilator capacity to Ach. The use of indomethacin, a nonselective inhibitor of COX isoforms, decreased vasodilation of non-IBD vessels to Ach by approximately 40%, while in IBD arterioles it resulted in frank vasoconstriction.[59] The mechanism of the impaired NO-mediated dilation may involve excess production of oxidative stress, as increased superoxide anion as well as other oxyradicals were measured by intravital dyes in IBD but not in control arterioles.[59]

This pattern of altered gut arteriolar physiology in IBD was recently reproduced in an animal model of chronic gut inflammation. Using the DSS-induced colonic inflammation in mice, Mori et al. reported a significant reduction (18–30%) in blood flow in small arterioles (<40 μm diameter) on days 4 through 6 of DSS colitis in response to bradykinin.[60] These patterns of microvascular dysfunction appeared to emerge over the time course of inflammation. The authors also found that NAD(P)H oxidase-derived superoxide plays a major role in the induction of the inflammation-induced endothelium-dependent arteriolar dysfunction.[60]

Loss of Endothelial Generation of NO in IBD Endothelial Cells

Early studies into the potential role of the endothelium in IBD pathogenesis focused on histological evaluation, characterizing the morphology of the microvasculature in chronically inflamed intestine. Dvorak et al. evaluated Crohn's disease intestinal specimens with transmission electron microscopy and demonstrated endothelial cell abnormalities, characterized by loss of monolayer integrity, tissue edema, extravasation of red blood cells, focal venular endothelial necrosis adjacent to areas of undamaged endothelial cells, and endothelial cell hypertrophy.[61,62] To more fully define the contribution of microvascular endothelial cells in chronic intestinal inflammation, HIMECs from small and large intestinal resected tissue were developed for *in vitro* studies.[4,63,64] Endothelial cultures were generated from areas of chronically inflamed and uninvolved Crohn's disease and ulcerative colitis intestine. HIMECs isolated from both chronically inflamed Crohn's disease and ulcerative colitis demonstrated a significantly enhanced capacity for leukocytes to adhere compared to control HIMECs cultures. The phenomenon of leukocyte "hyperadhesion" was only present in chronically inflamed IBD $himec_s$, as cultures derived from uninvolved areas in close proximity failed to demonstrate increased leukocyte binding.[5] The mechanisms underlying leukocyte hyperadhesion in the chronically inflamed IBD $himec_s$ did not involve altered patterns of CAM expression, but instead were linked to reduced NO production.[6,65] NO exerts a potent anti-inflammatory effect within the vasculature, downregulating the activation of vascular endothelial cells as well as their capacity to bind circulating leukocytes (normally an early, rate-limiting step in the inflammatory process).[66,67] Control $himec_s$ displayed distinct patterns of NO generation through both constitutive endothelial nitric oxide synthase (eNOS; NOS3) as well as inducible NOS (iNOS; NOS2). Inhibition of iNOS function in control HIMECs resulted in increased patterns of leukocyte binding that were similar to IBD $himec_s$. Investigation of the mechanisms of reduced NO generation in the IBD HIMEC confirmed that a loss of iNOS gene transcription and expression resulted from elevations in cytokines and LPS.

Enhanced Vasoconstrictor Products in IBD Intestine

Additional evidence for mucosal hypoperfusion in Crohn's disease and ulcerative colitis comes from studies investigating specific vasoconstrictor peptides. The endothelin peptides (ET-1, ET-2, and ET-3) are potent and long-acting vasoconstrictors that have been implicated as causative agents in a number of pathological states.[68,69] Because IBD microvessels often display heightened vasomotor tone, Murch *et al.* performed initial studies demonstrating increased levels of endothelins in IBD. Both ET-1 and ET-2 were found to be increased in the colonic mucosa in patients with Crohn's disease and ulcerative colitis.[70] This observation provided an important link between the hypotheses that immunological hypersensitivity[71] and vascular abnormalities[72,73] contribute to the pathophysiology of IBD. Interestingly, several of the proinflammatory cytokines[74,75] can stimulate production of endothelins.[76,77] Klemm *et al.* show that administration of tumor necrosis factor-alpha and interleukin-2 to anesthetized rats caused a marked elevation in the circulating plasma level of ET-1 and a very pronounced ET-1-dependent coronary vasoconstriction. In addition, rats suffering from adjuvant polyarthritis, in which there is marked joint inflammation and associated cytokine production, had dramatic increases in coronary perfusion pressure that were absent when the rats were treated with an endothelin receptor antagonist.

Despite these observations, other investigators have not confirmed an increase in tissue ET-1 and ET-2 in human IBD, and indeed Rachmilewtz *et al.* actually reported reduced levels of both mediators in ulcerative colitis.[78] These observations suggest that cytokines can significantly alter production of endothelin and that levels of these vasoconstrictor substances may vary during the course of disease. Further studies are required to define the presence and role of individual endothelin isopeptides within the human gastrointestinal tract.

Thromboxane A2 is a proinflammatory eicosanoid derived from isomerization of prostaglandin H2 by thromboxane synthase. Thromboxane A2 has a very short half-life and is rapidly metabolized to the more stable product, thromboxane B2.[79] Mucosal production of thromboxane is increased, both in the spontaneous model of colitis[80,81] and in colitis induced by exogenous agents.[82–84] In human IBD, thromboxane production in cultured isolated intestinal epithelial cells from patients with ulcerative colitis and those with Crohn's disease is increased.[85,86] In addition, in active colonic tissue homogenates from patients with ulcerative colitis[87,88] and in cultured biopsies from patients with both ulcerative colitis or Crohn's disease, excess thromboxane production is observed.[89–91] Moreover, rectal dialysis in patients with ulcerative colitis and Crohn's disease shows increased rectal mucosal production of thromboxane in active disease *in vivo.*[92–95] *In vitro* studies have shown that thromboxane has proinflammatory actions. It induces the activation of neutrophils[96] and the production of leukotriene B4,[97] and it enhances neutrophil adhesion to the endothelium[98] with subsequent diapedesis.[99] Furthermore, it induces apoptosis,[100] modulates T cell function,[101] and induces vasoconstriction[102] and platelet aggregation.[79] Platelet aggregates have been identified in the capillaries of inflamed rectal biopsy specimens in IBD,[103] and microvascular thrombosis has been proposed as an early pathogenic factor in Crohn's disease.[73] Thromboxane can thus perpetuate ischemic injury, thereby possibly playing a key role in the pathogenesis of IBD.

Therapeutic trials that have specifically targeted thromboxane, a mechanism of microvascular dysfunction in IBD, have been carried out. A series of trials targeting excess thromboxane in ulcerative colitis were completed, using a selective thromboxane antagonist, ridogrel (Janssen Research Foundation, Beerse, Belgium). Ridogrel was administered to ulcerative colitis patients both as an oral agent as well as an enema in placebo-controlled trials,[104,105] but failed to demonstrate efficacy and meet specified trial end points. Given that microvascular dysfunction appears to play a critical role in the process of chronic intestinal inflammation, the potential for agents targeting mechanisms of microvascular dysfunction may undergo further evaluation as adjuvant strategies, potentially targeting endothelin, thromboxane, or excess superoxide anion generation.

ANGIOGENESIS AS A THERAPEUTIC TARGET IN IBD

Angiogenesis and Repair Mechanisms in IBD-Associated Mucosal Healing

Angiogenesis is defined as a growth of new capillary blood vessels from preexisting vasculature.[106] This is of key importance in numerous physiologic and pathologic processes, including embryogenesis, tissue growth, wound healing, and the female reproductive cycle. Angiogenesis may also contribute to the pathologic processes of diseases such as cancer, psoriasis, tissue damage during reperfusion after ischemia or cardiac failure, diabetic retinopathy, and chronic inflammatory diseases in joints or gut.[107–110] Inflammation may promote angiogenesis in a number of ways.[108–111–115] Inflammatory tissue is often hypoxic, and hypoxia can induce angiogenesis through upregulation of factors such as vascular endothelial growth factor, fibroblast growth factor-1, tumor necrosis factor alpha, hypoxia-inducible factor-1, and other factors.[116–120] Extravasated plasma fibrinogen can stimulate neovascularization.[121–123] Inflammatory cells, such as macrophages, lymphocytes, mast cells, and fibroblasts, can stimulate vessel growth by producing angiogenic factors.[124–128] Increased blood flow itself may stimulate angiogenesis through shear stress on the endothelium.[129–131]

The most compelling evidence for the presence of angiogenesis in IBD includes neovascularization on the serosal surfaces of the bowel in chronically inflamed gut.[132] Additional supporting evidence includes upregulation of proangiogenic factors[133,134] and Doppler ultrasound findings of increased vessel density in inflamed bowel loops.[135,136] However, the increased vascular perfusion identified with transabdominal Doppler ultrasound may actually reflect the thickened bowel wall and creeping fat, which accompanies IBD, and not increased vessel density at the mucosal surfaces. Recent studies by Danese and colleagues have demonstrated angiogenic activity in a murine model of IBD, with additional demonstration of biologically active angiogenic cytokines being released from tissue biopsy from IBD patient's material.[137] Further studies have suggested that the IL-10 knockout mouse will demonstrate clinical improvement when treated with novel angiogenesis inhibitors, which have also demonstrated benefit in models of rheumatoid arthritis.[137]

Direct evidence for the development of therapeutic strategies targeting angiogenesis in chronic inflammatory disease remains limited, with the most promising studies emerging in the treatment of rheumatoid arthritis. Angiogenesis is felt to play a central role in the development of pannus formation in the inflamed synovium in joints affected by rheumatoid arthritis.[138] Therefore, the ability to restore joint architecture is integrally linked to inhibiting and reversing pannus formation. Emerging data also strongly suggest that angiogenesis and chronic inflammation are integrally linked, but the pathophysiologic relevance of angiogenesis in the perpetuation of chronic inflammation has been limited to animal studies.[138–141] Emerging studies in murine models of rheumatoid arthritis suggest that antiangiogenic agents, such as endostatin, may exert benefit in the ability to halt progression of joint destruction.[142] Further studies are warranted to define the role of angiogenesis in tissue remodeling and chronic inflammation in human IBD.

SUMMARY

The intestinal microvasculature serves essential functions in multiple physiological and pathophysiological conditions, including innate immunity and antimicrobial defense, as well as wound healing and angiogenesis. Various vascular mechanisms have been identified, which may contribute to the pathogenesis as well as to the perpetuation of chronic inflammation in human IBD. These include altered patterns of leukocyte recruitment with altered patterns of mucosal addressin expression in the chronically inflamed bowel. Microvascular dysfunction represents a key event in the pathogenesis of IBD, where impaired vasomotor responses hamper appropriate tissue perfusion rates and leukocyte emigration. Finally, angiogenesis appears to be integrally linked to chronic inflammation, including chronic gut inflammation, which is associated with tissue remodeling in the IBD-involved bowel. Treatment approaches targeting the dysregulated microvasculature in human IBD are presently emerging and will likely increase in the near future. These strategies will likely include biological agents targeting microvascular adhesion molecules and chemokines, as well as adjuvant strategies, which will target microvascular dysfunction and angiogenesis in attempts to improve mucosal healing and restoration of bowel architecture.

REFERENCES

1. PANES, J. & D.N. GRANGER. 1998. Leukocyte-endothelial cell interactions: molecular mechanisms and implications in gastrointestinal disease. Gastroenterology 114: 1066–1190.
2. FIOCCHI, C. 1993. Cytokines and animal models: a combined path to inflammatory bowel disease pathogenesis. Gastroenterology 104: 1202–1205.
3. YOUNGMAN, K.R. et al. 1993. Localization of intestinal interleukin 1 activity and protein and gene expression to lamina propria cells. Gastroenterology 104: 749–758.
4. BINION, D.G. et al. 1997. Enhanced leukocyte binding by intestinal microvascular endothelial cells in inflammatory bowel disease. Gastroenterology 112: 1895–1907.
5. BINION, D.G. et al. 1998. Acquired increase in leucocyte binding by intestinal microvascular endothelium in inflammatory bowel disease. Lancet 352: 1742–1746.
6. BINION, D.G. et al. 2000. Deficient iNOS in inflammatory bowel disease intestinal microvascular endothelial cells results in increased leukocyte adhesion. Free Radic. Biol. Med. 29: 881–888.

7. SALMI, M. *et al.* 1994. Aberrant binding of lamina propria lymphocytes to vascular endothelium in inflammatory bowel diseases. Gastroenterology **106**: 596–605.
8. BURGIO, V.L. *et al.* 1995. Peripheral monocyte and naive T-cell recruitment and activation in Crohn's disease. Gastroenterology **109**: 1029–1038.
9. BURNS, R.C. *et al.* 2001. Antibody blockade of ICAM-1 and VCAM-1 ameliorates inflammation in the SAMP-1/Yit adoptive transfer model of Crohn's disease in mice. Gastroenterology **121**: 1428–1436.
10. RIVERA-NIEVES, J. *et al.* 2005. L-selectin, alpha 4 beta 1, and alpha 4 beta 7 integrins participate in CD4+ T cell recruitment to chronically inflamed small intestine. J. Immunol. **174**: 2343–2352.
11. LEY, K. & G.S. KANSAS. 2004. Selectins in T-cell recruitment to non-lymphoid tissues and sites of inflammation. Nat. Rev. Immunol. **4**: 325–335.
12. BACHMANN, C. *et al.* 2006. Targeting mucosal addressin cellular adhesion molecule (MAdCAM)-1 to noninvasively image experimental Crohn's disease. Gastroenterology **130**: 8–16.
13. TEDDER, T.F. *et al.* 1995. The selectins: vascular adhesion molecules. FASEB J. **9**: 866–873.
14. TEDDER, T.F., D.A. STEEBER & P. PIZCUETA 1995. L-selectin-deficient mice have impaired leukocyte recruitment into inflammatory sites. J. Exp. Med. **181**: 2259–2264.
15. PANES, J. *et al.* 1995. Regional differences in constitutive and induced ICAM-1 expression *in vivo*. Am. J. Physiol. **269**(6 Pt 2): H1955–H1964.
16. PODOLSKY, D.K. *et al.* 1993. Attenuation of colitis in the cotton-top tamarin by anti-alpha 4 integrin monoclonal antibody. J. Clin. Invest. **92**: 372–380.
17. KOIZUMI, M. *et al.* 1992. Expression of vascular adhesion molecules in inflammatory bowel disease. Gastroenterology **103**: 840–847.
18. SANS, M. *et al.* 1999. VCAM-1 and ICAM-1 mediate leukocyte-endothelial cell adhesion in rat experimental colitis. Gastroenterology **116**: 874–883.
19. SORIANO, A. *et al.* 2000. VCAM-1, but not ICAM-1 or MAdCAM-1, immunoblockade ameliorates DSS-induced colitis in mice. Lab. Invest. **80**: 1541–1551.
20. CONNER, E.M. *et al.* 1997. Proteasome inhibition attenuates nitric oxide synthase expression, VCAM-1 transcription and the development of chronic colitis. J. Pharmacol. Exp. Ther. **282**: 1615–1622.
21. KAWACHI, S. *et al.* 2000. Cytokine and endothelial cell adhesion molecule expression in interleukin-10-deficient mice. Am. J. Physiol. Gastrointest. Liver Physiol. **278**: G734–G743.
22. VAN ASSCHE, G. & P. RUTGEERTS. 2002. Antiadhesion molecule therapy in inflammatory bowel disease. Inflamm. Bowel Dis. **8**: 291–300.
23. DUSTIN, M.L. *et al.* 1986. Induction by IL 1 and interferon-gamma: tissue distribution, biochemistry, and function of a natural adherence molecule (ICAM-1). J. Immunol. **137**: 245–254.
24. ROTHLEIN, R. *et al.* 1986. A human intercellular adhesion molecule (ICAM-1) distinct from LFA-1. J. Immunol. **137**: 1270–1274.
25. MARLIN, S.D. & T.A. SPRINGER. 1987. Purified intercellular adhesion molecule-1 (ICAM-1) is a ligand for lymphocyte function-associated antigen 1 (LFA-1). Cell **51**: 813–819.
26. DIAMOND, M.S. *et al.* 1990. ICAM-1 (CD54): a counter-receptor for Mac-1 (CD11b/CD18). J. Cell. Biol. **111**(6 Pt 2): 3129–3139.

27. KAVANAUGH, A.F. *et al.* 1994. Treatment of refractory rheumatoid arthritis with a monoclonal antibody to intercellular adhesion molecule 1. Arthritis Rheum. **37:** 992–999.
28. BENNETT, C.F. *et al.* 1994. Inhibition of endothelial cell adhesion molecule expression with antisense oligonucleotides. J. Immunol. **152:** 3530–3540.
29. NESTLE, F.O. *et al.* 1994. Cationic lipid is not required for uptake and selective inhibitory activity of ICAM-1 phosphorothioate antisense oligonucleotides in keratinocytes. J. Invest. Dermatol. **103:** 569–575.
30. CHIANG, M.Y. *et al.* 1991. Antisense oligonucleotides inhibit intercellular adhesion molecule 1 expression by two distinct mechanisms. J. Biol. Chem. **266:** 18162–18171.
31. HOKE, G.D. *et al.* 1991. Effects of phosphorothioate capping on antisense oligonucleotide stability, hybridization and antiviral efficacy versus herpes simplex virus infection. Nucleic Acids Res. **19:** 5743–5748.
32. WICKSTROM, E. 1986. Oligodeoxynucleotide stability in subcellular extracts and culture media. J. Biochem. Biophys. Methods **13:** 97–102.
33. YACYSHYN, B.R. *et al.* 1998. A placebo-controlled trial of ICAM-1 antisense oligonucleotide in the treatment of Crohn's disease. Gastroenterology **114:** 1133–1142.
34. SCHREIBER, S. *et al.* 2001. Absence of efficacy of subcutaneous antisense ICAM-1 treatment of chronic active Crohn's disease. Gastroenterology **120:** 1339–1346.
35. VAN DEVENTER, S.J., J.A. TAMI & M.K. WEDEL. 2004. A randomised, controlled, double blind, escalating dose study of alicaforsen enema in active ulcerative colitis. Gut **53:** 1646–1651.
36. DIGNASS, A. *et al.* 1994. Trefoil peptides promote epithelial migration through a transforming growth factor beta-independent pathway. J. Clin. Invest. **94:** 376–383.
37. SANDBORN, W.J. & T.A. YEDNOCK. 2003. Novel approaches to treating inflammatory bowel disease: targeting alpha-4 integrin. Am. J. Gastroenterol. **98:** 2372–2382.
38. GHOSH, S. *et al.* 2003. Natalizumab for active Crohn's disease. N. Engl. J. Med. **348:** 24–32.
39. SANDBORN, W.J. *et al.* 2005. Natalizumab induction and maintenance therapy for Crohn's disease. N. Engl. J. Med. **353:** 1912–1925.
40. FEAGAN, B.G. *et al.* 2005. Treatment of ulcerative colitis with a humanized antibody to the alpha4beta7 integrin. N. Engl. J. Med. **352:** 2499–2507.
41. PAPADAKIS, K.A. & S.R. TARGAN. 2000. The role of chemokines and chemokine receptors in mucosal inflammation. Inflamm. Bowel Dis. **6:** 303–313.
42. PAPADAKIS, K.A. 2004. Chemokines in inflammatory bowel disease. Curr. Allergy Asthma Rep. **4:** 83–89.
43. PAPADAKIS, K.A. *et al.* 2003. CC chemokine receptor 9 expression defines a subset of peripheral blood lymphocytes with mucosal T cell phenotype and Th1 or T-regulatory 1 cytokine profile. J. Immunol. **171:** 159–165.
44. PAPADAKIS, K.A. *et al.* 2001. CCR9-positive lymphocytes and thymus-expressed chemokine distinguish small bowel from colonic Crohn's disease. Gastroenterology **121:** 246–254.
45. PAPADAKIS, K.A. *et al.* 2000. The role of thymus-expressed chemokine and its receptor CCR9 on lymphocytes in the regional specialization of the mucosal immune system. J. Immunol. **165:** 5069–5076.

46. QIUPING, Z. *et al.* 2004. CC chemokine ligand 25 enhances resistance to apoptosis in CD4+ T cells from patients with T-cell lineage acute and chronic lymphocytic leukemia by means of living activation. Cancer Res. **64:** 7579–7587.

47. ZHENG WEI, L.E., T. BAUMGART, W. RUBAS, *et al.* 2005. Cc chemokine receptor 9 (ccr9) antagonist ameliorates experimental ileitis and colitis. Gastroenterology **128:** A–204–205.

48. FUNAYAMA, Y. *et al.* 1999. Remodeling of vascular wall in Crohn's disease. Dig. Dis. Sci. **44:** 2319–2323.

49. WAKEFIELD, A.J. *et al.* 1991. Granulomatous vasculitis in Crohn's disease. Gastroenterology **100**(5 Pt 1): 1279–1287.

50. HULTEN, L. *et al.* 1977. Regional intestinal blood flow in ulcerative colitis and Crohn's disease. Gastroenterology **72:** 388–396.

51. ANGERSON, W.J. *et al.* 1993. Neoterminal ileal blood flow after ileocolonic resection for Crohn's disease. Gut **34:** 1531–1534.

52. TATEISHI, S., S. ARIMA & K. FUTAMI. 1997. Assessment of blood flow in the small intestine by laser Doppler flowmetry: comparison of healthy small intestine and small intestine in Crohn's disease. J. Gastroenterol. **32:** 457–463.

53. BOGER, R.H. *et al.* 1998. Restoring vascular nitric oxide formation by L-arginine improves the symptoms of intermittent claudication in patients with peripheral arterial occlusive disease. J. Am. Coll. Cardiol. **32:** 1336–1344.

54. KERSTEIN, M.D. 1996. The non-healing leg ulcer: peripheral vascular disease, chronic venous insufficiency, and ischemic vasculitis. Ostomy Wound Manage. **42**(10A Suppl): 19S–35S.

55. MONTORI, V.M. *et al.* 2002. Intermittent compression pump for nonhealing wounds in patients with limb ischemia. The Mayo Clinic experience (1998–2000). Int. Angiol. **21:** 360–366.

56. FLYNN, M.D. & J.E. TOOKE. 1992. Aetiology of diabetic foot ulceration: a role for the microcirculation? Diabet. Med. **9:** 320–329.

57. VEVES, A. *et al.* 1998. Endothelial dysfunction and the expression of endothelial nitric oxide synthetase in diabetic neuropathy, vascular disease, and foot ulceration. Diabetes **47:** 457–463.

58. WHEATCROFT, S.B. *et al.* 2003. Pathophysiological implications of insulin resistance on vascular endothelial function. Diabet. Med. **20:** 255–268.

59. HATOUM, O.A. *et al.* 2003. Acquired microvascular dysfunction in inflammatory bowel disease: loss of nitric oxide-mediated vasodilation. Gastroenterology **125:** 58–69.

60. MORI, M. *et al.* 2005. Colonic blood flow responses in experimental colitis: time course and underlying mechanisms. Am. J. Physiol. Gastrointest. Liver Physiol. **289:** G1024–G1029.

61. DVORAK, A.M., A.B. CONNELL & G.R. DICKERSIN. 1979. Crohn's disease: a scanning electron microscopic study. Hum. Pathol. **10:** 165–177.

62. DVORAK, A.M. & G.R. DICKERSIN. 1979. Crohn's disease: electron microscopic studies. Pathol. Annu. **14**(Pt 2): 259–306.

63. HARALDSEN, G. *et al.* 1995. Isolation and longterm culture of human intestinal microvascular endothelial cells. Gut **37:** 225–234.

64. HARALDSEN, G. *et al.* 1996. Cytokine-regulated expression of E-selectin, intercellular adhesion molecule-1 (ICAM-1), and vascular cell adhesion molecule-1 (VCAM-1) in human microvascular endothelial cells. J. Immunol. **156:** 2558–2565.

65. BINION, D.G. *et al.* 1998. iNOS expression in human intestinal microvascular endothelial cells inhibits leukocyte adhesion. Am. J. Physiol. **275**(3 Pt 1): G592–G603.
66. KUBES, P., M. SUZUKI & D.N. GRANGER. 1991. Nitric oxide: an endogenous modulator of leukocyte adhesion. Proc. Natl. Acad. Sci. USA **88:** 4651–4655.
67. KUBES, P. & D.M. MCCAFFERTY. 2000. Nitric oxide and intestinal inflammation. Am. J. Med. **109:** 150–158.
68. HAYNES, W.G., A.P. DAVENPORT & D.J. WEBB. 1993. Endothelin: progress in pharmacology and physiology. Trends Pharmacol. Sci. **14:** 225–228.
69. RUBANYI, G.M. & M.A. POLOKOFF. 1994. Endothelins: molecular biology, biochemistry, pharmacology, physiology, and pathophysiology. Pharmacol. Rev. **46:** 325–415.
70. MURCH, S.H. *et al.* 1992. High endothelin-1 immunoreactivity in Crohn's disease and ulcerative colitis. Lancet **339:** 381–385.
71. BECK, P.L. & D.K. PODOLSKY. 1999. Growth factors in inflammatory bowel disease. Inflamm. Bowel Dis. **5:** 44–60.
72. HAMILTON, M.I. *et al.* 1995. Is proximal demarcation of ulcerative colitis determined by the territory of the inferior mesenteric artery? Lancet **345:** 688–690.
73. WAKEFIELD, A.J. *et al.* 1989. Pathogenesis of Crohn's disease: multifocal gastrointestinal infarction. Lancet **2:** 1057–1062.
74. NIELSEN, O.H. *et al.* 2000. Established and emerging biological activity markers of inflammatory bowel disease. Am. J. Gastroenterol **95:** 359–367.
75. BREESE, E.J. *et al.* 1994. Tumor necrosis factor alpha-producing cells in the intestinal mucosa of children with inflammatory bowel disease. Gastroenterology **106:** 1455–1466.
76. KLEMM, P. *et al.* 1995. Endothelin-1 mediates coronary vasoconstriction caused by exogenous and endogenous cytokines. J. Cardiovasc. Pharmacol. **26(Suppl 3):** S419–S421.
77. WARNER, T.D. & P. KLEMM. 1996. What turns on the endothelins? Inflamm. Res. **45:** 51–53.
78. RACHMILEWITZ, D. *et al.* 1992. Colonic endothelin–1 immunoreactivity in active ulcerative colitis. Lancet **339:** 1062.
79. HAMBERG, M., J. SVENSSON & B. SAMUELSSON. 1975. Thromboxanes: a new group of biologically active compounds derived from prostaglandin endoperoxides. Proc. Natl. Acad. Sci. USA **72:** 2994–2998.
80. CLAPP, N. *et al.* 1993. Inflammatory mediator changes in cotton-top tamarins (CTT) after SC-41930 anti-colitic therapy. Agents Actions **39**(Spec. No. regular weight): C8–C10.
81. CLAPP, N. *et al.* 1993. Anti-colitic efficacy of SC-41930 in colitic cotton-top tamarins. Agents Actions **39**(Spec. No. regular weight): C36–C38.
82. SHARON, P. & W.F. STENSON. 1985. Metabolism of arachidonic acid in acetic acid colitis in rats: similarity to human inflammatory bowel disease. Gastroenterology **88**(1 Pt 1): 55–63.
83. VILASECA, J. *et al.* 1990. Participation of thromboxane and other eicosanoid synthesis in the course of experimental inflammatory colitis. Gastroenterology **98:** 269–277.
84. KITSUKAWA, Y. *et al.* 1992. Effect of ingestion of eicosapentaenoic acid ethyl ester on carrageenan-induced colitis in guinea pigs. Gastroenterology **102:** 1859–1866.

85. ZIFRONI, A. *et al.* 1983. Prostanoid synthesis by cultured intestinal epithelial and mononuclear cells in inflammatory bowel disease. Gut **24:** 659–664.
86. RAMPTON, D.S. & C.E. COLLINS. 1993. Review article: thromboxanes in inflammatory bowel disease: pathogenic and therapeutic implications. Aliment. Pharmacol. Ther. **7:** 357–367.
87. BOUGHTON-SMITH, N.K., C.J. HAWKEY & B.J. WHITTLE. 1983. Biosynthesis of lipoxygenase and cyclo-oxygenase products from [^{14}C]-arachidonic acid by human colonic mucosa. Gut **24:** 1176–1182.
88. BOUGHTON-SMITH, N.K. & B.J. WHITTLE. 1983. Stimulation and inhibition of prostacyclin formation in the gastric mucosa and ileum in vitro by anti-inflammatory agents. Br. J. Pharmacol. **78:** 173–180.
89. HAWKEY, C.J., N.K. BOUGHTON-SMITH & B.J. WHITTLE. 1985. Modulation of human colonic arachidonic acid metabolism by sulfasalazine. Dig. Dis. Sci. **30:** 1161–1165.
90. HAWKEY, C.J. & D.S. RAMPTON. 1985. Prostaglandins and the gastrointestinal mucosa: are they important in its function, disease, or treatment? Gastroenterology **89:** 1162–1188.
91. HAWKEY, C.J. 1993. Gastroduodenal problems associated with non-steroidal, anti-inflammatory drugs (NSAIDs). Scand. J. Gastroenterol. **200**(Suppl): 94–95.
92. LAURITSEN, K. *et al.* 1988. Use of colonic eicosanoid concentrations as predictors of relapse in ulcerative colitis: double blind placebo controlled study on sulphasalazine maintenance treatment. Gut **29:** 1316–1321.
93. LAURITSEN, K. & J. RASK–MADSEN. 1988. Prostaglandin analogues. Baillieres Clin. Gastroenterol. **2:** 621–628.
94. LAURITSEN, K. *et al.* 1988. Longterm olsalazine treatment: pharmacokinetics, tolerance and effects on local eicosanoid formation in ulcerative colitis and Crohn's colitis. Gut **29:** 974–982.
95. LAURITSEN, K. *et al.* 1988. In vivo profiles of eicosanoids in ulcerative colitis, Crohn's colitis, and *Clostridium difficile* colitis. Gastroenterology **95:** 11–17.
96. KITCHEN, E.A., J.R. BOOT & W. DAWSON. 1978. Chemotactic activity of thromboxane B2, prostaglandins and their metabolites for polymorphonuclear leucocytes. Prostaglandins **16:** 239–244.
97. GOLDMAN, G. *et al.* 1991. Thromboxane A2 induces leukotriene B4 synthesis that in turn mediates neutrophil diapedesis via CD 18 activation. Microvasc. Res. **41:** 367–375.
98. WILES, M.E. *et al.* 1991. Thromboxane-induced neutrophil adhesion to pulmonary microvascular and aortic endothelium is regulated by CD18. Inflammation **15:** 181–199.
99. DOUKAS, J., H.B. HECHTMAN & D. SHEPRO. 1988. Endothelial-secreted arachidonic acid metabolites modulate polymorphonuclear leukocyte chemotaxis and diapedesis in vitro. Blood **71:** 771–779.
100. USHIKUBI, F. *et al.* 1993. Thromboxane A2 receptor is highly expressed in mouse immature thymocytes and mediates DNA fragmentation and apoptosis. J. Exp. Med. **178:** 1825–1830.
101. KELLY, J.P., M.C. JOHNSON & C.W. PARKER. 1979. Effect of inhibitors of arachidonic acid metabolism on mitogenesis in human lymphocytes: possible role of thromboxanes and products of the lipoxygenase pathway. J. Immunol. **122:** 1563–1571.

102. ZIPSER, R.D. *et al.* 1985. Hypersensitive prostaglandin and thromboxane response to hormones in rabbit colitis. Am. J. Physiol. **249**(4 Pt 1): G457–G463.
103. DHILLON, A.P. *et al.* 1992. Mucosal capillary thrombi in rectal biopsies. Histopathology **21**: 127–133.
104. AUWERDA, J.J. *et al.* 2001. Ridogrel enemas in distal ulcerative colitis. Eur. J. Gastroenterol. Hepatol. **13**: 397–400.
105. TYTGAT, G.N. *et al.* 2002. Efficacy and safety of oral ridogrel in the treatment of ulcerative colitis: two multicentre, randomized, double-blind studies. Aliment. Pharmacol. Ther. **16**: 87–99.
106. RISAU, W. 1997. Mechanisms of angiogenesis. Nature **386**: 671–674.
107. FOLKMAN, J. 1985. Tumor angiogenesis. Adv. Cancer Res. **43**: 175–203.
108. WALSH, D.A. 1999. Angiogenesis and arthritis. Rheumatology (Oxford) **38**: 103–112.
109. FOLKMAN, J. 1995. Angiogenesis in cancer, vascular, rheumatoid and other disease. Nat. Med. **1**: 27–31.
110. HANAHAN, D. & J. FOLKMAN. 1996. Patterns and emerging mechanisms of the angiogenic switch during tumorigenesis. Cell **86**: 353–364.
111. POLVERINI, P.J. 1997. Role of the macrophage in angiogenesis-dependent diseases. EXS **79**: 11–28.
112. CARMELIET, P. *et al.* 1999. Targeted deficiency or cytosolic truncation of the VE-cadherin gene in mice impairs VEGF-mediated endothelial survival and angiogenesis. Cell **98**: 147–157.
113. CARMELIET, P. *et al.* 1999. Impaired myocardial angiogenesis and ischemic cardiomyopathy in mice lacking the vascular endothelial growth factor isoforms VEGF164 and VEGF188. Nat. Med. **5**: 495–502.
114. CARMELIET, P. & D. COLLEN. 1999. Role of vascular endothelial growth factor and vascular endothelial growth factor receptors in vascular development. Curr. Top. Microbiol. Immunol. **237**: 133–158.
115. FERRARA, N. & K. ALITALO. 1999. Clinical applications of angiogenic growth factors and their inhibitors. Nat. Med. **5**: 1359–1364.
116. QU, Z. *et al.* 1995. Expression of basic fibroblast growth factor in synovial tissue from patients with rheumatoid arthritis and degenerative joint disease. Lab. Invest. **73**: 339–346.
117. QU, Z. *et al.* 1995. Mast cells are a major source of basic fibroblast growth factor in chronic inflammation and cutaneous hemangioma. Am. J. Pathol. **147**: 564–573.
118. WALSH, D.A. *et al.* 1998. Focally regulated endothelial proliferation and cell death in human synovium. Am. J. Pathol. **152**: 691–702.
119. WALSH, D.A. & P.I. MAPP. 1998. Joint physiology and synovial cell proliferation. Br. J. Rheumatol. **37**: 1032–1033.
120. WALSH, D.A., H.A. RODWAY & A. CLAXSON. 1998. Vascular turnover during carrageenan synovitis in the rat. Lab. Invest. **78**: 1513–1521.
121. JONES, A.L. *et al.* 2005. Histidine-rich glycoprotein specifically binds to necrotic cells via its amino-terminal domain and facilitates necrotic cell phagocytosis. J. Biol. Chem. **280**: 35733–35741.
122. HATTON, M.W. *et al.* 2004. Fibrinogen catabolism within the procoagulant VX-2 tumor of rabbit lung *in vivo*: effluxing fibrin(ogen) fragments contain antiangiogenic activity. J. Lab. Clin. Med. **143**: 241–254.
123. DALY, M.E. *et al.* 2003. Hemostatic regulators of tumor angiogenesis: a source of antiangiogenic agents for cancer treatment? J. Natl. Cancer Inst. **95**: 1660–1073.

124. SCAPINI, P. *et al.* 2002. Generation of biologically active angiostatin kringle 1-3 by activated human neutrophils. J. Immunol. **168:** 5798–5804.
125. COLLIN-OSDOBY, P. *et al.* 2002. Basic fibroblast growth factor stimulates osteoclast recruitment, development, and bone pit resorption in association with angiogenesis *in vivo* on the chick chorioallantoic membrane and activates isolated avian osteoclast resorption in vitro. J. Bone Miner. Res. **17:** 1859–1871.
126. OGAWA, H. *et al.* 2005. Mechanisms of MAdCAM-1 gene expression in human intestinal microvascular endothelial cells. Am. J. Physiol. Cell. Physiol. **288:** C272–C281.
127. OKADA, F. 2002. Inflammation and free radicals in tumor development and progression. Redox. Rep. **7:** 357–368.
128. CRIVELLATO, E. & D. RIBATTI. 2005. Involvement of mast cells in angiogenesis and chronic inflammation. Curr. Drug Targets Inflamm. Allergy **4:** 9–11.
129. MILKIEWICZ, M. *et al.* 2001. Association between shear stress, angiogenesis, and VEGF in skeletal muscles *in vivo*. Microcirculation **8:** 229–241.
130. CULLEN, J.P. *et al.* 2002. Pulsatile flow-induced angiogenesis: role of G(i) subunits. Arterioscler. Thromb. Vasc. Biol. **22:** 1610–1616.
131. SCHAPER, W. & D. SCHOLZ. 2003. Factors regulating arteriogenesis. Arterioscler. Thromb. Vasc. Biol. **23:** 1143–1151.
132. CONTRAN, R.S.1994. Robbins Pathologic Basis of Disease. 5th Ed. W. B. Saunders. Philadelphia.
133. SAITO, S. *et al.* 2003. Expression of platelet-derived endothelial cell growth factor in inflammatory bowel disease. J. Gastroenterol. **38:** 229–237.
134. KANAZAWA, S. *et al.* 2001. VEGF, basic-FGF, and TGF-beta in Crohn's disease and ulcerative colitis: a novel mechanism of chronic intestinal inflammation. Am. J. Gastroenterol. **96:** 822–828.
135. ROBOTTI, D. *et al.* 2004. Activity of Crohn disease: value of Color-Power-Doppler and contrast-enhanced ultrasonography. Abdom. Imaging **29:** 648–652.
136. DI SABATINO, A., E. ARMELLINI & G.R. CORAZZA. 2004. Doppler sonography in the diagnosis of inflammatory bowel disease. Dig. Dis. **22:** 63–66.
137. DANESE, S.S.M., D. SPENCER, I. BECK, *et al.* 2005. Starving the inflamed gut: angiogenesis blocked as a novel therapeutic approach to experimental colitis. Gastroenterology **128:** A–40.
138. STUPACK, D.G., C.M. STORGARD & D.A. CHERESH. 1999. A role for angiogenesis in rheumatoid arthritis. Braz. J. Med. Biol. Res. **32:** 573–581.
139. JACKSON, J.R. *et al.* 1997. Modulation of angiogenesis in a model of chronic inflammation. Inflamm. Res. **46**(Suppl 2): S129–S130.
140. HIRATA, S. *et al.* 1989. Inhibition of *in vitro* vascular endothelial cell proliferation and *in vivo* neovascularization by low-dose methotrexate. Arthritis Rheum. **32:** 1065–1073.
141. ROCCARO, A.M. *et al.* 2005. Antiangiogenesis for rheumatoid arthritis. Curr. Drug Targets Inflamm. Allergy **4:** 27–30.
142. MATSUNO, H. *et al.* 2002. Treatment with the angiogenesis inhibitor endostatin: a novel therapy in rheumatoid arthritis. J. Rheumatol. **29:** 890–895.

Novel Signal Transduction Pathways

Analysis of STAT-3 and Rac-1 Signaling in Inflammatory Bowel Disease

R. ATREYA, I. ATREYA, AND M.F. NEURATH

Laboratory of Immunology, Department of Medicine, University of Mainz, Mainz, Germany

ABSTRACT: Although the precise etiology of inflammatory bowel disease still remains unclear, considerable progress has been made in the identification of novel signal transduction pathways that elucidate the immunopathogenesis involved in the perpetuation of the inflammatory process. Augmented T cell resistance against apoptosis is regarded as a pivotal factor in the pathogenesis, as it impairs mucosal homeostasis and leads to unrestrained accumulation of activated T cells, which subsequently lead to the amplification of the inflammatory response. Therefore novel therapeutic strategies aim at restoring mucosal T cell susceptibility to apoptosis through targeting of signal transduction pathways that are elemental for augmented resistance of T lymphocytes against apoptosis. For example, a newly developed humanized anti-IL-6R monoclonal antibody that induces intestinal T cell apoptosis showed clinical efficacy in patients with active Crohn`s disease. Moreover, recent data that relate the immunosuppressive effects of azathioprine in inflammatory bowel disease to its apoptosis-inducing potential, have important implications for the design of a more specific therapeutic approach. The examination of these novel signal transduction pathways has elucidated the pathogenetic mechanisms involved in inflammatory bowel disease and gives hope for the development of new strategies that may result in a more effective and less toxic therapeutic procedure.

KEYWORDS: Inflammatory bowel disease; signal transduction; apoptosis; IL-6R-antibody; azathioprine

INTRODUCTION

Inflammatory bowel disease (IBD) comprises Crohn's disease and ulcerative colitis, which are defined as relapsing inflammations of the gastrointesti-

Address for correspondence: Markus F. Neurath, Laboratory of Immunology, Department of Medicine, University of Mainz, Langenbeckstrasse 1, 55101 Mainz, Germany. Voice: 49-6131-172374; fax: 49-6131-175508.

e-mail: neurath@1-med.klinik.uni-mainz.de

Ann. N.Y. Acad. Sci. 1072: 98–113 (2006). © 2006 New York Academy of Sciences.
doi: 10.1196/annals.1326.001

nal tract not due to specific pathogens.[1] Although the precise etiology still remains unclear, considerable progress has been made in the identification of important pathophysiological mechanisms. The discovery of novel signal transduction pathways has further clarified the immunopathogenetic mechanisms involved. At present it is a consensus that the major contributory factors to the etiopathogenesis of inflammatory bowel disease are genetic susceptibility, environmental triggers, and mucosal imbalance, with ongoing activation of the intestinal immune system that leads to the perpetuation of the inflammatory cascade.[2]

Current concepts on the pathogenesis of inflammatory bowel disease are based on a genetic predisposition that is modulated by various environmental factors.[3] This leads to alterations in the epithelial mucosal barrier, which result in an augmented intestinal permeability that exposes the mucosal immune system to luminal bacterial antigens from the commensal flora. In patients with inflammatory bowel disease, this results in a dysregulation of the host immune response, leading to an inappropriate activation of the intestinal immune system. This ultimately causes pathogenic gastrointestinal inflammation and tissue damage.[4] Nevertheless, the exact pathogenetic mechanisms involved are still incompletely understood and therapeutic strategies have thus far been limited to mostly evidence-based principles.

Inflammatory bowel disease has conventionally been treated using corticosteroids, aminosalicylates, and immunosuppressive agents, such as azathioprine or cyclosporine, which are assumed to target the inflammatory process rather broadly.[5] The moderate efficacy in a subgroup of patients and the possible association with serious and irreversible side effects show the necessity for a more sustained therapeutic response, which can only be the result of a more comprehensive approach in targeting critical points of signal transduction pathways involved in the inflammatory cascade.[6]

Direct therapeutic implications are derived from increasing evidence that excessive CD4+ T cell activation is the central pathogenic mechanism involved in the initiation and perpetuation of the inflammatory process.[7,8] The distinct characteristics of lamina propria T cells in inflammatory bowel disease are an increase in T lymphocyte proliferation and trafficking into the intestinal mucosa,[9] as well as an excessive production of proinflammatory cytokines.[2] Furthermore, augmented T cell resistance against apoptosis represents a potential key factor in the pathogenesis, as it impairs mucosal homeostasis and leads to the unrestrained accumulation of activated CD4+ T cells, which subsequently results in the amplification of the inflammatory response.[9] As these findings have elucidated the pathogenetic mechanisms involved in inflammatory bowel disease, there is hope for the development of new therapeutic strategies that are based on a sound pathophysiological rationale.[5]

RESULTS AND DISCUSSION

Targeting Inflammatory Bowel Disease by Inducing T Lymphocyte Apoptosis

It is now well recognized that downregulation of intestinal T lymphocyte activation is essential for the maintenance of mucosal homeostasis, as the mucosal immune system is constantly exposed to a high amount of luminal antigens. The peripheral T lymphocyte tolerance is normally ensured by anergy of the central immunoregulatory cells, cytokine-dependent downregulation, and, importantly, by the concept of activation-induced cell death.[10]

The loss of tolerance and hyperresponsiveness of the intestinal immune system in inflammatory bowel disease leads to the uncontrolled activation of central immune cell populations (T lymphocytes, macrophages) and consecutive dysregulation of mucosal homoeostasis. This results in the production of proinflammatory cytokines that contribute to the inflammatory process, which is moreover aggravated by increased resistance of mucosal T lymphocytes against apoptosis.[3,4,11] While normal intestinal lamina propria T cells are highly susceptible to apoptosis, mucosal lymphocytes in Crohn's disease are less vulnerable to Fas-mediated apoptosis, which corresponds with an increased concentration of the antiapoptotic protein Bcl-xl.[12,13] Accordingly, recent data also revealed diminished expression of Fas on intestinal T cells and macrophages from patients with inflammatory bowel disease, reflecting lessened apoptosis via the Fas/FasL pathway.[14]

Therefore novel therapeutic strategies aim at restoring intestinal T cell susceptibility to apoptosis through targeting signal transduction pathways that are elemental for augmented apoptosis resistance in inflammatory bowel disease. Because cytokines have key immunoregulatory and effector roles in the inflammatory process, with consistent elevation of proinflammatory cytokines, they have been regarded as ideal targets for forthcoming immunomodulatory therapies.[15] This attractive therapeutic approach is implemented in the administration of a neutralizing anti-IL-12 antibody in an experimental model of colitis, exhibiting a Th-1 cytokine-mediated inflammation.[16] The application of the antibody led to the induction of apoptosis of intestinal CD4+ T cells and to consecutive abrogation of mucosal inflammation. This induction of apoptosis was Fas-mediated, although the precise pathways involved are not yet fully understood.[17] A recent study report showed that treatment with a monoclonal antibody against IL-12 induced clinical response and remission in patients with Crohn's disease.[18] The therapeutic rationale of the already established treatment with antibodies to TNF in active Crohn's disease also seems to be due to rapid and augmented induction of intestinal T lymphocyte apoptosis.[19] Furthermore, *ex vivo* treatment of blood monocytes from patients with Crohn's disease showed signs of caspase-dependent apoptosis after treatment with the chimeric anti-TNF-α monoclonal antibody.[20] This induction of apoptosis is mediated by outside-to-inside (reverse) signaling through trans-membrane TNF-α (mTNF), as its bipolar function enables mTNF to act as a ligand and as a receptor.[21]

In the following section, therapeutic implications of recent advances made in the understanding of the immunopathogenesis of inflammatory bowel disease are presented and their possible relevance in potential future therapeutic strategies is discussed.

Interleukin(IL)-6 Signaling Pathway and Associated Transcription Factors

In contrast to the predominant paradigm of Th1/Th2 differentiation in Crohn's disease and ulcerative colitis,[22] recent data clearly indicate a predominant role of the proinflammatory cytokine IL-6 in the pathogenesis of both entities of inflammatory bowel disease.

In patients with active Crohn's disease, marked elevations of serum IL-6 levels were repeatedly demonstrated.[23–26] These data correspond with results of increased IL-6 mRNA levels in colonic mucosal biopsy specimens[27] and heightened *in vitro* IL-6 production of lamina propria mononuclear cells from patients with acute Crohn's disease.[28,29] Similar results could also be found in ulcerative colitis, where elevated IL-6 mRNA expression in inflamed mucosa[27] and increased IL-6 production of cultivated lamina propria mononuclear cells were perceived.[29,30] Moreover, IL-6 concentrations also turned out to be a clinically relevant parameter for Crohn's disease and ulcerative colitis, as they positively correlated with inflammatory activity. [31,32] Intestinal CD4+ T cells and macrophages were subsequently found to be the main producers of IL-6.[33]

The biological function of IL-6 in inflammatory bowel disease is not mediated through a membrane-bound receptor for IL-6 (IL-6R) that consists of a ligand-binding subunit (pg 80) and signal-transducing subunit (gp130), as most lamina propria T cells of inflammatory bowel disease patients did not express this form of receptor.[33] Instead IL-6 exerts its effects through binding to a soluble form of its corresponding receptor (sIL-6R).[34] The sIL6R is generated either by translation from an alternatively spliced mRNA or by limited proteolysis of the membrane-bound form (shedding) and is mainly produced by macrophages.[35,36] Lipopolysaccharide has been shown to enhance IL-6 production in ulcerative colitis lamina propria mononuclear cells[32] mediated by the macrophage migration inhibitory factor,[37] and bacterial toxins trigger the process of shedding.[38] In conclusion, it is probable that these processes are triggered in inflammatory bowel disease due to the permanent exposure of the intestinal immune system to bacterial antigens.[3] Consistently, the soluble IL-6R (sIL-6R) and circulating sIL-6R/IL-6 concentrations in the serum are elevated in inflammatory bowel disease[39] and increased *in vitro* sIL-6R production by intestinal mononuclear cells was also noticed.[33,40] The complex of IL-6/sIL-6R

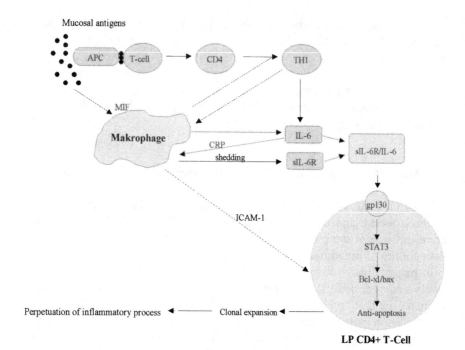

FIGURE 1. Model of IL-6 transsignaling in the immunopathology of IBD. Continuous stimulation by mucosal antigens (LPS, bacterial toxins) leads to ongoing activation of the mucosal immune system. Mediated by MIF there is augmented production of IL-6 by intestinal macrophages and CD4+ T cells. Moreover, the concentration of the soluble receptor sIL-6R, which is generated through shedding of the membrane-bound receptor from the surface of intestinal macrophages by proteolytic cleavage, is similarly increased. The IL-6/sIL-6R complexes that interact with gp130 on the membrane of CD4+ T cells lead to increased expression and nuclear translocation of STAT-3. This causes the induction of antiapoptotic genes, such as Bcl-xl resulting in an augmented resistance of lamina propria T cells against apoptosis. The ensuing T cell expansion contributes to the perpetuation of the chronic intestinal inflammation.

then associates with gp130 on intestinal cells lacking the IL-6R.[34] In consequence, IL-6 uses this alternative pathway through the sIL-6R to activate target cells lacking the membrane-bound form of the IL-6R. This process has been classified as transsignaling and plays a crucial role in IL-6-modulated signal transduction.[41] This signaling pathway leads to increased expression and nuclear translocation of signal transducer and activator of transcription (STAT)-3 and subsequently to considerable induction of the antiapoptotic genes Bcl-2 and Bcl-xl,[33] whereas the expression of the STAT-3 independent proapoptotic gene Bax is not altered.[42] This imbalance of the Bcl-xl/Bax ratio evokes intestinal T cell resistance to apoptosis in inflammatory bowel disease (FIG. 1).[33] To examine the functional impact of blockade of this IL-6-mediated STAT-3 pathway, lamina propria mononuclear cells were treated with a neutralizing

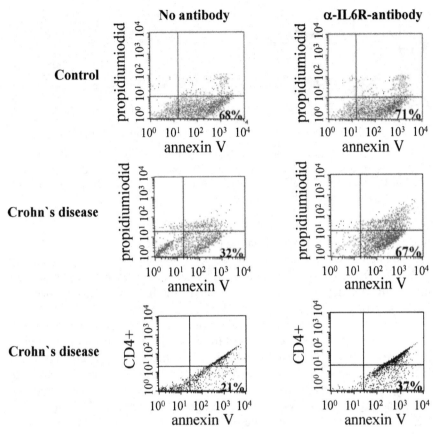

FIGURE 2. Induction of T cell apoptosis in IBD after treatment with α-IL-6R antibody. Lamina propria mononuclear cells were stimulated for 2 days with PMA, PHA, and CRP, and then analyzed by annexinV-FITC/propidiumiodid staining or antibodies against CD4. AnnexinV-positive/propidiumiodid-negative cells represent early apoptotic cells. There is induction of apoptosis and of annexin-positive lamina propria CD4+ T cells in Crohn's disease after treatment with the α-IL-6R antibody, but not in comparable controls.

antibody against the sIL-6R. Consistently, we found that this led to enhanced apoptosis in intestinal cells from patients with Crohn's disease, but not from controls (FIG. 2).[33]

In addition, application of the antibody in diverse murine models of chronic intestinal inflammation suppressed or reduced inflammatory activity. This therapeutic effect was established in enterocolitis in T cell–reconstituted SCID mice, IL-10 knockout mice, colitis induced by the hapten trinitrobenzene sulphonic acid (TNBS), and colitis occurring in severe combined immunodeficiency (SCID) mice upon transfer of naive (CD 62 L[+] CD45 Rb[hi]) T cells, thereby confirming the role of sIL-6R in mucosal inflammation *in vivo*.[33,43] Moreover, the curative impact of the antibody was based upon induction of

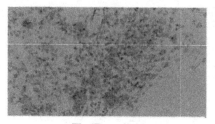 

α-IL-6R-antibody   no antibody

FIGURE 3. Apoptosis induction in colitic mice after treatment with the α-IL-6R antibody. The experimental colitis of the IL-10 knockout mouse model was treated with 1 mg of the α-IL-6R-Ak. Considerable induction of apoptosis was detected 7 days after treatment in colonic sections analyzed by TUNEL assays.

intestinal T cell apoptosis, elucidating the pathogenic role of IL-6 transsignaling and implicating the therapeutic potential of blocking the IL-6 transsignaling pathway (FIG. 3).[33] Further studies to directly demonstrate an essential pathogenic function for the sIL-6R-mediated transsignaling in an enterocolitis model *in vivo* were performed in an adoptive transfer model in SCID mice. In this model IL-6 was required in the development of the Th1 T cell–mediated disease, as antibody treatment against the IL-6R led to the prevention of colitis by macroscopic and histologic criteria. The treatment led to reduction of both colonic- and splenic-transferred CD4+ T cell expansion, as it suppressed the accumulation of ICAM-1-positive cells in the lamina propria and the expression of ICAM-1 and VCAM-1 in the intestinal vascular endothelium. The treatment further reduced colonic expression of TNF-α and IFN-γ mRNA without affecting the production of TGF-β.[43]

Therefore blocking the IL-6 signaling pathway is considered as a new therapeutic strategy in Crohn's disease. Recently, a clinical trial with a humanized anti-IL-6R monoclonal antibody for active Crohn's disease was carried out and efficacy of the treatment, with consecutive normalization of the acute-phase response, suggested an overall therapeutic benefit.[44] Further efforts to establish the safety and efficacy of the antibody in larger trials of patients with Crohn's disease are under way. It is tempting to speculate that specific targeting of the IL-6 transsignaling pathway could lead to a more selective therapeutic approach in inflammatory bowel disease, resulting in a more effective treatment regimen.

Because most cytokines exert their biological properties through a downstream pathway that involves activation of corresponding signal transducers and activators of transcription (STAT), recent research has focused on these signaling pathways. Cytokines bind to their respective receptor, which induces dimerization of the receptor and activation of cytoplasmic Janus-activated kinases (JAKs), which in turn phosphorylate the receptor. This enables the STAT proteins to bind to intracellular domains of the receptor, which are in turn phosphorylated by JAKs. This leads to dimerization and migration of the STAT proteins to the nucleus, where gene transcription is subsequently controlled.[45] Several transcription factors have been identified to play a central role in the inflammatory cascade in inflammatory bowel disease. Consistent with the model of an IL-6 transsignaling-mediated disease progression, activated STAT-3 was upregulated in isolated lamina propria mononuclear cells from inflamed tissue of inflammatory bowel disease patients in comparison to corresponding controls.[46,47] Furthermore, overexpression of STAT-4 in transgenic mice leads to the development of chronic enterocolitis and to increased production of IFN-γ and TNF-α.[48] The transcriptional factor NF-κB, which initiates the transcription of various cytokine,[49] is assumed to have a pivotal pathogenic role among the transcriptional factors. Increased expression of NF-κB p65 in isolated lamina propria mononuclear cells in patients with Crohn's disease has been described along with augmented production of proinflammatory cytokines.[50] After application of an antisense oligodeoxynucleotide that binds to NF-κB p65, attenuation of the chronic inflammatory process was achieved in several models of intestinal inflammation.[51] Moreover, the transcription factor T bet has been detected to induce IFN-γ production and Th-1 development in Crohn's disease. Adoptive transfer experiments also revealed a key regulatory role of T bet in the pathogenesis of T cell–mediated colitis, as T bet–deficient T cells failed to induce experimental colitis in the CD4+ CD62L+ transfer model.[52] In conclusion, specific therapy aiming at the transcriptional level may represent a hopeful strategy to establish a novel treatment for patients with IBD.

Molecular Mechanism of Action of Azathioprine: Rac1 GTPase Inhibition

Azathioprine is considered as first-line therapy for the maintenance of steroid-free remission in patients with inflammatory bowel disease.[53,54] Although azathioprine has been in clinical use for several decades and has proven its clinical efficacy in multiple studies,[55] its precise mechanism of action in inflammatory bowel disease was still unclear. The molecular targets and associated intracellular signal transduction pathways, which are modulated by azathioprine and its metabolites, have only recently been discovered and help explain the observed immunosuppressive effects.[56] The therapeutic concept of restoring T cell susceptibility to apoptosis in inflammatory bowel disease also seems to be elemental in the immunmodulatory effects of azathioprine. Azathioprine-induced apoptosis in blood and lamina propria T cells from patients with inflammatory bowel disease is solely detectable after CD28 costimulation (FIGS. 4 and 5). Therefore azathioprine-mediated effects are confined to highly activated lamina propria T cells, which subsequently cause the chronic inflammatory process in inflammatory bowel disease. Functional studies focusing on the mechanics of azathioprine revealed activation of a mitochondrial pathway of T cell apoptosis.[56] The molecular interaction between the

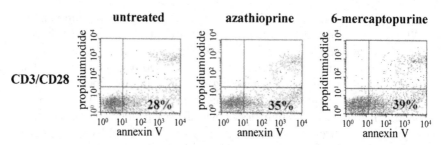

FIGURE 4. Azathioprine/6-mercaptopurine treatment induces T cell apoptosis. CD4$^+$ T lymphocytes were isolated from human blood, stimulated with recombinant Il-2 and anti-CD3 plus anti-CD28 antibodies. Cells were treated with azathioprine (5μM) or 6-mercaptopurine (5 μM) on day 0. On day 5 apoptotic cells were analyzed by annexinV-FITC/propidiumiodid staining. AnnexinV-positive/propidiumiodid-negative cells represent early apoptotic cells. There is induction of apoptosis after treatment with azathioprine/6-mercaptopurine.

azathioprine metabolites 6-thio-GTP and the small GTPase Rac1 are pivotal for these phenomena. GTPases are guanine nucleotide-binding proteins that are characterized by their ability to bind to guanosine diphosphate (GDP) or guanosine triphosphate (GTP) according to their respective state of activation. GTP-bound GTPases are classified as activated forms, which are able to interact with further intracellular signaling effector proteins and therefore initiate signaling cascades that regulate various biological processes.[57] The GDP/GTP exchange of the GTPases are mediated by guanosine exchange factors (GEFs). One of the several GEFs for Rac is Vav.[58] Only tyrosine-phosphorylated Vav is able to catalyze the dissociation of GDPs from inactivated Rac and therefore augment the exchange activity of GDPs against GTPs at Rac.[59] Increased and relatively long-lasting tyrosine phosphorylation of Vav was detected in CD28 costimulated cells.[57] Recently, it has been shown that specific blockade of CD28-mediated Rac activation is achieved through binding of the azathioprine metabolite 6-thio-GTP to Rac instead of GTP.[56] The azathioprine-mediated inhibition of Rac activation has several consequences, as activated Rac-GTP plays a crucial role in various intracellular signaling pathways. Rac-GTP is known to bind and activate STAT-3[60] and NF-κB,[61] which regulate the expression of the antiapoptotic protein Bcl-xl.[62,63] Consequently, azathioprine is able to suppress activation of NF-κB and inhibit the expression of Bcl-xl by 6-thio-GTP-mediated blocking of Rac activation.[56]

Taken together these data indicate that activation of the costimulatory molecule CD28 leads to enhanced survival of activated T cells in inflammatory bowel disease, as the CD28-initiated upregulation of Vav leads to augmented supply of activated Rac-GTP. This in turn leads to activation of NFκ-B and STAT-3 and hence to increased Bcl-xl levels, which counteract the mitochondrial-mediated apoptosis. The azathioprine metabolite 6-thio-GTP specifically targets Rac activation through binding to Rac instead of GTP,

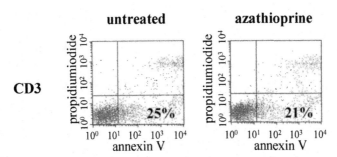

FIGURE 5. Azathioprine-induced apoptosis is dependent on costimulation with CD28. CD4$^+$ T lymphocytes were isolated from human blood, and stimulated with recombinant Il-2 and anti-CD3. Cells were treated with azathioprine (5 μM) on day 0. On day 5 apoptotic cells were analyzed by annexinV-FITC/propidiumiodid staining. AnnexinV-positive/propidiumiodid-negative cells represent early apoptotic cells. Without CD28 costimulation there is no induction of apoptosis after treatment with azathioprine.

which inhibits STAT-3 and NF-κB activation. The resulting inhibition of Bcl-xl expression explains the observed mitochondrial induction of apoptosis in azathioprine-treated T lymphocytes.[56] Azathioprine thus converts the primary costimulatory CD28 signal into an apoptotic signal by modulating Rac activity (FIG. 6). Further studies revealed that first signs of *in vitro* apoptosis of T lymphocytes of inflammatory bowel disease patients were detected 5 days after prior treatment with azathioprine.[56] These experimental observations are consistent with clinical practice, where a delayed onset of the therapeutic efficacy of azathioprine has been noted.[64] The reason for this delayed therapeutic property may be explainable through the, in comparison to GTP, lower affinity of 6-thio-GTP to Rac, resulting in the requirement of high intracellular 6-thio-GTP levels before therapeutic effects can be achieved. These considerations may also have direct implications in optimizing the therapeutic progress through improved monitoring of azathioprine therapy in patients with inflammatory bowel disease. At present the level of thiopurine methyl transferase (TPMT) activity, which among other enzymes catalyzes the conversion of azathioprine to 6-thio-guanine, has been considered responsible for the variation in the therapeutic efficacy and toxicity of thiopurine drugs.[65] Consequently, monitoring of azathioprine treatment is based primarily on the study of TPMT genetic polymorphism or in the corresponding intracellular activity. Recent studies focusing on patients with inflammatory bowel disease treated with azathioprine revealed no correlation between TPMT activity and clinical response or drug toxicity.[66] Furthermore, even the measurement of 6-thio-guanine nucleotide (6-TGN) levels to optimize azathioprine treatment proved to be an ineffective prognostic parameter.[67]

    In regard to the recent data elucidating the central role of 6-thio-GTP in azathioprine treatment, monitoring of 6-thio-GTP levels in patients treated with azathioprine may reveal a direct correlation between clinical efficacy and

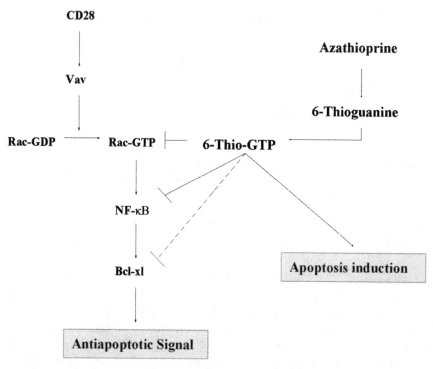

FIGURE 6. Model of the molecular mechanism of action of azathioprine. CD28 co-stimulation of the cell leads to long-lasting tyrosine phosphorylation of Vav, which mediates the dissociation of GDPs from inactivated Rac-GDP and thus initiates the exchange of GDP against GTP at Rac, leading to the formation of Rac-GTP. Rac-GTP activates the transcriptional factors STAT-3 and NF-κB, which regulate the expression of the antiapoptotic protein Bcl-xl. The azathioprine metabolite 6-thio-GTP specifically targets Rac activation through binding to Rac instead of GTP, which in turn inhibits STAT-3 and NF-κB activation. The resulting inhibition of Bcl-xl expression leads to mitochondrial induction of apoptosis in azathioprine-treated cells

induction of remission and may allow identifying patients for whom azathioprine treatment is futile and alternative therapeutic options are required. Taken together the therapeutic effect of azathioprine in inflammatory bowel disease lies in its capability to induce apoptosis in intestinal T cells, remaining consistent with the hypothesis of enhanced lamina propria CD4+ T cell resistance to apoptosis being the central pathogenic factor in these diseases. This perception harbors important implications for the design of more specific therapeutic approaches, as azathioprine derivates with higher affinity to Rac may allow an even more efficient immunosuppressive effect. Furthermore, there is recent evidence that a RhoA-dependent signaling pathway also plays a central role in inflammatory bowel disease, as RhoA and its corresponding effector are activated in Crohn's disease and in experimental colitis. Specific blockade of Rho kinase significantly reduced intestinal inflammation in rats with TNBS-induced colitis, as inhibition of proinflammatory cytokine production via inhibition of NF-κB activation was achieved.[68] Therefore blockade of Rho kinase may be a further therapeutic alternative in the treatment of inflammatory bowel disease. The specific inhibition of different Rho GTPases, like Rac1 and Rho, could have important implications in the treatment of IBD, as possible synergetic effects could enable an even more effective therapeutic approach.

CONCLUSION

The forthcoming challenge lies in the translation of the considerable progress in understanding the pathophysiology of inflammatory bowel disease into the development of novel disease specific therapies. The unraveling of immunopathogenetic mechanisms has already led to the evolution of new potential biological therapies that are expanding the range of treatment options for inflammatory bowel disease. This development is best exemplified by the emergence of anti-TNF-α agents, which have been the major advance in inflammatory bowel disease therapeutics over the past few years.[69-71] The efficacy of this drug in patients that are otherwise refractory to conventional therapies clearly underlines the importance for further available therapeutic alternatives in the treatment of inflammatory bowel disease. Moreover, additional new biological therapies, like the human anti-IL-6 receptor monoclonal antibody[33] or new insights regarding the molecular actions of the immunosuppressive agent azathioprine[56] are promising first results of the extensive endeavors taken in the research of the signal transduction pathways that are involved in inflammatory bowel disease. These drugs, whose mode of action is based on restoring intestinal T cell susceptibility to apoptosis, reflect our increased understanding of disease pathophysiology. Furthermore, it is tempting to speculate that combinations of drugs that alter T lymphocyte apoptosis through different mechanisms may become even more effective through probable synergistic effects (e.g., combining azathioprine and anti-TNF therapies). It is therefore becoming a realistic and achievable aim to base future therapeutic strategies on a more effective and, it is hoped, less toxic therapeutic rationale.

REFERENCES

1. PODOLSKY, D.K. 1991. Inflammatory bowel disease. N. Engl. J. Med. **325:** 928–937.
2. PODOLSKY, D.K. 2002. Inflammatory bowel disease. N. Engl. J. Med. **347:** 417–429.
3. DUCHMANN, R. *et al.* 1999. Crohn's disease. *In* Mucosal Immunology. P. L. Ogra, *et al.*, Eds.: 1055–1080. Academic Press, San Diego.
4. FIOCCHI, C. 1998. Inflammatory bowel disease: etiology and pathogenesis. Gastroenterology **115:** 182–205.

5. SCHÖLMERICH, J. *et al*. 1998. Which immunosuppressors do you use to treat Crohn's disease and ulcerative colitis? In which order of priority and how worried are you about toxicity? Inflamm. Bowel Dis. **4:** 248–252.

6. SHANAHAN, F. 2002. Crohn's disease. Gastroenterology **120:** 622–635.

7. NEURATH, M.F. *et al*. 2002. The role of Th1/Th2 polarization in mucosal immunity. Nat. Med. **8:** 567–573.

8. SARTOR, R.B. 1994. Cytokines in intestinal inflammation: pathophysiologic and clinical considerations. Gastroenterology **106:** 533–539.

9. RUTGEERTS, P. *et al*. 2003. The expanding role of biological agents in the treatment of inflammatory bowel disease—focus on selective adhesion molecule inhibition. Aliment. Pharmacol. Ther. **17:** 1435–1450.

10. INA, K. *et al*. 1995. Crohn's disease (CD) mucosal T-cells are resistant to apoptosis. Gastroenterology **108:** A841.

11. NEURATH, M.F. *et al*. 2001. Regulation of T-cell apoptosis in inflammatory bowel disease: to die or not to die, that is the mucosal question. Trends Immunol. **22:** 21–26.

12. BOIRIVANT, M. *et al*. 1999. Lamina propria T cells in Crohn's disease and other gastrointestinal inflammation show defective CD2 pathway-induced apoptosis. Gastroenterology **116:** 557–565.

13. INA, K. *et al*. 1999. Resistance of Crohn's disease T cells to multiple apoptotic signals is associated with a Bcl-2/Bax mucosal imbalance. J. Immunol. **163:** 1081–1090.

14. SOUZA, H.S.P. *et al*. 2005. Apoptosis in the intestinal mucosa of patients with inflammatory bowel disease: evidence of altered expression of FasL and perforin cytotoxic pathways. Int. J. Colorectal Dis. **20:** 277–286.

15. SHANAHAN, F. 2001. Inflammatory bowel disease: immunodiagnostics, immunotherapies, and ecotherapeutics. Gastroenterology **120:** 622–635.

16. NEURATH, M.F. *et al*. 1995. Antibodies to interleukin 12 abrogate established experimental colitis in mice. J. Exp. Med. **182:** 1281–1290.

17. FUSS, I.J. *et al*. 1999. Anti-interleukin 12 treatment regulates apoptosis of Th1 T cells in experimental colitis in mice. Gastroenterology **117:** 1078–1088.

18. MANNON, P.J. *et al*. 2004. Anti-interleukin-12 antibody for active Crohn's Disease. N. Engl. J. Med. **351:** 2069–2079.

19. VAN DEN BRANDE, J.M.H. *et al*. 2003. Gastroenterology **124:** 1774–1785.

20. LUGERING, A. *et al*. 2001. Infliximab induces apoptosis in monocytes from patients with chronic active Crohn's disease by using a caspase-dependent pathway. Gastroenterology **121:** 1145–1157.

21. MITOMA, H. *et al*. 2005. Infliximab induces potent anti-inflammatory responses by outside-to-inside signals through transmembrane TNF-α. Gastroenterology **128:** 376–392.

22. FUSS, I.J. *et al*. 1996. Disparate CD4+ lamina propria (LP) lymphokine secretion profiles in inflammatory bowel disease. Crohn's disease LP cells manifest increased secretion of IFN-gamma, whereas ulcerative colitis LP cells manifest increased secretion of IL-5. J. Immunol. **157:** 1261–1270.

23. HOLUB, M.C. *et al*. 1998. Increased interleukin-6 levels, interleukin-6 receptor and gp130 expression in peripheral lymphocytes of patients with inflammatory bowel disease. Scand. J. Gastroenterol. Supplement **228:** 47–50.

24. HYAMS, J.S. *et al*. 1993. Relationship of functional and antigenic interleukin 6 to disease activity in inflammatory bowel disease. Gastroenterology **104:** 1285–1292.

25. GROSS, V. *et al.* 1992. Evidence for continuous stimulation of interleukin-6 production in Crohn's disease. Gastroenterology **102:** 514–519.
26. MAHIDA, Y. *et al.* 1991. High circulating concentrations of interleukin-6 in active Crohn's disease but not ulcerative colitis. Gut **32:** 1531–1534.
27. ISAACS, K.L. *et al.* 1992. Cytokine messenger RNA profiles in inflammatory bowel disease mucosa detected by polymerase chain reaction amplification. Gastroenterology **103:** 1587–1595.
28. DAIG, R. *et al.* 2000. Human intestinal epithelial cells secrete interleukin-1 receptor antagonist and interleukin-8 but not interleukin-1 or interleukin-6. Gut **46:** 350–358.
29. REINECKER, H.C. *et al.* 1993. Enhanced secretion of tumour necrosis factor-alpha, IL-6, and IL-1 beta by isolated lamina propria mononuclear cells from patients with ulcerative colitis and Crohn's disease. Clin. Exp. Immunol. **94:** 174–181.
30. JONES, S.C. *et al.* 1994. Mucosal interleukin-6 secretion in ulcerative colitis: effects of anti-inflammatory drugs and T-cell stimulation. Scan. J. Gastroenterol. **29:** 722–728.
31. REINISCH, W. *et al.* 1999. Clinical relevance of serum interleukin-6 in Crohn's disease: single point measurements, therapy monitoring, and prediction of clinical relapse. Am. J. Gastroenterol. **94:** 2156–2164.
32. ISHIGURO, Y. 1999. Mucosal proinflammatory cytokine production correlates with endoscopic activity of ulcerative colitis. J. Gastroenterol. **34:** 66–74.
33. ATREYA, R. *et al.* 2000. Blockade of interleukin 6 trans signaling suppresses T-cell resistance against apoptosis in chronic intestinal inflammation: evidence in Crohn's disease and experimental colitis in vivo. Nat. Med. **6:** 583–588.
34. TAGA, T. *et al.* 1989. Interleukin-6 (IL-6) triggers the association of its receptor (IL-6-R) with a possible signal transducer, gp130. Cell **58:** 573–581.
35. HEINRICH, P. *et al.* 1998. Interleukin-6-type cytokine signalling through the gp130/Jak/STAT pathway. Biochem. J. **334:** 297–314.
36. HOSOKAWA, T. *et al.* 1999. Interleukin-6 and soluble interleukin-6 receptor in the colonic mucosa of inflammatory bowel disease. J. Gastroenterol. Hepatol. **14:** 987–996.
37. DE JONG, Y.P. *et al.* 2001. Development of chronic colitis is dependent on the cytokine MIF. Nat. Immunol. **2:** 1061–1066.
38. WALEV, I. *et al.* 1996. Pore-forming toxins trigger shedding of receptors for interleukin 6 and lipopolysaccharide. Proc. Natl. Acad. Sci. USA **93:** 7882–7887.
39. MITSUYAMA, K. *et al.* 1995. Soluble interleukin-6 receptors in inflammatory bowel disease: relation to circulating interleukin-6. Gut **36:** 45–49.
40. HOSOKAWA, T. *et al.* 1999. Interleukin-6 and soluble interleukin-6 receptor in the colonic mucosa of inflammatory bowel disease. J. Gastroenterol. Hepatol. **14:** 987–996.
41. ROSE-JOHN, S. *et al.* 1994. Soluble receptors for cytokines and growth factors: generation and biological function. Biochem. J. **300:** 281–290.
42. ITOH, J. *et al.* 2001. Decreased bax expression by mucosal T cells favors resistance to apoptosis in Crohn's disease. Gut **49:** 35–41.
43. YAMAMOTO, M. *et al.* 2000. IL-6 is required for the development of TH1 cell-mediated murine colitis. J. Immunol. **164:** 4878–4882.
44. ITO, H. *et al.* 2004. A pilot randomized trial of a human anti-interleukin-6 receptor monoclonal antibody in active Crohn's disease. Gastroenterology **126:** 989–996.
45. GREENALGH, J.C. *et al.* 2002. Suppressors of cytokine signaling; relevance to gastrointestinal function and disease. Gastroenterology **123:** 2064–2081.

46. MUDTER, J. *et al.* 2005. Activation pattern of signal transducers and activators of transcription (STAT) factors in inflammatory bowel diseases. Am. J. Gastroenterol. **100:** 64–72.

47. LOVATO, P. *et al.* 2003. Constitutive activation in intestinal T cells from patients with Crohn's disease. J. Biol. Chem. **278:** 16777–16781.

48. WIRTZ, S. *et al.* 1999. Cutting edge: chronic intestinal inflammation in STAT-4 transgenic mice: characterization of disease and adoptive transfer by TNF-plus IFN-gamma-producing CD4+T cells that respond to bacterial antigens. J. Immunol. **162:** 1884–1488.

49. BAUERLE, P.A., *et al.* 1997. NF-κB as a frequent target for immunosuppressive and anti-inflammatory molecules. Adv. Immunol. **65:** 111–137.

50. NEURATH, M.F. *et al.* 1998. Cytokine gene transcription by NF-kappa B family members in patients with inflammatory bowel disease. Ann. N. Y. Acad. Sci. **859:** 149–159.

51. NEURATH, M.F. *et al.* 1996. Local administration of antisense phosphorothioate oligonucleotides to the p65 subunit of NF-kappa B abrogates established experimental colitis in mice. Nat. Med. **9:** 998–1004.

52. NEURATH, M.F. *et al.* 2002. The transcription factor T-bet regulates mucosal T cell activation in experimental colitis and Crohn's disease. J. Exp. Med. **195:** 1129–1143.

53. PRESENT, D.H. *et al.* 1980. Treatment of Crohn's disease with 6-mercaptopurine: a long-term, randomized, double-blind study. N. Engl. J. Med. **302:** 981–987.

54. LEWIS, J.D., J.S. SCHWARTZ & G.R. LICHTENSTEIN. 2000. Azathioprine for maintenance of remission in Crohn's disease: benefits outweigh the risk of lymphoma. Gastroenterology **118:** 1018–1024.

55. FRASE, A.G. *et al.* 2002. The efficacy of azathioprine for the treatment of inflammatory bowel disease: a 30 year review. Gut **50:** 485–489.

56. TIEDE, I. *et al.* 2003. CD28-dependent Rac1 activation is the molecular target of azathioprine in primary human CD4+ T lymphocytes. J. Clin. Invest. **111:** 1133–1145.

57. CANTRELL, D.A. 2003. GTPases and T cell activation. Immunol. Rev. **192:** 122–130.

58. MOVILLA, N. *et al.* 2001. How Vav proteins discriminate the GtPases Rac1 and RhoA from Cdc42. Oncogene **20:** 8057–8065.

59. CRESPO, P. *et al.* 1997. Phosphotyrosine-dependent activation of Rac-1 GDP/GTP exchange by the vav proto-oncogene product. Nature **385:** 169–172.

60. SIMON, A.R. *et al.* 2000. Regulation of STAT3 by direct binding to the Rac1 GTPase. Science **290:** 144–147.

61. FANGER, G.R. *et al.* 1997. MEK kinases are regulated by EGF and selectively interact with Rac/Cdc42. EMBO J. **16:** 4961–4972.

62. KHOSHNAN, A. *et al.* 2000. The NF-kappa B cascade is important in Bcl-xL expression and for the anti-apoptotic effects of the CD28 receptor in primary human CD4+ lymphocytes. J. Immunol. **165:** 1743–1754.

63. GRAD, J.M. *et al.* 2000. Regulation of Bcl-xL: a little bit of this and a little bit of STAT. Curr. Opin. Oncol. **12:** 543–549.

64. PRESENT, D.H. *et al.* 1980. Treatment of Crohn's disease with 6-mercaptopurine: a long-term, randomized, double-blind study. N. Engl. J. Med. **302:** 981–987.

65. CARA, C.J. *et al.* 2004. Reviewing the mechanism of action of thiopurine drugs: towards a new paradigm in clinical practice. Med. Sci. Monit. **10:** RA 247–254.

66. LOWRY, P.W. *et al.* 2001. Measurement of thiopurine methyltransferase activity and azathioprine metabolites in patients with inflammatory bowel disease. Gut **49:** 665–670.

67. CUFFARI, C. *et al.* 2001. Utilisation of 6-thioguanine metabolite levels to optimize azathioprine therapy in patients with inflammatory bowel disease. Gut **48:** 642–646.

68. SEGAIN, J.P. *et al.* 2003. Rho kinase blockade prevents inflammation via nuclear factor κB Inhibition: evidence in Crohn's disease and experimental colitis. Gastroenterology **124:** 1180–1187.

69. HANAUER, S.B. *et al.* 2002. Maintenance infliximab for Crohn's disease: the ACCENT I randomised trial. Lancet **359:** 1541–1549.

70. TARGAN, S.R. *et al.* 1997. A short-term study of chimeric monoclonal antibody cA2 to tumor necrosis factor alpha for Crohn's disease. Crohn's Disease cA2 Study Group. N. Engl. J. Med. **337:** 1029–1035.

71. VAN DULLEMEN, H.M. *et al.* 1995. Treatment of Crohn's disease with anti-tumor necrosis factor chimeric monoclonal antibody (cA2). Gastroenterology **109:** 129–135.

NF-κB Signaling

Pros and Cons of Altering NF-κB as a Therapeutic Approach

LAURENCE J. EGAN[a] AND MURAT TORUNER[b]

[a]Department of Pharmacology and Therapeuticity, Clinical Science Institute, University College Hospital, Galway, Ireland

[b]Department of Gastroenterology, Ankara University Medical School, Sihhiye - 06100 Anakara, Turkey

ABSTRACT: The transcription factor, nuclear factor-κB (NF-κB), is a dominant regulator of the expression of hundreds of genes, many of which play important roles in the regulation of inflammation and programmed cell death (apoptosis). Since the discovery of NF-κB in the mid 1980s, this transcription factor has been the subject of intense investigation. Excess or inappropriate activation of NF-κB has been observed in human inflammatory bowel disease and in a host of other inflammatory diseases and type of cancer. Functional studies in animals have shed light on the role of NF-κB in broader pathophysiological contexts. From such studies, it has become quite clear that NF-κB plays unique and distinct functions in different cell types. Because of the importance of NF-κB in signaling inflammation, and in inhibiting programmed cell death, many pharmaceutical companies are developing small-molecule inhibitors of this pathway. In this article, we evaluate the relative pros and cons of blocking NF-κB as a therapeutic approach for inflammatory bowel disease. On the basis of the results of studies in animals that have primarily used genetic approaches to inhibit NF-κB activity, we suggest that there are certain niche indications for blocking NF-κB in inflammatory bowel disease that offer particular promise.

KEYWORDS: nuclear factor-kappa B; inflammatory bowel disease

INTRODUCTION

Nuclear factor-κB (NF-κB) was first described in 1986 as a protein binding to the κ enhancer in B lymphocytes.[1] However, subsequent studies revealed

Address for correspondence: Laurence J. Egan, M.D., Clinical Science Institute, University College Hospital, Galway, Ireland. Voice: +353-91-495370; fax: +353-91-495572.
e-mail: laurence.egan@nuigalway.ie

Ann. N.Y. Acad. Sci. 1072: 114–122 (2006). © 2006 New York Academy of Sciences.
doi: 10.1196/annals.1326.009

that NF-κB is in fact primarily a cytoplasmic factor that is expressed by almost all cell types.[2] Moreover, the function of NF-κB as a transcription factor can be induced by a wide variety of cellular stimuli that induce the nuclear translocation and sequence-specific DNA binding of NF-κB proteins. These stimuli most commonly include inflammatory cytokines, such as interleukin-1 or tumor necrosis factor-α (TNF-α),[3] infection with invasive microbes, such as *Salmonella*[4] or viruses, bacterial cell wall products, such as lipopolysaccharide, peptidoglycan, and by other forms of cellular stress including oxidative stress and DNA double-strand breaks.[5] The expression of over 150 genes has shown to be upregulated by NF-κB. The encoded products of those genes are proteins that play important roles in immunity, apoptosis, and cellular proliferation.[6]

NF-κB IN INFLAMMATORY BOWEL DISEASE

Pathways to NF-κB Activation

Two principal signaling pathways have been identified that control the activity of NF-κB.[6] The best studied of these pathways positions the kinase IKKβ (inhibitor of NF-κB kinase beta, also known as IKK2) as the focus point of signals emanating from a variety of sources including certain cell surface cytokine receptors (e.g., TNF-α receptor type I) and bacterial pattern-recognition receptors (e.g., toll-like receptor 4), intracellular redox sensing mechanisms, and nuclear DNA damage signaling proteins (e.g., ATM). IKKβ is one component of the multisubunit IKK complex and, when activated, catalyzes the serine phosphorylation of IκBα on residues 32 and 36.[7] IκBα retains NF-κB proteins, principally the p50 and p65 subunits, in the cytoplasm. Upon phosphorylation by IKKβ, IκBα is targeted for degradation by a ubiquitin–proteasomal pathway. This event represents the key cellular control point for the activation of the important NF-κB p50/p65 heterodimer. For this reason, IKKβ has emerged as an attractive therapeutic target for the inhibition of NF-κB.[8]

The more recently described alternative pathway to NF-κB activation appears to be most important in lymphocytes. This pathway is stimulated by specific lymphoid cytokines including BAFF, CD40 ligand, and lymphotoxin-β and leads to the IKKα-dependent proteolytic processing of NF-κB p100 into the active p52 form.[9] p52 usually dimerizes with another NF-κB protein RelB and translocates to the nucleus to induce expression of a set of genes important in lymphoid structure and function.

NF-κB Is Inappropriately Activated in Inflammatory Bowel Disease Mucosa

When it was recognized that NF-κB is important for controlling the expression of many genes involved in signaling inflammation, investigators searched for evidence of NF-κB activation in numerous inflammatory diseases, including inflammatory bowel disease. Several papers have documented excess or inappropriate NF-κB activation both in ulcerative colitis and Crohn's disease and in animal models of inflammatory bowel disease.[10–12] NF-κB activity has been observed in lamina propria mononuclear cells and in epithelial cells of the inflamed gut. The importance of NF-κB activity in the pathogenesis of inflammatory bowel disease has also been hinted at by the fact that certain anti-inflammatory drugs commonly used for inflammatory bowel disease appear to inhibit NF-κB. Thus, corticosteroids have been shown to block nuclear translocation of NF-κB polypeptides and also to increase expression of IκBα, the chief endogenous inhibitor of NF-κB within cells.[13] Moreover, sulfasalazine and 5-aminosalicylic acid drugs have also been shown to block NF-κB activation through inhibiting the activity of the IKK complex[14] and also by blocking functionally important posttranslational modifications of the p65 NF-κB subunit.[15]

CELL TYPE–SPECIFIC FUNCTIONS OF NF-κB

Functional Studies of NF-κB in Mice

The overall importance of NF-κB as an inhibitor of apoptosis was revealed by gene knockout studies. Mice that were engineered to lack expression of the p65 NF-κB subunit or the essential subunits of the IKK complex, IKKβ[16,17] or IKK-γ[18] (also known as NF-κB essential modulator, NEMO) all exhibit a very similar phenotype of embryonic lethality at day 13.5. This is due to massive hepatocyte apoptosis caused by TNF-α signaling. To further probe the *in vivo* functions of NF-κB, a number of laboratories have generated conditional knockout mice that lack the ability to activate NF-κB in specific cell types using bone marrow chimeras or cre/*loxP* technology. Below we highlight some of the important results from studies of mice engineered to lack IKKβ expression and hence NF-κB activity, in cell types that are important in inflammatory bowel disease: lymphocytes, monocyte/macrophages, and intestinal epithelial cells.

Lymphocyte-Specific IKK-β Knockout Mice

Mice have been engineered to lack IKKβ expression in both T lymphocytes and B lymphocytes. Deletion of IKKβ severely impairs NF-κB activation in T lymphocytes.[19] This is accompanied by slightly lower overall levels of T lymphocytes in both spleen and lymph nodes. However, more strikingly, there are defects in the maturation of those cells in the absence of IKKβ, as evidenced by greatly lower numbers of regulatory T cells and memory T cells.[20] At the functional level, IKKβ was shown to be important for the inhibition of T lymphocyte apoptosis induced by stimulation with TNF-α.[19] B lymphocytes that lack IKKβ survive poorly, as reflected by overall lower numbers of immature B cells, follicular B cells, and marginal zone B cells compared to IKKβ-sufficient cells.[21] This is functionally important because IKKβ-deficient B lymphocytes do not mount robust T cell–dependent or T cell–independent antibody responses upon antigenic stimulation.[22] Thus, these observations indicate important roles for the IKK- NF-κB system in the survival, maturation, and activation of lymphocytes, in their resistance to apoptosis, and in the generation of robust antibody responses. Recent data suggest that T lymphocytes from certain patients with inflammatory bowel disease might have acquired resistance to apoptotis.[23,24] It is unknown whether NF-κB is involved in mediating this apoptotis resistance.

Monocyte and Macrophages

Monocytes and macrophages are important cells that link innate immune responses to the adaptive immune system, primarily by the secretion of cytokines that act upon lymphocytes. NF-κB can be robustly activated within monocytes and macrophages by many stimuli that are important in the pathogenesis of inflammatory bowel disease, such as bacteria-derived lipopolysaccharide, peptidoglycan, and immunostimulatory DNA. The importance of NF-κB in monocyte activation by those factors was revealed by the dramatically lower levels of interleukin-6 and interleukin-12 secretion by IKKβ-deficient monocytes after stimulation by those factors.[25] Moreover, the chemokines MIP-2 and KC are also strongly under the control of IKKβ in monocytes.[26] The functional importance of monocyte NF-κB activation was revealed in experiments of colitis-associated colon cancer in mice. Those studies revealed a very strong role for monocyte NF-κB in their promotion of tumor growth.[26] Thus, in monocytes and macrophages, the IKK–NF-κB system is essential for production of proinflammatory cytokines, prostaglandins, and in tumor promotion in the colon.

Epithelial Cells

Intestinal epithelial cells constitute a single cell barrier that separates the host from the contents of the intestinal lumen and whose integrity is vital for health. The intestinal epithelial cells, while playing important protective and absorptive functions, can also participate actively in mucosal immunity by the elaboration of cytokines and chemokines. Numerous studies in cell lines and in genetically engineered mice have revealed a very important role for IKKβ and NF-κB in the expression of inflammatory cytokines, such as TNF-α, enzymes such as cyclo-oxygenase-2 and chemokines, such as interleukin-8 by these cells.[27–29] Moreover, NF-κB activation in intestinal epithelial cells can be triggered by numerous forms of cellular stress typical of human disease, such as ischemia/reperfusion, radiation injury, and chronic inflammation. Functional studies in mice have clearly revealed a very important role for IKKβ in blocking apoptosis of intestinal epithelial cells under all of those conditions.[26,30,31] This is reflected in worse mucosal injury in animal models of colitis and ischemia/reperfusion in the absence of NF-κB activation.[26,32] Although a failure to activate NF-κB in intestinal epithelium is associated with worse morphologic injury in these disease models, the development of colon cancer was strongly inhibited. Thus, the IKK–NF-κB system in intestinal epithelial cells is important for the elaboration of inflammatory cytokines, the inhibition of apoptosis, promotion of ulcer healing, and carcinogenesis.

PROS AND CONS OF NF-κB INHIBITION IN INFLAMMATORY BOWEL DISEASE

Considering the results of the aforementioned studies, NF-κB has emerged as an exciting potential therapeutic target. The predicted effects of blocking NF-κB in different cell types within the context of inflammatory bowel disease are summarized in TABLE 1. NF-κB inhibition would be predicted to decrease the overactive state of the mucosal immune system in inflammatory bowel disease, by inactivating or killing lymphocytes and macrophages. In view of the relative resistance of lymphocytes to apoptosis in inflammatory bowel disease, blockade of NF-κB should restore apoptotis sensitivity in those cells, an effect that is especially appealing. This beneficial effect may be partially offset by immune suppression and the risks of opportunistic infections. The net effect of blocking NF-κB in intestinal epithelial cells is difficult to predict and may depend on clinical factors, such as the presence of ulceration. It is likely that NF-κB inhibitors would decrease cytokine release from the epithelium, but would also predispose cells to apoptosis, which might harm effective mucosal barrier functions and delay ulcer healing. However, induction of intestinal epithelial cell death by NF-κB blockade probably underlies the anticancer effects of this strategy, which would be a distinct benefit.

TABLE 1. Predicted cell type–specific effects, beneficial and harmful of inhibition of NF-κB, in patients with inflammatory bowel disease

Cell type	Benefit	Harm
T lymphocyte	⇓ activation ⇓ cytokine expression ⇑ apoptosis susceptibility	Immune suppression
B lymphocyte	⇓ antibody production	Immune suppression
Monocyte/macrophage	⇓ cytokine expression	Immune suppression
Intestinal epithelial cell	⇓ cytokine expression ⇑ apoptosis susceptibility	⇓ ulcer healing
Keratinocyte		⇑ risk of malignant transformation
Osteoclast	⇓ activation	

While substantial evidence indicates a procarcinogenic role for NF-κB in many epithelia, including those throughout the gastrointestinal tract, this is not true in the skin. In fact, NF-κB activity in keratinocytes appears to prevent the development of squamous cell carcinomas.[33] Although the molecular mechanisms of this effect have not been fully elucidated, these findings suggest that NF-κB inhibitors might increase susceptibility to squamous cell skin cancer.

THERAPEUTIC NICHES FOR NF-κB INHIBITION IN INFLAMMATORY BOWEL DISEASE

1. *Prevention of colonic neoplasia*: 5-Aminosalicylic acid drugs are cornerstones of inflammatory bowel disease therapy. The use of these agents has been shown in some epidemiological studies to be associated with lower rates of colonic neoplasia development in patients with inflammatory bowel disease.[34] This fact, combined with powerful results from genetic studies indicating an essential role for NF-κB activation in the development of colitis-associated neoplasia[26] suggests strongly that NF-κB–inhibiting drugs could be used to prevent or treat early-stage colitis-associated neoplasia. Thus, inflammatory bowel disease patients at especially high risk for colonic neoplasia, including those with very long-standing disease, a prior history of indefinite dysplasia, or with coexisting primary sclerosing cholangitis, might be good candidates for NF-κB–inhibiting therapy.

2. *Maintenance of remission*: The intestines of mice lacking the ability to activate NF-κB in lymphocytes, monocytes/macrophages, or intestinal epithelial cells are normal. This indicates that NF-κB in these cell types does not have an important homeostatic role for intestinal morphogenesis or overall health. Early stages of inflammatory bowel disease activity are characterized by the expression in excess quantities of numerous cytokines, whose expression is controlled by NF-κB. Therefore, the use of NF-κB inhibition to prevent relapses of inflammatory bowel disease would be a rational objective that would not be hampered by the potential for NF-κB inhibition to slow ulcer healing, a potentially detrimental effect.

3. *Treatment of inflammatory bowel disease: associated inflammatory arthritis*–In addition to the aforementioned functional roles, several studies have pointed toward the importance of NF-κB in osteoclastogenesis.[35,36] In the absence of functional NF-κB signaling, stimulators of bone resorption, such as the RANK ligand, are unable to initiate the activation of osteoclasts, which are the cells that are important for bone resorption. Thus, patients with inflammatory bowel disease that is associated with destructive arthritis, such as ankylosing spondylitis or inflammatory oligoarthritis might especially benefit from administration of a systemic NF-κB inhibitor.

CONCLUSIONS

At present, our prediction of the effects of systemic NF-κB inhibition on normal physiological processes and within the context of disease pathophysiology requires us to piece together information derived from cell type–specific knockout mice and studies in cell lines. However, with the advent of potent and specific IKK-β inhibitors, which are under development by many pharmaceutical companies, we should be able to more accurately obtain information regarding the overall functional effects of NF-κB inhibition in disease models, and eventually in patients. There is much to be learned. In particular, significant effort will have to be focused on studying the benefits and adverse effects of IKKβ inhibitors in animal models and linking the inhibition of IKKβ to molecular effects, such as gene expression, and to cell biological events, such as cell migration, proliferation, and death. Furthermore, it is likely that as the molecular subclassification of inflammatory bowel disease progresses, we will be able to identify subgroups of inflammatory bowel disease patients who might benefit especially from therapeutic strategies directed at selectively inhibiting NF-κB.

REFERENCES

1. SEN, R. & D. BALTIMORE. 1986. Multiple nuclear factors interact with the immunoglobulin enhancer sequences. Cell **46:** 705–716.
2. SEN, R. & D. BALTIMORE. 1986. Inducibility of kappa immunoglobulin enhancer-binding protein Nf-kappa B by a posttranslational mechanism. Cell **47:** 921–928.
3. OSBORN, L., S. KUNKEL & G.J. NABEL. 1989. Tumor necrosis factor alpha and interleukin 1 stimulate the human immunodeficiency virus enhancer by activation of the nuclear factor kappa B. Proc. Natl. Acad. Sci. USA **86:** 2336–2340.
4. ELEWAUT, D. et al. 1999. NF-kappa B is a central regulator of the intestinal epithelial cell innate immune response induced by infection with enteroinvasive bacteria. J. Immunol. **163:** 1457–1466.
5. LI, N. & M. KARIN. 1998. Ionizing radiation and short wavelength UV activate NF-kappaB through two distinct mechanisms. Proc. Natl. Acad. Sci. USA **95:** 13012–13017.
6. HAYDEN, M.S. & S. GHOSH. 2004. Signaling to NF-kappaB. Genes Dev. **18:** 2195–2224.
7. ZANDI, E. et al. 1997. The IkappaB kinase complex (IKK) contains two kinase subunits, IKKalpha and IKKbeta, necessary for IkappaB phosphorylation and NF-kappaB activation. Cell **91:** 243–252.
8. KARIN, M., Y. YAMAMOTO & Q.M. WANG. 2004. The IKK NF-kappa B system: a treasure trove for drug development. Nat. Rev. Drug Discov. **3:** 17–26.
9. SENFTLEBEN, U. et al. 2001. Activation by IKKalpha of a second, evolutionary conserved, NF-kappa B signaling pathway. Science **293:** 1495–1499.
10. ROGLER, G. et al. 1998. Nuclear factor kappaB is activated in macrophages and epithelial cells of inflamed intestinal mucosa. Gastroenterology **115:** 357–369.

11. SCHREIBER, S., S. NIKOLAUS & J. HAMPE. 1998. Activation of nuclear factor kappa B inflammatory bowel disease. Gut **42:** 477–484.

12. NEURATH, M.F. *et al.* 1996. Local administration of antisense phosphorothioate oligonucleotides to the p65 subunit of NF-kappa B abrogates established experimental colitis in mice. Nat. Med. **2:** 998–1004.

13. AUPHAN, N. *et al.* 1995. Immunosuppression by glucocorticoids: inhibition of NF-kappa B activity through induction of I kappa B synthesis. Science **270:** 286–290.

14. WAHL, C. *et al.* 1998. Sulfasalazine: a potent and specific inhibitor of nuclear factor kappa B. J. Clin. Invest. **101:** 1163–1174.

15. EGAN, L.J. *et al.* 1999. Inhibition of interleukin-1-stimulated NF-kappaB RelA/p65 phosphorylation by mesalamine is accompanied by decreased transcriptional activity. J. Biol. Chem. **274:** 26448–26453.

16. LI, Z.W. *et al.* 1999. The IKKbeta subunit of IkappaB kinase (IKK) is essential for nuclear factor kappaB activation and prevention of apoptosis. J. Exp. Med. **189:** 1839–1845.

17. LI, Q. *et al.* 1999. Severe liver degeneration in mice lacking the IkappaB kinase 2 gene. Science **284:** 321–325.

18. MAKRIS, C. *et al.* 2000. Female mice heterozygous for IKK gamma/NEMO deficiencies develop a dermatopathy similar to the human X-linked disorder incontinentia pigmenti. Mol. Cell. **5:** 969–979.

19. SENFTLEBEN, U. *et al.* 2001. IKKbeta is essential for protecting T cells from TNFalpha-induced apoptosis. Immunity **14:** 217–230.

20. SCHMIDT-SUPPRIAN, M. *et al.* 2003. Mature T cells depend on signaling through the IKK complex. Immunity **19:** 377–389.

21. PASPARAKIS, M., M. SCHMIDT-SUPPRIAN & K. RAJEWSKY. 2002. IkappaB kinase signaling is essential for maintenance of mature B cells. J. Exp. Med. **196:** 743–752.

22. LI, Z.W. *et al.* 2003. IKK beta is required for peripheral B cell survival and proliferation. J. Immunol. **170:** 4630–4637.

23. ITOH, J. *et al.* 2001. Decreased Bax expression by mucosal T cells favours resistance to apoptosis in Crohn's disease. Gut **49:** 35–41.

24. INA, K. *et al.* 1999. Resistance of Crohn's disease T cells to multiple apoptotic signals is associated with a Bcl-2/Bax mucosal imbalance. J. Immunol. **163:** 1081–1090.

25. CHU, W. *et al.* 2000. DNA-PKcs is required for activation of innate immunity by immunostimulatory DNA. Cell **103:** 909–918.

26. GRETEN, F.R. *et al.* 2004. IKKbeta links inflammation and tumorigenesis in a mouse model of colitis-associated cancer. Cell **118:** 285–296.

27. BERIN, M.C. *et al.* 2002. Role of EHEC O157:H7 virulence factors in the activation of intestinal epithelial cell NF-kappaB and MAP kinase pathways and the upregulated expression of interleukin 8. Cell. Microbiol. **4:** 635–648.

28. BERIN, M.C. *et al.* 2001. Regulated production of the T helper 2-type T-cell chemoattractant TARC by human bronchial epithelial cells in vitro and in human lung xenografts. Am. J. Respir. Cell. Mol. Biol. **24:** 382–389.

29. ECKMANN, L. *et al.* 2000. Analysis by high density cDNA arrays of altered gene expression in human intestinal epithelial cells in response to infection with the invasive enteric bacteria *Salmonella*. J. Biol. Chem. **275:** 14084–14094.

30. EGAN, L.J. *et al.* 2004. IkappaB-kinasebeta-dependent NF-kappaB activation provides radioprotection to the intestinal epithelium. Proc. Natl. Acad. Sci. USA **101:** 2452–2457.
31. CHEN, L.W. *et al.* 2003. The two faces of IKK and NF-kappaB inhibition: prevention of systemic inflammation but increased local injury following intestinal ischemia-reperfusion. Nat. Med. **9:** 575–581.
32. EGAN, L.J. *et al.* 2003. Nuclear factor-kappa B activation promotes restitution of wounded intestinal epithelial monolayers. Am. J. Physiol. Cell. Physiol. **285:** C1028–C1035.
33. DAJEE, M. *et al.* 2003. NF-kappaB blockade and oncogenic Ras trigger invasive human epidermal neoplasia. Nature **421:** 639–643.
34. BERNSTEIN, C.N. *et al.* 2002. Cancer prevention in inflammatory bowel disease and the chemoprophylactic potential of 5-aminosalicylic acid. Inflamm. Bowel Dis. **8:** 356–361.
35. JIMI, E. *et al.* 2004. Selective inhibition of NF-kappa B blocks osteoclastogenesis and prevents inflammatory bone destruction in vivo. Nat. Med. **10:** 617–624.
36. RUOCCO, M.G. *et al.* 2005. I{kappa}B kinase (IKK){beta}, but not IKK{alpha}, is a critical mediator of osteoclast survival and is required for inflammation-induced bone loss. J. Exp. Med. **201:** 1677–1687.

Role of the Melanocortin System in Inflammation

CHRISTIAN MAASER, KLAUS KANNENGIESSER, AND
TORSTEN KUCHARZIK

Department of Medicine B, University of Muenster, Muenster, Germany

ABSTRACT: In recent years, scientific interest in melanocortins (MC) has progressively increased due to their wide range of effects and expression on various tissues.primarily discovered as mediators of skin pigmentation, recent research has shown their important roles in various body functions, such as energy homeostasis, sexual function, and inflammation. The anti-inflammatory and immunomodulatory properties discovered so far have led to the hypothesis that alpha-melanocyte-stimulating hormone (MSH) and its cognate receptors might present potential anti-inflammatory treatment options.

KEYWORDS: colitis; MSH; melanocortin; KPV; intestinum

INTRODUCTION

The melanocortin system is best known for its role in melanogenesis and more recently for the regulation of energy homeostasis. However, the discovery of various anti-inflammatory and immunomodulatory functions has led to the suggestion that alpha-melanocyte-stimulating hormone, its related peptides, and its cognate receptors responsibile for transmitting these effects might present potential treatment options for inflammatory diseases.[1,2] This review describes the players of the melanocortin system and their function in inflammation, with a focus on organ systems exposed to the external environment.

MELANOCORTINS

The melanocortin (MC) peptides, which include adrenocorticotropic hormone (ACTH), α-melanocyte-stimulating hormone (MSH), β-MSH, and γ-MSH, are derived from a 31- to 36-kDa precursor protein named proopiomelanocortin (POMC). One of the main players of the MC system is

Address for correspondence: Christian Maaser, Albert-Schweitzer Str. 33, 48129 Muenster, Germany. Voice: +49-251-834-7661; fax: +49-251-834-7576.
e-mail: maaser@uni-muenster.de

Ann. N.Y. Acad. Sci. 1072: 123–134 (2006). © 2006 New York Academy of Sciences.
doi: 10.1196/annals.1326.016

alpha-melanocyte-stimulating hormone, which is a neuroimmunomodulatory, 13–amino acid peptide sharing its sequence with the N-terminal amino acids of ACTH (FIG. 1). It is derived from its precursor molecule POMC by posttranslational modification depending on the prohormone convertase (PC) present in the specific cell. Thus, the generation of biologically active α-MSH depends on two main components: the polypeptide precursor molecule and the proteolytic enzyme. To date seven precursor convertases have been identified, of which PC2 appears to be required for the production of α-MSH, while PC1 is required for ACTH. The activity of these convertases is tissue specific.[3] While α-MSH has originally been discovered to be expressed in the pituitary gland, it has subsequently been detected in various different cell types, for example, melanocytes, monocytes, B cells, natural killer cells, a subset of cytotoxic T cells, and epithelial cells.[4–11]

MC RECEPTORS

The actions of α-MSH are transmitted via specific MC receptors, of which five different ones have been identified, so far termed *MC-1* to *MC-5* receptor (FIG. 2). All five receptors are G-protein-coupled, seven-transmembrane receptors, which intracellularly mediate their effects by activating cAMP-dependent pathways. The seven-transmembrane receptors show different affinities to the different MC peptides and tissue-specific expression levels.

MC1 Receptor(R)

MC1R was the first MC receptor to be cloned.[12,13] Its main function was primarily thought to be the regulation of skin physiology and melanogenesis.[11] However, the expression of MC1R by macrophage/monocytic cells,[14] lymphocytes with antigen-presenting and cytotoxic functions,[10] neutrophils,[15] and dendritic cells[16] in addition to keratinocytes and melanocytes suggests a role of MC1R in inflammation. Supporting this, the expression of MC1R, for example, on monocytes was shown to be upregulated by endotoxins and proinflammatory cytokines.[17] Among all known MC peptides, α-MSH has the highest affinity to MC1R.[18] In inflammatory cells activation of MC1R has been shown to cause a marked reduction of activation and translocation of the nuclear transcription factor NF-κB.[19] It has therefore been suggested, that α-MSH potentially exerts its anti-inflammatory effect in part through binding to and activation of MC1R. Evidence about the important role of MC1R in human disease was recently shown in mice with a nonfunctional MC1R.[20] These mice revealed dramatic worsening of experimental colitis, indicating the importance of MC1R in intestinal homeostasis.

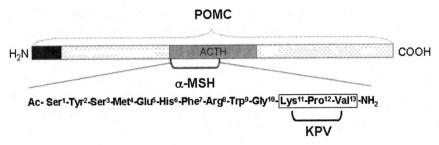

FIGURE 1. POMC and its derivates.

MC2 Receptor

The MC2R, which is mainly expressed in the zona fasciculata and zona glomerulosa of the adrenal cortex,[12] mediates physiological influences of ACTH in the production and release of steroids in the adrenal cortex.[21,22] While ACTH preferentially binds to MC2R, the other MCs show no significant affinity to MC2R. Hereditary isolated glucocorticoid deficiency, a rare autosomal disorder, is caused by mutations in the MC2R gene.[23]

MC3 Receptor

The MC3R has similar binding affinities to all MC peptides. Activation of this receptor can lead to signaling via cAMP as well as inositol–phospholipid pathways.[24] In the periphery, it is expressed in the placenta, ovary, mammary gland, testis, gastrointestinal tract, and the heart.[13,25,26] Furthermore, expression was detected within the central nervous system, for example, within the hypothalamus, thalamus, hippocampus, anterior amygdala, and cortex.

MCR Subtype	Ligand affinity	mRNA expression	Function
MC1R	α-MSH=ACTH> β-MSH>γ-MSH	e.g. melanocytes, endothelial cells, astrocytes, macrophages, neutrophils	pigmentation, immunomodulation
MC2R	ACTH	adrenal cortex	steroidogenesis
MC3R	α-MSH=β-MSH=γ-MSH=ACTH	e.g. CNS, placenta, duodenum, stomach, pancreas	regulation of cardiovascular functions and feeding behaviour, thermoregulation, immunomodulation
MC4R	α-MSH=ACTH>β-MSH>>γ-MSH	CNS	regulation of feeding behaviour and energy homeostasis, erectile function, pain
MC5R	α-MSH>ACTH=β-MSH>>γ-MSH	e.g. skin, adrenal gland, thymus, testis, ovary, stomach, lymphocytes, CNS	regulation of exocrine functions, immunomodulation

ACTH= Adrenocorticotropic hormone, MSH= Melanocyte stimulating hormone, CNS= central nervous system

FIGURE 2. The MC receptor family.

Regarding its function it is likely to play an important role in the regulation of cardiovascular functions, thermoregulation, and feeding behavior.[2,27] For example, MC3R-deficient mice show increased fat mass, reduced lean mass, and higher weight gain per food intake.[28] However, in recent years MC3R has also been suggested to play an important role in mediating some of the anti-inflammatory effects of α-MSH.[2,29,30] The receptor in this regard is expressed by residential macrophages, and natural as well as synthetic agonists of MC3R have been shown to possess anti-inflammatory properties.[31,32]

MC4 Receptor

MC4R is believed to play a major role in the regulation of feeding behavior and energy homeostasis. Mutations of the receptors have been associated with severe obesity and a binge eating phenotype.[33,34] Furthermore, murine gene disruption experiments of the MC4R gene resulted in obesity, hyperphagia, and hyperinsulinemia.[35] In addition, these mice are unresponsive to the anorectic effects of α-MSH.[36]

Similar to MC1R, the MC4R shows the highest affinity for α-MSH and ACTH. Interestingly, the MC4R has been found in various regions of the brain and spinal cord, but several studies have failed to show its expression in the periphery.[26,37,38] In addition to the function of MC4R in energy homeostasis MC4R has been shown to also participate in sexual functions; for example, it seems to modulate sexual behavior and erectile function.[39]

MC5 Receptor

Murine studies indicate a potential role of the MC5R in thermoregulation and the regulation of sebaceous gland secretion. Mice with a disruption of the MC5R gene, for example, show a defective water repulsion and thermoregulation as well as a reduced sebaceous gland secretion.[40] High expression levels of MC5R can be found in exocrine glands in addition to various other tissue types.[40] Its expression by B and T cells, in which binding of its ligand α-MSH leads to activation of the JAK/STAT pathway, suggests an additional role in immunomodulation.[41]

GENERAL MECHANISMS OF ANTI-INFLAMMATORY ACTION

In vitro various anti-inflammatory effects have been shown for α-MSH. Binding of α-MSH to its MC receptors leads to downregulation of various proinflammatory cytokines, such as IL-1, IL-6, TNF-α, IL-2, IFN-γ, IL-4, and IL-13.[42–44] In murine macrophages, α-MSH inhibits inflammation-related nitric oxide (NO) production by inhibiting the expression of inducible NO synthase.[14] Becher *et al.* demonstrated that costimulatory molecules like CD86 and

CD49 are downregulated on antigen-presenting dendritic cells in the presence of α-MSH.[16] Furthermore, α-MSH appears to inhibit IL-8-mediated biological responses in neutrophils by downregulating CXCR1 and CXCR2 through inhibition of serine proteases.[45] In contrast, the production of the cytokine synthesis inhibitor IL-10 is upregulated by α-MSH.[44]

At the molecular level, part of the anti-inflammatory effects seem to be mediated by inhibition of nuclear factor (NF)-κB activation; for example, α-MSH inhibits lipopolysaccharide (LPS)-induced NF-κB activation in the human monocytic cell line U937 as well as in human microvascular endothelial cells (HMEC-1), leading to the downregulation of adhesion molecule expression in the latter.[19,46] Peripheral inhibition of NF-κB by central administration of α-MSH has been demonstrated to lead to a reduction in proinflammatory cytokine expression due to the protection of IκBα.[47] In addition to central effects, α-MSH appears to exert some of its anti-inflammatory functions in an autocrine way.[14,48]

Interestingly, some of the anti-inflammatory actions of α-MSH might be due to the C-terminal tripeptide KPV, which corresponds to α-MSH11–13. While some researchers suggest that KPV as α-MSH exerts its anti-inflammatory effect via binding to MC1R, others rather see KPV as an IL-1 receptor antagonist.[43,49,50]

MC and Anti-microbial Functions

α-MSH and its C-terminal peptide Lys-Pro-Val (KPV) exert antimicrobial effects. Both peptides significantly inhibited *Staphylococcus aureus* colony formation and reduced viability and germ tube formation of the yeast *Candida albicans*. Antimicrobial effects occurred over a wide range of concentrations, including the one at physiological picomolar range.[50] Furthermore, in humans, different plasma levels of α-MSH have been detected in patients recovering from septic shock compared to those who later died. Taken together with *in vitro* results showing an inhibitory effect of α-MSH on TNFα and IL-1β release of LPS-stimulated blood samples from these patients led to the hypothesis that α-MSH might be a potential tool to treat sepsis syndrome in humans.[50,51]

ANTI-INFLAMMATORY EFFECTS OF THE MC SYSTEM IN ORGAN SYSTEMS EXPOSED TO THE EXTERNAL ENVIRONMENT

Skin

The skin represents one of the well-known extrapituitary sites of α-MSH expression and secretion. In addition to its role in melanogenesis, elevated α-MSH levels have been reported in several cutaneous inflammatory disorders.[52–54] Furthermore, potent anti-inflammatory properties of α-MSH have been demonstrated in murine models of delayed-type hypersensitivity and hapten-specific tolerance. In this model, epicutaneous application of α-MSH inhibited both the induction as well as elicitation phase of contact hypersensitivity response in mice.[55,56] Systemically administered α-MSH similarly promoted induction of hapten-specific tolerance.[55] *In vivo* tolerance by α-MSH could be abrogated by the administration of an IL-10 antibody at the site of sensitization, indicating that the α-MSH-induced hapten-specific tolerance in mice is mediated by IL-10 release.[55]

Lung

In addition to skin, the airway represents another primary site at which the organism itself is in direct contact with the external environment. In contrast to skin, relatively little is known about the potential role of the MC system in lung inflammatory physiology and pathophysiology. Ichiyama *et al.* reported that transfection of human pulmonary epithelial cells (A549) led to inhibition of NF-κB activation.[57] *In vivo* Raap *et al.* detected α-MSH in bronchial lavage fluids of mice, showing increased production in response to aerosol challenges in nonsensitized animals. Looking at a murine model of allergic airway inflammation this rapid increase of α-MSH in bronchoalveolar fluid was absent in allergic animals, while treatment of these mice with α-MSH resulted in a significant suppression of allergen-specific IgE production and eosinophil influx. Similar to the findings by Grabbe *et al.* regarding hapten-specific tolerance in mice, the effects in the murine allergic airway inflammation model appear to be mediated via IL-10, as IL-10 knockout mice were resistant to α-MSH treatment.[55,58]

Intestinal Tract

The third major organ site at which the organism is in direct contact with the external environment is the gastrointestinal tract. Although some significant advancements in the understanding of the anti-inflammatory role of MC system in various cell types and organs have been made in recent years, relatively little is known on the expression and functional role of the different MC family members in the intestinal tract, as with the lung.

Studying duodenal biopsy tissue by immunohistochemistry, Colombo and colleagues have detected MC1R protein expression mainly in goblet cells in both celiac and normal subjects. Furthermore, α-MSH expression was shown in the same set of biopsy samples in endocrine-like cells as well as scattered cells in the lamina propria. A more intense staining for α-MSH and MC1R in tissue of celiac patients and a marked downregulation of gliadin-induced IL-6 release by duodenal specimens in response to incubation with α-MSH led the authors to the conclusion that treatment of selected cases of refractory celiac disease with peptides such as α-MSH might present a potential therapeutic strategy.[59]

Mesenteric ischemic reperfusion is a common clinical problem in the settings of shock and sepsis for which currently there are still a considerable morbidity and mortality and hardly any direct therapeutic options. Hassoun *et al*. have been able to show that administration of α-MSH to rats that underwent a temporal mesenteric artery occlusion followed by reperfusion led to intestinal transit times and histological injury scores comparable to those of sham-operated controls. Furthermore, as one would expect from the *in vitro* findings for α-MSH signaling modulation, the addition of α-MSH to the mesenteric ischemic reperfusion injury model caused a significant downregulation of intestinal NF-κB activity.[60,61] Similarly, San *et al*. detected an anti-inflammatory effect for α-MSH in endotoxin-induced intestinal injury. In their model, rats were injected intravenously (i.v.) with LPS from *S. enteritidis*, leading to diffuse mucosal changes characterized by altered villus structure and epithelial desquamanation in all intestinal segments of endotoxin-treated control animals. In contrast, treatment with α-MSH reversed the extent of lesions in the distal ileum, whereas no significant changes could be detected in the jejunal and mid-ileal segments. In addition, α-MSH led to a marked decrease of neutrophil infiltration in the distal ileum compared to controls. The anti-inflammatory mechanism of α-MSH in this endotoxin-induced injury model thereby appears to involve NO, as pretreatment with the nonselective COX inhibitor indomethacin reversed the effect of α-MSH on neutrophil migration.[62]

Given the various anti-inflammatory functions of α-MSH and the unspecific, often side-effect-associated current medical treatment of inflammatory bowel disease, this peptide might present an effective therapeutic option. This hypothesis is supported by data from Rajora *et al*., who studied the effect of α-MSH on experimental inflammatory bowel disease. In their hands daily intraperitoneal (i.p.) application of α-MSH to mice subjected to a dextran-sodium sulfate-induced colitis led to a reduced appearance of fecal blood by over 80%, significantly inhibited weight loss, and prevented disintegration of the general condition of the animals. This effect appeared in part to result from inhibition of TNF-α and NO.[63] Furthermore, Oktar *et al*. described reduced colonic macroscopic lesions in rats undergoing a trinitrobenzene sulfonic acid–induced colitis when treated with α-MSH i.p twice daily as compared to untreated controls in both acute and chronic inflammation.[64]

As at least part of the anti-inflammatory effects of α-MSH are mediated through the three C-terminal amino acids Lys-Pro-Val (KPV), we tested the hypothesis that similar effects in experimental colitis can be detected by treatment of mice with this tripeptide. In addition to reduced production costs, applying this tripeptide instead of α-MSH might go along with less side effects, especially regarding influences on melanogenesis. Similarly as for α-MSH, application of KPV to DSS-treated mice led to a significant inhibition of weight loss and signs of histological inflammation in colonic tissue. These anti-inflammatory effects could be reproduced in a therapeutic setup using the CD45Rb high transfer colitis, in which KPV was applied after the induction of colitis (Maaser *et al.*, unpublished findings).

As α-MSH and MC1R are thought to exert their anti-inflammatory effects in an autoregulatory loop, we further studied whether disruption of this system would lead to worsening of inflammation, taking advantage of mice with a frameshift mutation of the MC1R gene (MC1Re/e) and leading to a nonfunctioning receptor.[65] While the colon of untreated MC1Re/e mice appears normal, the course of DSS colitis in MC1Re/e mice is dramatically aggravated with a significantly higher weight loss and marked histological changes compared to C57BL/6WT. Furthermore, results from experiments with MC1Re/e-C57BL/6 bone marrow chimeras suggest that mesenchymal cell–expressed MC1R is required to effectively exert its anti-inflammatory functions for recovery of intestinal inflammation. More detailed analysis revealed epithelial cells expressed MC1R as one of the potential cell population that is required for maintaining intestinal homeostasis.[20]

CONCLUSION

The presence of α-MSH in skin, lung, and gut, three organ systems that are in direct contact with the external environment, suggests that this molecule may be a component of the innate host defense. The findings of a potent anti-inflammatory potential of α-MSH and its tripeptide KPV in different models of intestinal inflammation as well as dramatic worsening of colitis in mice with nonfunctional MC1R encourages the development of α-MSH-like peptides and the use of MC1R as potential targets for the treatment of IBD.

ACKNOWLEDGMENT

This work was supported by a grant from the Eli and Edythe L. Broad Foundation (IBD-0038).

REFERENCES

1. CATANIA, A., S. GATTI, G. COLOMBO, *et al.* 2004. Targeting melanocortin receptors as a novel strategy to control inflammation. Pharmacol. Rev. **56**: 1–29.
2. GETTING, S.J. 2002. Melanocortin peptides and their receptors: new targets for anti-inflammatory therapy. Trends Pharmacol. Sci. **23**: 447–449.
3. PRITCHARD, L.E., A.V. TURNBULL & A. WHITE. 2002. Pro-opiomelanocortin processing in the hypothalamus: impact on melanocortin signalling and obesity. J. Endocrinol. **172**: 411–421.

4. THODY, A.J., K. RIDLEY, R.J. PENNY, *et al.* 1983. MSH peptides are present in mammalian skin. Peptides **4**: 813–816.
5. WINTZEN, M. & B.A. GILCHREST. 1996. Proopiomelanocortin, its derived peptides, and the skin. J. Invest. Dermatol. **106**: 3–10.
6. LUGER, T.A., T. BRZOSKA, T.E. SCHOLZEN, *et al.* 2000. The role of alpha-MSH as a modulator of cutaneous inflammation. Ann. N. Y. Acad. Sci. **917**: 232–238.
7. BHARDWAJ, R.S. & T.A. LUGER. 1994. Proopiomelanocortin production by epidermal cells: evidence for an immune neuroendocrine network in the epidermis. Arch. Dermatol. Res. **287**: 85–90.
8. BOTCHKAREV, V.A., N.V. BOTCHKAREVA & A. SLOMINSKI. 1999. Developmentally regulated expression of alpha-MSH and MC-1 receptor in C57BL/6 mouse skin suggests functions beyond pigmentation. Ann. N. Y. Acad. Sci. **885**: 433–439.
9. SCHOLZEN, T.E., D.H. KALDEN & T. BRZOSKA. 2000. Expression of proopiomelanocortin peptides in human dermal microvascular endothelial cells: evidence for a regulation by ultraviolet light and interleukin-1. J. Invest. Dermatol. **115**: 1021–1028.
10. NEUMANN ANDERSEN, G., O. NAGAEVA, I. MANDRIKA, *et al.* 2001. MC(1) receptors are constitutively expressed on leucocyte subpopulations with antigen presenting and cytotoxic functions. Clin. Exp. Immunol. **126**: 441–446.
11. SLOMINSKI, A., J. WORTSMAN, T. LUGER, *et al.* 2000. Corticotropin releasing hormone and proopiomelanocortin involvement in the cutaneous response to stress. Physiol. Rev. **80**: 979–1020.
12. MOUNTJOY, K.G., L.S. ROBBINS, M.T. MORTRUD, *et al.* 1992. The cloning of a family of genes that encode the melanocortin receptors. Science **257**: 1248–1251.
13. CHHAJLANI, V. & J.E. WIKBERG. 1992. Molecular cloning and expression of the human melanocyte stimulating hormone receptor cDNA. FEBS Lett. **309**: 417–420.
14. STAR, R.A., N. RAJORA, J. HUANG, *et al.* 1995. Evidence of autocrine modulation of macrophage nitric oxide synthase by alpha-melanocyte–stimulating hormone. Proc. Natl. Acad. Sci. USA **92**: 8016–8020.
15. CATANIA, A., N. RAJORA, F. CAPSONI, *et al.* 1996. The neuropeptide alpha-MSH has specific receptors on neutrophils and reduces chemotaxis in vitro. Peptides **17**: 675–679.
16. BECHER, E., K. MAHNKE, T. BRZOSKA, *et al.* 1999. Human peripheral blood-derived dendritic cells express functional melanocortin receptor MC-1R. Ann. N. Y. Acad. Sci. **885**: 188–195.
17. LUGER, T.A., T. SCHOLZEN, T. BRZOSKA, *et al.* 1998. Cutaneous immunomodulation and coordination of skin stress responses by alpha-melanocyte–stimulating hormone. Ann. N. Y. Acad. Sci. **840**: 381–394.
18. MOUNTJOY, K.G. 1994. The human melanocyte stimulating hormone receptor has evolved to become "super-sensitive" to melanocortin peptides. Mol. Cell. Endocrinol. **102**: R7–R11.
19. MANNA, S.K. & B.B. AGGARWAL. 1998. Alpha-melanocyte-stimulating hormone inhibits the nuclear transcription factor NF-kappa B activation induced by various inflammatory agents. J. Immunol. **161**: 2873–2880.
20. MAASER, C., K. KANNENGIESSER, C. SPECHT, *et al.* 2006. Crucial role of the melanocortin receptor MC1R in experimental colitis. Gut. E-publication ahead of print.

21. XIA, Y. & J.E. WIKBERG. 1996. Localization of ACTH receptor mRNA by in situ hybridization in mouse adrenal gland. Cell. Tissue. Res. **286**: 63–68.
22. BUCKLEY, D.I. & J. RAMACHANDRAN. 1981. Characterization of corticotropin receptors on adrenocortical cells. Proc. Natl. Acad. Sci. USA **78**: 7431–7435.
23. TSIGOS, C., K. ARAI, W. HUNG, et al. 1993. Hereditary isolated glucocorticoid deficiency is associated with abnormalities of the adrenocorticotropin receptor gene. J. Clin. Invest. **92**: 2458–2461.
24. KONDA, Y., I. GANTZ, J. DELVALLE, et al. 1994. Interaction of dual intracellular signaling pathways activated by the melanocortin-3 receptor. J. Biol. Chem. **269**: 13162–13166.
25. GANTZ, I., Y. KONDA, T. TASHIRO, et al. 1993. Molecular cloning of a novel melanocortin receptor. J. Biol. Chem. **268**: 8246–8250.
26. CHHAJLANI, V. 1996. Distribution of cDNA for melanocortin receptor subtypes in human tissues. Biochem. Mol. Biol. Int. **38**: 73–80.
27. LOW, M.J. 2004. Role of proopiomelanocortin neurons and peptides in the regulation of energy homeostasis. J. Endocrinol. Invest. **27**(6 Suppl): 95–100.
28. CHEN, A.S., D.J. MARSH, M.E. TRUMBAUER, et al. 2000. Inactivation of the mouse melanocortin-3 receptor results in increased fat mass and reduced lean body mass. Nat. Genet. **26**: 97–102.
29. GETTING, S.J., H.C. CHRISTIAN, R.J. FLOWER, et al. 2002. Activation of melanocortin type 3 receptor as a molecular mechanism for adrenocorticotropic hormone efficacy in gouty arthritis. Arthritis. Rheum. **46**: 2765–2775.
30. GETTING, S.J., H.C. CHRISTIAN, C.W. LAM, et al. 2003. Redundancy of a functional melanocortin 1 receptor in the anti-inflammatory actions of melanocortin peptides: studies in the recessive yellow (e/e) mouse suggest an important role for melanocortin 3 receptor. J. Immunol. **170**: 3323–3330.
31. GETTING, S.J., G.H. ALLCOCK, R. FLOWER, et al. 2001. Natural and synthetic agonists of the melanocortin receptor type 3 possess anti-inflammatory properties. J. Leukoc. Biol. **69**: 98–104.
32. GETTING, S.J., L. GIBBS, A.J. CLARK, et al. 1999. POMC gene-derived peptides activate melanocortin type 3 receptor on murine macrophages, suppress cytokine release, and inhibit neutrophil migration in acute experimental inflammation. J Immunol **162**: 7446–7453.
33. FAROOQI, I.S., J.M. KEOGH, G.S. YEO, et al. 2003. Clinical spectrum of obesity and mutations in the melanocortin 4 receptor gene. N. Engl. J. Med. **348**: 1085–1095.
34. BRANSON, R., N. POTOCZNA, J.G. KRAL, et al. 2003. Binge eating as a major phenotype of melanocortin 4 receptor gene mutations. N. Engl. J. Med. **348**: 1096–1103.
35. HUSZAR, D., C.A. LYNCH, V. FAIRCHILD-HUNTRESS, et al. 1997. Targeted disruption of the melanocortin-4 receptor results in obesity in mice. Cell **88**: 131–141.
36. MARSH, D.J., G. HOLLOPETER, D. HUSZAR, et al. 1999. Response of melanocortin-4 receptor-deficient mice to anorectic and orexigenic peptides. Nat. Genet. **21**: 119–122.
37. MOUNTJOY, K.G., M.T. MORTRUD, M.J. LOW, et al. 1994. Localization of the melanocortin-4 receptor (MC4-R) in neuroendocrine and autonomic control circuits in the brain. Mol. Endocrinol. **8**: 1298–1308.
38. GANTZ, I., H. MIWA, Y. KONDA, et al. 1993. Molecular cloning, expression, and gene localization of a fourth melanocortin receptor. J. Biol. Chem. **268**: 15174–15179.
39. VAN DER PLOEG, L.H., W.J. MARTIN, A.D. HOWARD, et al. 2002. A role for the melanocortin 4 receptor in sexual function. Proc. Natl. Acad. Sci. USA **99**: 11381–11386.

40. CHEN, W., M.A. KELLY, X. OPITZ-ARAYA, *et al.* 1997. Exocrine gland dysfunction in MC5-R-deficient mice: evidence for coordinated regulation of exocrine gland function by melanocortin peptides. Cell **91**: 789–798.

41. BUGGY, J.J. 1998. Binding of alpha-melanocyte-stimulating hormone to its G-protein-coupled receptor on B-lymphocytes activates the Jak/STAT pathway. Biochem. J. **331**: 211–216.

42. ADACHI, S., T. NAKANO, H. VLIAGOFTIS, *et al.* 1999. Receptor-mediated modulation of murine mast cell function by alpha-melanocyte stimulating hormone. J. Immunol. **163**: 3363–3368.

43. LUGER, T.A., T.E. SCHOLZEN, T. BRZOSKA, *et al.* 2003. New insights into the functions of alpha-MSH and related peptides in the immune system. Ann. N. Y. Acad. Sci. **994**: 133–140.

44. LUGER, T.A., R.S. BHARDWAJ, S. GRABBE, *et al.* 1996. Regulation of the immune response by epidermal cytokines and neurohormones. J. Dermatol. Sci. **13**: 5–10.

45. MANNA, S.K., A. SARKAR & Y. SREENIVASAN. 2006. Alpha-melanocyte-stimulating hormone down-regulates CXC receptors through activation of neutrophil elastase. Eur. J. Immunol.

46. KALDEN, D.H., T. SCHOLZEN, T. BRZOSKA, *et al.* 1999. Mechanisms of the antiinflammatory effects of alpha–MSH: role of transcription factor NF-kappa B and adhesion molecule expression. Ann. N. Y. Acad. Sci. **885**: 254–261.

47. ICHIYAMA, T., T. SAKAI, A. CATANIA, *et al.* 1999. Inhibition of peripheral NF-kappaB activation by central action of alpha-melanocyte-stimulating hormone. J. Neuroimmunol. **99**: 211–217.

48. ICHIYAMA, T., I.L. CAMPBELL, S. FURUKAWA, *et al.* 1999. Autocrine alpha-melanocyte-stimulating hormone inhibits NF-kappaB activation in human glioma. J. Neurosci. Res. **58**: 684–689.

49. GETTING, S.J., H.B. SCHIOTH & M. PERRETTI. 2003. Dissection of the antiinflammatory effect of the core and C-terminal (KPV) alpha-melanocyte-stimulating hormone peptides. J. Pharmacol. Exp. Ther. **306**: 631–637.

50. CUTULI, M., S. CRISTIANI, J.M. LIPTON, *et al.* 2000. Antimicrobial effects of alpha-MSH peptides. J. Leukoc. Biol. **67**: 233–239.

51. CATANIA, A., M. CUTULI, L. GAROFALO, *et al.* 2000. Plasma concentrations and anti-L-cytokine effects of alpha-melanocyte stimulating hormone in septic patients. Crit. Care. Med. **28**: 1403–1407.

52. SLOMINSKI, A., J. WORTSMAN, J.E. MAZURKIEWICZ, *et al.* 1993. Detection of proopiomelanocortin-derived antigens in normal and pathologic human skin. J. Lab. Clin. Med. **122**: 658–666.

53. SLOMINSKI, A., R. PAUS & J. WORTSMAN. 1993. On the potential role of proopiomelanocortin in skin physiology and pathology. Mol. Cell. Endocrinol. **93**: C1–C6.

54. BAYERL, C., J. LAUK, I. MOLL, *et al.* 1997. Immunohistochemical characterization of HSP, alpha-MSH, Merkel cells and neuronal markers in acute UV dermatitis and acute contact dermatitis in vivo. Inflamm. Res. **46**: 409–411.

55. GRABBE, S., R.S. BHARDWAJ, K. MAHNKE, *et al.* 1996. Alpha-melanocyte-stimulating hormone induces hapten-specific tolerance in mice. J. Immunol. **156**: 473–478.

56. RHEINS, L.A., A.L. COTLEUR, R.S. KLEIER, *et al.* 1998. Alpha-melanocyte stimulating hormone modulates contact hypersensitivity responsiveness in C57/BL6 mice. J. Invest. Dermatol. **93**: 511–517.

57. ICHIYAMA, T., K. OKADA, I.L. CAMPBELL, *et al.* 2000. NF-kappaB activation is inhibited in human pulmonary epithelial cells transfected with alpha–melanocyte-stimulating hormone vector. Peptides **21**: 1473–1477.
58. RAAP, U., T. BRZOSKA, S. SOHL, *et al.* 2003. Alpha-melanocyte-stimulating hormone inhibits allergic airway inflammation. J. Immunol. **171**: 353–359.
59. COLOMBO, G., R. BUFFA, M.T. BARDELLA, *et al.* 2002. Anti-inflammatory effects of alpha-melanocyte-stimulating hormone in celiac intestinal mucosa. Neuroimmunomodulation **10**: 208–216.
60. HASSOUN, H.T., L. ZOU, F.A. MOORE, *et al.* 2002. Alpha-melanocyte-stimulating hormone protects against mesenteric ischemia-reperfusion injury. Am. J. Physiol. Gastrointest. Liver Physiol. **282**: G1059–G1068.
61. ZOU, L., B. ATTUWAYBI & B.C. KONE. 2003. Effects of NF-kappa B inhibition on mesenteric ischemia-reperfusion injury. Am. J. Physiol. Gastrointest. Liver Physiol. **284**: G713–G721.
62. SAN, T., B.K. OKTAR, E. SALIK, *et al.* 2001. The effect of alpha-melanocyte stimulating hormone on endotoxin-induced intestinal injury. Peptides **22**: 2077–2082.
63. RAJORA, N., G. BOCCOLI, A. CATANIA, *et al.* 1997. Alpha-MSH modulates experimental inflammatory bowel disease. Peptides **18**: 381–385.
64. OKTAR, B.K., F. ERCAN, B.C. YEGEN, *et al.* 2000. The effect of alpha-melanocyte stimulating hormone on colonic inflammation in the rat. Peptides **21**: 1271–1277.
65. ROBBINS, L.S., J.H. NADEAU, K.R. JOHNSON, *et al.* 1993. Pigmentation phenotypes of variant extension locus alleles result from point mutations that alter MSH receptor function. Cell **72**: 827–834.

Immunology of Crohn's Disease

HENRI BRAAT,[a] MAIKEL P. PEPPELENBOSCH,[b]
AND DAAN W. HOMMES[c]

[a]Laboratory of Experimental Internal Medicine, Academic Medical Center,
University of Amsterdam, Meibergdreef 9, NL-1105 AZ Amsterdam,
the Netherlands

[b]Department of Cell Biology, University Medical Center Groningen,
University of Groningen, 9713 AV Groningen, the Netherlands

[c]Department of Gastroenterology, Academic Medical Center, University of
Amsterdam, Meibergdreef 9, NL-1105 AZ Amsterdam, the Netherlands

ABSTRACT: The immense microbiological load of the gastrointestinal
tract poses a daunting challenge for the mucosal immune system: whereas
it should tolerate the vast number of commensal bacteria, it should adequately attack pathogenic organisms. Millions of years of co-evolution
have produced an intricate system in which interactions between the
endogenous flora and mucosal immune system manage to perform this
difficult balancing act. When components of this interaction are defective, for instance by mutation, inflammatory bowel disease may result.
In the present review, we comprehensively discuss the mucosal immune
system in the context of Crohn's disease (CD) and its genetic risk factors, describe the clinical management of the disease, and discuss how
knowledge of the mucosal immune system may yield novel therapeutical
avenues for dealing with this debilitating disease.

KEYWORDS: Crohn's disease; mucosal immunology; dendritic cells; pattern recognition and host bacterial cells

CURRENT TREATMENT OF CD

Induction and Maintenance of Remission

Crohn's disease (CD) is an uncontrolled chronic mucosal inflammation in
the susceptible host (FIG. 1). Most patients with CD are referred to the hospital with severe complaints resulting from established chronic inflammation,
tissue destruction, and even sometimes perforating or stenosing disease with

Address for correspondence: Maikel P. Peppelenbosch, Department of Cell Biology, University
Medical Center Groningen, University of Groningen, 9713 AV Groningen, the Netherlands. Voice:
+31-50-363-2522; fax: +31-50-363-2512.
e-mail: m.peppelenbosch@med.umcg.nl

Ann. N.Y. Acad. Sci. 1072: 135–154 (2006). © 2006 New York Academy of Sciences.
doi: 10.1196/annals.1326.039

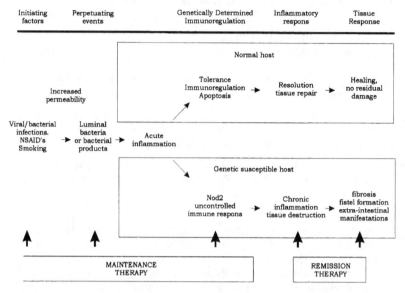

FIGURE 1. Initiating events increase intestinal permeability, and subsequently luminal bacteria or bacterial products disseminate in the mucosal compartment. In normal individuals these small inflamatory events reside subclinically; inflammation is controlled via tolerogenic immune responses that finally result in healing. The pattern recognition receptor NOD2, which is involved in the recognition of bacterial components and initiation of innate- and adaptive immune responses, is crucial in this process. Mutations within the Nod2 gene are associated with uncontrolled gastrointestinal immune responses that finally result in signs of chronic inflammation. Currently many therapies for induction of remission are interfering with processes late in the inflammatory cascade, and the challenge of contemporary research is to develop maintenance strategies that are aimed at early intervention in this cascade.

extra-intestinal manifestations. Histological examination will reveal ulceration with transmural nodular lymphoid aggregates. The presence of granulomas is a strong evidence for CD but may be absent with only non-specific transmural inflammation. In this stage of disease, perpetuating events (activation T cells and epithelial destruction) are more pronounced than initiating events (inability to recognize conserved microbial patterns and uncontrolled immunity). Therefore, general immunosuppressive drugs and targeting T-cell activation/apoptosis are the most important initial strategies. Corticosteroids are the most commonly used to induce remission in patients with CD; up to 60 mg oral per day or intravenously in severely ill patients. Corticosteroids should be continued only when needed to control acute inflammation, as they have no maintenance benefit and serious side effects. For some patients, the side effects may be partially circumvented by the use of topical corticosteroids, but no evidence exists that prolonged intake does not induce systemic side effects. Furthermore, 6-mercaptopurine, azathioprine, and methotrexate can be used for induction of remission.[1,2]

TABLE 1. Characteristics of current therapies

	Remission Induction	Remission Maintenance	Mucosal Healing	Steroid Sparing	Disease Modifying
Mesalazine	±	±	−	−	−
Prednisone	++	−	−	−	−
Azathioprine	±	+	+	+	?
Methotrexate	+	±	?	+	?
Infliximab	++	+	++	+	?

When CD was first described in 1952,[3] mortality was one of the main issues in its management. Improvement of surgical techniques and the use of potent anti-inflammatory therapies have reduced complications and prolonged periods of remission in CD significantly. The main challenge of developing new therapies for CD is now focused on maintenance of remission instead of remission induction. During early phases of CD, inflammation is limited to the mucosal and submucosal compartment and typical aphthous ulcers and limited numbers of lymphocytes and antigen-presenting cells (APCs) are present. It is very likely that a small infectious event precedes these early histological changes and that the subsequent disrupted intestinal barrier further diminishes the fragile tolerogenic balance that exists against the autologous flora in a susceptible host. New maintenance drugs should interfere with processes in the early phase of disease development, i.e., preventing potential pathogenic colonization, preventing disruption in barrier integrity, or actively inducing the development of tolerogenic immunity. Although corticosteroids are very efficient in inducing remission in patients with active disease, both systemic and local administration of corticosteroids in patients with quiescent disease does not reduce the risk of relapse over a follow-up period of 24 and 12 months, respectively. Azathioprine, methotrexate, and anti-TNF-α are effective in maintaining remission, with a possible steroid-sparing effect for azathioprine and anti-TNF-α, but not for methotrexate. However, the long-term toxicity of these drugs is not thoroughly investigated, and certainly both methotrexate and azathioprine need close monitoring and the need for intravenous administration of anti-TNF hampers the long-term use of this compound. Therefore, the current maintenance therapies for CD are to certain extent effective, but certainly do not modify disease susceptibility, and other long-term maintenance strategies are needed (TABLE 1).

PATHOGENIC FACTORS IN CD

Innate and Adaptive Immunity

The systemic, immune-associated complications occurring during the course of CD, the efficacy of immunosuppressive drugs, and the pathological features of Crohn's lesions clearly indicate the involvement of the immune system.[4] Interestingly, allogenic stem cell transplantation can lead to the development of CD in the human situation, indicating an important role (but not an exclusive one) of hematopoietic cells in disease development.[5] Of all body surfaces, the gastrointestinal tract constitutes the largest area in contact with the exterior milieu; the gastrointestinal barrier is continuously exposed to a wide variety of different potential pathogenic microorganisms and it requires efficient strategies to prevent infectious events. The continuous lining of intestinal epithelial cells with its tight junctions and brush border is important in the innate defense mechanism. Furthermore, intestinal epithelial cells (especially Paneth cells) are important for the secretion of many antimicrobial substances (mucus, s-IgA,[6] defensins,[7] and lysozymes) and danger signals (chemokines, prostaglandins, heat-shock proteins, and cytokines) that induce the recruitment and differentiation of innate immune cells. They can also act as non-professional APCs.

Pattern-Recognition Receptors

Recognition of pathogens by epithelial cells, neutrophils, macrophages, and dendritic cells (DCs) is mediated by germ-line encoded pattern-recognition receptors (PRRs). Several groups can be distinguished including (C-type) lectins, mannose receptors, complement receptors, scavenger receptors, Nod proteins, and toll-like receptors (TLRs). These receptors have evolved by natural selection and are specific for a limited amount of highly conserved microbial motifs (pathogen-associated molecular patterns or PAMPs).[8,9] TLRs belong to the cytokine receptor family, and so far 10 different TLRs have been described (TABLE 2). Their extracellular domains contain leucine-rich repeats (LRRs) that participate in ligand recognition; the intracellular domains contain regions that are highly similar to the intracellular domain of the IL-1 receptor. After activation, all TLRs finally activate NF-κB, but important differences remain. TLR4 is activated when the LPS–LPS binding protein complex is transferred from the CD14 receptor.[10,11] Binding of LPS to a TLR4 heterodimer–MD2 complex results in the activation of different domains of the intracellular region. Roughly, an early MyD88-dependent and late MyD88-independent pathway can be distinguished.[12] The term "pathogen-associated molecular patterns" suggests that only pathogens are recognized by PRRs; however, non-pathogenic microorganisms and self-proteins also are able to activate PRRs (TABLE 2).

Dendritic Cells

Although the recognition of PAMPs by the innate immune system leads to a rather temporal and localized response, activation of PRRs on DCs leads

TABLE 2. The toll-like receptor family

Name	Ligand	Reference
TLR1/	Ara-lipoarabinomannan	
TLR2	Tri-acyl lipopeptides	13
	Lysophosphatidylserine	14
	Lipoarabinomannan	15
TLR2	Lipoproteins	16
	Porin	17
	Zymosan	18
TLR2/	Modulin	19
TLR6	Peptidoglycan	20
	Di-acyl lipopeptides	16,21
TLR3	Double-stranded RNA	22
	Mannuronic acid polymers	23
TLR4	Teichuronic acid	24
	Glucuronoxylomannan	25
	Heat-shock proteins	26
TLR5	Flagellin	27
TLR7	Imidazoquinolines	
	GU-rich s-RNA	28,29
TLR8	Imidazoquinolines	29
	GU-rich s-RNA	
TLR9	CpG repeats	30

to differentiation, migration, and antigen presentation in secondary lymphoid structures, where they initiate prolonged and dispersed immune responses. In this way, dendritic cells continuously provide specific immune cells with information to acquire memory and specificity after repeated exposure.[31] DCs share much homology with mononuclear phagocytes of the innate immune system, but they are highly specialized in antigen presentation and therefore are a critical link between innate and adaptive immunity and provide the organism with an immunological advantage in combating recurrent infections.[32] Depending on their stage of differentiation, DCs are situated in the mucosal lining of the body or are present within secondary lymphoid organs. Immature DCs are solitary, situated in mucosal surfaces, and function as sentinels, continuously sampling the environment for danger signals.[33] Upon exposure to PAMPs and inflammatory mediators, immature DCs undergo a maturation process involving several functional and morphological changes. Endocytosis is downregulated, the expression of co-stimulatory molecules enhanced, MHC II-peptide complexes transported to the cell surface,[34] and peptide-specific antigens presented. Upon arrival in secondary lymphoid tissue, dendritic cells interact with lymphoid cells to induce adaptive immune responses.[34-35] Adequate stimulation of naive T cells is dependent on three distinctive signals: antigen-specific peptide presentation via MHC molecules, co-stimulation within the direct surrounding of MCH-TCR complex, and the cytokine environment, respectively. The combination of these three factors will finally determine the differentiation

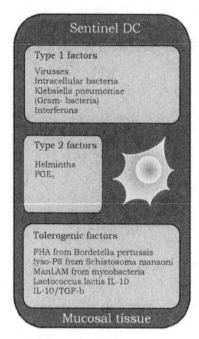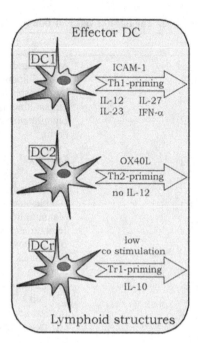

FIGURE 2. The type of T cell response generated is fully dependent on the phenotype of effector DCs, which undergo a very flexible program of maturation upon activation by pathogenic motifs and/or environmental signals. Type 1 factors present in the mucosal tissue activate sentinel DCs to become effector DCs with Th1 polarizing capacity (DC1), that is, the expression of ICAM-1 and the secretion of IL-12, IL-23, IL-27 and IFN-α. Type 2 factors present in the mucosal tissue activate sentinal DCs to become DC2 and tolerogenic factors will generate regulatory DCs, which are of therapeutic interest in autoimmune disease.

and fate of naive CD4$^+$ T lymphocytes, such as Th$_1$-, Th$_2$-, or T$_{reg}$- immune responses[38] (FIG. 2).

There are several arguments to adduce that dendritic cells play a pivotal role in active immunity against and tolerance toward gastrointestinal microorganisms. DCs are not just passive sentinels, but actively form transepithelial dendrites, which enable the cells to directly sample luminal bacteria.[39] After phagocytosis, DCs retain small numbers of live bacteria for several days to induce local immune responses[40] and systemic T-cell responses that regulate active immunity and tolerance toward gastrointestinal microorganisms.[41] Besides functional instruction, DCs induce the expression of gut-homing receptors (CCR9 and α4β7) that promote recirculation of T cells to the gastrointestinal mucosa (gut tropism).[42] Appropriate function of dendritic cells is dependent on the functionality of PRRs, and several reports have shown that CD is associated with genetic mutations of these receptors.[43–45] Two distinctive mucosal DC subsets have been described that differ in their expression of DC-sign and CD83, localization, and cytokine production. DC-sign+ DCs are present in the subepithelial compartment and submucosa in normal subjects, but are more pronounced, have a normal expression of CD80, and produce both interleukin-12 (IL-12) and interleukin-18 (IL-18) in CD.[46,47] The abundance of DCs within the mucosal compartment explains the significant numbers of T lymphocytes. Both immunohistochemistry and *ex vivo* experiments with lamina propria lymphocytes have identified a typical T helper 1 (Th1) immune response in CD with mainly CD4[+], interferon-γ (IFN)-γ-producing T cells.[48-50] The transcription factors T-bet and Stat4 are involved in the differentiation of Th1 lymphocytes and development of experimental colitis.[51-54] T-bet activation is induced upon co-stimulatory signals and results in upregulation of IL-12R and IFN-γ production,[52,55] and subsequently Stat4 can be activated by IL-12, which in turn results in final Th1 differentiation.[56]

Regulatory Cells

The regulation of immune responses involves maintenance of self-tolerance while retaining the ability to mount effective immune responses against invading microorganisms. Several types of regulatory T cells have been described, and it is important to distinguish natural and adaptive regulatory T cells on the basis of their origin, specificity, and mechanism of action[57] (TABLE 3). Although the bacterial flora is an important trigger for the development of CD, the role of natural regulatory T cells should not be neglected. Experimental colitis induced by the injection of naive T cells in severely combined immunodeficient

TABLE 3. A comparison of natural and adaptive regulatory cells

Feature	Natural T_{reg} cells	Adaptive T_{reg} cells
Site of induction	Thymus	Periphery
Differentiation characteristics		
Negative selection	Yes	Yes
Positive selection	Yes	Yes
Central tolerance	Yes	No
Peripheral tolerance	Possible	Yes
Mechanism of induction		
CD28-CD80/CD86	Yes	No
IL-2	Yes	Yes
Phenotype		
CD25 expression	Yes (high)	Variable
GITR	Yes	No
CTLA-4	Yes	Variable
FoxP3	Yes	No
Specificity	Self-antigens expressed in thymus	Tissue-specific antigens and foreign antigens
Mechanism of suppression		
Contact-dependent	Yes	Yes
Cytokine dependent	No	Yes

mice can be prevented by coinjection with $CD4^+CD25^+$ thymic-derived regulatory T cells.[58,59] The activation of fork head transcription factor *foxp3* and its gene product scurfin are required for the development of these natural regulatory T cells.[60,61] In contrast to naturally occurring regulatory T cells, two types of adaptive regulatory T cells have been described on the basis of phenotype and mechanisms of action. These include type 1 regulatory T cells (Tr1), which secrete high levels of interleukin-10 and low to moderate levels of TGF-beta and type 3 T regulatory cells (Th3), which primarily secrete TGF-β. The generation of Tr1 cells from naive or resting CD4+ T cells can be achieved by repetitive exposure to IL-10 and antigen; Tr1 cells mainly produce IL-10 but no IL-2 or IL-4.[62] Th3 cells were originally identified in mice after oral tolerance induction to myelin basic protein (MBP)[63] and have suppressive properties against Th1 and Th2 cells via the secretion of TGF-β.[64]

Danger Theory

It is remarkable that the immune system is able to distinguish between the endless diversity of molecules and how the decision is made to provoke an inflammatory response with often-substantial collateral damage to neighboring tissue. The "danger model" proposes that APCs are activated not only by foreign molecules, but also by danger signals from injured or distressed cells, and that especially the combination of exogenous foreign molecules and endogenous danger signals will lead to immunity (FIG. 3). Interestingly, there are now some reports showing that activation of APCs by exogenous pathogenic motifs in the absence of danger signals will lead to the development of immunoregulation. Antigen delivery of DCs via a monoclonal antibody directed against a DC-restricted endocytic receptor (DEC-205) in the absence of endogenous danger signals induces transient antigen-specific T-cell activation and subsequent T-cell deletion and unresponsiveness.

Nod2 Gene

The description of a genetic variation in Nod2 and its association with the occurrences of CD and Blau syndrome has increased the interest in this group of PRRs.[43,65,66] The Nod family shares a nucleotide-binding oligomerization domain, are localized within the cytosol, and often contain a C-terminal LRR and/or an N-terminal caspase-recruitment domain (CARD), suggesting that these receptors play a role in pattern recognition and apoptosis.[67] The Nod2 protein is expressed in myelomonocytic cells and has two N-terminal CARDs able to activate NF-κB via the intermediation of RICK.[68] Interestingly, proinflammatory mediators can induce the expression of Nod2 in intestinal epithelial cells,[69,70] and its overexpression in epithelial cells prevents intracellular survival of *Salmonella typhimurium*.[71] The expression of Nod2 in Paneth cells

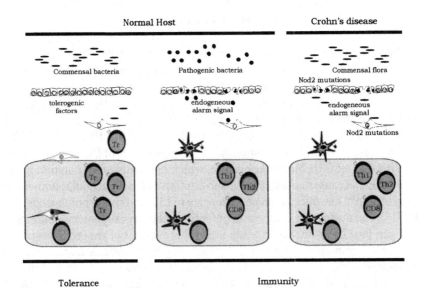

FIGURE 3. In a normal host there is adequate recognition of the normal commensal flora, and tolerogenic factors within the mucosal compartment will lead to the induction of regulatory DCs and Treg cells. Only pathogenic bacteria, possessing virulent factors, are able to disrupt the intestinal barrier significantly. In response several endogenous danger signals will lead to active immunity. In patients with CD the commensal flora is inadequately recognized and as a result endogenous danger signals will disrupt the induction of regulatory immune responses. Active immunity is insufficiently downregulated, and perpetuating events continuously activate the mucosal immune system, leading to chronic intestinal inflammation.

might be important for the secretion of defensins, influencing the establishment of a "healthy" commensal flora.[72,73] Initially Nod2 was regarded as an intracellular receptor for PGN, but biochemical and functional analysis showed that only a small part of PGN (a muramyl dipeptide) mediates activation of this receptor.[74,75] It is intriguing that a mutation in a receptor that activates NF-κB is involved in the pathogenesis of CD, while NF-κB is known to be overexpressed in inflamed tissue of CD patients. An explanation could be that Nod2 is a negative regulator of other PRR signaling[76]; however, a molecular mechanism was not eluded and other reports failed to substantiate these findings.[77] It should be noted that both authors adapted Nod2 mice and this could be an important difference compared to the human situation where a mutated Nod2 is present. In this light, studies with mice carrying a mutated Nod2 might be more representative of the human situation,[78] which suggests a gain-of-function instead of defective inhibitory function of Nod2. Clearly, Nod2 is involved in the response to muramyl dipeptides, but knowledge about its exact role in CD is lacking and important reports are conflicting. So far, it seems most reasonable to hypothesize that defective Nod2 signaling is a predisposing rather than an initiating factor for CD.

The Tlr4 Gene

There are three single nucleotide polymorphisms (SNPs) described for the *Tlr4* gene, each responsible for a different amino acid substitution: two are located in the extracellular domain, and one in the intracellular domain of the receptor. Persons with the allelic Asp299Gly and Thr399Ile substitution had decreased airway responsiveness after LPS inhalation, but only the Asp299Gly substitution was shown to be responsible for decreased NF-κB activation.[79] The possible relevance of *Tlr4* mutations for the development of CD is indicated by the *Tlr4* mutant C3H/HeJ mouse strain, which has a missense mutation in the *Tlr4* gene that causes an amino acid substitution in the intracellular domain of the receptor.[80] The mice are hyporesponsive to LPS and show spontaneous colitis.[80,81] The inadequate response to potential pathogenic organisms containing LPS can thus be protective in acute infectious events, but are predisposing to chronic inflammatory conditions. Altogether, genetic defects underlying CD are located within genes involved in recognition of conserved microbial motifs of the gastrointestinal flora and CD as a normal adaptive immune response to a deregulated innate immune system.

HOST BACTERIAL INTERACTION IN CD

Mucosal contact with luminal contents is essential for recurrent disease because mucosal inflammation is not present when the fecal stream is diverted by an ostomy proximal to anastomoses, but ulceration promptly recurs after restoration of bowel continuity.[82] This idea was further substantiated in a study in which a bypassed quiescent ileal segment was infused with ileostomy content; within 8 days after the start of infusion there were signs of inflammation on routine histological examination.[83] A comparable study was performed in which 22-nm ultra-filtrated ileostomy content was used to infuse the bypassed bowel segment. In this way it was established that especially bacteria or large food particles are responsible for recurrence of disease.[84] Higher concentrations of bacteria are present at the mucosal surface compared to healthy controls, and in addition these bacteria have the tendency to reside within epithelial cells and macrophages, more often indicating that the mucosal immune system of patients with CD is not capable of containing bacterial invasion.[85–87] Most likely, not one but multiple bacteria within the normal commensal intestinal flora are involved in the inflammatory response in CD. Although much effort has been put into the identification of a single causative microbial agent, not one single pathogen has shown to be exclusively related to CD.

Protective Microorganisms

The composition of the colonic flora with its more than 500 mainly strictly anaerobic species and its spatial and temporal complexity renders this a difficult ecosystem to study. The number of bacteria is lowest in the stomach, and also remains low in the small intestine. Microbial cells quickly rise to 10^{13} in the distal ileum and colon, exceeding the total number of eukaryotic cells in the human body.[88] Although the gastrointestinal microflora displays a remarkable functional stability, the composition is dynamic, containing native species that occupy a continuous niche as well as a variable set of transient species that only temporarily fill an empty niche, exhibiting complex behavior.[89] Bacterial cell-to-cell communication is known as "quorum sensing" and mediates bacterial behavior, such as biofilm formation, expression of virulence factors, sporulation, and motility.[90] Quorum-sensing is achieved via production and release of small soluble mediators, and detection can only take place when sufficient bacteria (a quorum) are present. The existence of competitive mechanisms between different bacterial species is a very attractive field of research; the identification of signaling molecules used by bacteria to prevent biofilm formation, invasive gene expression, and colonization could be employed for the development of new therapies of chronic infectious disease.[91] Not only is inter-bacterial signaling important for persistence of certain species, but also cross-talk between bacteria and their hosts provides species with an advantage in niche colonization.[92] Several symbiotic mechanisms have been described between plants and bacteria, and often this kind of regulation results in the development of visible structures (i.e., nodules and rhizobia). The formation of these structures appears to be mediated via signals secreted by the root, which induce bacteria to produce factors that elicit organogenesis in plants via PRRs.[93–95] These symbiotic processes are subjected to negative control mechanisms to sustain the delicate balance between hosts and microbes, and, of interest, PRRs containing LRR are involved in this process.[93,96] Comparable bacterial–bacterial and host–bacterial interactions occur in the human gastrointestinal tract, although quorum-sensing and biofilm formation have not been reported to exist within the gut.[97] Epithelial cells produce glycoconjugates favoring the colonization and growth of certain bacterial species that, in turn, influence epithelial gene expression,[98] including the expression of the antimicrobial substance angiogenin.[99] After initial colonization, bacterial activity will shape a metabolic environment that allows a more diverse composition of bacterial species.

Role of Bacteria in Promoting Immune Function

The development of the mucosa-associated immunity is functionally dependent on the presence of the bacterial microflora.[100,101] The composition and activity of the intestinal bacterial community has a significant impact on the health of the host because of its influence on nutrition, bowel habit, epithelial cell physiology, and the mucosal immune system,[88] and it is an important factor in colorectal cancer[102] and inflammatory bowel diseases.[103]

At the start of the 20th century, Metchnikoff postulated that the well-being of humans could be promoted through maintaining an intestinal microflora of correctly "balanced" composition. Because lactic acid–producing bacteria were able to inhibit the growth of proteolytic bacteria, one reasoned that domination of these bacteria in the intestinal microflora could protect against autointoxication from proteolytic bacterial products. Later, these protective bacteria were called *probiotics* and defined as living microorganisms that upon ingestion in specific numbers exert health benefits beyond those of inherent basic nutrition.[104] Like any bacteria, protective bacteria struggle for survival in a very complex microenvironment with multiple competitors residing in the same niche. In general, protective bacteria achieve their persistence in the gastrointestinal tract through secretion of antimicrobial substances and through symbiotic cross-talk with host cells. The secretion of antimicrobial substances and epithelial adherence might prevent small pathogenic events that often precede exacerbations of CD,[105,106] while symbiotic properties of protective bacteria promote epithelial physiology[107,108] and immune reactivity.[109,110]

Although there appears to be a sound rationale for the use of protective bacteria in the treatment of CD, large randomized controlled studies have not been reported, and smaller trials show contradictionary results.[111] Apparently, there is insufficient knowledge about the exact properties of currently available protective bacteria for effective drug design. Pathogenic bacteria use various evolutionarily adapted mechanisms to infect the host;[112] these virulence factors are necessary to penetrate natural barriers and spread within the host. However, for maintenance of infection it is crucial that the bacterium is able to avoid clearance by the host immune system. Therefore, several pathogenic bacteria produce immune-modulating factors or contain outer-membrane components that are able to subvert innate and adaptive immune responses.[113] *Yersinia enterocolitica* and *pseudotuberculosis* are highly virulent enteropathogens able to cause chronic infections, and, as their survival in nature is dependent on fecal transmission, their persistence within the gastrointestinal system is essential. *Yersinia* contains several strategies to infect a host, but the low calcium response protein V (LcrV) is of interest in this context. There, it prevents clearance by the immune system.[114–116] *Bordetella pertussis* is a Gram-negative bacterium that causes whooping cough, a protracted respiratory disease in young children. The protractive course of whooping cough is due to several strategies of *B. pertussis* to circumvent protective immune responses.[117] Filamentous haemagglutinin (FHA) functions primarily as a virulence factor, but it is also involved in the immune evasion of *B. pertussis*. FHA is able to induce IL-10 and inhibit LPS-induced IL-12 production by DCs, and the respiratory challenge of FHA leads to the induction of suppressor T cells that produce high amounts of IL-10 and inhibit protective Th1 responses against *B. pertussis*.[118] Inhibition of protective immune responses and the presence of suppressor T cells after *B. pertussis* infection appeared to be dependent on the presence of a functional TLR4 receptor.[119] FHA and LcrV are examples of bacterial-derived products involved in both virulence and immune evasion. It is likely that other microorganisms contain comparable compounds that provide the organism with an advantage in the establishment and persistence of infection. The identification and isolation of these microbial products could contribute to the development of potential new therapies for chronic inflammatory disease.

Bacteria as Delivery System

Topical treatment of disease has many advantages compared to systemic treatment, including the lower toxicity and higher biological availability of the active compound. Topical application of proteins is hampered by the large proteolytic activity present within the gut. Alternative strategies to circumvent this problem are gene therapy and genetic manipulation of certain microbial species that are able to (temporarily) reside at the mucosal surface. Bacteria can be genetically modified for the production of certain human proteins. *Lactococcus lactis* has been used for thousands of years for fermentation milk products and is therefore generally regarded as safe (GRAS). It has become possible to use this organism as an expression vector of human proteins. Despite its lack of invasiveness, *L. lactis* is able to deliver proteins to the mucosal immune system after oral ingestion, and treatment of colitogenic mice with IL-10–producing *L. lactis* has shown to be successful.[120] An ingenious suicidal system has been designed which does not allow the bacteria to multiply and/or survive in an environment that is lacking thymidine.[121] Hence bacteria, while ultimately being the cause of CD, as they trigger the exaggerated immune response underlying Crohn's disease, may also hold an important key to its treatment.

REFERENCES

1. SANDBORN, W., L. SUTHERLAND, D. PEARSON, *et al.* 2000. Azathioprine or 6-mercaptopurine for inducing remission of Crohn's disease. Cochrane Database Syst. Rev: CD000545.
2. ALFADHLI, A.A., J.W. MCDONALD & B.G. FEAGAN. 2003. Methotrexate for induction of remission in refractory Crohn's disease. Cochrane Database Syst. Rev: CD003459.
3. CROHN, B.B., L. GINZBURG & G.D. OPPENHEIMER. 1952. Regional ileitis: a pathologic and clinical entity. Am. J. Med. **13:** 583–590.
4. BOUMA, G. & W. STROBER. 2003. The immunological and genetic basis of inflammatory bowel disease. Nat. Rev. Immunol. **3:** 521–533.
5. SONWALKAR, S.A., R.M. JAMES, T. AHMAD, *et al.* 2003. Fulminant Crohn's colitis after allogeneic stem cell transplantation. Gut **52:** 1518–1521.
6. MACPHERSON, A.J., D. GATTO, E. SAINSBURY, *et al.* 2000. A primitive T cell-independent mechanism of intestinal mucosal IgA responses to commensal bacteria. Science **288:** 2222–2226.

7. GANZ, T. 2003. Microbiology: gut defence. Nature **422:** 478–479.
8. BARTON, G.M. & R. MEDZHITOV. 2002. Toll-like receptors and their ligands. Curr. Top. Microbiol. Immunol. **270:** 81–92.
9. JANEWAY, C.A. JR. & R. MEDZHITOV. 2002. Innate immune recognition. Annu. Rev. Immunol. **20:** 197–216.
10. JIANG, Q., S. AKASHI, K. MIYAKE, *et al.* 2000. Cutting edge: lipopolysaccharide induces physical proximity between CD14 and toll-like receptor 4 (TLR4) prior to nuclear translocation of NF-{kappa}B. J. Immunol. **165:** 3541–3544.
11. CHOW, J.C., D.W. YOUNG, D.T. GOLENBOCK, *et al.* 1999. Toll-like receptor-4 mediates lipopolysaccharide-induced signal transduction. J. Biol. Chem. **274:** 10689–10692.
12. PALSSON-MCDERMOTT, E.M. & L.A. O'NEILL. 2004. Signal transduction by the lipopolysaccharide receptor, toll-like receptor-4. Immunology **113:** 153–162.
13. SANDOR, F., E. LATZ, F. RE, *et al.* 2003. Importance of extra- and intracellular domains of TLR1 and TLR2 in NFkappa B signaling. J. Cell. Biol. **162:** 1099–1110.
14. VAN DER KLEIJ, D., E. LATZ, J.F. BROUWERS, *et al.* 2002. A novel host-parasite lipid cross-talk: schistosomal lyso-phosphatidylserine activates toll-like receptor 2 and affects immune polarization. J. Biol. Chem. **277:** 48122–48129.
15. MEANS, T.K., E. LIEN, A. YOSHIMURA, *et al.* 1999. The CD14 ligands lipoarabinomannan and lipopolysaccharide differ in their requirement for toll-like receptors. J. Immunol. **163:** 6748–6755.
16. NAKAO, Y., K. FUNAMI, S. KIKKAWA, *et al.* 2005. Surface-expressed TLR6 participates in the recognition of diacylated lipopeptide and peptidoglycan in human cells. J. Immunol. **174:** 1566–1573.
17. BUWITT-BECKMANN, U., H. HEINE, K.H. WIESMULLER, *et al.* 2005. Toll-like receptor 6-independent signaling by diacylated lipopeptides. Eur. J. Immunol. **35:** 282–289.
18. GANTNER, B.N., R.M. SIMMONS, S.J. CANAVERA, *et al.* 2003. Collaborative induction of inflammatory responses by dectin-1 and toll-like receptor 2. J. Exp. Med. **197:** 1107–1117.
19. HAJJAR, A.M., D.S. O'MAHONY, A. OZINSKY, *et al.* 2001. Cutting edge: functional interactions between toll-like receptor (TLR) 2 and TLR1 or TLR6 in response to phenol-soluble modulin. J. Immunol. **166:** 15–19.
20. OZINSKY, A., D.M. UNDERHILL, J.D. FONTENOT, *et al.* 2000. The repertoire for pattern recognition of pathogens by the innate immune system is defined by cooperation between toll-like receptors. Proc. Natl. Acad. Sci. USA **97:** 13766–13771.
21. FUJITA, M., T. INTO, M. YASUDA, *et al.* 2003. Involvement of leucine residues at positions 107, 112, and 115 in a leucine-rich repeat motif of human toll-like receptor 2 in the recognition of diacylated lipoproteins and lipopeptides and *Staphylococcus aureus* peptidoglycans. J. Immunol. **171:** 3675–3683.
22. ALEXOPOULOU, L., A.C. HOLT, R. MEDZHITOV, *et al.* 2001. Recognition of double-stranded RNA and activation of NF-kappaB by toll-like receptor 3. Nature **413:** 732–738.
23. FLO, T.H., L. RYAN, E. LATZ, *et al.* 2002. Involvement of toll-like receptor (TLR) 2 and TLR4 in cell activation by mannuronic acid polymers. J. Biol. Chem. **277:** 35489–35495.

24. YANG, S., S. SUGAWARA, T. MONODANE, *et al.* 2001. *Micrococcus luteus* teichuronic acids activate human and murine monocytic cells in a CD14- and toll-like receptor 4-dependent manner. Infect. Immun. **69:** 2025–2030.
25. SHOHAM, S., C. HUANG, J.M. CHEN, *et al.* 2001. Toll-like receptor 4 mediates intracellular signaling without TNF-alpha release in response to *Cryptococcus neoformans* polysaccharide capsule. J. Immunol. **166:** 4620–4626.
26. ZAMZE, S., L. MARTINEZ-POMARES, H. JONES, *et al.* 2002. Recognition of bacterial capsular polysaccharides and lipopolysaccharides by the macrophage mannose receptor. J. Biol. Chem. **277:** 41613–41623.
27. SMITH, K.D., E. ANDERSEN-NISSEN, F. HAYASHI, *et al.* 2003. Toll-like receptor 5 recognizes a conserved site on flagellin required for protofilament formation and bacterial motility. Nat. Immunol. **4:** 1247–1253.
28. LUND, J.M., L. ALEXOPOULOU, A. SATO, *et al.* 2004. Recognition of single-stranded RNA viruses by toll-like receptor 7. Proc. Natl. Acad. Sci. USA **101:** 5598–5603.
29. HEIL, F., H. HEMMI, H. HOCHREIN, *et al.* 2004. Species-specific recognition of single-stranded RNA via toll-like receptor 7 and 8. Science **303:** 1526–1529.
30. LATZ, E., A. SCHOENEMEYER, A. VISINTIN, *et al.* 2004. TLR9 signals after translocating from the ER to CpG DNA in the lysosome. Nat. Immunol. **5:** 190–198.
31. BANCHEREAU, J. & R.M. STEINMAN. 1998. Dendritic cells and the control of immunity. Nature **392:** 245–252.
32. MOSER, M. & K.M. MURPHY. 2000. Dendritic cell regulation of TH1-TH2 development. Nat. Immunol. **1:** 199–205.
33. WILSON, N.S., D. EL-SUKKARI, G.T. BELZ, *et al.* 2003. Most lymphoid organ dendritic cell types are phenotypically and functionally immature. Blood **102:** 2187–2194.
34. CHOW, A., D. TOOMRE, W. GARRETT, *et al.* 2002. Dendritic cell maturation triggers retrograde MHC class II transport from lysosomes to the plasma membrane. Nature **418:** 988–994.
35. KADOWAKI, N., S. HO, S. ANTONENKO, *et al.* 2001. Subsets of human dendritic cell precursors express different toll-like receptors and respond to different microbial antigens. J. Exp. Med. **194:** 863–870.
36. HUANG, Q., D. LIU, P. MAJEWSKI, *et al.* 2001. The plasticity of dendritic cell responses to pathogens and their components. Science **294:** 870–875.
37. LANZAVECCHIA, A. & F. SALLUSTO. 2000. From synapses to immunological memory: the role of sustained T cell stimulation. Curr. Opin. Immunol. **12:** 92–98.
38. KAPSENBERG, M.L. 2003. Dendritic-cell control of pathogen-driven T-cell polarization. Nat. Rev. Immunol. **3:** 984–993.
39. NIESS, J.H., S. BRAND, X. GU, *et al.* 2005. CX3CR1-mediated dendritic cell access to the intestinal lumen and bacterial clearance. Science **307:** 254–258.
40. MACPHERSON, A.J. & T. UHR. 2004. Induction of protective IgA by intestinal dendritic cells carrying commensal bacteria. Science **303:** 1662–1665.
41. ALPAN, O., G. RUDOMEN & P. MATZINGER. 2001. The role of dendritic cells, B cells, and M cells in gut-oriented immune responses. J. Immunol. **166:** 4843–4852.
42. JOHANSSON-LINDBOM, B., M. SVENSSON, M.A. WURBEL, *et al.* 2003. Selective generation of gut tropic T cells in gut-associated lymphoid tissue (GALT): requirement for GALT dendritic cells and adjuvant. J. Exp. Med. **198:** 963–969.

43. HUGOT, J.P., M. CHAMAILLARD, H. ZOUALI, et al. 2001. Association of NOD2 leucine-rich repeat variants with susceptibility to Crohn's disease. Nature 411: 599–603.

44. FRANCHIMONT, D., S. VERMEIRE, H. EL HOUSNI, et al. 2004. Deficient host-bacteria interactions in inflammatory bowel disease? The toll-like receptor (TLR)-4 Asp299gly polymorphism is associated with Crohn's disease and ulcerative colitis. Gut 53: 987–992.

45. VERMEIRE, S., G. WILD, K. KOCHER, et al. 2002. CARD15 genetic variation in a Quebec population: prevalence, genotype-phenotype relationship, and haplotype structure. Am. J. Hum. Genet. 71: 74–83.

46. TE VELDE, A., Y. VAN KOOYK, H. BRAAT, et al. 2003. Increased expression of DC-SIGN+IL-12+IL-18+ and CD83+IL-12-IL-18- dendritic cell populations in the colonic mucosa of patients with Crohn's disease. Eur. J. Immunol. 33: 143–151.

47. BECKER, C., S. WIRTZ, M. BLESSING, et al. 2003. Constitutive p40 promoter activation and IL-23 production in the terminal ileum mediated by dendritic cells. J. Clin. Invest. 112: 693–706.

48. CAMOGLIO, L., A.A. TE VELDE, A.J. TIGGES, et al. 1998. Altered expression of interferon-gamma and interleukin-4 in inflammatory bowel disease. Inflamm. Bowel Dis. 4: 285–290.

49. PARRONCHI, P., P. ROMAGNANI, F. ANNUNZIATO, et al. 1997. Type 1 T-helper cell predominance and interleukin-12 expression in the gut of patients with Crohn's disease. Am. J. Pathol. 150: 823–832.

50. FUSS, I.J., M. NEURATH, M. BOIRIVANT, et al. 1996. Disparate CD4+ lamina propria (LP) lymphokine secretion profiles in inflammatory bowel disease. Crohn's disease LP cells manifest increased secretion of IFN-gamma, whereas ulcerative colitis LP cells manifest increased secretion of IL-5. J. Immunol. 157: 1261–1270.

51. NEURATH, M.F., B. WEIGMANN, S. FINOTTO, et al. 2002. The transcription factor T-bet regulates mucosal T cell activation in experimental colitis and Crohn's disease. J. Exp. Med. 195: 1129–1143.

52. IIJIMA, H., M.F. NEURATH, T. NAGAISHI, et al. 2004. Specific regulation of T helper cell 1-mediated murine colitis by CEACAM1. J. Exp. Med. 199: 471–482.

53. SIMPSON, S.J., S. SHAH, M. COMISKEY, et al. 1998. T cell-mediated pathology in two models of experimental colitis depends predominantly on the interleukin 12/signal transducer and activator of transcription (Stat)-4 pathway, but is not conditional on interferon gamma expression by T cells. J. Exp. Med. 187: 1225–1234.

54. WIRTZ, S., S. FINOTTO, S. KANZLER, et al. 1999. Cutting edge: chronic intestinal inflammation in STAT-4 transgenic mice: characterization of disease and adoptive transfer by TNF- plus IFN-gamma-producing CD4+ T cells that respond to bacterial antigens. J. Immunol. 162: 1884–1888.

55. MULLEN, A.C., F.A. HIGH, A.S. HUTCHINS, et al. 2001. Role of T-bet in commitment of TH1 cells before IL-12-dependent selection. Science 292: 1907–1910.

56. AGNELLO, D., C.S. LANKFORD, J. BREAM, et al. 2003. Cytokines and transcription factors that regulate T helper cell differentiation: new players and new insights. J. Clin. Immunol. 23: 147–161.

57. BLUESTONE, J.A. & A.K. ABBAS. 2003. Natural versus adaptive regulatory T cells. Nat. Rev. Immunol. 3: 253–257.

58. ASSEMAN, C., S. READ & F. POWRIE. 2003. Colitogenic Th1 cells are present in the antigen-experienced T cell pool in normal mice: control by CD4+ regulatory T cells and IL-10. J. Immunol. **171:** 971–978.
59. MALOY, K.J., L. SALAUN, R. CAHILL, *et al.* 2003. CD4+CD25+ T(R) cells suppress innate immune pathology through cytokine-dependent mechanisms. J. Exp. Med. **197:** 111–119.
60. KHATTRI, R., T. COX, S.A. YASAYKO, *et al.* 2003. An essential role for Scurfin in CD4+CD25+ T regulatory cells. Nat. Immunol. **4:** 337–342.
61. FONTENOT, J.D., M.A. GAVIN & A.Y. RUDENSKY. 2003. Foxp3 programs the development and function of CD4+CD25+ regulatory T cells. Nat. Immunol. **4:** 330–336.
62. GROUX, H., A. O'GARRA, M. BIGLER, *et al.* 1997. A CD4+ T-cell subset inhibits antigen-specific T-cell responses and prevents colitis. Nature **389:** 737–742.
63. GONNELLA, P.A., Y. CHEN, J. INOBE, *et al.* 1998. In situ immune response in gut-associated lymphoid tissue (GALT) following oral antigen in TCR-transgenic mice. J. Immunol. **160:** 4708–4718.
64. CHEN, Y., V.K. KUCHROO, J. INOBE, *et al.* 1994. Regulatory T cell clones induced by oral tolerance: suppression of autoimmune encephalomyelitis. Science **265:** 1237–1240.
65. HAMPE, J., A. CUTHBERT, P.J. CROUCHER, *et al.* 2001. Association between insertion mutation in NOD2 gene and Crohn's disease in German and British populations. Lancet **357:** 1925–1928.
66. OGURA, Y., D.K. BONEN, N. INOHARA, *et al.* 2001. A frameshift mutation in NOD2 associated with susceptibility to Crohn's disease. Nature **411:** 603–606.
67. INOHARA, N. & G. NUNEZ. 2001. The NOD: a signaling module that regulates apoptosis and host defense against pathogens. Oncogene **20:** 6473–6481.
68. OGURA, Y., N. INOHARA, A. BENITO, *et al.* 2001. Nod2, a Nod1/Apaf-1 family member that is restricted to monocytes and activates NF-kappaB. J. Biol. Chem. **276:** 4812–4818.
69. GUTIERREZ, O., C. PIPAON, N. INOHARA, *et al.* 2002. Induction of Nod2 in myelomonocytic and intestinal epithelial cells via nuclear factor-kappa B activation. J. Biol. Chem. **277:** 41701–41705.
70. ROSENSTIEL, P., M. FANTINI, K. BRAUTIGAM, *et al.* 2003. TNF-alpha and IFN-gamma regulate the expression of the NOD2 (CARD15) gene in human intestinal epithelial cells. Gastroenterology **124:** 1001–1009.
71. HISAMATSU, T., M. SUZUKI, H.C. REINECKER, *et al.* 2003. CARD15/NOD2 functions as an antibacterial factor in human intestinal epithelial cells. Gastroenterology **124:** 993–1000.
72. OGURA, Y., S. LALA, W. XIN, *et al.* 2003. Expression of NOD2 in Paneth cells: a possible link to Crohn's ileitis. Gut **52:** 1591–1597.
73. LALA, S., Y. OGURA, C. OSBORNE, *et al.* 2003. Crohn's disease and the NOD2 gene: a role for Paneth cells. Gastroenterology **125:** 47–57.
74. INOHARA, N., Y. OGURA, A. FONTALBA, *et al.* 2003. Host recognition of bacterial muramyl dipeptide mediated through NOD2: implications for Crohn's disease. J. Biol. Chem. **278:** 5509–5512.
75. GIRARDIN, S.E., I.G. BONECA, J. VIALA, *et al.* 2003. Nod2 is a general sensor of peptidoglycan through muramyl dipeptide (MDP) detection. J. Biol. Chem. **278:** 8869–8872.

76. WATANABE, T., A. KITANI, P.J. MURRAY, et al. 2004. NOD2 is a negative regulator of toll-like receptor 2-mediated T helper type 1 responses. Nat. Immunol. **5:** 800–808.

77. KOBAYASHI, K.S., M. CHAMAILLARD, Y. OGURA, et al. 2005. Nod2-dependent regulation of innate and adaptive immunity in the intestinal tract. Science **307:** 731–734.

78. MAEDA, S., L.C. HSU, H. LIU, et al. 2005. Nod2 mutation in Crohn's disease potentiates NF-kappaB activity and IL-1beta processing. Science **307:** 734–738.

79. ARBOUR, N.C., E. LORENZ, B.C. SCHUTTE, et al. 2000. TLR4 mutations are associated with endotoxin hyporesponsiveness in humans. Nat. Genet. **25:** 187–191.

80. POLTORAK, A., X. HE, I. SMIRNOVA, et al. 1998. Defective LPS signaling in C3H/HeJ and C57BL/10ScCr mice: mutations in Tlr4 gene. Science **282:** 2085–2088.

81. HOSHINO, K., O. TAKEUCHI, T. KAWAI, et al. 1999. Cutting edge: toll-like receptor 4 (TLR4)-deficient mice are hyporesponsive to lipopolysaccharide: evidence for TLR4 as the Lps gene product. J. Immunol. **162:** 3749–3752.

82. RUTGEERTS, P., K. GOBOES, M. PEETERS, et al. 1991. Effect of faecal stream diversion on recurrence of Crohn's disease in the neoterminal ileum. Lancet **338:** 771–774.

83. D'HAENS, G.R., K. GEBOES, M. PEETERS, et al. 1998. Early lesions of recurrent Crohn's disease caused by infusion of intestinal contents in excluded ileum. Gastroenterology **114:** 262–267.

84. HARPER, P.H., E.C. LEE, M.G. KETTLEWELL, et al. 1985. Role of the faecal stream in the maintenance of Crohn's colitis. Gut **26:** 279–284.

85. SWIDSINSKI, A., A. LADHOFF, A. PERNTHALER, et al. 2002. Mucosal flora in inflammatory bowel disease. Gastroenterology **122:** 44–54.

86. GLASSER, A.L., J. BOUDEAU & N. BARNICH. 2001. Adherent invasive *Escherichia coli* strains from patients with Crohn's disease survive and replicate within macrophages without inducing host cell death. Infect. Immun. **69:** 5529–5537.

87. DARFEUILLE-MICHAUD, A., C. NEUT & N. BARNICH. 1998. Presence of adherent *Escherichia coli* strains in ileal mucosa of patients with Crohn's disease. Gastroenterology **115:** 1405–1413.

88. HOOPER, L.V., T. MIDTVEDT, & J.I. GORDON. 2002. How host-microbial interactions shape the nutrient environment of the mammalian intestine. Annu. Rev. Nutr. **22:** 283–307.

89. FALK, P.G., L.V. HOOPER, T. MIDTVEDT, et al. 1998. Creating and maintaining the gastrointestinal ecosystem: what we know and need to know from gnotobiology. Microbiol. Mol. Biol. Rev. **62:** 1157–1170.

90. TAGA, M.E. & B.L. BASSLER. 2003. Chemical communication among bacteria. Proc. Natl. Acad. Sci. USA 100: 14549–14554.

91. HENTZER, M. & M. GIVSKOV. 2003. Pharmacological inhibition of quorum sensing for the treatment of chronic bacterial infections. J. Clin. Invest. **112:** 1300–1307.

92. SPAINK, H.P. 2002. Plant-microbe interactions: a receptor in symbiotic dialogue. Nature **417:** 910–911.

93. KRUSELL, L., L.H. MADSEN, S. SATO, et al. 2002. Shoot control of root development and nodulation is mediated by a receptor-like kinase. Nature **420:** 422–426.

94. MADSEN, E.B., L.H. MADSEN, S. RADUTOIU, *et al.* 2003. A receptor kinase gene of the LysM type is involved in legume perception of rhizobial signals. Nature **425:** 637–640.
95. RADUTOIU, S., L.H. MADSEN, E.B. MADSEN, *et al.* 2003. Plant recognition of symbiotic bacteria requires two LysM receptor-like kinases. Nature **425:** 585–592.
96. NISHIMURA, R., M. HAYASHI, G.J. WU, *et al.* 2002. HAR1 mediates systemic regulation of symbiotic organ development. Nature **420:** 426–429.
97. HOOPER, L.V. & J.I. GORDON. 2001. Commensal host-bacterial relationships in the gut. Science **292:** 1115–1118.
98. HOOPER, L.V., M.H. WONG, A. THELIN, *et al.* 2001. Molecular analysis of commensal host-microbial relationships in the intestine. Science **291:** 881–884.
99. HOOPER, L.V., T.S. STAPPENBECK & C.V. HONG. 2003. Angiogenins: a new class of microbicidal proteins involved in innate immunity. Nat. Immunol. **4:** 269–273.
100. YAMANAKA, T., L. HELGELAND, I.N. FARSTAD, *et al.* 2003. Microbial colonization drives lymphocyte accumulation and differentiation in the follicle-associated epithelium of Peyer's patches. J. Immunol. **170:** 816–822.
101. RHEE, K.J., P. SETHUPATHI, A. DRIKS, *et al.* 2004. Role of commensal bacteria in development of gut-associated lymphoid tissues and preimmune antibody repertoire. J. Immunol. **172:** 1118–1124.
102. KADO, S., K. UCHIDA, H. FUNABASHI, *et al.* 2001. Intestinal microflora are necessary for development of spontaneous adenocarcinoma of the large intestine in T-cell receptor beta chain and p53 double-knockout mice. Cancer Res. **61:** 2395–2398.
103. SARTOR, R.B. 2004. Therapeutic manipulation of the enteric microflora in inflammatory bowel diseases: antibiotics, probiotics, and prebiotics. Gastroenterology **126:** 1620–1633.
104. GUARNER, F. & G.J. SCHAAFSMA. 1998. Probiotics. Int. J. Food Microbiol. **39:** 237–238.
105. FORESTIER, C., C. DE CHAMPS, C. VATOUX, *et al.* 2001. Probiotic activities of *Lactobacillus casei* rhamnosus: in vitro adherence to intestinal cells and antimicrobial properties. Res. Microbiol. **152:** 167–173.
106. MACK, D.R., S. MICHAIL, S. WEI, *et al.* 1999. Probiotics inhibit enteropathogenic *E. coli* adherence in vitro by inducing intestinal mucin gene expression. Am. J. Physiol. **276:** G941-G950.
107. BANASAZ, M., E. NORIN, R. HOLMA, *et al.* 2002. Increased enterocyte production in gnotobiotic rats mono-associated with *Lactobacillus rhamnosus* GG. Appl. Environ. Microbiol. **68:** 3031–3034.
108. GARCIA-LAFUENTE, A., M. ANTOLIN, F. GUARNER, *et al.* 2001. Modulation of colonic barrier function by the composition of the commensal flora in the rat. Gut **48:** 503–507.
109. KALLIOMAKI, M., S. SALMINEN, H. ARVILOMMI, *et al.* 2001. Probiotics in primary prevention of atopic disease: a randomised placebo-controlled trial. Lancet **357:** 1076–1079.
110. SCHIFFRIN, E.J., D. BRASSART, A.L. SERVIN, *et al.* 1997. Immune modulation of blood leukocytes in humans by lactic acid bacteria: criteria for strain selection. Am. J. Clin. Nutr. **66:** 515S-520S.
111. PRANTERA, C., M.L. SCRIBANO, G. FALASCO, *et al.* 2002. Ineffectiveness of probiotics in preventing recurrence after curative resection for Crohn's disease: a randomised controlled trial with *Lactobacillus* GG. Gut **51:** 405–409.

112. GALAN, J.E. & J.B. BLISKA. 1996. Cross-talk between bacterial pathogens and their host cells. Annu. Rev. Cell. Dev. Biol. **12:** 221–255.
113. HORNEF, M.W., M.J. WICK, M. RHEN, *et al.* 2002. Bacterial strategies for overcoming host innate and adaptive immune responses. Nat. Immunol. **3:** 1033–1040.
114. CORNELIS, G.R. 2002. The *Yersinia* Ysc-Yop 'type III' weaponry. Nat. Rev. Mol. Cell. Biol. **3:** 742–752.
115. SING, A., D. ROST, N. TVARDOVSKAIA, *et al.* 2002. *Yersinia* V-antigen exploits toll-like receptor 2 and CD14 for interleukin 10-mediated immunosuppression. J. Exp. Med. **196:** 1017–1024.
116. SING, A., A. ROGGENKAMP, A.M. GEIGER, *et al.* 2002. *Yersinia* enterocolitica evasion of the host innate immune response by V antigen-induced IL-10 production of macrophages is abrogated in IL-10-deficient mice. J. Immunol. **168:** 1315–1321.
117. MILLS, K.H. 2001. Immunity to *Bordetella pertussis*. Microbes Infect. **3:** 655–677.
118. McGUIRK, P., C. McCANN & K.H. MILLS. 2002. Pathogen-specific T regulatory 1 cells induced in the respiratory tract by a bacterial molecule that stimulates interleukin 10 production by dendritic cells: a novel strategy for evasion of protective T helper type 1 responses by *Bordetella pertussis*. J. Exp. Med. **195:** 221–231.
119. HIGGINS, S.C., E.C. LAVELLE, C. McCANN, *et al.* 2003. Toll-like receptor 4-mediated innate IL-10 activates antigen-specific regulatory T cells and confers resistance to *Bordetella pertussis* by inhibiting inflammatory pathology. J. Immunol. **171:** 3119–3127.
120. STEIDLER, L., W. HANS, L. SCHOTTE, *et al.* 2000. Treatment of murine colitis by *Lactococcus lactis* secreting interleukin- 10. Science **289:** 1352–1355.
121. STEIDLER, L., S. NEIRYNCK, N. HUYGHEBAERT, *et al.* 2003. Biological containment of genetically modified *Lactococcus lactis* for intestinal delivery of human interleukin 10. Nat. Biotechnol. **21:** 785–789.

Role of CEACAM1 as a Regulator of T Cells

TAKASHI NAGAISHI, HIDEKI IIJIMA, ATSUSHI NAKAJIMA,
DAOHONG CHEN, AND RICHARD S. BLUMBERG

*Gastroenterology Division, Brigham and Women's Hospital, Harvard Medical
School, Boston, Massachusetts 02115, USA*

ABSTRACT: A major inmmunological attribute of inflammatory bowel
disease (IBD) is the presence of unrestrained activation of T cells that
produce a variety of inflammatory cytokines and other mediators. Gaining an understanding of T cell regulation is therefore fo major importance to IBD. Carcinoembryonic antigen-related cell adhesion molecule
1 CEACAM1) is a novel protein that has been recently recognized as
being expressed by immune cells and T lymphocytes, in particular; this
protein appears to function as a coinhibitory receptor after T cell activation. Ligation of CEACAM1 on T cells induces a signal cascade that
leads inhibition of T cell cytokine production and IBD. CEACAM1 is
thus a novel potential therapeutic target in the treatment of IBD.

KEYWORDS: T lymphocytes; receptors; inhibition; inflammatory bowel
disease

INTRODUCTION

Inflammatory bowel disease (IBD) represents a dysregulated response of
the immune system associated within mucosal tissues to an environmental
antigen, which is most likely a component of the normal resident microbiota,
in a genetically susceptible host.[1] It is clear from numerous studies of human
tissues with IBD as well as in animal models that this dysregulated immune response is due to either an inappropriate drive to immune cell activation and/or
inadequate regulation of the immune system together with altered intestinal
epithelial cell (IEC) barrier function. The drivers of inflammation are mainly
derived from the interactions between antigen-presenting cells (APCs), most
importantly dendritic cells (DCs), and T cells through their inappropriate response to normal microbial antigens leading to the exaggerated upregulation

Address for correspondence: Richard S. Blumberg, Gastroenterology Division, Brigham and
Women's Hospital, Harvard Medical School, Boston, Massachusetts 02115 USA. Voice: 617-732-
6917; fax: 617-264-5185.
e-mail: rblumberg@partners.org

Ann. N.Y. Acad. Sci. 1072: 155–175 (2006). © 2006 New York Academy of Sciences.
doi: 10.1196/annals.1326.004

of a variety of cell surface molecules on the APC and T cells. These inter-actions distill into one of two final common pathways, which are associated with excess T helper 1 (Th1) and/or excess Th2 cytokines. At its origins, IBD thus evolves from dysregulated innate and adaptive immune responses to the mucosal microbiota that are presumably defined by the genetic composition of the host.

The major regulators of inflammation that have generated the most atten-tion and definition to date are those associated with a variety of T regulatory subsets that are either evolved from the thymus (CD4$^+$CD25$^+$ T cells) or that evolve in the periphery within mucosal tissues (T regulatory 1 cells or Tr1 and Th3 cells).[2] These cells have as a major feature the ability to secrete IL-10 and TGF-β and exhibit contact-dependent (perhaps through cell surface TGF-β) interactions that impose a profound suppression on the major drivers of immune response.[1,2] It has been recently and increasingly appreciated that regulation of inflammation and the inflammation of IBD, in particular, has many additional layers. These include the regulatory properties of B cells that have the ability to secrete IL-10[3,4] and the possibility that regulatory CD8$^+$ cells exist within the epithelial compartment.[5] Moreover, regulation of im-mune activation and thus IBD occurs at other levels of the immune response through a variety of mediators (FIG. 1). These include those that inhibit the inflammatory cascade and stimulate repair (e.g., cannabinoids, opioids, re-solvins, and lipoxins),[6–8] mediators that inhibit leukocyte extravasation (e.g., apoA-IV),[9] or intracellular signaling molecules that block proinflammatory cytokine and signaling cascades (e.g., PPAR γ and suppressors of cytokine synthesis).[10,11] Given these latter experimental observations, it has become clear that regulation of the immune response and, consequently, inflammation is a broadly expressed fabric of inhibitory networks that affect virtually all aspects of the cascade of events that extends from the initial antigen encounter to the production of inflammatory mediators.

Especially interesting are those negative regulators that impose themselves at the earliest time points of the immune response that take place when antigen recognition by the TCR/CD3 complex occurs. It has become clear that TCR/CD3 complex–mediated signaling is regulated both positively, by a variety of so-called costimulatory molecules, and negatively, by a variety of coinhibitory molecules. The costimulatory molecules that have been most well described include CD28 and CD28-related molecules such as ICOS, and a number of other non-CD28 family members.[12] Fewer examples of coin-hibitory molecules have been described for T lymphocytes and have mainly been shown to be CD28-related family members, such as CTLA-4 and PD-1.[13–14] Whereas costimulatory molecules facilitate TCR/CD3 complex sig-naling and thus T cell activation, coinhibitory molecules inhibit TCR/CD3 complex signaling. Molecules such as CTLA-4 and PD-1 are functionally related to a variety of other inhibitory receptors that have previously been de-scribed on B lymphocytes, such as inhibitory Fcγ receptors (FcγRIIb)[15] and inhibitory receptors on natural killer (NK) cells (killer inhibitory receptors).[16]

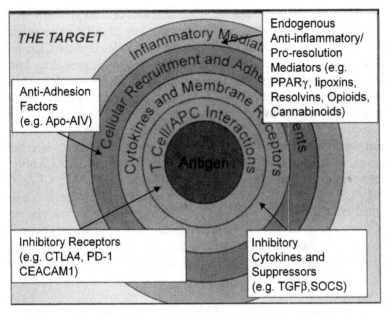

FIGURE 1. Layers of events in initiating an immune response as therapeutic target. *Boxes* highlight potential mechanisms of inhibition.

A common feature of these coinhibitory receptors is their expression within the cytoplasmic (cyt) tail of a characteristic motif, a so-called immunoreceptor tyrosine-based inhibitory motif (ITIM).[17] This motif, which consists of a characteristic amino acid sequence of I/VxYxxL/V, in single-letter amino acid code where x represents any amino acid, functions in a characteristic pathway that is notable for the recruitment of *Src* homology domain phosphatases (SHP)-1, SHP-2, or SHiP after phosphorylation of the tyrosine residue within the ITIM by *Src* family member-related kinases (SFKs). The relevance of these inhibitory pathways to immunobiology is best defined by the fact that lack of these inhibitory molecules, such as CTLA-4, leads to hyperproliferation of T cells and potentially autoimmunity.[18] Recently, our work has identified a potential novel function for carcinoembryonic antigen–related cell adhesion molecule 1 (CEACAM1) as a non-CD28-related coinhibitory molecule in T lymphocytes. Moreover, these studies have shown a role for this inhibitory function in the intestinal inflammation associated with IBD.

CEACAM1

Introduction

CEACAM1 is a member of the carcinoembryonic antigen (CEA) family, which engages in intercellular binding interactions affecting a wide variety of normal and pathogenic processes associated with cellular growth and differentiation. In humans, the CEA family is encoded by 29 different genes closely situated in chromosome 19q13.2. These are subdivided into the CEA-related cellular adhesion molecules (CEACAMs; FIG. 1) and the pregnancy-specific glycoproteins (PSGs) on the basis of protein homologies, developmental expression patterns, and that CEACAMs are typically cell surface–anchored, whereas PSGs are exclusively secreted. Individual CEACAMs are differentially expressed on various human cell types, such that one or more are present on most cells (FIG. 1). CEACAMs generally mediate intercellular adhesion via homophilic (CEACAM1, CEACAM5, and CEACAM6) and/ or heterophilic (CEACAM1–CEACAM5 [CEA], CEACAM5–CEACAM6, and CEACAM6–CEACAM8) binding.[19–22] While important studies have established critical roles for various CEA family members in vascular neogenesis,[23] insulin metabolism,[24] tissue architecture,[25,26] tumor development,[27] apoptosis,[26–28] and as receptors for pathogenic bacteria and viruses,[29,30] the impact of CEACAM1 on immune cell function has only recently been recognized.

CEACAM1 Expression, Structure, and Function

While not being ubiquitous, CEACAM1 (previously called biliary glycoprotein [BGP], C-CAM1, or CD66a) has the broadest tissue distribution among the CEA family (FIG. 2). In normal tissues, CEACAM1 is expressed by certain epithelial, endothelial, lymphoid, and myeloid cells.[31] CEACAM1 is the most

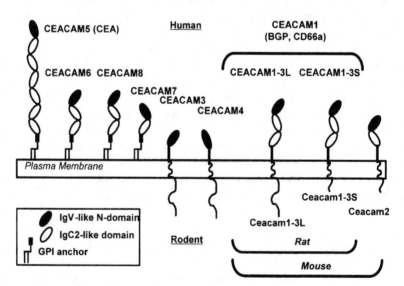

FIGURE 2. Model of carcinoembryonic antigen (CEA)–related molecules in humans and rodents. (Adapted from Öbrink.[31]).

highly conserved member of the CEA family, and appears to be the primordial CEACAM, given that it is the only member with obvious orthologues from rodents to man. The full-length protein consists of a membrane-distal Ig variable domain (IgV)-like amino (N)-terminal domain region that is highly conserved among all CEA family members, followed by up to three membrane-proximal C2-type Ig constant domain-related sequences. The N-domain consists of two stacked, anti-parallel β-sheets, which are held in apposition by a salt bridge. This domain mediates homophilic intercellular adhesion, and is the target for various bacterial and viral adhesins. The ligand-binding face is free of glycans, consistent with the protein–protein nature of these interactions. Unique among the Ig superfamily is an extended hairpin-like structure within the N-domain, which is formed by two (C and C′) β-strands folding back upon the ligand-binding surface.[32] This rigid, convoluted loop forms the receptor site for the murine hepatitis virus (MHV) spike protein, and contains residues involved in homophilic intercellular, and bacterial binding.

In humans, 11 different CEACAM1 splice variants have been detected from the single CEACAM1 gene that are named for the number of extracellular domains and the type of cytoplasmic tail.[33] The individual CEACAM1 isoforms differ with respect to the number of extracellular IgC2-like domains present,

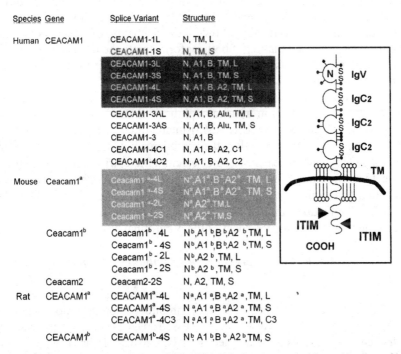

Species	Gene	Splice Variant	Structure
Human	CEACAM1	CEACAM1-1L	N, TM, L
		CEACAM1-1S	N, TM, S
		CEACAM1-3L	N, A1, B, TM, L
		CEACAM1-3S	N, A1, B, TM, S
		CEACAM1-4L	N, A1, B, A2, TM, L
		CEACAM1-4S	N, A1, B, A2, TM, S
		CEACAM1-3AL	N, A1, B, Alu, TM, L
		CEACAM1-3AS	N, A1, B, Alu, TM, S
		CEACAM1-3	N, A1, B
		CEACAM1-4C1	N, A1, B, A2, C1
		CEACAM1-4C2	N, A1, B, A2, C2
Mouse	Ceacam1^a	Ceacam1^a-4L	N^a,A1^a,B^a,A2^a,TM, L
		Ceacam1^a-4S	N^a,A1^a,B^a,A2^a,TM, S
		Ceacam1^a-2L	N^a,A2^a,TM,L
		Ceacam1^a-2S	N^a,A2^a,TM,S
	Ceacam1^b	Ceacam1^b-4L	N^b,A1^b,B^b,A2^b,TM, L
		Ceacam1^b-4S	N^b,A1^b,B^b,A2^b,TM, S
		Ceacam1^b-2L	N^b,A2^b,TM, L
		Ceacam1^b-2S	N^b,A2^b,TM, S
	Ceacam2	Ceacam2-2S	N, A2, TM, S
Rat	CEACAM1^a	CEACAM1^a-4L	N^a,A1^a,B^a,A2^a,TM, L
		CEACAM1^a-4S	N^a,A1^a,B^a,A2^a,TM, S
		CEACAM1^a-4C3	N^a,A1^a,B^a,A2^a,TM, C3
	CEACAM1^b	CEACAM1^b-4S	N^b,A1^b,B^b,A2^b,TM, S

FIGURE 3. Alternate splicing of CEACAM1 in humans and rodents. Naming of isoforms is according to Beauchemin *et al.*[33].

membrane anchorage, and/or the length of their cyt tail (long, L; short, S) (FIG. 3). In mice, only the CEACAM1-4L, -4S, -3L, and -3S have been detected. While the functional differences between CEACAM1 isoforms containing different numbers of extracellular domains remain unclear, the differential splicing of cytoplasmic domains have pronounced effects on the cellular response to CEACAM1 binding. Eight of the isoforms are anchored via a single hydrophobic membrane-spanning region followed by either a short (10–12 aa) or long (71–73 aa) cyt tail, while the other CEACAM1 variants lack a transmembrane domain and are thereby secreted. The long cyt tail contains two ITIMs. The short cytoplasmic domain-containing isoforms of CEACAM1 lack ITIM sequences.

Critically, the abundance of CEACAM1 protein and relative ratio of long and short isoforms are not static, and can vary significantly according to the cell type, its phase of growth, and activation state.[34] When at the cell surface, CEACAM1 appears to exist largely as a *cis*-homodimer.[31,35] Since the dimeric state has been proposed to regulate the receptor's ability to recruit effectors, including the SFKs and tyrosine phosphatases,[31] the equilibrium between monomeric and dimeric forms undoubtedly affects cellular responses to CEACAM1 binding. Dimerization is affected by intracellular calcium concentrations, as the binding of calcium-loaded calmodulin to membrane-proximal sequences within the receptor's cytoplasmic domain causes dissolution of the *cis*-dimers.[31] CEACAM1-L and CEACAM1-S splice variants can both undergo dimerization, presumably allowing the formation of dimers consisting of either one or a combination of both isoforms, with the balance presumably reflecting their relative expression levels. Given that both forms bind calmodulin, each dimer would be susceptible to intracellular calcium fluxes.

In addition to its propensity to exist as a *cis*-dimer within the cell membrane, CEACAM1 also engages in transhomophilic (CEACAM1–CEACAM1) and -heterophilic (CEACAM1–CEACAM5) intercellular binding as monomers. This monomeric state may reflect the arrangement of CEACAM1 at an immunological synapse (see below), since calcium fluxes triggered upon immune cell activation should cause calmodulin-dependent dissociation of *cis*-dimers. As with interactions between Ig family members, such as CD2,[36] CEACAM1-mediated interactions involve anti-parallel protein–protein interactions between the nonglycosylated β-sheet of the N-terminal domain.[37,38]

CEACAM1 Expression on Lymphoid Cell Types

CEACAM1 is an activation-induced cell surface molecule on T cells (see below) and NK cells, on which it is likely inhibitory through homophilic interactions.[39,40] Similarly, CEACAM1 is expressed on DCs[41] although the function in this context remains to be defined. Finally, CEACAM1 has been shown to be constitutively expressed on primary spleen B cells in the mouse.[42] Mouse B cells express both the 4 and 2 extracellular domain isoforms of CEACAM1 with equal ratios of the long and short cyt tails. The function of CEACAM1 on B cells has been reported to be either coinhibitory or costimulatory in *in vitro* studies.[43,44]

CEACAM1 EXPRESSION AND FUNCTION ON T CELLS

Introduction

Although early studies on mouse T cells suggested that CEACAM1 is not expressed on the cell surface, transcripts for CEACAM1 could be detected in resting T cells at low levels.[42] Consistent with this, we observed that CEACAM1 protein was expressed intracellularly in primary mouse spleen T cells and rapidly upregulated on the cell surface of CD4[+] and CD8[+] T cells after mitogen stimulation.[45] These studies indicate that CEACAM1 is an activation-induced cell surface molecule on T cells that, like CTLA-4,[14] may be rapidly mobilized from an intracellular compartment.

CEACAM1 is also an activation-induced cell surface molecule on human T cells. CEACAM1 is expressed at low levels on resting CD4[+] T cells but not on CD8[+] or $\alpha\beta^+$ T cells, such as intraepithelial lymphocytes (IEL).[46-49] After activation, CEACAM1 is rapidly and strongly upregulated on all classes of human T cells.[46,47,49-51] T cells express CEACAM1 *in vivo* in human tissues of the lamina propria of small intestine in celiac disease[49] and the large intestine of inflammatory bowel disease,[51] suggesting a functional role for CEACAM1 in immune-mediated diseases of the intestines (*vide infra*). Importantly, human IEL[49] and peripheral blood T (PBT) cells[47] do not express any CEACAM-related family member other than CEACAM1 after stimulation, suggesting a unique role for CEACAM1 in T cell function.

Although human CEACAM1 exhibits complex splicing to generate 11 alternative isoforms (FIG. 2), only a limited number have been detected in primary PBT cells by reverse-transcriptase (RT) polymerase chain reaction (PCR) amplification since no antibodies can distinguish between the various splice products. Resting (unstimulated) human T cells only express the CEACAM1-4L and -3L isoforms.[47,52] Upon stimulation, primary human PBT cells upregulate CEACAM1-L isoforms[47] without clear evidence of CEACAM1-S isoform expression.[52] Established T cell clones have been suggested to show qualitative evidence of CEACAM1-4L, -3L, -4S, and -3S transcripts, suggesting that long-term activation may increase CEACAM1-S expression.[51] Quantification of these transcript levels has not been performed. However, it would be predicted that CEACAM1-L isoforms are expressed predominantly over CEACAM1-S isoforms, extrapolating from rodent T cells.[52] These studies suggest that CEACAM1-S isoforms may play a role in regulating the function of CEACAM1-L isoforms in T cells, making it imperative to understand CEACAM1-S ratios in T cells.

Previous studies in epithelial model systems have indicated that CEACAM1-L-isoforms are commonly downregulated during neoplastic transformation[53] and inhibit *in vivo* growth of mouse breast, mouse IECs, mouse prostate, and human pancreatic cell tumors[54–57] in a process that is dependent upon SFKs, the ITIM domains, and SHP-1.[58,59] Consistent with this, several studies have suggested an inhibitory function for CEACAM1 isoforms expressing a long cyt tail in mouse and human T cells when stimulated with T cell–specific stimuli, resulting in inhibition of cytokine production, proliferation, and cytotoxicity.[45,47,49,50,60–63] In addition, human CEACAM1-4L has been shown to cocap with CD3 and SHP-1 and induce increased TCR/CD3 complex association with ZAP70 and calmodulin, suggesting entry of CEACAM1 into the immune synapse.[61]

However, two studies have suggested that ligation of CEACAM1 on PBMCs and established T cell clones under cross-linking conditions in the presence of anti-CD3 induces T cell activation.[47,51] Whether this is due to removal of CEACAM1 from the immune synapse under cross-linking conditions or some other mechanism is unknown. Another possibility is that CEACAM1-S isoforms may be activating and/or inhibitory to CEACAM1-L isoform function. CEACAM1-S isoform expression in T cells is controversial and requires further investigation, as noted above.[47,51,52] The human CEACAM1-4S isoform can induce apoptosis of human mammary epithelial cells consistent with an activating function for these isoforms.[64] As discussed below, in transiently transfected Jurkat T cells, human CEACAM1-3S alone, a model of the nonphysiologic situation, costimulated anti-CD28–induced activation in the presence of anti-CD3, and diminished the inhibitory function of concomitantly expressed CEACAM1-3L, a model of the physiologic context.[62] The mechanistic basis for this relationship between CEACAM1-L and CEACAM1-S isoforms is yet to be defined, but draws similarities between CEACAM1 splice variants and killer inhibitory/activating receptors,[65,66] which are also, interestingly, encoded on human chromosome 19.[66] They suggest that CEACAM1 is predominantly inhibitory on account of the overexpression of CEACAM1-L isoforms, but is a tunable signal transduction system because of the possible coexpression of CEACAM1-S isoforms.

Activation-Induced Expression of CEACAM1 on Mouse T Cells

We observed that whereas CD3$^+$ cells in the spleen showed little evidence of CEACAM1 expression on the cell surface, after activation with mitogens or other stimuli, CEACAM1 was rapidly upregulated on the cell surface within 30 min such that, by 24 h, virtually all T cells expressed this surface molecule. CEACAM1 expression was mainly detectable on blast cells and correlated kinetically with the expression of CD69. Upregulation of CEACAM1 was prior to that of CTLA-4 and not blocked by either cyclohexamide, actinomycin-D, or brefeldin, suggesting that CEACAM1 expression did not require either new RNA production or protein synthesis. Consistent with this, Western blotting or immunohistochemistry of purified T cells showed evidence of CEACAM1 protein expression intracellularly. To investigate this regulated expression of CEACAM1 on the cell surface, the interaction between the cyt tail of CEACAM1 and adaptor protein (AP)-1 and -2 was evaluated. Whereas AP-1 regulates protein transport between the trans-Golgi network in the endolysosomal system, AP-2 regulates protein sorting from the cell surface membrane to endolysosomal compartments. For these purposes, we generated a glutathione S-transferase (GST)- fusion protein of the mouse CEACAM1 long cyt tail. We further generated GST-cyt tail fusion proteins that were either phosphorylated on tyrosine residues or nonphosphorylated to pull down protein lysates from a variety of sources. By these approaches, we showed that the long cyt tail of CEACAM1 could bind to AP-1 and AP-2 when nonphosphorylated, but bind SHP-1 when phosphorylated. Finally, the expression of CEACAM1 on the cell surface of mouse T cells was presumed to be functional since a mAb that was specific for mouse CEACAM1 (CC1) (kindly provided by Kathryn V. Holmes, Colorado Health Sciences Center, Denver, CO)[67] could inhibit an allogeneic mixed lymphocyte reaction (MLR) between spleen mononuclear cells from Balb/c and C57BL/6 (B6) mice as well as inhibit the activation of spleen mononuclear cells when stimulated with anti-CD3 and anti-CD28. Moreover, administration of the CC1 antibody was able to inhibit a delayed-type hypersensitivity (DTH) response to oxazolone in the skin. These studies show that, like human T cells, CEACAM1 is expressed on the cell surface after activation and is functionally associated with T cell inhibition.

Characterization of CEACAM1 Effects upon Th1 and Th2 Cytokine Production

We generated a model transfection system with either the human CEACAM1-3L (3L) or CEACAM1-3S (3S) isoforms, which represent a model of a CEACAM1 isoform containing a long and a short cyt tail, respectively, but yet contain the same number of extracellular domains.[62] These isoforms were engineered into an expression vector that allowed for transient transfections in Jurkat cells that were stably transfected with the SV40-large T antigen (Jurkat-T). Jurkat cells do not normally express CEACAM1.[51] In these studies, Jurkat-T cells were transiently transfected with either the empty vector, 3S, 3L, 3L with mutated ITIM domains (3L-YY) or both the 3L plus 3S isoforms. The latter was performed to model the events that might occur in a normal T cell wherein both long and short isoforms are expressed. These studies showed that, in comparison to the vector control, the 3L isoform, but not the 3S isoform, inhibited both Th1 (interferon-γ or IFN-γ) and Th2 (IL-4) cytokine secretion. This inhibition of Th1 and Th2 cytokine secretion by the 3L isoform was decreased by deletion of the two ITIM domains, silencing of SHP-1 expression using small inhibitory (si) RNAs, or cotransfection with the 3S isoform. These studies show that the 3L isoform can inhibit Th1 and Th2 expression in a model T cell line when overexpressed and that this inhibition is dependent upon the ITIM domains and the ability of the CEACAM1 isoform to interact with SHP-1. Interestingly, the release of inhibition mediated by the 3L isoform by cotransfection with the 3S isoform has several potential interpretations. These included either a dominant-negative effect through dimerization with the 3L isoform, thus diluting its potential inhibitory properties or a direct stimulatory effect of the 3S isoform. Although both interpretations remain possible, other studies performed suggest that CEACAM1 isoforms expressing a short cyt tail may, in fact, have the property of costimulating T cell function, suggesting that CEACAM1 isoforms may be a tunable system that is regulated by the ratio of short and long cyt tail domain-containing isoforms.[57]

In a related group of studies, the effects of CEACAM1 ligation on Th1 and Th2 cytokine production was also examined with primary mouse T cells.[60] To perform these studies, we took advantage of the known heterophilic ligation of CEACAM1 by the MHV spike glycoprotein that binds the N-domain.[30,67] MHV spike glycoprotein (kindly provided by Dr. K. V. Holmes) was added to primary spleen T cells either during T cell differentiation under Th1 (in the presence of anti-CD3 and -CD28 plus IL-12, IL-2, and anti-IL-4) or Th2-inducing (anti-CD3 and anti-CD28 plus IL-4 and anti-IL-12) conditions. Alternatively, the MHV spike glycoprotein was added to T cells that had been differentiated into Th1- or Th2-deviated cells and restimulated with anti-CD3 and anti-CD28. This approach allowed an analysis of the effects of CEACAM1 ligation on the differentiation of T cells into Th1 or Th2 effectors or the ability of differentiated Th1 or Th2 effectors to secrete their respective cytokines. These studies showed that, in contrast to overexpression of human CEACAM1 on a model human T cell line, ligation of endogenous CEACAM1 on a primary mouse T cell resulted in inhibition of Th1 (IFN-γ but not Th2 (IL-4) differentiation and secretion. Moreover, the specific effect of CEACAM1 ligation on Th1, but not Th2, pathways on primary mouse spleen T cells was, interestingly, consistent with the effects of CEACAM1 ligation *in vivo* during the course of either trinitrobenzene sulfate (TNBS) or oxazolone-induced colitis wherein *in vivo* treatment of mice with either a heterophilic (CEACAM1-specific antibody) or homophilic (N-domain Fc fusion protein) ligand led to amelioration of colitis in association with a specific decrease of Th1 (IFN-γ, but not Th2 (IL-4), cytokine secretion. Whether these differences in effects between CEACAM1 ligation and Th1 and Th2 cytokine differentiation and secretion are due to the relative levels of CEACAM1 that are achieved on transfected cells versus endogenously activated cells, they do suggest that Th1 pathways may be more sensitive to inhibition than Th2 pathways. Such a hypothesis is consistent with prior studies on another inhibitory receptor that is expressed on T cells, PD-1, which shows increased sensitivity of Th1 relative to the Th2 pathways.[68]

CEACAM1 Ligation with a CEACAM1-Fc Fusion Protein is Associated with T Cell Inhibition

We generated a CEACAM1-Fc fusion protein expressing three extracellular domains of CEACAM1 as would be contained in the CEACAM1-3L isoform. These constructs were expressed in CHO cells and the CEACAM1-Fc fusion proteins purified with protein A. This CEACAM1-Fc fusion protein potently inhibited a human allogeneic MLR at doses between 1 and 2 μg/mL; concentrations that were nearly as inhibitory as CTLA-4-Ig (inhibition between 0.25–1 μg/mL). These studies show that homophilic ligation of CEACAM1 as modeled with a CEACAM1-Fc fusion protein can mediate T cell inhibition. Similar observations were made with a 4-domain CEACAM1-Fc fusion protein modeling CEACAM1-4L (unpublished observations in collaboration with Dr. Nalan Utku, Berlin; see letter of collaboration). Moreover, as will be discussed in some detail below, this homophilic ligation is clinically relevant since a mouse N-domain CEACAM1-Fc fusion protein (kindly provided by Dr. Thomas Gallagher, Loyola University, Chicago, IL)[69] was able to mediate suppression of oxazolone colitis in association with specific inhibition of Th1 cytokine production (see below).

Characterization of the Homophilic-Binding Sites in the N-Domain of CEACAM1 for Lymphocyte Interactions

Over the past several years, CEACAM1 has been characterized on NK cells.[38,39,40] These studies have shown that after activation-induced expression of CEACAM1 on NK cells, CEACAM1 mediates inhibition of NK cell function independently of MHC class I. These studies have shown how CEACAM1 through homophilic ligation with CEACAM1 on either a normal or transformed cell type can ligate CEACAM1 on the activated NK cell and inhibit this function. This inhibition has also been shown to be mediated by the cyt tail of CEACAM1.

It was specifically shown that critical residues ([43]Arg and [44]Gln) within the N-domain and adjacent to the C-C′ loop (see FIG. 3) and thus the homophilic-binding site as described by the crystallographic solution of the mouse N-domain,[32] is also involved in homophilic interactions between CEACAM1 on an NK cell and another CEACAM1 molecule in trans on an apposing cell as modeled with a CEACAM1-Fc fusion protein.[30] Mutation of the critical [43]Arg and [44]Gln residues abrogated this homophilic interaction and the ability of the CEACAM1-Fc fusion protein to induce inhibition of NK cell function. Thus, [43]Arg and [44]Gln residues are critical for CEACAM1 homophilic binding and CEACAM1-mediated inhibition of NK cell cytotoxicity.

These studies show how critical residues within the N-domain may mediate homophilic ligation of CEACAM1. Moreover, it is highly interesting that the homophilic-binding region of CEACAM1 is also shared with the heterophilic binding of both mouse hepatitis virus (MCV)[67] and antibodies that are functionally important in regulating lymphocyte function. In this regard, in collaboration with Dr. Sue Watt (MRC Hematology Unit, Oxford, UK), we have shown that the 5F4 monoclonal antibody, which was originally generated by us,[49] binds in the functionally important regions of the N-domain around the C-C' loop.[37] Specifically, in the studies with Dr. Watt using mutated human CEACAM1-Fc fusion proteins, it was shown that binding of the 5F4 monoclonal antibody to the N-domain of CEACAM1 was abrogated by mutations, such as 39Val, which are directly adjacent to the C-C' loop and predicted to unfold this critical domain (see FIG. 3). In total, these studies show that homophilic and heterophilic ligation of CEACAM1 in critical regions within the N-domain mediates inhibition of multiple lineages of lymphocytes, including NK and presumably T cells *in vitro*.

Intracellular Signaling Mechanisms Associated with CEACAM1 Long Isoform Function

To model CEACAM1 long cyt tail–containing isoform function and its relationship to isoforms expressing a short cyt tail, a Jurkat-T cell transfection model was established, as briefly summarized in FIGURE 4. Jurkat-T cells were transiently transfected with an NFAT-AP1 luciferase reporter construct together

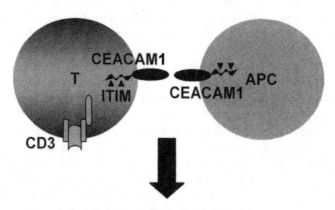

Inhibition of T cell signaling
→ ITIM → SHP-1
→ MAPK → ↓ t-bet/GATA3
→ ↓ Th1/Th2

FIGURE 4. Mechanism of inhibition mediated by CEACAM1 after homophilic adhesion. Details are in text.

with the wild-type human 3L, wild-type human 3S, or human 3L isoform in which either the intracellular cyt tail membrane proximal tyrosine (459Tyr) or membrane distal cyt tail tyrosine (486Tyr), as part of the two ITIM domains, were mutated. In these studies, after transient transfection, Jurkat-T cells were subjected to either no stimulation or stimulation with anti-CD3 plus anti-CD28. It was observed that the 3L isoform potently inhibited the TCR/CD3-induced activation as manifest by a dramatic diminution in relative luciferase activity. Interestingly and notably, the CEACAM1-3S isoform stimulated NFAT-AP1 luciferase reporter activity, even in the resting state in the absence of anti-CD3 and anti-CD28 stimulation, and partially reversed the inhibitory functions of the 3L splice variant when cotransfected together with this isoform. As suggested above, and to be described in more detail below, this is consistent with a presumed weak costimulatory effect of the 3S splice variant as opposed to a dominant-negative effect of the 3S splice variant on the function of 3L.

This ability of the 3L splice variant to inhibit anti-CD3 plus anti-CD28-induced activation of Jurkat-T cells was not abrogated by mutation of either 459Tyr or 486Tyr individually. However, when both tyrosine residues and, therefore, both ITIM domains were mutated, the ability of the 3L isoform to inhibit was almost completely lost. The 3L isoform was also unable to inhibit in the absence of SHP-1 expression, as achieved by silencing SHP-1 with siRNA. The 3L isoform was also able to inhibit anti-CD3 and anti-CD28–induced activation of MAPK pathways, specifically the phosphorylation of C-Jun N-terminal kinase (JNK) and extracellular response kinase (ERK), but not p38. This ability of the 3L splice variant to inhibit phosphorylation of JNK and ERK was also dependent upon the presence of SHP-1 and the two ITIM domains since silencing of SHP-1 or mutation of the two tyrosine residues reversed the inhibition of the MAPK pathway. This inhibition of JNK and ERK is consistent with the inhibition of Th1 and Th2 cytokine production by CEACAM1 ligation, given the relationship between JNK and ERK with Th1 and Th2 cytokine pathways, respectively.[70] Moreover, given that the only source of ligand in these studies was the transfected CEACAM1 on the Jurkat-T cells, and given that Jurkat cells do not normally express CEACAM1 unless transfected,[51] these studies indicate that it is the homophilic ligation of CEACAM1 on the Jurkat-T cells after transfection that likely provides the inhibitory signal and has implications for understanding T–T interactions.

Regulation of Murine Colitis by CEACAM1

Since CEACAM1 is an activation-induced molecule, we reasoned that ligation of CEACAM1 and, therefore, mediation of its inhibitory functions may be most appreciable during an ongoing immune response. Therefore, the effects of CEACAM1 ligation on the development of colitis was tested in a model system wherein a CEACAM1-specific mAb (CC1) or control antibody was administered before the sensitization phase (skin-painting) or the rectal challenge phase during the evolution of hapten-mediated colitis models as previously described by us and others[71,72] (FIG. 5). These studies showed that the CC1 mAb was able to inhibit TNBS colitis when administered prior to the rectal challenge (effector) phase, but not the sensitization (skin-painting) phase. This amelioration of colitis was specifically associated with inhibition of Th1 (IFN-γ) but not Th2 (IL-4) cytokine production by lamina propria lymphocytes (LPLs). In a similar manner, the CC1 mAb also inhibited the development of oxazolone colitis, in association with specific inhibition of Th1, but not Th2, cytokine production. Proof that this was associated with specific inhibition of Th1 cytokine production *in vitro* was provided by evidence that this was associated with decreased nuclear translocation of T-bet, the master transcription factor for Th1 pathways,[71] but not GATA-3. During the course of these studies, we further observed that the oxazolone colitis model in the B6 genetic background was a mixed Th1Th2 colitis, in that the colitis could be ameliorated by deletion of the IFN-γ or IL-4 genes, respectively.[60]

The specific inhibition of Th1, but not Th2, cytokines *in vitro* by ligation of CEACAM1 *in vivo* with the CC1 mAb, was consistent with *in vitro* studies of purified T cells wherein ligation with a natural heterophilic ligand for CEACAM1, the MHV spike glycoprotein,[67] also specifically inhibited Th1, but not Th2, cytokines.[55] Similar observations were made when the natural ligand for CEACAM1 was tested in the oxazolone colitis model. Specifically, administration of an N-domain Fc fusion protein of mouse CEACAM1 (kindly provided by Dr. Thomas Gallagher, Loyola University, Chicago, IL)[69] also inhibited colitis clinically and pathologically in association with specific inhibition of Th1, but not Th2, cytokines.

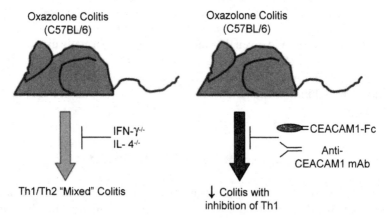

FIGURE 5. *In vivo* effects of CEACAM1 ligation in oxazolone-treated colitis. Details are in text.

Together, these studies lead to the exciting possibility that CEACAM1-specific reagents can inhibit diseases marked by T cell activation. These include colitis and, as shown in other studies performed in collaboration with Dr. Nalan Utku (Charité Humboldt Hospital, Berlin, Germany), CEACAM1 ligation with a homophilic ligand (human CEACAM1 4-domain-Fc fusion protein) inhibits collagen-induced arthritis (a model of rheumatoid arthritis) and experimental allergic encephalitis (a model of multiple sclerosis) (unpublished observations). Because CEACAM1 expression is induced by activation on T cells, CEACAM1-mediated inhibitory signaling may be most evident after the cell is stimulated, which, together with the broad expression of CEACAM1 on hematopoietic cells, makes CEACAM1 an interesting experimental target in immune-mediated diseases, such as colitis.

HYPOTHETICAL MODEL OF CEACAM1 FUNCTION ON T CELLS

As described in preliminary studies and the studies of others, in a resting T cell, CEACAM1 is likely expressed as CEACAM1-L *cis*-dimers[47,52,61] that exist intracellularly with very low levels on the cell surface. (FIG. 6)[45,47] Given the association between the long cyt tail of mouse CEACAM1 and AP-1 and AP-2,[45] CEACAM1 may be a rapidly recycling molecule that exists preferentially in lipid rafts.[61] With TCR activation, the predominantly *cis*-dimeric structure of CEACAM1 would be predicted to favor association

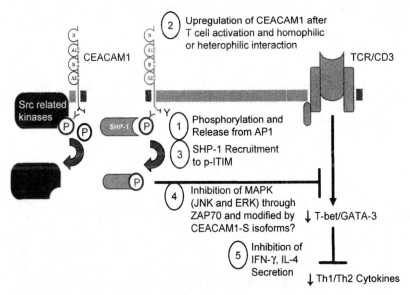

FIGURE 6. Model of signaling mediated by CEACAM1 that are related to inhibitory functions. Details are in text.

and phosphorylation by the *src*-kinases, *lck,* and *fyn*, which are known to phosphorylate the long CEACAM1 cyt tail *in vitro*.[73] Tyrosine phosphorylation of the YxxΦ motif of CEACAM1 would release it from internalization by AP-2 and allow for stabilization on the cell surface;[74] similar to that proposed for CTLA-4 release to the cell surface.[74] Moreover, the elevated calcium levels intracellularly induced by PLC activation would favor calmodulin-induced dissociation of CEACAM1-L *cis*-dimers.[35] The formation of CEACAM1-L monomers would favor and be further promoted by the cell–cell contact induced by TCR signaling and the allowance for homophilic ligation if the APC is a CEACAM1-bearing cell (e.g., a B cell, macrophage, or DC).[41,42] CEACAM1 ligation is predicted to occur in trans (between two cell types) under the monomeric state.[75–77]

TCR signaling will also activate Rho-GTPases downstream of the *syk*-related tyrosine kinase, ZAP70, leading to cytoskeletal rearrangements.[78] CEACAM1-L isoform localization to the points of cell–cell contact are known to be regulated by Rho, Rac, and Pak1-induced cytoskeletal rearrangements in fibroblasts and epithelial cells[79,80] consistent with the association of CEACAM1-L cyt tail association with actin.[81] This makes it possible that similar processes downstream of TCR signaling will have a similar consequence leading to the entry of CEACAM1 into the TCR signalosome.[82] Indeed, CEACAM1 cocapping with CD3 is supportive of this, as noted.[61] This would place CEACAM1 in a critical location to regulate TCR/CD3 complex function. At this location, association of SHP-1 with the phosphorylated ITIM domains of CEACAM1, which is known to functionally occur in human, and, probably, mouse T cells *in* vitro on the basis of our preliminary studies,[61,62] would be further predicted to result in dephosphorylation of *src*- and *syk*-kinases, which are known to associate with TCR signaling.[83] Most important among these is the *syk*-related kinase, ZAP70. The possibility that SHP-1 in association with CEACAM1 might dephosphorylate ZAP70 is very important since ZAP70 is critical to the integration of TCR signaling and mobilization of intracellular calcium, cytoskeletal rearrangements and mitogen-activated protein kinase (MAPK) pathway activation.[78]

CONCLUSION

The identification of CEACAM1 as a novel non-CD28-related coinhibitory receptor that may mediate inhibition of TCR/CD3 complex function and, consequently, intestinal inflammation has highly significant implications for understanding T cell regulation and the treatment of colitis. Elucidating the molecular mechanisms of the apparent T cell inhibition by CEACAM1-L, the relationship between the long and short cyt tails of CEACAM1 and the possibility that T cell expression of CEACAM1 may mediate T–T regulation are major areas for future study.

ACKNOWLEDGMENTS

This work was funded by NIH grants: DK44319, DK5136, and DK53056; The Crohn's and Colitis Foundation of America; and The Harvard Digestive Diseases Center.

REFERENCES

1. STROBER, W., I.J. FUSS & R.S. BLUMBERG. 2002. The immunology of mucosal models of inflammation. Annu. Rev. Immunol. **20:** 495–549.
2. UHLIG, H.H. & F. POWRIE. 2005. The role of mucosal T lymphocytes in regulating intestinal inflammation. Springer Semin. Immunopathol. **27:** 167–180.
3. VELAZQUEZ, P., B. WEI & J. BRAUN. 2005. Surveillance B lymphocytes and mucosal immunoregulation. Springer Semin. Immunopathol. **26:** 453–462.
4. MIZOGUCHI, A., E. MIZOGUCHI, *et al.* 2002. Chronic intestinal inflammatory condition generates IL-10 producing regulatory B cell subset characterized by CD1d upregulation. Immunity **16:** 219–230.
5. BRIMNES, J., M. ALLEZ, *et al.* 2005. Defects in CD8+ regulatory T cells in the lamina propria of patients with inflammatory bowel disease. J. Immunol. **174:** 5814–5822.
6. KUNOS, G. & P. PACHER. 2004. Cannabinoids cool the intestine. Nat. Med. **10:** 678–679.
7. FIORUCCI, S., J.L. WALLACE, *et al.* 2004. A beta-oxidation-resistant A4 analog treats hapten-induced colitis by attenuating inflammation and immune dysfunction. Proc. Natl. Acad. Sci. USA **101:** 15736–15741.
8. MAKOTO, A., M. YOSHIDA, *et al.* 2005. Resolvin E1, an endogenous lipid mediator derived from omega-3 eicosapentaenoic acid, protects against 2,4,6-trinitrobenzene sulfonic acid-induced colitis. Proc. Natl. Acad. Sci. USA **102:** 7671–7676.
9. VOWINKEL, T., M. MORI, *et al.* 2004. Apolipoprotein A-IV inhibits experimental colitis. J. Clin. Invest. **114:** 260–269.
10. WADA, K., A. NAKAJIMA & R.S. BLUMBERG. 2001. PPARγ and inflammatory bowel disease: a new therapeutic target for ulcerative colitis and Crohn's disease. Trends Molec. Med. **7:** 329–331
11. NAKAJIMA, A., K. WADA, H. MIKI, *et al.* 2001. Endogenous PPARγ mediates anti-inflammatory activity in murine ischemia-reperfusion injury. Gastroenterology **120:** 460–469.
12. KEIR, M.E. & A.H. SHARPE. 2005. Th B7/CD28 costimulatory family in autoimmunity. Immunol. Rev. **204:** 128–143.
13. VON BOEHMER, H. 2005. Mechanisms of suppression by suppressor T cells. Nat. Immunol. **6:** 338–344.
14. GREENWALD, R.J., G.J. FREEMAN & A.H. SHARPE. 2005. The B7 family revisited. Annu. Rev. Immunol. **23:** 515–548.
15. MCGAHA, T.L., B. SORRENTINO & J.V. RAVETCH. 2005. Restoration of tolerance in lupus by targeted inhibitory receptor expression. Science **307:** 590–593.
16. HSU, K.C. & B. DUPONT. 2005. Natural killer cell receptors: regulating innate immune responses to hematologic malignancy. Semin. Hematol. **42:** 91–103.
17. TAYLOR, L.S., S.P. PAUL & D.W. MCVICAR. 2000. Paired inhibitory and activating receptor signals. Rev. Immunogenet. **2:** 204–219.

18. NEEL, B.G., H.J. GU & L. PAO. 2003. The 'Shp'ing news: SH2 domain-containing tyrosine phosphatases in cell signaling. Trends Biochem. Science **28:** 284–293.
19. BENCHIMOL, S. *et al.* 1989. Carcinoembryonic antigen, a human tumor marker, functions as an intercellular adhesion molecule. Cell **57:** 327–334.
20. ROBITAILLE, J. *et al.* 1999. Comparison of expression patterns and cell adhesion properties of the mouse biliary glycoproteins Bbgp1 and Bbgp2. Eur. J. Biochem. **264:** 534–544.
21. OIKAWA, S. *et al.* 1991. A specific heterotypic cell adhesion activity between members of carcinoembryonic antigen family, W272 and NCA, is mediated by N-domains. J. Biol. Chem. **266:** 7995–8001.
22. STERN, N. *et al.* 2005. Carcinoembryonic antigen (CEA) inhibits NK killing via interaction with CEA-related cell adhesion molecule 1. J. Immunol. **174:** 6692–6701.
23. WAGENER, C. & S. ERGUN. 2000. Angiogenic properties of the carcinoembryonic antigen-related cell adhesion molecule 1. Exp. Cell. Res. **261:** 19–24.
24. NAJJAR, S.M. 2002. Regulation of insulin action by CEACAM1. Trends Endocrinol. Metab. **13:** 240–245.
25. ILANTZIS, C., L. DEMARTE, *et al.* 2002. Deregulated expression of the human tumor marker CEA and CEA family member CEACAM6 disrupts tissue architecture and blocks colonocyte differentiation. Neoplasia **4:** 151–163.
26. KIRSHNER, J., C.J. CHEN, P. LIU, *et al.* 2003. CEACAM1-4S, a cell-cell adhesion molecule, mediates apoptosis and reverts mammary carcinoma cells to a normal morphogenic phenotype in a 3D culture. Proc. Natl. Acad. Sci. USA **100:** 521–526.
27. FOURNES, B., S. SADEKOVA, C. TURBIDE, *et al.* 2001. The CEACAM1-L Ser503 residue is crucial for inhibition of colon cancer cell tumorigenicity. Oncogene **20:** 219–230.
28. NITTKA, S., J. GUNTHER, C. EBISCH, *et al.* 2004. The human tumor suppressor CEA-CAM1 modulates apoptosis and is implicated in early colorectal tumorigenesis. Oncogene **23:** 9306–9313.
29. GRAY-OWEN, S.D. 2003. Neisserial Opa proteins: impact on colonization, dissemination and immunity. Scand. J. Infect. Dis. **35:** 614–618.
30. HEMMILA, E. *et al.* 2004. Ceacam1a-/- mice are completely resistant to infection by murine coronavirus mouse hepatitis virus a59. J. Virol. **78:** 10156–10165.
31. ÖBRINK, B. 1997. CEA adhesion molecules: multifunctional proteins with signal-regulatory properties. Curr. Opin. Cell. Biol. **9:** 616–626.
32. TAN, K. *et al.* 2002. Crystal structure of murine sCEACAM1a[1,4]: a coronavirus receptor in the CEA family. EMBO J. **21:** 2076–2086.
33. BEAUCHEMIN, N., P. DRABER, G. DVEKSLER, *et al.* 1999. Nomenclature announcement: redefined nomenclature for members of the carcinoembryonic antigen family. Exp. Cell. Res. **252:** 243–249.
34. SINGER, B.B., I. SCHEFFRAHN & B. ÖBRINK. 2000. The tumor growth-inhibiting cell adhesion molecule CEACAM1 (C-CAM) is differently expressed in proliferating and quiescent epithelial cells and regulates cell proliferation. Cancer Res. **60:** 1236–1244.
35. EDLUND, M., I. BLIKSTAD & B. ÖBRINK. 1996. Calmodulin binds to specific sequences in the cytoplasmic domain of C-CAM and down-regulates C-CAM self-association. J. Biol. Chem. **271:** 1393–1399.
36. CHOTHIA, C. & E.Y. JONES. 1997. The molecular structure of cell adhesion molecules. Annu. Rev. Biochem. **66:** 823–862.

37. WATT, S.M. *et al.* 2001. Homophilic adhesion of human CEACAM1 involves N-terminal domain interactions: structural analysis of the binding site. Blood **98:** 1469–1479.

38. MARKEL, G. *et al.* 2004. The critical role of residues 43R and 44Q of carcinoembryonic antigen cell adhesion molecules-1 in the protection from killing by human NK cells. J. Immunol. **173:** 3732–3739.

39. MARKEL, G. *et al.* 2004. The mechanisms controlling NK cell autoreactivity in TAP2-deficient patients. Blood **103:** 1770–1778.

40. MARKEL, G. *et al.* 2002. CD66A interactions between human melanoma and NK cells: a novel class I MHC-independent inhibitory mechanism of cytotoxicity. J. Immunol. **168:** 2803–2810.

41. KAMMERER, R., D. STOBER, B.B. SINGER, *et al.* 2001. Carcinoembryonic antigen-related cell adhesion molecule 1 on murine dendritic cells is a potent regulation of T cell stimulation. J. Immunol. **166:** 6537–6544.

42. COUTELIER, J.-P. *et al.* 1994. B lymphocyte and macrophage expression of carcinoembryonic antigen-related adhesion molecules that serve as receptors for murine coronavirus. Eur. J. Immunol. **24:** 1383–1390.

43. GREICIUS, G., E. SEVERINSON, N. BEAUCHEMIN, *et al.* 2003. CEACAM1 is a potent regulator of B cell receptor complex-induced activation. J. Leukocyte Biol. **74:** 126–134.

44. CHIEN, T. *et al.* 2001. Biliary glycoprotein (BGPa, CD66a, CEACAM1) mediates inhibitory signals. J. Leukocyte Biol. **70:** 335–340.

45. NAKAJIMA, A. *et al.* 2002. Activation-induced expression of carcinoembryonic antigen-cell adhesion molecule 1 regulates mouse T lymphocyte function. J. Immunol. **168:** 1028–1035.

46. MÖLLER, M.J., R. KAMMERER, *et al.* 1996. Biliary glycoprotein (BGP) expression on T cells and on a natural-killer-cell sub-population. Int. J. Cancer. **65:** 740–745.

47. KAMMERER, R., S. HAHN, *et al.* 1998. Biliary glycoprotein (CD66a), a cell adhesion molecule of the immunoglobulin superfamily, on human lymphocytes: structure, expression and involvement in T cell activation. Eur. J. Immunol. **28:** 3664–3674.

48. GUY-GRAND, D. & P. VASSALLI. 2002. Gut intraepithelial lymphocyte development. Curr. Opin. Immunol. **14:** 255–259.

49. MORALES, V.M. *et al.* 1999. Regulation of human intestinal intraepithelial lymphocyte cytolytic function by biliary glycoprotein (CD66a). J. Immunol. **163:** 1363–1370.

50. BOULTON, I.C. & S.D. GRAY-OWEN. 2002. Neisserial binding to CEACAM1 arrests the activation and proliferation of CD4$^+$ lymphocytes. Nat. Immunol. **3:** 229–236.

51. DONDA, A. *et al.* 2000. Locally inducible CD661 (CEACAM1) as an amplifier of the human intestinal T cell response. Eur. J. Immunol. **30:** 2593–2603.

52. SINGER, B.B. *et al.* 2002. Carcinoembryonic antigen-related cell adhesion molecule 1 expression and signaling in human, mouse, and rat leukocytes: evidence for replacement of the short cytoplasmic domain isoform by glycosylphosphatidylinositol-linked proteins in human leukocytes. J. Immunol. **168:** 5139–5146.

53. TANAKA, K., Y. HINODA, H. TAKAHASHI, *et al.* 1997. Decreased expression of biliary glycoprotein in hepatocellular carcinomas. Int. J. Cancer **20:** 15–19.

54. LUO, W., C.G. WOOD, K. EARLEY, *et al.* 1997. Suppression of tumorigenicity of breast cancer cells by an epithelial cell adhesion molecule (C-CAM1): the

adhesion and growth suppression are mediated by different domains. Oncogene **14:** 1697–1704.

55. KUNATH, T., C. ORDOÑEZ-GARCIA, *et al.* 1995. Inhibition of colonic tumor cell growth by biliary glycoprotein. Oncogene **11:** 2375–2382.

56. TURBIDE, C., T. KUNATH, *et al.* 1997. Optimal ratios of biliary glycoprotein isoforms required for inhibition of colonic tumor cell growth. Cancer Res. **57:** 2781–2788.

57. HSIEH, J.-T. *et al.* 1995. Tumor suppressive role of an androgen-regulated epithelial cell adhesion molecule (C-CAM) in prostate carcinoma cell revealed by sense and antisense approaches. Cancer Res. **55:** 190–197.

58. HUBER, M. *et al.* 1999. The carboxyl-terminal region of biliary glycoprotein controls its tyrosine phosphorylation and association with protein-tyrosine phosphatases SHP-1 and SHP-2 in epithelial cells. J. Biol. Chem. **274:** 335–344.

59. BRÜMMER, J., M. NEUMAIER, *et al.* 1995. Association of $pp60^{c-src}$ with biliary glycoprotein (CD66a), an adhesion molecule of the carcinoembryonic antigen family downregulated in colorectal carcinomas. Oncogene **11:** 1649–1655.

60. IIJIMA, H. *et al.* 2004. Specific regulation of T helper cell 1-mediated murine colitis by CEACAM1. J. Exp. Med. **199:** 471–482.

61. CHEN, C.-J. & J.E. SHIVELY. 2004. The cell-cell adhesion molecule carcinoembryonic antigen-related cellular adhesion molecule 1 inhibits IL-2 production and proliferation in human T cells by association with Src homology protein-1 and down-regulates IL-2 receptor. J. Immunol. **172:** 3544–3552.

62. CHEN, D. *et al.* 2004. Carcinoembryonic antigen-related cellular adhesion molecule 1 isoforms alternatively inhibit and costimulate human T cell function. J. Immunol. **172:** 3535–3543.

63. MARKEL, G. *et al.* 2002. Pivotal role of CEACAM1 protein in the inhibition of activated decidual lymphocyte functions. J. Clin. Invest. **110:** 943–953.

64. KIRSHNER, J., C.-J. CHEN, *et al.* 2003. CEACAM1-4S, a cell-cell adhesion molecule, mediates apoptosis and reverts mammary carcinoma cells to a normal morphogenic phenotype in a 3D culture. Proc. Natl. Acad. Sci. USA **100:** 521–526.

65. VÉLY, F. & E. VIVIER. 1999. Conservation of structural features reveals the existence of a large family of inhibitory cell surface receptors and noninhibitory/activatory counterparts. J. Immunol. **159:** 2075–2077.

66. HSU, K.C., S. CHIDA, *et al.* 2002. The killer cell immunoglobulin-like receptor (KIR) genomic region: gene-order, haplotypes and allelic polymorphism. Immunol. Rev. **190:** 40–52.

67. WILLIAMS, W.K., Gui-S. JIANG & K.V. HOLMES. 1991. Receptor for mouse hepatitis virus is a member of the carcinoembryonic antigen family of glycoproteins. Proc. Natl. Acad. Sci. USA **88:** 5533–5536.

68. LATCHMAN, Y. *et al.* 2001. PD-L2 is a second ligand for PD-1 and inhibits T cell activation. Nat. Immunol. **2:** 261–268.

69. GALLAGHER, T.M. 1997. A role for naturally occurring variation of the murine coronavirus spike protein in stabilizing association with the cellular receptor. J. Virol. **71:** 3129–3137.

70. KAMINSKA, B. 2005. MAPK signalling pathways as molecular targets for anti-inflammatory therapy—from molecular mechanisms to therapeutic benefits. Biochim. Biophys. Acta **175:** 253–262.

71. NEURATH, M.F., B. WEIGMANN, S. FINOTTO, *et al.* 2002. The transcription factor T-bet regulates mucosal T cell activation in experimental colitis and Crohn's disease. J. Exp. Med. **195:** 1129–1143.

72. HELLER, F., I.J. FUSS, E.E. NIEUWENHUIS, *et al.* 2002. Oxazolone colitis, a Th2 colitis model resembling ulcerative colitis, is mediated by IL-13-producing NK-T cells. Immunity **17:** 629–638.

73. BRÜMMER, J. *et al.* The CD66 complex: activation of tyrosine kinases of the Src family. *In* VIth Leukocyte Culture Conference: CD66 Family Workshop.

74. BRADSHAW, J.D. *et al.* 1997. Interaction of the cyt tail of CTLA-4 CD152 with a clathrin-associated protein is negatively regulated by tyrosine phosphorylation. Biochemistry **36:** 15975–15982.

75. ÖBRINK, B. *et al.* 2002. Computational analysis of isoform-specific signal regulation by CEACAM1: a cell adhesion molecule expressed in PC12 cells. Ann. N.Y. Acad. Sci. **971:** 597–602.

76. OLSSON, H., K. WIKSTRÖM, *et al.* 1995. Cell adhesion activity of the short cytoplasmic domain isoform of C-CAM (C-CAM2) in CHO cells. FEBS Lett. **365:** 51–56.

77. OIKAWA, S., K. MOTOMU, *et al.* 1992. Homotypic and heterotypic Ca^{++} independent cell adhesion activities of biliary glycoprotein, a member of carcinoembryonic antigen family, expressed on CHO cell surface. Biochem. Biophys. Res. Comm. **186:** 881–887.

78. ABRAHAM, R.T. & A. WEISS. 2004. Jurkat T cells and development of the T-cell receptor signalling paradigm. Nat. Rev. Immunol. **4:** 301–308.

79. SADEKOVA, S., N. LAMARCHE-VANE, *et al.* 2000. The CEACAM1-L glycoprotein associates with the actin cytoskeleton and localizes to cell-cell contact through activation of Rho-like GTPases. Molec. Biol. Cell. **11:** 65–77.

80. FOURNÈS, B., J. FARRAH, M. OLSON, *et al.* 2003. Distinct Rho GTPase activities regulate epithelial cell localization of the adhesion molecule CEACAM1: involvement of the CEACAM1 transmembrane domain. Molec. Cell. Biol. **23:** 7291–7304.

81. SCHUMANN, D., C.-J. CHEN, *et al.* 2001. Carcinoembryonic antigen cell adhesion molecule 1 directly associates with cytoskeleton proteins actin and tropomyosin. J. Biol. Chem. **276:** 47421–47433.

82. VAN DER MERWE, P.A., S.J. DAVIS, *et al.* 2000. Cytoskeletal polarization and redistribution of cell-surface molecules during T cell antigen recognition. Semin. Immunol. **12:** 5–21.

83. VEILLETTE, A., S. LATOUR & D. DAVIDSON. 2002. Negative regulation of immunoreceptor signaling. Annu. Rev. Immunol. **20:** 669–707.

Therapeutic Drug Delivery by Genetically Modified *Lactococcus lactis*

LOTHAR STEIDLER[a] AND PIETER ROTTIERS[b]

[a]*Alimentary Pharmabiotic Centre, Transgenic Bacteriology, University College Cork, Western Road, Cork, Ireland*

[b]*Department for Molecular Biomedical Research, Flanders Interuniversity Institute for Biotechnology (VIB) and Ghent University, Ghent, Belgium*

ABSTRACT: Food-grade bacteria have been consumed throughout history without associated pathologies and are, therefore, absolutely safe to ingest. Unexpectedly, *Lactococcus lactis (L. lactis)*, known from cheese production, can be genetically engineered to constantly secrete satisfactory amounts of bioactive cytokines. Both of these features enabled the development of a new kind of topical delivery system: topical and active delivery of therapeutic proteins by genetically modified micro-organisms. The host organism's record inspired the development of applications that target intestinal diseases. In a variety of mouse models, chronic colon inflammation can be successfully treated with (interleukin) IL-10–secreting *L. lactis*. Trefoil factor (TFF) producer strains have also been shown to be very effective in the treatment of acute colitis. Such novel therapeutic strains are textbook examples of genetically modified (GM) organisms. There are legitimate concerns with regard to the deliberate release of GM micro-organisms. On development of these applications, therefore, we have engineered these bacteria in such a way that biological containment is guaranteed. The essential gene *thyA*, encoding thymidylate synthase, has been exchanged for IL-10. This makes the GM strain critically dependent on thymidine. Lack of thymidine, for example, resulting from thymidine consumption by *thyA*-deficient strains–will irreversibly lead to induced "thymidine-less death." This accomplishment has created the possibility of using this strategy for application in human medicine.

KEYWORDS: lactococcus; containment; delivery; colitis; expression

INTRODUCTION

Food preservation and flavor development can be achieved by bacterial and fungal fermentation of raw nutrient materials. Food-grade bacteria, many of

Address for correspondence: Lothar Steidler, Alimentary Pharmabiotic Centre, Transgenic Bacteriology, University College Cork, Western Road, Cork, Ireland. Voice: +353-21-490-1383; fax: +353-21-490-1377.

e-mail: l.steidler@ucc.ie

Ann. N.Y. Acad. Sci. 1072: 176–186 (2006). © 2006 New York Academy of Sciences.

doi: 10.1196/annals.1326.031

which are lactic acid bacteria (LAB), have been extensively consumed by both humans and livestock. Accordingly, the impact of these organisms on health is very well documented and is monitored systematically with the industrialization of food and feed production. As concerns associated with their consumption are extremely unusual, LAB use in nutrition is therefore rarely disputed. One intrinsic advantage of food-grade LAB therefore lies in the knowledge that they are not pathogenic, not even when given overt opportunity, as would be the case in an ongoing disease. For this reason numerous LAB species are granted a "Generally Regarded As Safe" (GRAS) status by the U.S. Food and Drug Administration.

Many LAB are normal constituents of the microflora in the intestine of mammals. It was not until recently that the effects of the enteric microflora on the well-being of the host have been recognized. Much effort is now focused on isolating specific strains of LAB that can be used to reestablish optional intestinal function on both a digestive and an immunological level. These specific strains, which provide lactic acid bacterium particular health benefits beyond their mere nutritive value, are called probiotics.

Lactococcus lactis (*L. lactis*) is a noncolonizing that cannot, on ingestion, invade the tissues, nor does it ever cause infection. It also does not convey any health benefit as such and is therefore not classed as a probiotic. The species has been used in industry for many years where it is essential in a large number of dairy and other food fermentations, in particular in the production of cheese. *L. lactis* can nowadays be genetically engineered quite efficiently. Many elaborate and highly effective tools have become available over the last 15 years,[1,2] the major driving force residing in the desire to understand dairy production. A particularly useful aspect is the ability to use genetic modification (GM) tools for heterologous gene expression. Following the pioneering work of Wells and co-workers, much effort has been directed to the use of LAB as delivery vehicles for foreign antigens at mucosal surfaces (for a review see Refs. 3 and 4). Oral as well as intranasal inoculation with *L. lactis* that express tetanus toxin fragment C (TTFC) leads to the induction of high-serum antibody levels, protective against tetanus toxin.[5,6,7] GM lactococci can also be used to raise protective responses toward streptococcal infection. Mice vaccinated with recombinant *L. lactis* that express the conserved C-repeat region of *Streptococcus pyogenes* M protein were protected against pharyngeal infection following a nasal challenge with *S. pyogenes*.[8]

FAVORABLE TOOLS: CYTOKINES AND SINGLE-CHAIN ANTIBODIES

In addition to cell–cell contact, the immune system relies heavily for its "long distance communication" on relatively small (roughly 10 to 20 kDa) and simple messenger proteins: cytokines, interferons, growth factors, and chemokines. Induction of a specific cytokine pattern drives cellular immunity and will lead to either destruction of invading pathogens, immune suppression, the establishment of memory, and so on. Our main research focuses on the design of *L. lactis* for the expression and secretion of cytokines[9,10,11,12] and in the use of such recombinant strains for the redirection of the immune system.

Cytokines in general display fairly simple structures. Their biological activity does not depend on complex glycosylation or other secondary modifications and in most cases access, binding, and activation of their receptors is straightforward. Many of them, however, critically depend on correct disulfide bridge formation. This dependence is well established for interleukin-2 (IL-2),[13] IL-6,[14] IL-10,[15] and trefoil factors (TFFs).[16] Because bioactivity of the recombinant proteins has been shown both *in vitro* and *in vivo*, mouse (m)IL-2, mIL-6,[10] mIL-10,[11] human IL-10,[17] and TFFs[18] represent excellent proof that lactococci are capable of correct disulfide bridge formation in the processing of unfamiliar proteins.

Given our ample experience with cytokine expression from *Escherichia coli*,[19,20,21] we were particularly surprised to find that continuous synthesis of bioactive cytokines by *L. lactis* had no negative effects on its growth rate.[9,22] This observation fired our imagination, especially in view of the very high biological activity of these immune messengers, to further develop an entirely new category of therapeutics. We first investigated *in situ* cytokine delivery to the nasal mucosa. As stated previously, high, specific antibody titers can be detected in the serum of mice following intranasal inoculation with TTFC-expressing *L. lactis*.[5,6,7] Intranasal immunization of mice with *L. lactis* strains that coexpressed either mIL-2 or mIL-6 together with TTFC produced significantly higher antibody titers against the antigen than did the parental strain expressing TTFC alone.[10] Bacteria-expressing TTFC in combination with mIL-6 were also capable of eliciting serum anti-TTFC IgA responses. The boosting effect was completely lost when the bacteria were killed prior to immunization, indicating that viable bacteria that actively secrete the cytokines *in situ* are essential to the mechanism. Delivery to the intestinal mucosa, however, has now become the focus of our research.

The widespread success of neutralizing antibodies is hardly met by any other class of biologicals. Directed toward a pathogen, toxin, cytokine, or basically any other agent, they have proven to be very valuable and specific medicinal tools. Biotechnology has provided single-chain (ScFv) antibody technology and so has allowed it to be possible to produce such neutralizing antibodies from GM bacteria. Most efforts in the field have focussed on bulk production of the antibody, downstream processing, and use as an injectable purified protein. However, very unfavorable pharmacokinetic profiles have seriously hampered their medical use. Suitable delivery systems are therefore key for future medical use. A number of applications use GM bacteria for *in situ* production of the antibody fragment. In particular, so-called "passive immunization," immune therapy to control pathogens, is now well developed.

IN SITU DELIVERY OF THERAPEUTICS BY GM BACTERIA

Our reports have opened the whole field of GM micro-organisms applied as delivery tools for the localized, mucosal administration of cytokines and other bioactive proteins. It has now become clear that one can construct GM bacteria–*L. lactis*, *Streptococcus gordonii* (*S. gordonii*), *Lactobacillus* species–that constitutively secrete high-quality, correctly processed, bioactive molecules derived from a eukaryotic background.

The "safe" nature of LAB on one hand and the gradual availability of tools for genetic modification on the other have prompted many to speculate on novel medical applications. As an example, Drouault *et al.*[23] used GM *L. lactis* to try to enhance lipid digestion. They expressed *Staphylococcus hyicus* lipase in the cytoplasm of *L. lactis* and demonstrated that, when this strain was used, fat absorption was higher in pigs with ligated pancreatic ducts. This approach has the potential to improve the treatment of pancreatic insufficiency in humans. Chang and colleagues[24] showed, *in vitro*, that *Lactobacillus jensenii*, a natural human vaginal isolate secreting two-domain CD4 proteins, can inhibit HIV-1 entry into HeLa cells.

Bermudez-Humaran and co-workers[25] were able to secrete a heterodimeric cytokine, mIL-12 in *L. lactis*. The researchers expressed mIL-12 as two separate polypeptides (p35 and p40) or as a single polypeptide by linking the p35 to the p40 subunit. The single-chain mIL-12 showed higher biological activity. Expression of the two genes separately resulted in the formation of the heterodimeric polypeptide, p70, as well as the antagonistic homodimer, p80 (p40–p40).[26] Intranasal coadministration of the single-chain mIL-12–secreting strain alongside *L. lactis* that produces the E7 antigen of human papillomavirus type 16 resulted in enhanced levels of the Th1 cytokines mIL-2 and mIFNγ. Thus, switching the Th2 response, the preferred default route after intranasal immunization with the E7 antigen, toward a Th1 response may be possible. This capacity for immune modulation can be ingeniously enhanced by the appropriate choice of host organisms. Coadministration in a mouse model for birch pollen allergy of either one of two wild-type LAB, *L. lactis,* or *Lactobacillus plantarum*, and the main allergen of birch pollen allergy prior to or after sensitization, induced a shift toward Th1 immune responses.[27] This offers the possibility of vaccinating against type I allergy. The capacity of these wild-type LAB may be further enhanced by designing them to secrete appropriate cytokines, such as IL-12.

Shortcomings of neutralizing ScFv antibodies may be met by the use of localized delivery by GM producer strains. A number of applications are now emerging in which the expressor strain itself is used for the *in situ* production of the antibody fragment. Especially, the control of colonization by pathogens has led to a number of applications. It had been observed that dental caries can be reduced by the oral administration of antibodies that recognize *Streptococcus mutans* (*S. mutans*).[28,29] *Lactobacillus zeae* was therefore engineered to produce a single-chain antibody fragment against streptococcal antigen III adhesion molecule of *S. mutans*.[30] When these bacteria were used in a rat model for caries, both *S. mutans* counts and caries scores were markedly reduced. This approach may be of interest for *in vivo* immunotherapy.

A more elaborate approach has been used to combat *Candida albicans* (*C. albicans*), one of the most frequent causative agents of mucosal inflammation in humans.[31] Infections are seen in the mouth and esophagus of immune-compromised persons, such as HIV-infected subjects. *C. albicans* also causes acute vaginitis in otherwise healthy women. There exists a real need for new therapeutics in this area because few adequate drugs are known, resistance is increasing, and vaccines are not available. Beninati and co-workers have made a recombinant *S. gordonii*, a species with good vaginal colonization and heterologous expression potential *in vivo*,[32,33,34] for the eradication of *C. albicans* infections.[35] Anti-idiotypic ScFv were produced, the surface of which resembled the structure of a wide-spectrum killer toxin (KT) of *Pichia anomala*.[36,37] Two *S. gordonii* strains were constructed: one that expressed the ScFv at its surface and a second that secreted the ScFv. Similarity in structure with KT could be shown by cross reactivity with specific monoclonal antibodies. Both surface-bound and secreted ScFv showed candidacidal activity over a wide concentration range. Both *S. gordonii* strains successfully colonized the vagina and cleared experimental *C. albicans* infection in rats, dependent on the presence of this ScFv. The secretor, however, reduced the pathogenic load 7 days faster, a result comparable with a full-course treatment using the antifungal fluconazole. This work shows that local production of a designer microbicide is a valid approach for the treatment of a very common mucosal pathology. Thus the expression of single-chain antibodies by bacteria opens up the possible application range to a wide range of diseases.

INTESTINAL IL-10 DELIVERY BY GM *L. LACTIS*

Inflammatory bowel disease (IBD) most likely occurs as a consequence of the breakdown of immune tolerance toward intestinal microflora. The cytokine IL-10 is a powerful anti-inflammatory and is a central factor in induction and maintenance of immune tolerance.[38,39] Although IL-10 is a very attractive therapeutic for intestinal inflammation, correct targeting of the compound was its Achilles heel. Braat and co-workers have recently reviewed the use of IL-10 in IBD treatment.[40] Attempts have been made to administer recombinant IL-10 to IBD patients by injection. Moderate side effects are observed when IL-10 is administered through the systemic route.[41,42] The clinical result being unsatisfactory,[43] this route has now been abandoned altogether. More important, however, injection of IL-10 leads to the induction of the proinflammatory IFNγ.[44] Long-term, high-dose injection of IL-10 has thereby become pointless. Therapeutic targeting could solve that problem but oral administration is hampered by the extremely acid sensitivity of IL-10 and, to date, no oral formulation for IL-10 is known.

We tried to address all these problems by constructing an IL-10–secreting *L. lactis*.[11] Daily oral dosage of this strain efficiently cures chronic murine DSS colitis. The observed healing is comparable to systemic treatment with prominent anti-inflammatory drugs, such as dexamethasone and anti-IL-12. When given systemically, recombinant IL-10 also decreases inflammation to the same level as IL-10–producing *L. lactis*, but the amount of IL-10 required to achieve this effect is 1000-fold higher. This indicates that greatly improved IL-10 delivery has been achieved by using GM *L. lactis*.

Daily treatment with IL-10–producing *L. lactis* leads to the prevention of colitis, normally associated with the IL-10$^{-/-}$ genotype in 129 Sv/Ev mice. When left untreated, 129 Sv/Ev IL10$^{-/-}$ mice developed colitis from week 3 on. Treatment with IL-10–producing *L. lactis* stalled the development of intestinal inflammation. More recently, Foligné and co-workers have shown the validity of this approach in TNBS colitis.[45]

Ultraviolet light (UV) killing of the IL-10–producing bacteria prior to inoculation abrogated their curative effect. This shows that *in situ* production of IL-10 is an essential feature of the mechanism of action. We therefore think that following oral administration these recombinant bacteria travel through the gut with the flow of the matrix, arrive at the affected area, and produce the therapeutic agent. Because of this localized production it can be speculated that side effects associated with systemic administration of IL-10 can be reduced or even avoided.

INTESTINAL DELIVERY OF TFF BY GM *L. LACTIS*

Treatment of acute intestinal inflammation may be a means to prevent the onset of IBD, but the number of therapeutic strategies for acute colitis is rather limited. TFF1, 2, and 3 form a class of nonmitogenic peptides that are important in the protection and repair of the intestinal epithelium.[46] Accordingly, they are promising tools for treatment of acute colitis that is characterized by extensive epithelial ruptures. Despite extreme resistance of TFFs to acid and enzymatic degradation, no successful oral TFF formulation is yet at our disposal. The main reason for this is that luminally administered TFFs stick to the bowel mucus and are removed from the lumen at the cecum.[47] Topical and active delivery of TFFs in the colon by localized synthesis from *L. lactis* circumvents this problem.

GM *L. lactis* are able to produce and secrete biologically active murine TFFs in suitable quantities. Oral application of these strains subsequently results in adequate production of the TFF *in situ*.[18] Daily intragastric administration of the TFF-secreting strains, prior to or during disease induction, resulted in significant protection against DSS colitis as observed by reduced mortality, reduced loss of body weight, substantial improvement of colon histology, and the reduction of inflammatory infiltrate. The protective effect requires *de novo* TFF synthesis by live *L. lactis*. Oral administration of high amounts of purified mTFF1 did not ameliorate acute colitis, whereas rectal administration did, albeit much less effectively than orally administered mTFF-secreting *L. lactis*. Basolateral contact between colonocytes and the GM *L. lactis* cells probably enables TFFs to accumulate out of reach of complexing mucins and allows them to interact with the putative basolateral TFF receptors on enterocytes.[48]

Ptgs2, a known TFF target gene,[49,50] is strongly induced in the intestine of mice treated with mTFF-secreting *L. lactis*. This strongly suggests that recombinant TFFs were biologically active *in situ* in the colon. Ptgs2 contributes to the healing and downregulation of the inflammatory responses in the gastrointestinal tract.[51,52] Inhibition of Ptgs2 by meloxicam substantially abrogated the prophylactic effect of mTFF-producing *L. lactis* and, so, Ptgs2 induction forms a major part of the mechanism of action.

PROSPECTS

The use of GM bacteria that secrete any of the vast numbers of immune mediators described to date offers fascinating possibilities for medicine. The deliberate release of live GM bacteria, as would occur following medical application, however, raises legitimate concerns. These GM strains will necessarily have to be redesigned to reconcile medical effectiveness and biological safety before they can be applied "in the real world."

We established adequate means for inheritable growth control of engineered *L. lactis* by genetically exchanging the chromosomal thymidylate synthase gene *thyA* for the IL-10 gene.[17] Thymidylate synthase is a mandatory enzyme in the synthesis of the DNA constituents thymidine and thymine. The resulting GM *L. lactis*, Thy12, no longer carries its GM traits on a plasmid, nor does it require antibiotic selection for their stable inheritance. More importantly, Thy12 is strictly dependent on the presence of thymidine or thymine for its growth and survival. In contrast to deprivation of any other metabolic mutant of its complementing metabolite, thymidine starvation of Thy12 leads to induced cell death due to increased DNA damage and subsequent induction of SOS repair genes and fragmentation of the DNA. This phenomenon was first reported almost 50 years ago and is known as thymine-less death.[53] Readily amenable systems based on this phenomenon have, however, not been described up to now. This approach has received approval from the Dutch authorities for the conduct of the first clinical trial ever that uses a live GM bacterium as a therapeutic agent. It may well be that the conduct of this clinical trial leads us into the development of a completely novel pharmacology: GM bacterial therapeutics.

ACKNOWLEDGMENTS

This research was in part supported by the Flanders Interuniversity Institute for Biotechnology and Ghent University (GOA Projects No, 12050700 and 12051501). The Science Foundation Ireland (SFI(01(F.1(B036) partly supported the contribution of L.S.

REFERENCES

1. AHMED, F.E. 2003. Genetically modified probiotics in foods. Trends Biotechnol. **21:** 491–497.
2. KLEEREBEZEM, M. & J. HUGENHOLTZ. 2003. Metabolic pathway engineering in lactic acid bacteria. Curr. Op. Biotechnol. **14:** 232–237.
3. SEEGERS, J.F. 2002. Lactobacilli as live vaccine delivery vectors: progress and prospects. Trends Biotechnol. **20:** 508–515.
4. NOUAILLE, S., L.A. RIBEIRO, A. MIYOSHI, *et al.* 2003. Heterologous protein production and delivery systems for *Lactococcus lactis*. Genet. Mol. Res. **2:** 102–111.
5. WELLS, J.M., P.W. WILSON, P.M. NORTON, *et al.* 1993. *Lactococcus lactis*: high-level expression of tetanus toxin fragment C and protection against lethal challenge. Mol. Microbiol. **8:** 1155–1162.
6. NORTON, P.M., J.M. WELLS, H.W. BROWN, *et al.* 1997. Protection against tetanus toxin in mice nasally immunized with recombinant *Lactococcus lactis* expressing tetanus toxin fragment C. Vaccine **15:** 616–619.
7. ROBINSON, K., L.M. CHAMBERLAIN, K.M. SCHOFIELD, *et al.* 1997. Oral vaccination of mice against tetanus with recombinant *Lactococcus lactis*. Nat. Biotechnol. **15:** 653–657.
8. MANNAM, P., K.F. JONES & B.L. GELLER. 2004. Mucosal vaccine made from live, recombinant *Lactococcus lactis* protects mice against pharyngeal infection with streptococcus pyogenes. Infect. Immun. **72:** 3444–3450.
9. STEIDLER, L., J.M. WELLS, A. RAEYMAEKERS, *et al.* 1995. Secretion of biologically active murine interleukin-2 by *Lactococcus lactis* subsp. lactis. Appl. Environ. Microbiol. **61:** 1627–1629.
10. STEIDLER, L., K. ROBINSON, L. CHAMBERLAIN, *et al.* 1998. Mucosal delivery of murine interleukin-2 (IL-2) and IL-6 by recombinant strains of *Lactococcus lactis* coexpressing antigen and cytokine. Infect. Immun. **66:** 3183–3189.
11. STEIDLER, L., W. HANS, L. SCHOTTE, *et al.* 2000. Treatment of murine colitis by *Lactococcus lactis* secreting interleukin-10. Science **289:** 1352–1355.
12. SCHOTTE, L., L. STEIDLER, J. VANDEKERCKHOVE, *et al.* 2000. Secretion of biologically active murine interleukin-10 by *Lactococcus lactis*. Enzyme Microb. Technol. **27:** 761–765.
13. RONG, Y., N. LEE & S.M. LIANG. 1992. Analysis of IL-2 functional structure by multiple cysteine substitutions. Biochem. Biophys. Res. Commun. **188:** 949–955.
14. ZHANG, J.G., J.M. MATTHEWS, L.D. WARD, *et al.* 1997. Disruption of the disulfide bonds of recombinant murine interleukin-6 induces formation of a partially unfolded state. Biochemistry **36:** 2380–2389.

15. WINDSOR, W.T., R. SYTO, A. TSARBOPOULOS, et al. 1993. Disulfide bond assignments and secondary structure analysis of human and murine interleukin 10. Biochemistry 32: 8807–8815.
16. CHADWICK, M.P., F.E. MAY & B.R. WESTLEY. 1995. Production and comparison of mature single-domain 'trefoil' peptides pNR-2/pS2 Cys58 and pNR-2/pS2 Ser58. Biochem. J. 308: 1001–1007.
17. STEIDLER, L., S. NEIRYNCK, N. HUYGHEBAERT, et al. 2003. Biological containment of genetically modified Lactococcus lactis for intestinal delivery of human interleukin 10. Nat. Biotechnol. 21: 785–789.
18. VANDENBROUCKE, K., W. HANS, J. VAN HUYSSE, et al. 2004. Active delivery of trefoil factors by genetically modified Lactococcus lactis prevents and heals acute colitis in mice. Gastroenterology 127: 502–513.
19. MERTENS, N., E. REMAUT & W. FIERS. 1995. Tight transcriptional control mechanism ensures stable high-level expression from T7 promoter-based expression plasmids. Biotechnology 13: 175–179.
20. GUISEZ, Y., J. DEMOLDER, N. MERTENS, et al. 1993. High-level expression, purification, and renaturation of recombinant murine interleukin-2 from Escherichia coli. Protein Expr. Purif. 4: 240–246.
21. DERYNCK, R., E. REMAUT, E. SAMAN, et al. 1980. Expression of human fibroblast interferon gene in Escherichia coli. Nature 287: 193–197.
22. STEIDLER, L., W. FIERS & E. REMAUT. 1996. Expression of human and murine interleukins in Lactococcus lactis. In Metabolism and Application of Lactic Acid Bacteria. B. Ray & F. Bozoglu, Eds.: 63–79. Springer-Verlag. Berlin-Heidelberg, New York.
23. DROUAULT, S., C. JUSTE, P. MARTEAU, et al. 2002. Oral treatment with Lactococcus lactis expressing Staphylococcus hyicus lipase enhances lipid digestion in pigs with induced pancreatic insufficiency. Appl. Environ. Microbiol. 68: 3166–3168.
24. CHANG, T.L., C.H. CHANG, D.A. SIMPSON, et al. 2003. Inhibition of HIV infectivity by a natural human isolate of Lactobacillus jensenii engineered to express functional two-domain CD4. Proc. Natl. Acad. Sci. USA 100: 11672–11677.
25. BERMUDEZ-HUMARAN, L.G., P. LANGELLA, N.G. CORTES-PEREZ, et al. 2003. Intranasal immunization with recombinant Lactococcus lactis secreting murine interleukin-12 enhances antigen-specific Th1 cytokine production. Infect. Immun. 71: 1887–1896.
26. LING, P., M.K. GATELY, U. GUBLER, et al. 1995. Human IL-12 p40 homodimer binds to the IL-12 receptor but does not mediate biologic activity. J. Immunol. 154: 116–127.
27. REPA, A., C. GRANGETTE, C. DANIEL, et al. 2003. Mucosal co-application of lactic acid bacteria and allergen induces counter-regulatory immune responses in a murine model of birch pollen allergy. Vaccine 22: 87–95.
28. LEHNER, T., J. CALDWELL & R. SMITH. 1985. Local passive immunization by monoclonal antibodies against streptococcal antigen I(II in the prevention of dental caries. Infect. Immun. 50: 796–799.
29. MICHALEK, S.M., R.L. GREGORY, C.C. HARMON, et al. 1987. Protection of gnotobiotic rats against dental caries by passive immunization with bovine milk antibodies to Streptococcus mutans. Infect. Immun. 55: 2341–2347.
30. KRUGER, C., Y. HU, Q. PAN, et al. 2002. In situ delivery of passive immunity by lactobacilli producing single-chain antibodies. Nat. Biotechnol. 20: 702–706.

31. FIDEL, P.L., JR. & J.D. SOBEL. 1996. Immunopathogenesis of recurrent vulvovaginal candidiasis. Clin. Microbiol. Rev. **9:** 335–348.
32. MEDAGLINI, D., C.M. RUSH, P. SESTINI, *et al.* 1997. Commensal bacteria as vectors for mucosal vaccines against sexually transmitted diseases: vaginal colonization with recombinant streptococci induces local and systemic antibodies in mice. Vaccine **15:** 1330–1337.
33. MEDAGLINI, D., M.R. OGGIONI & G. POZZI. 1998. Vaginal immunization with recombinant gram-positive bacteria. Am. J. Reprod. Immunol. **39:** 199–208.
34. DI FABIO, S., D. MEDAGLINI, C.M. RUSH, *et al.* 1998. Vaginal immunization of cynomolgus monkeys with *Streptococcus gordonii* expressing HIV-1 and HPV 16 antigens. Vaccine **16:** 485–492.
35. BENINATI, C., M.R. OGGIONI, M. BOCCANERA, *et al.* 2000. Therapy of mucosal candidiasis by expression of an anti-idiotype in human commensal bacteria. Nat. Biotechnol. **18:** 1060–1064.
36. MAGLIANI, W., S. CONTI, F. DE BERNARDIS, *et al.* 1997. Therapeutic potential of antiidiotypic single chain antibodies with yeast killer toxin activity. Nat. Biotechnol. **15:** 155–158.
37. POLONELLI, L. & G. MORACE. 1987. Production and characterization of yeast killer toxin monoclonal antibodies. J. Clin. Microbiol. **25:** 460–462.
38. THOMPSON, C. & F. POWRIE. 2004. Regulatory T cells. Curr. Opin. Pharmacol. **4:** 408–414.
39. BLUESTONE, J.A. & A.K. ABBAS. 2003. Natural versus adaptive regulatory T cells. Nat. Rev. Immunol. **3:** 253–257.
40. BRAAT, H., M.P. PEPPELENBOSCH & D.W. HOMMES. 2003. Interleukin-10-based therapy for inflammatory bowel disease. Exp. Op. Biol. Ther. **3:** 725–731.
41. FEDORAK, R.N., A. GANGL, C.O. ELSON, *et al.* 2000. Recombinant human interleukin 10 in the treatment of patients with mild to moderately active Crohn's disease. The Interleukin 10 Inflammatory Bowel Disease Cooperative Study Group. Gastroenterology **119:** 1473–1482.
42. SCHREIBER, S. 2000. Genetics of inflammatory bowel disease: a puzzle with contradictions? Gut **47:** 746–747.
43. VAN DEVENTER, S.J., C.O. ELSON & R.N. FEDORAK. 1997. Multiple doses of intravenous interleukin 10 in steroid-refractory Crohn's disease. Crohn's Disease Study Group. Gastroenterology **113:** 383–389.
44. TILG, H., H. ULMER, A. KASER, *et al.* 2002. Role of IL-10 for induction of anemia during inflammation. J.Immunol. **169:** 2204–2209.
45. FOLIGNE, B., S. NUTTEN, L. STEIDLER, *et al.* 2006. Recommendations for improved use of the murine TNBS-induced colitis model in evaluating anti-inflammatory properties of lactic acid bacteria: technical and microbiological aspects. Dig. Dis. Sci. **51:** 390–400.
46. TAUPIN, D. & D.K. PODOLSKY. 2003. Trefoil factors: initiators of mucosal healing. Nat. Rev. Mol. Cell. Biol. **4:** 721–732.
47. POULSEN, S.S., J. THULESEN, L. CHRISTENSEN, *et al.* 1999. Metabolism of oral trefoil factor 2 (TFF2) and the effect of oral and parenteral TFF2 on gastric and duodenal ulcer healing in the rat. Gut **45:** 516–552.
48. THIM, L. & E. MORTZ. 2000. Isolation and characterization of putative trefoil peptide receptors. Regul. Pept. **90:** 61–68.
49. TAN, D., H. CHEN, P. LIU, *et al.* 2000. Prostanoids mediate the protective effect of trefoil factor 3 in oxidant-induced intestinal epithelial cell injury: role of cyclooxygenase-2. J. Cell. Sci. **113:** 2149–2155.

50. RODRIGUES, S., E. VAN AKEN, S. VAN BOCXLAER, *et al.* 2003. Trefoil peptides as proangiogenic factors in vivo and in vitro: implication of cyclooxygenase-2 and EGF receptor S. signaling. FASEB J. **17:** 7–16.

51. MIZUNO, H., C. SAKAMOTO, K. MATSUDA, *et al.* 1997. Induction of cyclooxygenase 2 in gastric mucosal lesions and its inhibition by the specific antagonist delays healing in mice. Gastroenterology **112:** 387–397.

52. EHRLICH, K., S. PLATE, T. STROFF, *et al.* 1998. Peptidergic and cholinergic neurons and mediators in peptone-induced gastroprotection: role of cyclooxygenase-2. AJP Gastrointest. Liver Physiol. **274:** G955–G964.

53. AHMAD, S.I., S.H. KIRK & A. EISENSTARK. 1998. Thymine metabolism and thymineless death in prokaryotes and eukaryotes. Annu. Rev. Microbiol. **52:** 591–625.

Role of Lymphotoxins in the Development of Peyer's Patches and Mesenteric Lymph Nodes

Relevance to Intestinal Inflammation and Treatment

THOMAS W. SPAHN,[a,b] MICHAEL K. MÜLLER,[b]
WOLFRAM DOMSCHKE,[a] AND TORSTEN KUCHARZIK[a]

[a]Department of Medicine B, Münster University Hospital, Münster, Germany

[b]Department of General Internal Medicine and Gastroenterology,
Marienhospital Osnabrück, Johannisfreiheit 2-4, D-49074 Osnabrück, Germany

ABSTRACT: Hallmarks of the adaptive immune system are antigen-specific cellular and humoral immune responses. Secondary lymphoid organs serve as sites of contact between antigen-presenting cells (APCs) and immune effector T and B lymphocytes. The gut-associated lymphatic system (GALT) as the intestinal branch of the immune system provides different mechanisms to protect organisms against pathogens. Simultaneously, immune activation secondary to genetic factors and/or environmental signals can induce detrimental autoimmunity. The effector pathways in host defense and autoimmunity use similar cytokines and chemokines. Unlike few other cytokines, lymphotoxin (LT) α/β regulates the development of intestinal lymphoid organs, including Peyer's patches (PPs) and mesenteric lymph nodes (MLNs). In addition, intestinal inflammation is suppressed by inhibition of LTβ signalling, an observation which has initiated clinical studies using this treatment principle. Conversely, the course of *Citrobacter rodentium*–induced infectious colitis is more severe in mice with impaired LTβ-receptor-mediated signalling. This report provides an overview on the role of the different organs of the GALT in intestinal inflammation. Moreover, it describes the role of the LTβ-receptor-mediated signalling in intestinal inflammation as encountered in autoimmune and infectious pathology. The contribution of LT to the delicate balance of immune effector functions in host defense and autoimmunity is discussed.

KEYWORDS: inflammatory bowel disease; lymphotoxin; immune regulation; infectious disease

Address for correspondence: Thomas W. Spahn, M.D., Department of General Internal Medicine and Gastroenterology, Marienhospital Osnabrück, Johannisfreiheit 2-4, D-49074 Osnabrück, Germany. Voice: 49-541-326-0; fax: 49-541-326-4656.
e-mail: spahn@uni-muenster.de

Ann. N.Y. Acad. Sci. 1072: 187–193 (2006). © 2006 New York Academy of Sciences.
doi: 10.1196/annals.1326.029

THE LYMPHOTOXIN AND LIGHT LIGAND /RECEPTOR SYSTEM AND ITS ROLE IN LYMPHOID ORGAN ARCHITECTURE AND AUTOIMMUNE DISEASES

Ligands and Receptors

Lymphotoxin (LT) is a tumor necrosis factor (TNF)-family cytokine. FIGURE 1 describes the LT/LIGHT ligands and receptors. Soluble $LT\alpha_3$ is a secreted protein and interacts with the TNF receptors I (55kD) and II (75kD). $LT\alpha$ is coexpressed with the membrane protein $LT\beta$ as $LT\alpha\beta$ heterodimers, which are tethered to the cell membrane. $LT\alpha1\beta2$ binds to a TNF-family receptor known as $LT\beta R$. LT-related inducible ligand (LIGHT) is a second ligand interacting with the $LT\beta R$. Activated lymphocytes and a subset of resting B cells express

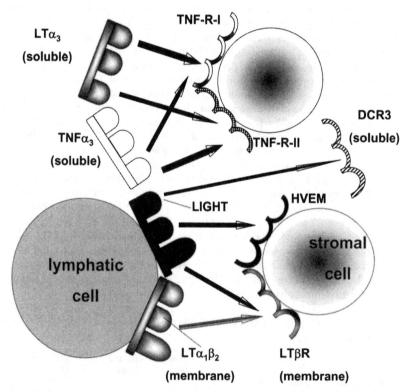

FIGURE 1. LT/LIGHT ligands and receptors. Soluble $LT\alpha3$ interacts with the TNF-receptors I (55kD) and II (75kD) whereas membrane-bound $LT\alpha1\beta2$ heterodimers interact with the membrane molecule $LT\beta R$. LIGHT is a second ligand of the $LT\beta R$, which also binds to the soluble decoy receptor (DCR3) and the herpes virus entry mediator (HVEM).

LT. The LTβR is expressed mainly on nonhematopoietic and myeloid lineage cells. [1]

Inhibition of LTβR-*Mediated Signalling: Modulation of the Lymphoid Microenvironment Alters Inflammatory Responses*

The role of the LT/LIGHT ligands and receptors has been characterized in gene-deficient mice (reviewed in Refs. 2 and 3). Deletion of the *lt*α and *lt*β*r* genes in LTα[−/−] and LTβR[−/−] mice is associated with the loss of all lymph nodes (LNs), Peyer's patches (PPs), and changes to the lymphoid architecture of the spleen. Targeted disruption of the *lt*β gene results in loss of peripheral LNs, whereas the mucosa draining cervical and mesenteric LNs are retained. Treatment with soluble LTβR-IgG fusion protein (LTβRIgG) similarly blocks the interaction of LTαβ and LIGHT with the LTβR. Gestational treatment with LTβRIgG prevents the formation of PPs and LNs. Postgestational LTβR signalling during the first 6 weeks after birth is critical for the development of intestinal lamina propria B cells, IgA secretion, and isolated lymphoid follicles (ILFs) of the intestine. The lymphoid microenvironment is defined as the local interplay between mobile lymphocytes and the fixed reticular/stromal cells, and includes cell adhesion, trafficking, chemokine function, and cellular positioning.[1] Secondary lymphoid organs are structures with a high degree of plasticity. Inhibition of LTβR signalling in adult mice alters the lymphoid microenvironment. Permanent LTβR-mediated signalling is required for the structural integrity of follicular dendritic cell (FDC) networks and splenic marginal zones (MZs). Inhibition of the LTβR also blocks the migration or maturation of certain dendritic cells (DCs).[4] PPs, isolated ILFs, cryptopatches, and colonic patches are organized lymphoid aggregates of the intestine. The number and cellular content of these aggregates is reduced in adult mice undergoing anti-LTβR treatment.[5] The potential mode of action in anti-LTβR treatment is to impair immune function by preventing proper placement of T cells, B cells, and antigen-presenting cells (APCs) in secondary lymphoid organs and thus preventing the induction of appropriate antigen-specific immune responses. A number of human inflammatory and autoimmune disorders are associated with the formation of ectopic lymphoid structures at the site of the inflamed organ which resemble secondary lymphoid organs.[6] It is likely that immune responses to self-antigens expand in these *de novo* lymphoid organs, as they allow colocalization of antigen-specific T and B cells with APCs. In mice, ectopic lymphoid structures can be induced by transgenic overexpression of LTα [7] and are called tertiary lymphoid tissues. Data from animal models of autoimmune diseases associated with the formation of ectopic lymphoid tissue indicate that autoimmunity is less severe, cured, or prevented if the LTβR is blocked in these conditions (reviewed in Ref. 1). FIGURE 2 provides an overview of the effects of LTβR blocking on autoimmunity and host defense.

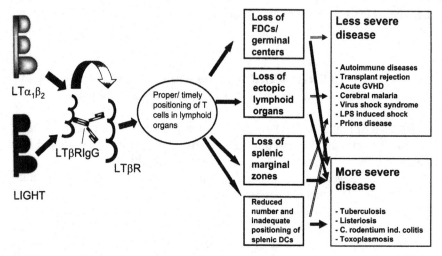

FIGURE 2. Biological effects of inhibition of LTα1β2/LIGHT-LTβR interaction in autoimmune and infectious diseases. Soluble LTβRIgG fusion protein blocks LTβR-mediated signaling, causing a loss of proper and timely positioning of T cell in lymphoid organs and thus changing lymphoid organ formation and microarchitecture (4 boxes). The altered lymphoid organs are associated with changes in the course of autoimmune and infectious inflammatory diseases.

THE ROLE OF GALT ORGANS IN INTESTINAL INFLAMMATION: IBD IS FOCUSED AT SITES OF HIGHLY CONCENTRATED LYMPHOID TISSUE

There is a striking focus of intestinal inflammation in the ileocecal region, a site with highly concentrated aggregation of secondary lymphoid tissue. In humans, ileocecal colitis is common in inflammatory bowel disease (IBD), such as Crohn's disease (CD) or backwash ileitis in ulcerative colitis (UC). However, infectious agents such as *Yersinia enterocolitica* and *Mycobacteria* also cause pseudoappendicitis and mesenteric lymphadenitis.[8,9] The terminal ileum is also a preferential site of inflammation in several animal models of IBD.[10,11] Circumstantial evidence indicates that the appendix plays a pivotal role in the development of CD and UC. There is a negative association between appendectomy and the onset and severity of these two diseases.[12,13]

ROLE OF LTα$_1$β$_2$–LTβR INTERACTIONS, GALT ORGANS IN DEVELOPMENT AND OUTCOME OF MURINE INTESTINAL INFLAMMATION

Experimental colitis induced by transfer of T$_H$1-type CD45RBhi cells or reconstitution of Tg$_ε$26 mice with wild-type (wt) bone marrow is attenuated by LTβRIgG treatment during disease induction.[14] The effect of LTβRIgG treatment on these two models of T_H1-mediated colitis was similar to that of anti-TNF treatment. As a consequence of this study anti-LTβ-directed treatment of CD is currently investigated. The course of TNBS colitis in mice made deficient in PPs and colonic ILFs secondary to gestational inhibition of $LT\alpha_1\beta_2$–LTβR interactions was investigated.[5] Mice deficient in colonic patches developed focal ulcers with T_H1-type responses whereas lesions in normal mice were of a diffuse mucosal type with both T_H1- and T_H2-type cytokine production.[5] Thus colonic ILFs and PPs provide help to control intestinal inflammation in TNBS-induced colitis. γ-IFN$^{-/-}$ mice undergoing such treatment were protected from TNBS colitis. Thus T_H2-type colitis is dependent on the presence of colonic patches or of $LT\alpha_1\beta_2$–LTβR interactions. It is of interest that both T_H1-type and T_H2-type cytokine-mediated types of experimental colitis can be controlled by inhibition of the $LT\alpha_1\beta_2$–LTβR pathway though the mechanism might vary in the different disease models. We have recently described more severe DSS-induced colitis in mice deficient in both PPs and LN (PP/LN null; LTα$^{-/-}$ mice and in PP/LN null mice secondary to gestational treatment with LTβRIgG and TNFRIgG).[15] There was hyperplasia and induction of colonic ILFs in LTα$^{-/-}$ mice and PP/LN null mice, suggesting a LT-independent pathway of formation of colonic lymphoid tissue induced during colonic inflammation. Clinically, DSS-induced colitis was similar in wild-type and mice without PP but with mesenteric lymph nodes (MLNs) (PP null/LN+ mice), although there also was induction of colonic lymphoid tissue in PP null/LN+ mice. Thus, PPs alone do not regulate DSS-induced colitis, whereas the presence of MLNs is critical in this regard.

The role of LT in host defense has been investigated in various animal models of infectious diseases (reviewed in Ref. 16). Mice undergoing oral pretreatment with streptomycin develop infectious colitis following oral infection with *Salmonella enterica* serovar Typhimurium, which resembles human *S. enterica*–induced colitis. The development of *S. enterica*–induced colitis was not affected by the presence of PPs, MLNs, or the LTβR because the course of this infection was similar in wild-type and LTβR$^{-/-}$ mice without PP and MLN. Infection of mice with *S. enterica* without antibiotic treatment induced a typhoid type of disease with bacterial expansion in PP and MLN. Interestingly, the typhoid type of *S. enterica* infection was also similar in wild-type and LTβR$^{-/-}$ mice without gut-associated lymphatic system (GALT) organs.[17] Infection of mice with *Citrobacter (C.) rodentium* serves as an animal model of human infection with enteropathogenic *Escherichia coli* (EPEC).[18] *C. rodentium*–induced colitis was more severe in LTβRIgG-treated mice and in LTα$^{-/-}$, LTβ$^{-/-}$, and LTβR$^{-/-}$ mice, suggesting a critical role for $LT\alpha_1\beta_2$– LTβR interactions in anti-*Citrobacter* immunity. In mice with disrupted LTβR signalling there were fewer splenic CD11c$^+$ DCs, and FDCs were absent in the spleen. These observations indicate that the loss of local intestinal lymphoid organs and changes to antigen-presenting functions of the spleen are associated with impaired immunity against this noninvasive pathogen.

SUMMARY—GALT ORGANS AND LT REGULATING INTESTINAL INFLAMMATION

Recent studies have shed new light on the mechanisms underlying the development of the organized GALT. TNF-family cytokine members are among the master regulators of intestinal lymphoid development. Gestational $LT\alpha1\beta2$–$LT\beta R$ interactions are critical for the development of PPs whereas blockade of the $LT\alpha_1\beta_2$–$LT\beta R$ pathway in adolescence is pivotal for lamina propria (LP) B-cell development. GALT organs are the intestinal branch of the organized lymphoid system. PPs are sites of IgA production and thus contribute to local and systemic immunity against intestinal antigens. We assume that MLNs serve as a site where DCs prime T cells for antiinflammatory T cell responses, as the course of acute DSS-colitis was more severe in mice without MLNs than in those with MLN. Human IBD and experimental colitis in mice are associated with immune activation in all GALT organs. Similar to MLNs the appendix seems to be critical for the development of both IBD and experimental colitis in animals since appendectomy attenuates both conditions. Inhibition of $LT\alpha_1\beta_2$–$LT\beta R$ signalling in T_H1- and T_H2-mediated experimental colitis suppresses intestinal inflammation. The effects of such treatment are secondary to changes to the lymphoid microenvironment and have also been demonstrated in the spleen of nonhuman primates.[19] Conversely, the course of experimental infectious colitis and tuberculosis are more severe in mice with disrupted $LT\beta R$-mediated signalling.[20,21] Bearing in mind the substantial differences between the human and murine immune systems and different modes of action in experimental murine infections and spontaneous infections of humans, immunity against infectious colitis induced by EPEC might be impaired in humans undergoing anti-$LT\beta R$ treatment. $LT\beta R$-blockade might be a potent biological tool that has to be carefully tested in clinical trials, considering the delicate balance between sufficient host defense and the suppression of autoimmunity.

REFERENCES

1. GOMMERMAN, J. & J.L. BROWNING. 2003. Lymphotoxin/LIGHT, lymphoid microenvironments and autoimmune disease. Nat. Rev. Immunol. **3:** 642–655.
2. CYSTER, J.G. 2003. Lymphoid organ development and cell migration. Immunol. Rev. **195:** 5–14.
3. SPAHN, T.W. & T. KUCHARZIK. 2004. Modulating the intestinal immune system: the role of lymphotoxin and GALT organs. Gut **53:** 456–465.

4. MACKAY, F. *et al.* 1997. Lymphotoxin but not tumor necrosis factor functions to maintain splenic architecture and humoral responsiveness in adult mice. Eur. J. Immunol. **27:** 2033–2042.

5. DOHI, T. *et al.* 2001. Elimination of colonic patches with lymphotoxin beta receptor-Ig prevents Th2 cell-type colitis. J. Immunol. **167:** 2781–2790.

6. RUDDLE, N.H. 1999. Lymphoid neo-organogenesis: lymphotoxin's role in inflammation and development. Immunol. Res. **19:** 119–125.

7. KRATZ, A. *et al.* 1996. Chronic inflammation caused by lymphotoxin is lymphoid neogenesis. J. Exp. Med. **183:** 1461–1472.

8. BOTTONE, E.J. 1999. *Yersinia enterocolitica*: overview and epidemiologic correlates. Microbes. Infect. **1:** 323–333.

9. HORVATH, K.D. & R.L. WHELAN. 1998. Intestinal tuberculosis: return of an old disease. Am. J. Gastroenterol. **93:** 692–696.

10. KONTOYIANNIS, D. *et al.* 1999. Impaired on/off regulation of TNF biosynthesis in mice lacking TNF AU-rich elements: implications for joint and gut-associated immunopathologies. Immunity **10:** 387–398.

11. SUNDBERG, J.P. *et al.* 1994. Spontaneous, heritable colitis in a new substrain of C3H/HeJ mice. Gastroenterology **107:** 1726–1735.

12. RADFORD-SMITH, G.L. *et al.* 2002. Protective role of appendicectomy on onset and severity of ulcerative colitis and Crohn's disease. Gut **51:** 808–813.

13. COSNES, J. *et al.* 2002. Effects of appendicectomy on the course of ulcerative colitis. Gut. **51:** 803–807.

14. MACKAY, F. *et al.* 1998. Both the lymphotoxin and tumor necrosis factor pathways are involved in experimental murine models of colitis. Gastroenterology **115:** 1464–1475.

15. SPAHN, T.W. *et al.* 2002. Induction of colitis in mice deficient of Peyer's patches and mesenteric lymph nodes is associated with increased disease severity and formation of colonic lymphoid patches. Am. J. Pathol. **161:** 2273–2282.

16. SPAHN, T.W. *et al.* 2005. The role of lymphotoxin in experimental models of infectious diseases: potential benefits and risks of a therapeutic inhibition of the lymphotoxin-receptor pathway. Infect. Immun. **73:** 7077–7088.

17. BARTHEL, M. *et al.* 2003. Pretreatment of mice with streptomycin provides a *Salmonella enterica* serovar typhimurium colitis model that allows analysis of both pathogen and host. Infect. Immun. **71:** 2839–2858.

18. LEVINE, M.M. 1987. *Escherichia coli* that cause diarrhea: enterotoxigenic, enteropathogenic, enteroinvasive, enterohemorrhagic, and enteroadherent. J. Infect. Dis. **155:** 377–389.

19. GOMMERMAN, J.L. *et al.* 2002. Manipulation of lymphoid microenvironments in nonhuman primates by an inhibitor of the lymphotoxin pathway. J. Clin. Invest. **110:** 1359–1369.

20. SPAHN, T.W. *et al.* 2004. The lymphotoxin-beta receptor is critical for control of murine *Citrobacter rodentium*-induced colitis. Gastroenterology **127:** 1463–1473.

21. ROACH, D.R. *et al.* 2001. Secreted lymphotoxin-alpha is essential for the control of an intracellular bacterial infection. J. Exp. Med. **193:** 239–246.

Immunomodulatory Roles of the Carcinoembryonic Antigen Family of Glycoproteins

LING SHAO, MATTHIEU ALLEZ, MEE-SOOK PARK, AND LLOYD MAYER

Center for Immunobiology, The Mount Sinai School of Medicine, 1 Gustave L. Levy Place, New York, New York 10029, USA

ABSTRACT: One of the most remarkable aspects of the immune system is its ability to fashion an immune response most appropriate to the activating stimulus. Although the immune system possesses a number of adaptations to accomplish this, an important theme is local immune regulation by site-specific expression of receptors and ligands. One family of molecules that is gaining attention as modulators of the immune system is the carcinoembryonic antigen cell-adhesion molecule family (CEACAM). Functionally, the carcinoembryonic antigen family can mediate cell–cell contact, host–pathogen interactions, and immune regulation. For example, biliary glycoprotein (CEACAM1) can have direct activity on T cells, leading to the inhibition of helper or cytotoxic T cell function. The expression of carcinoembryonic antigen (CEACAM5) on intestinal epithelial cells is involved in the activation of populations of regulatory CD8$^+$ T cells, while a distinct subset of regulatory CD8$^+$ T cells is activated by nonspecific cross-reacting antigen (CEACAM6) on placental trophoblasts. Interestingly, the function and phenotype of these cells depend upon the specific member of the carcinoembryonic antigen family expressed, as well as the antigen-presenting molecule with which it associates. Thus, these glycoproteins comprise a family of molecules whose functions can depend on their nature and context.

KEYWORDS: mucosal immunity; regulatory T cells; carcinoembryonic antigen

INTRODUCTION

The immune system at mucosal surfaces, for example, in the intestine, is a product of the unusual microenvironment to which it is exposed. The indigenous microflora of the intestine poses a remarkable challenge to the

Address for correspondence: Lloyd Mayer, 1425 Madison Avenue, Box 1089, New York, NY 10029. Voice: 212-659-9261; fax: 212-987-5593.

e-mail: lloyd.mayer@mssm.edu

Ann. N.Y. Acad. Sci. 1072: 194–209 (2006). © 2006 New York Academy of Sciences.
doi: 10.1196/annals.1326.037

gut-associated lymphoid tissue (GALT). The antigen load represented by these commensal organisms is both exceedingly large ($> 10^{12}$ organisms per gram of colonic tissue) and extraordinarily diverse.[1–5] In addition, the GALT is faced with a large antigenic load from the normal diet. Yet in most cases, these types of antigens are well tolerated. Simultaneously, this nonpathogenic pool of antigens must be constantly surveyed to alert the GALT to the presence of pathogenic organisms. The resultant immunologic state in the intestine is markedly distinct from the systemic immune system and reflects these dichotomous characteristics.

The overarching immunologic tone of the GALT is one of hyporesponsiveness. This basal state of suppression prevents a pathologic response to the constant presence of commensal flora and dietary antigens. While systemic immunization characteristically activates cellular immune responses and production of immunoglobulins (Ig) IgG and IgM, oral administration of antigen leads to a blunting of systemic cellular immune responses and production of secretory IgA.[6,7]

The mechanisms underlying this unique response to antigen is complex and involves a number of cellular components. Antigen presentation in the gut can occur through several different pathways. Trafficking of antigen through M cells is critical for activating host–pathogen responses against viruses (e.g., polio) and important enteropathogenic bacteria (e.g., Salmonella).[8] Dendritic cells are also important antigen-presenting cells in the GALT and subpopulations of these cells are likely to play a role in tolerance.[9] Finally, intestinal epithelial cells can also process and present antigens and activate tolerogenic responses.

Our laboratory first described the ability of human intestinal epithelial cells to act as antigen-presenting cells for a subpopulation of CD8$^+$ T cells. These cells are CD28$^-$, express mucosal homing markers CD101 and CD103, and have contact-dependent regulatory activity independent of perforin, granzyme, and CTLA-4 (FIG. 1).[10] Surprisingly, further analysis of these CD8$^+$ T cells showed that they were not dependent on classical antigen-presenting molecules or costimulatory molecules for activation.

Intestinal epithelial cells harbor the capacity to present antigen through a surprisingly diverse set of antigen-presenting molecules. In addition to the expression of MHC class I and class II antigens, intestinal epithelial cells can express a wide variety of nonclassical MHC class I-like antigens.[11] Furthermore, intestinal epithelial cells lack the classical costimulatory molecules B7.1 and B7.2, but do express B7h and B7H1.[12] Indeed, a subpopulation of regulatory CD8$^+$ T cells in the gut are activated by a combination of the nonclassical MHC class I molecule CD1d and a novel costimulatory molecule termed gp180 (FIG. 1).

Further analysis of gp180 revealed a heavily glycosylated protein of approximately 180 kD that was expressed highly in the intestinal epithelium, but also by cortical thymic epithelial cells and trophoblasts in the placenta.

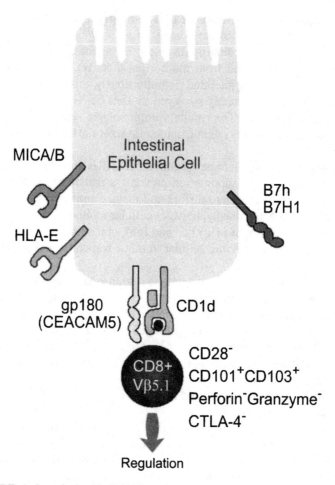

FIGURE 1. Intestinal epithelial cells activate and expand a subset of regulatory CD8+ T cells. Intestinal epithelial cells express a variety of classical and nonclassical MHC molecules. In addition, intestinal epithelial cells lack the expression of classical costimulatory molecules such as B7.1 and B7.2, but do express the novel costimulatory molecules B7h and B7H1. Intestinal epithelial cells can activate regulatory CD8+ T cells through a combination of the nonclassical MHC class I molecule, CD1d, and the costimulatory molecule gp180 (CEAMCAM5).

N-terminal sequencing of purified gp180 demonstrated sequence identity with carcinoembryonic antigen (CEA).

CARCINOEMBRYONIC ANTIGEN

Carcinoembryonic antigen (CEA) was first described in 1965 by Gold and Freedman as an antigen associated with intestinal malignancies. Since its first

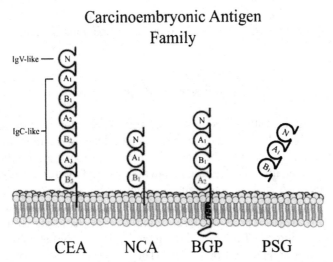

FIGURE 2. The carcinoembryonic antigen family. The carcinoembryonic antigen family consists of four major divisions: carcinoembryonic antigen (CEA, CEACAM5), nonspecific cross-reacting antigen (NCA, CEACAM6), biliary glycoprotein (BGP, CEACAM1), and the pregnancy-specific glycoproteins (PSG). Structurally, the family consists of an IgV-like N-domain and a variable number of IgC-like A and B domains. They may be tethered to the membrane by a GPI anchor (CEA and NCA), exist as transmembrane proteins (BGP), or be secreted (PSGs). The members of the family share a large degree of sequence homology in the N-domain, but differences in sequence and posttranslational modifications can give rise to functional differences.

description, a family of evolutionarily conserved members has been delineated. Among these are carcinoembryonic antigen (designated CEA-related cell–cell adhesion molecule 5, CEACAM5), nonspecific cross-reacting protein (CEACAM6), and biliary glycoprotein (CEACAM1). Additional related molecules exist in the family including the pregnancy-specific glycoproteins that are exclusively secreted by trophoblasts.

Structurally, the members of the CEA family have an IgV-like N-terminal domain, followed by a variable number of IgC-like A and B domains (FIG. 2). The N-domains of CEACAM1, -5, and -6, are approximately 90% identical, while the A and B domains are less homologous. These extracellular domains can be tethered to the membrane via a GPI anchor in the case of CEACAM5 and CEACAM6, or exist in a transmembrane form in the case of CEACAM1 (FIG. 2). Posttranslational modification of CEA can be extensive, leading to differences in function.[13]

Clinically, CEA is widely used as a marker of tumor progression in colonic and other gastrointestinal malignancies, ovarian, bladder, and breast cancers. Elevated CEA is associated with a larger tumor burden, and a poorer prognosis presurgically, and may indicate a recurrence of disease postsurgically.[14]

However, while CEA has been clinically studied for several decades, the functional properties that lead to its clinical associations have only recently been explored.

Adhesion Molecules

Some of the earliest reports on the function of CEA family members suggested a possible role as intercellular adhesion molecules, forming homotypic or heterotypic interactions.[15–18] These interactions occur through the highly conserved N-domain in a calcium-dependent fashion.[19] Interestingly, adhesion mediated by CEA may augment further interactions via classical integrins. Cross-linking CEA family members using an N-domain antibody enhances the adhesion of neutrophils to fibronectin.[20] Downstream signaling is also initiated following of CEA cross-linking, activating the tyrosine kinases lyn, hck, and src in human neutrophils.[20,21] These events can lead to neutrophil aggregation[22] or degranulation.[23] In epithelial cells, enhanced adhesion to the extracellular matrix mediated by CEACAM5 and CEACAM6 manifests as decreased apoptosis and anoikis,[24] while in endothelial cells, CEACAM1 stimulates angiogenesis.[25]

Pathogen Receptors

Several members of the CEA family are also known to serve as pathogen receptors. CEAMCAM1, CEACAM5, CEACAM6, and others can serve as ligands for the gonococcal opacity (Opa) proteins.[26–28] Internalization of *N. gonorrhoeae* by a human cell line is mediated in part by the CEA family.[29–32] CEACAM1, CEACAM5, and CEACAM6 can also serve as receptors for the Afa/Dr adhesions of *Escherichia coli*.[33]

Similar to homotypic or heterotypic cross-linking, interaction of CEA family members with the Opa proteins or Afa/Dr leads to a cascade of intracellular signaling.[29–33] Muenzer *et al.* demonstrated in epithelial cells that Opa signaling enhances integrin-dependent cell adhesion and upregulated the expression of the TGF-β1 receptor, CD105.[34] In contrast, proliferation and antibody production in CEACAM1-expressing B cells were decreased and the rate of apoptosis increased after interaction with Opa proteins.[35] Together, these results suggest an important role for CEA family members in host–pathogen interactions.

Immunoregulatory Ligands

Intercellular interactions, downstream signaling, and expression on a variety of immune cells strongly suggest a direct role for CEA in immune regulation. Indeed, evidence in mice suggests that CEACAM1 activation on murine dendritic cells causes IL-6 and IL-12 release.[36] Natural killer cell activity is inhibited by the interaction of surface CEACAM1 and either CEACAM5 or CEACAM1 on target cells.[37,38] Similarly, directly cross-linking CEACAM1 on murine T cells inhibited *in vitro* allogeneic mixed lymphocyte reactions, as well as *in vivo* delayed type hypersensitivity to oxazalone.[39] This inhibition was dependent upon the immunoreceptor tyrosine inhibitory motifs contained within the long intra-cytoplasmic tail of CEACAM1[40] and may involve the inhibition of IL-2 production.[41]

In addition to homotypic and heterotypic interactions, recent evidence has suggested that members of the CEA family may interact with the T cell receptor, albeit indirectly. Ideo *et al.* reported that galectin-4 bound to CEA with nanomolar affinity.[42] Galectin-4 has previously been shown to activate CD4$^+$ T cells through an MHC class II-dependent pathway in a murine model of colitis.[43] Taken together, these data suggest that members of the CEA family may directly and indirectly influence the development and propagation of the immune response.

In concert with these data, our laboratory has demonstrated the ability of gp180 (CEACAM5) to interact with the immune system via a novel interaction with CD8. Murine T cells transfected with human CD8 but not human CD4, efficiently adsorbed CEA from supernatants generated by PIPLC treatment of T84 adenocarcinoma cells that express gp180 endogenously (data not shown). Additionally, gp180 could induce the phosphorylation of p56^{lck} in 3G8 cells expressing human CD8, but not human CD4. Functionally, purified gp180 completely blocked flu-specific CTL induction (FIG. 3A), which may involve the ability of gp180 to block phosphatidyl-inositol-3-kinase activation in these cells (FIG. 3B). Interestingly, purified gp180 did not alter the effector phase of CTL function (FIG. 3C), suggesting that binding of gp180 to CD8 did not inhibit an interaction of CD8 with MHC class I. Indeed, we have previously shown that gp180 binds to CD8 on sites that are distinct from classical MHC class I binding.

ACTIVATION OF CD8$^+$ REGULATORY T CELLS

Immune Regulation in the Intestine

To study the interaction between gp180 (CEACAM5) and CD8, we generated a panel of monoclonal antibodies directed against gp180. Several antibodies directed against overlapping regions of the CEACAM5 N-domain were obtained. One antibody, termed B9, was selected for further study because of its unique ability to block the generation of regulatory CD8$^+$ T cells in cultures with freshly isolated human intestinal epithelial cells.

As alluded to above, these cells are activated by a combination of the nonclassical MHC class I molecule CD1d and the costimulatory molecule of the CEA

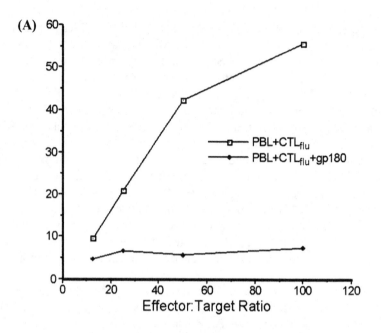

(B)   Allogeneic Mixed Lymphocyte Reaction

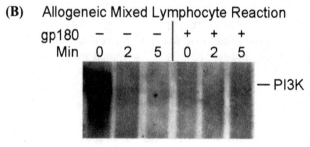

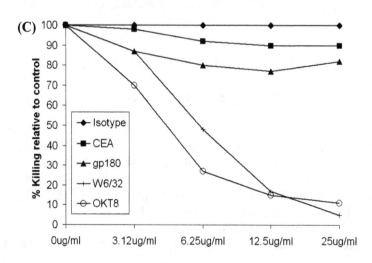

TABLE 1. Expansion of CD8⁺Vβ5.1⁺ T cells in Cocultures of Intestinal Epithelial Cells and Peripheral Blood T cells Compared to the Percentage of CD8⁺ Vβ5.1⁺ T cells in Freshly Isolated Normal and IBD Lamina Propria Lymphocytes

	IBD ($N = 5$)	Normal ($N = 8$)
In vitro (IEC:PB T coculture)		
%Vβ5.1/ IEC-activated CD8⁺ T cells (CFSE^{lo})	1.52 ± 1.33%*	4.36 ± 2.42%
In vivo (LPL) % Vβ5.1/CD8⁺ LPL	2.23 ± 1.04%**	4.72 ± 1.41%

Peripheral blood T cells labeled with CFSE were cocultured with intestinal epithelial cells (IEC) from patients with inflammatory bowel disease (IBD) or normal controls. Proliferation of CD8⁺Vβ5.1⁺ T cells was measured by flow cytometry (decreased CFSE intensity). Intestinal epithelial cells from IBD patients had a decreased ability to stimulate the expansion of CD8⁺Vβ5.1⁺ T cells compared to intestinal epithelial cells from normal controls. *In vivo*, lamina propria lymphocytes isolated from IBD patients had a decreased percentage of CD8⁺Vβ5.1⁺ T cells than normal controls.
*$P < 0.05$.
**$P < 0.01$.

family, gp180 (CEACAM5), and display a regulatory phenotype. Predictably, restriction of these cells by the nonpolymorphic antigen-presenting molecule CD1d, leads to the activation of a limited subset of T cells, in particular a population of T cells utilizing the T cell receptor gene Vβ5.1. Functionally, these cells can act as third-party suppressor cells in a mixed lymphocyte reaction and mitogen-stimulated immunoglobulin secretion. *In vivo* these cells are found in relatively high concentrations within the lamina propria. Interestingly, the presence of these cells is significantly decreased in patients with inflammatory bowel disease, suggesting a possible role for these cells in moderating intestinal inflammation (TABLE 1).

←————————————————————————————

FIGURE 3. (**A**) gp180 (CEACAM5) inhibits CTL induction but not CTL effector function. Influenza A infected peripheral blood lymphocytes (PBL) were used to generate flu-specific CTL in the absence (◇) or presence (■) of gp180. CTLs generated in the absence of gp180 efficiently killed flu-infected target cells in a chromium release assay. In contrast, preincubation with soluble gp180 completely blocked the generation of flu-specific CTLs. (**B**) Allogeneic mixed lymphocyte reactions were performed in the absence (lanes 1–3) or presence (lanes 4–6) of gp180 and probed by phosphotyrosine Western blot. Rapid and transient induction of PI3K was observed in allogeneic mixed lymphocyte reactions in the absence of gp180. Addition of gp180 completely abrogated the activation of PI3K. (**C**) Flu-specific CTLs were used to kill flu-infected targets in a chromium release assay. Flu-specific CTLs treated with an isotype control antibody, commercial CEA, or gp180 purified from PIPLC treated T84 cells (an adenocarcinoma cell line) did not block lysis. In contrast, flu-specific killing was inhibited by mABs against MHC class I (W6/32) or CD8 (OKT8). Taken together these data suggest that gp180 (CEACAM5) can block the induction of CTL, potentially through an inhibitory effect on PI3K. gp180 has no activity on CTL effector functions. Furthermore, the inability of gp180 to block CTL effector function suggests that its interaction with CD8 does not inhibit CD8 interactions with MHC class I.

Immune Regulation in the Placenta

The expression of CEA by other epithelial cells suggested the possibility that regulatory CD8$^+$ T cells might be activated at those sites as well. One such site might be at the maternal–fetal interface where an immune reaction against a semi-allogeneic fetus could be devastating. Similar to intestinal epithelial cells, trophoblasts form a single cell barrier between the immune system and an abundance of foreign antigen. Like intestinal epithelial cells, trophoblasts express a diverse array of nonclassical MHC class I molecules including CD1d (FIG. 4).

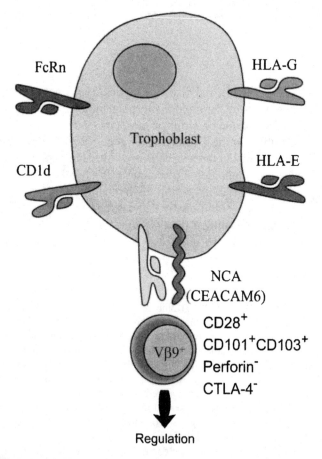

FIGURE 4. Trophoblasts Activate a Subset of Regulatory CD8$^+$ T cells. Trophoblasts lack the expression of classical restriction elements but do express a variety of nonclassical MHC class I molecules. Similar to intestinal epithelial cells, trophoblasts can activate a subset of regulatory CD8$^+$ T cells, but interestingly, these regulatory T cells require a different restriction element and costimulation by a distinct member of the carcinoembryonic antigen family, NCA (CEACAM6).

Indeed, we were able to demonstrate that trophoblasts were able to activate regulatory CD8$^+$ T cells.[44] Critically, while these regulatory CD8$^+$ T cells shared some similarities with those found in the intestine, a number of important differences exist. While intestinal CD8$^+$ regulatory T cells depend upon gp180 (CEACAM5) for activation, placental regulatory T cells depend upon costimulation by the closely related CEACAM6. This critical difference also manifests functionally, since placental regulatory CD8$^+$ T cells have restricted regulatory activity against immunoglobulin secretion and have no activity as third-party suppressor cells in an allogeneic mixed lymphocyte reaction. Furthermore, our data indicate that placental regulatory CD8$^+$ T cells are independent of CD1d and use a distinct T-cell repertoire (predominantly Vβ9), suggesting that CEACAM6 preferentially pairs with another nonclassical MHC class I molecule. We postulate that these cells may play a role in maternal tolerance of the semi-allogeneic fetus.

SUMMARY

The carcinoembryonic antigen family is a diverse set of glycoproteins with a multitude of functions including cell–cell adhesion, host–pathogen interactions, and immune modulation. Within the immune system, different members of the CEA family or different forms of the same protein (through posttranslational modification) can have disparate activities.

Members of the CEA family are highly expressed on epithelial cells of the intestine and placenta where they can participate in the activation of CD8$^+$ regulatory T cells. Importantly, differential expression of CEA family members contributes to functional differences in the regulatory T-cell populations activated at different sites. This supports a model in which distinct CEA family members act at different sites, forming complexes with distinct antigen-presenting molecules, leading to separate functional outcomes. This would allow for both flexibility and fine-tuning of the immune system based on the surrounding microenvironment.

METHODS

Cell Lines and Media

T84, HT29, and 293T cells were obtained from the ATCC (Manassas, VA). Murine T-cell transfectants 3G4 and 3G8, transfected with a full-length human CD4 or a full-length CD8α cDNA, respectively, were kind gifts from Dr. S. J. Burakoff (Dana-Farber Institute, Boston, MA). FO-1 cells (a human melanoma cell line) was a kind gift from Dr. R. Blumberg (Brigham and Women's Hospital, Boston, MA). 293T cells were transfected with full-length CEA pCDNA plasmid or vector control using Superfect (Invitrogen, Carlsbad CA) according to the manufacturer's instructions. Cell lines were grown in RPMI 1640 (Medi-atech Inc. Herndon VA) with 10% fetal calf serum (Omega Scientific, Tarzana CA) with 1% penicillin–streptomycin–glutamate (Invitrogen, Carlsbad CA). Freshly isolated peripheral blood mononuclear cells (PBMC) were cultured in serum-free media, AIM-V (Invitrogen) with 1% penicillin–streptomycin–glutamate.

Isolation of IECs and LPLs

Intestinal epithelial cells were isolated as described previously.[45] Briefly, surgical specimens were obtained in accordance with the Mount Sinai School of Medicine Internal Review Board guidelines and washed extensively in PBS. The mucosa was mechanically separated from the underlying submucosa and cut into 2×2-mm sections and treated with 1 mM DTT (Sigma-Aldrich, St. Louis, MO) for 15 min. The tissue was then washed in PBS and incubated twice for 30 min in medium containing 3 mg/mL Dispase II (Roche, Indianapolis, IN) at 37°C, 5% CO_2. The supernatant (released IECs) was collected and washed in medium twice. The viability of the isolated IECs was >95%.

Lamina propria lymphocytes (LPLs) were isolated from the tissue remain-ing after the dispase treatments. The tissue was incubated for 1 h at 37°C in medium containing 1 mg/mL collagenase (clostridiopeptidase A) and 5 μg/mL DNase I (both Sigma-Aldrich). The supernatant was collected and centrifuged on a discontinuous Percoll (Amersham Biosciences, Piscataway, NJ) density gradient and the LPLs were harvested from the 40–60% interface. Viability was >90%.

Isolation of Peripheral Blood T cells and Co-culture

Heparinized venous blood was collected from normal donors, diluted in a ratio of 1:3 with PBS, layered on a Ficoll-hypaque density gradient (Amersham Biosciences), and centrifuged for 30 min at 1800 rpm. PBMCs were collected from the interface and washed three times with PBS. Cells were resuspended in RPMI 1640 and the cell density was adjusted to 5×10^6 cells/mL. PBMCs were incubated with neuraminidase-treated sheep red blood cells overnight and then subjected to centrifugation over Ficoll-hypaque density gradient. Non-T cells were collected from the interface, washed with PBS, and resuspended in cul-ture medium (Aim V, 50 U/mL penicillin, 50 μg/mL streptomycin, 2 mmol/L glutamine). Rosetted T cells were treated with 0.75% ammonium chloride on ice for 5–10 min to lyse sheep red blood cells. The T-cell suspension was then washed with PBS. T cells (5×10^6/mL) were for stained with 1 mM CFSE (Molecular Probes, Eugene, OR) for 10 min at 37°C. T cells were then washed twice in RPMI. Mixed cell culture was performed using irradi-ated IECs (3,000 rad) as stimulator cells and allogeneic T cells as responder cells. CFSE-labeled T cells and IECs were cocultured at 1×10^6/mL and

0.5×10^6/mL, respectively, in culture medium at 37°C in a 5% CO_2 humidified incubator for 5–10 days.

Flow Cytometry and Sorting

Freshly isolated lamina propria lymphocytes or CFSE-labeled peripheral blood T-cell cocultured with intestinal epithelial cells were washed twice in PBS/1% BSA (Sigma). Cells were stained with monoclonal antibodies against CD3-PerCP, CD8-APC (BD Pharmingen), and Vβ5.1-PE (Immunotech, Marseille, France) for 30 min at 4°C then washed three times in PBS/1% BSA. Cells were analyzed on a FacsCalibur (BD Immunocytometry, San Jose, CA). T cells were first gated on CD3-PerCP. Proliferating cells were identified by a decreased CFSE intensity (CFSE^{lo}).

PIPLC Treatment, gp180 purification, and Absorption Studies

Ten to twenty million isolated T84 cells were harvested by nonenzyme cell dissociation solution (Sigma) and washed three times with PBS and treated with PIPLC (Sigma) at concentrations of 0.3–1 unit/mL RPMI at 37°C for 45 min. For some experiments purified gp180 was obtained by subjecting PIPLC supernatants to affinity chromatography using B9 mAb-conjugated recombinant protein G-Sepharose 4B (Amersham Biosciences) beads. The purity of gp180 after chromatography was confirmed by SDS-PAGE followed by silver staining. The cell-free supernatant from PIPLC treatment was collected and incubated with murine T cell hybridomas expressing human CD4 (3G4), CD8 (3G8), or an unrelated cell line control (FO-1). After incubation cells were lysed in Laemmli buffer and resolved on 10% SDS-PAGE and then transferred onto a nitrocellulose membrane at 15 V overnight in transfer buffer (20% methanol, 150mM glycine, 25mM Tris, pH 8.3). After transfer, the nitrocellulose sheet was blocked by 50mL of 5% nonfat milk in PBS. The nitrocellulose sheet was washed once with PBS and probed with either the Col-1 anti-CEA (CEACAM5) mAb (Sigma) or B9 mAb against gp180 (generated in our lab) in PBS/0.5% nonfat milk solution at 4°C overnight. After washing three to five times with 0.05% Tween 20 in PBS, horseradish peroxidase-conjugated goat anti-mouse IgG antibody (1–2 µg/mL) (BD Pharmingen) was added and incubated at room temperature for 1–2 h. Membranes were then washed three to five times with washing buffer and developed with Supersignal (Pierce, Rockford IL) chemiluminscence reagent.

T cell Stimulation and Phosphotyrosine Detection

Murine T cells (2×10^6) transfected with human CD4 (3G4) or human CD8 (3G8) were stimulated with either FFB2.3 mAb (anti-CD4), OKT8 (anti-CD8), or PIPLC supernatants from 293T cells transfected with full-length CEA or vector control for 0–15 min at 37°C. The stimulation was stopped by the addition of 1 mL of ice-cold stop buffer (100 μM Na_2VO_3 in PBS). The cells were centrifuged and the stop buffer was removed. Two hundred microliters of lysis buffer (1% Nonidet P-40, 100 μM Na_2VO_3, 1 mM PMSF, 5 mM iodoacetamide, 20 μg/mL aprotinin, 20 μg/mL leupeptin, 140 mM NaCl, 20 mM Tris–HCl, pH 7.4) was added into the cell pellet and kept on ice for 30 min, vortexing every 5–10 min. The cell lysate was centrifuged at 4°C for 10 min at 12,000 × g. The lysate was mixed with loading buffer containing 5% β-mercaptoethanol and boiled for 3 min. Lysates were resolved by SDS-PAGE and subjected to Western blot using an anti-phosphotyrosine mAb 4G10 (Upstate Biotechnology Inc., Lake Placid, NY) or anti-Ig heavy chain or β-actin as controls. Membranes were then probed with goat anti-mouse horseradish peroxidase conjugated IgG antibody (BD Pharmingen) and developed with Supersignal (Pierce) as detailed above.

CTL generation and Chromium Release Assays

Peripheral blood samples from normal volunteers were obtained by vein puncture and PBMC isolated by Ficoll (Pharmacia, Uppsala, Sweden) gradient separation. To generate effector cytotoxic T lymphocytes (CTL), PBMCs were stimulated *in vitro* with 10 μg/mL of specific CTL peptide derived from influenza A Puerto Rico isolate (PR8). In some experiments, CTLs were generated in the presence carcinoembryonic antigen (CEACAM6), purified gp180, or antibodies against human MHC class I (W6/32), CD8 (OKT8), or isotype controls. After 7 days, lines were stimulated with 2 × 10^6 irradiated (3,000 rad) autologous adherent cells pulsed for 2 h with peptide (10 μg/mL). CTL lines were fed by adding 1 mL of fresh media and 40 U/mL human recombinant IL2 (rh-IL2) (Endogen, Cambridge, MA) at days 3, 6, 9, and 12.

Seven days after the second *in vitro* stimulation, CTL lines were assayed for cytotoxicity. Autologous PBMCs (1×10^6) were infected overnight with PR8. Flu-infected PBMCs were labeled with ^{51}Cr (Perkin Elmer, Wellesley MA) for 4 h at room temperature.

Triplicate wells of effector CTLs were incubated with 5 × 10^3 ^{51}Cr-labeled targets in different ratios in V-bottom plates (Nalge Nunc, Rochester NY) for 4 h at 37°C, with 5% CO_2. In some experiments, effectors were preincubated with gp180 for 1 h prior to incubation with target cells. After incubation, 100 μL of culture supernatant was harvested and the amount of released ^{51}Cr in each triplicate sample was assayed by a gamma counter. Spontaneous release of ^{51}Cr was measured by incubating P815 cells alone, while maximal release was determined by solubilizing labeled P815 cells in 1% Triton-X100. Specific lysis was calculated by the formula:

$$\% \text{ specific lysis} = 100 \times \frac{(^{51}\text{Cr released} - \text{spontaneous } ^{51}\text{Cr release})}{(\text{maximal } ^{51}\text{Cr release} - \text{spontaneous } ^{51}\text{Cr release})}$$

Allogeneic Mixed Lymphocyte Reaction and Western Blot

Peripheral blood T cells and non-T cells were isolated as described above. T cells (2×10^6) and 1×10^6 irradiated (3,000 rads) non-T cells from unrelated donors were incubated for 0–5 min in the presence or absence of gp180. Cells were lysed in Laemmli buffer and resolved by SDS-PAGE. Proteins were transferred to nitrocellulose membranes and probed by and antibody against PI3K.

REFERENCES

1. HOLDEMAN, L.V., I.J. GOOD & W.E.C. MOORE. 1976. Human fecal flora: variation in bacterial composition within individuals and a possible effect of emotional stress. Appl. Environ. Microbiol. **31:** 359–375.
2. SAVAGE, D.C. 1977. Microbial ecology of the gastrointestinal tract. Annu. Rev. Microbiol. **31:** 107–133.
3. FINEGOLD, S.M., V.L. SUTTER & G.E. MATHISEN. 1983. Normal indigenous intestinal flora. In Human Intestinal Microflora in Health and Disease. Hentges, D. J. Ed.: 3–32. Academic Press. New York.
4. SAVAGE, D.C. 1986. Gastrointestinal microflora in mammalian nutrition. Annu. Rev. Nutr. **6:** 155–178.
5. SAVAGE, D.C. 1989. The normal human microflora composition. In The regulatory and protective role of the normal microflora. Grubb, R., T. Midvedt & E. Norin Eds.: 3–18. Stockton. London.
6. HUSBY, S., J. MESTECKY, Z. MOLDOVEANU, *et al.* 1994. Oral tolerance in humans. T cell but not B cell tolerance after antigen feeding. J. Immunol. **152:** 4663–4670.
7. KRAUS, T.A., L. TOY, L. CHAN, *et al.* 2004. Failure to induce oral tolerance to a soluble protein in patients with inflammatory bowel disease. Gastroenterology. **126:** 1771–1778.
8. KRAEHENBUHL, J.P. & M.R. NEUTRA. 2000. Epithelial M cells: differentiation and function. Annu. Rev. Cell Dev. Biol. **16:** 301–332.
9. DUBOIS, B., A. GOUBIER, G. JOUBERT, *et al.* 2005. Oral tolerance and regulation of mucosal immunity. Cell Mol. Life Sci. **62:** 1322–1332.
10. ALLEZ, M., J. BRIMNES, I. DOTAN, *et al.* 2002. Expansion of CD8+ T cells with regulatory function after interaction with intestinal epithelial cells. Gastroenterology. **123:** 1516–1526.
11. SHAO, L., O. KAMALU & L. MAYER. 2005. Non-classical MHC class I molecules on intestinal epithelial cells: mediators of mucosal crosstalk. Immunol. Rev. **206:** 160–176.
12. NAKAZAWA, A., I. DOTAN, J. BRIMNES, *et al.* 2004. The expression and function of costimulatory molecules B7H and B7-H1 on colonic epithelial cells. Gastroenterology. **126:** 1347–1357.
13. GRIMM, T., G. RIETHMULLER & J.P. JOHNSON. 1994. Characteristics of carcinoembryonic antigen (CEA) expressed in different cell types: evidence that CEA can function as an adhesion molecule and as a repulsion molecule. Biochem. Biophys. Res. Commun. **204:** 1225–1234.
14. CRAWFORD, N.P., D.W. COLLIVER & S. GALANDIUK. 2003. Tumor markers and colorectal cancer: utility in management. J. Surg. Oncol. **84:** 239–248.

15. BENCHIMOL, S., A. FUKS, S. JOTHY, et al. 1989. Carcinoembryonic antigen, a human tumor marker, functions as an intercellular adhesion molecule. Cell **57:** 327–334.

16. OIKAWA, S., C. INUZUKA, M. KUROKI, et al. 1989. Cell adhesion activity of non-specific cross-reacting antigen (NCA) and carcinoembryonic antigen (CEA) expressed on CHO cell surface: homophilic and heterophilic adhesion. Biochem. Biophys. Res. Commun. **164:** 39–45.

17. ROJAS, M., A. FUKS & C.P. STANNERS. 1990. Biliary glycoprotein, a member of the immunoglobulin supergene family, functions in vitro as a Ca2(+)-dependent intercellular adhesion molecule. Cell Growth Differ. **1:** 527–533.

18. OIKAWA, S., M. KUROKI, Y. MATSUOKA, et al. 1992. Homotypic and heterotypic Ca(++)-independent cell adhesion activities of biliary glycoprotein, a member of carcinoembryonic antigen family, expressed on CHO cell surface. Biochem. Biophys. Res. Commun. **186:** 881–887.

19. KUROKI, M., H. ABE, T. IMAKIIREI, et al. 2001. Identification and comparison of residues critical for cell-adhesion activities of two neutrophil CD66 antigens, CEACAM6 and CEACAM8. J. Leukoc. Biol. **70:** 543–550.

20. NAIR, K.S. & S.M. ZINGDE. 2001. Adhesion of neutrophils to fibronectin: role of the cd66 antigens. Cell Immunol. **208:** 96–106.

21. SKUBITZ, K.M., K.D. CAMPBELL, K. AHMED, et al. 1995. CD66 family members are associated with tyrosine kinase activity in human neutrophils. J. Immunol. **155:** 5382–5390.

22. KUIJPERS, T.W., C.E. VAN DER SCHOOT, M. HOOGERWERF, et al. 1993. Cross-linking of the carcinoembryonic antigen-like glycoproteins CD66 and CD67 induces neutrophil aggregation. J. Immunol. **151:** 4934–4940.

23. KLEIN, M.L., S.A. MCGHEE, J. BARANIAN, et al. 1996. Role of nonspecific cross-reacting antigen, a CD66 cluster antigen, in activation of human granulocytes. Infect. Immun. **64:** 4574–4579.

24. ORDONEZ, C., R.A. SCREATON, C. ILANTZIS, et al. 2000. Human carcinoembryonic antigen functions as a general inhibitor of anoikis. Cancer Res. **60:** 3419–3424.

25. WAGENER, C. & S. ERGUN. 2000. Angiogenic properties of the carcinoembryonic antigen-related cell adhesion molecule 1. Exp. Cell Res. **261:** 19–24.

26. CHEN, T. & E.C. GOTSCHLICH. 1996. CGM1a antigen of neutrophils, a receptor of gonococcal opacity proteins. Proc. Natl. Acad. Sci. USA. **93:** 14851–14856.

27. VIRJI, M., K. MAKEPEACE, D.J. FERGUSON, et al. 1996. Carcinoembryonic antigens (CD66) on epithelial cells and neutrophils are receptors for Opa proteins of pathogenic neisseriae. Mol. Microbiol. **22:** 941–950.

28. CHEN, T., F. GRUNERT, A. MEDINA-MARINO, et al. 1997. Several carcinoembryonic antigens (CD66) serve as receptors for gonococcal opacity proteins. J. Exp. Med. **185:** 1557–1564.

29. HAUCK, C.R., T.F. MEYER, F. LANG, et al. 1998. CD66-mediated phagocytosis of Opa52 Neisseria gonorrhoeae requires a Src-like tyrosine kinase- and Rac1-dependent signalling pathway. EMBO J. **17:** 443–454.

30. HAUCK, C.R., E. GULBINS, F. LANG, et al. 1999. Tyrosine phosphatase SHP-1 is involved in CD66-mediated phagocytosis of Opa52-expressing Neisseria gonorrhoeae. Infect. Immun. **67:** 5490–5494.

31. MUENZNER, P., M. NAUMANN, T.F. MEYER, et al. 2001. Pathogenic Neisseria trigger expression of their carcinoembryonic antigen-related cellular adhesion molecule 1 (CEACAM1; previously CD66a) receptor on primary endothelial cells by activating the immediate early response transcription factor, nuclear factor-kappaB. J. Biol. Chem. **276:** 24331–24340.

32. BILLKER, O., A. POPP, V. BRINKMANN, *et al.* 2002. Distinct mechanisms of internalization of *Neisseria gonorrhoeae* by members of the CEACAM receptor family involving Rac1- and Cdc42-dependent and -independent pathways. EMBO J. **21:** 560–571.

33. BERGER, C.N., O. BILLKER, T.F. MEYER, *et al.* 2004. Differential recognition of members of the carcinoembryonic antigen family by Afa/Dr adhesins of diffusely adhering *Escherichia coli* (Afa/Dr DAEC). Mol. Microbiol. **52:** 963–983.

34. MUENZNER, P., M. ROHDE, S. KNEITZ, *et al.* 2005. CEACAM engagement by human pathogens enhances cell adhesion and counteracts bacteria-induced detachment of epithelial cells. J. Cell Biol. **170:** 825–836.

35. PANTELIC, M., Y.J. KIM, S. BOLLAND, *et al.* 2005. *Neisseria gonorrhoeae* kills carcinoembryonic antigen-related cellular adhesion molecule 1 (CD66a)-expressing human B cells and inhibits antibody production. Infect. Immun. **73:** 4171–4179.

36. KAMMERER, R., D. STOBER, B.B. SINGER, *et al.* 2001. Carcinoembryonic antigen-related cell adhesion molecule 1 on murine dendritic cells is a potent regulator of T cell stimulation. J. Immunol. **166:** 6537–6544.

37. MARKEL, G., N. LIEBERMAN, G. KATZ, *et al.* 2002. CD66a interactions between human melanoma and NK cells: a novel class I MHC-independent inhibitory mechanism of cytotoxicity. J. Immunol. **168:** 2803–2810.

38. STERN, N., G. MARKEL, T.I. ARNON, *et al.* 2005. Carcinoembryonic antigen (CEA) inhibits NK killing via interaction with CEA-related cell adhesion molecule 1. J. Immunol. **174:** 6692–6701.

39. NAKAJIMA, A., H. IIJIMA, M.F. NEURATH, *et al.* 2002. Activation-induced expression of carcinoembryonic antigen-cell adhesion molecule 1 regulates mouse T lymphocyte function. J. Immunol. **168:** 1028–1035.

40. CHEN, D., H. IIJIMA, T. NAGAISHI, *et al.* 2004. Carcinoembryonic antigen-related cellular adhesion molecule 1 isoforms alternatively inhibit and costimulate human T cell function. J. Immunol. **172:** 3535–3543.

41. CHEN, C.J. & J.E. SHIVELY. 2004. The cell-cell adhesion molecule carcinoembryonic antigen-related cellular adhesion molecule 1 inhibits IL-2 production and proliferation in human T cells by association with Src homology protein-1 and down-regulates IL-2 receptor. J. Immunol. **172:** 3544–3552.

42. IDEO, H., A. SEKO, & K. YAMASHITA. 2005. Galectin-4 binds to sulfated glycosphingolipids and carcinoembryonic antigen in patches on the cell surface of human colon adenocarcinoma cells. J. Biol. Chem. **280:** 4730–4737.

43. HOKAMA, A., E. MIZOGUCHI, K. SUGIMOTO, *et al.* 2004. Induced reactivity of intestinal CD4(+) T cells with an epithelial cell lectin, galectin-4, contributes to exacerbation of intestinal inflammation. Immunity **20:** 681–693.

44. SHAO, L., A.R. JACOBS, V.V. JOHNSON, *et al.* 2005. Activation of CD8+ regulatory T cells by human placental trophoblasts. J. Immunol. **174:** 7539–7547.

45. MAYER, L. & R. SHLIEN. 1987. Evidence for function of Ia molecules on gut epithelial cells in man. J. Exp. Med. **166:** 1471–1483.

Induction of Intestinal Lymphoid Tissue

The Role of Cryptopatches

ANDREAS LÜGERING AND TORSTEN KUCHARZIK

Department of Medicine B, University of Münster, Albert-Schweitzer-Straße 33, 48129 Münster, Germany

ABSTRACT: The intestinal immune system includes several organized structures, such as Peyer's patches, isolated lymphoid follicles (ILFs), cryptopatches (CPs) as well as mesenteric lymph nodes (MLNs) that constitute an extensive network with other nonorganized parts, such as intraepithelial and lamina propria lymphocytes. CPs are small clusters of lymphoid cells with an immature lymphocyte phenotype and dendritic cells. Initial observations in transfer experiments suggested that the immature lymphocytes are T cell precursors and CPs a potential site of extrathymic intraepithelial lymphocyte (IEL) differentiation. This feature has recently been challenged particularly by the observation that CP cells express the orphan receptor RORγt and are phenotypically indistinguishable from lymphoid tissue-inducer (LTi) cells, suggesting that CP cells are the adult counterpart of fetal LTi cells. In addition, the chemokine receptor CCR6 is specifically expressed by precursor cells within CPs and its deletion inhibits the development of ILFs. Therefore, it is likely that ILFs derive from CPs under the control of CCR6 under inflammatory conditions and might constitute a valuable target for anti-inflammatory therapies.

KEYWORDS: lymphoid organogenesis; isolated lymphoid follicles; cryptopatches; lymphoid tissue-inducer cells; CCR6

HISTORY OF CRYPTOPATCHES (CPs)

Cryptopatches (CPs) were initially described in 1996 by Ishikawa and colleagues,[1] demonstrating that the murine gut harbors small clusters of lymphoid cells containing two different cellular subsets: the centrally located lymphocytes express c-kit, the interleukin-7 receptor a-chain, and CD44, but no markers specific for T-, B-, granulocyte, or macrophage lineages and therefore resemble early T cell precursors (lin- c-kit+ IL-7Rα+ CD44+; CP cells).

Address for correspondence: Andreas Lügering, Department of Medicine B, University of Münster, Albert-Schweitzer-Straße 33, 48129 Münster, Germany. Voice: +49-251-8347661; fax:+49-251-8356230.

e-mail: Andreas.Luegering@web.de

Ann. N.Y. Acad. Sci. 1072: 210–217 (2006). © 2006 New York Academy of Sciences.
doi: 10.1196/annals.1326.015

These clusters are surrounded by CD11c+ dendritic cells, which constitute the second main cell population found within these structures. CPs are not present until day 14 after birth and are found throughout the small and large intestine. Studies of variant knockout mice could show that CPs develop independently of T and B cells (present in SCID and RAG-2$^{-/-}$ mice) and do not depend on the NF-κB pathway. Recent studies could also demonstrate that intestinal CPs formation in mice—like ILFs and PP formation—requires lymphotoxin alpha and the lymphotoxin beta receptor as well as IL-7Rα and the common cytokine γ-chain.[2] However, CPs but not ILFs were found in the small intestine of NF-κB-inducing kinase-deficient alymphoplasia mice. The CP cells did not show signs of apoptosis and only a limited amount of RAG activity was detected.

In subsequent papers the same group isolated CP cells by microscopic dissection and flow cytometry followed by transfer into immunodeficient mice.[3-5] Interestingly, the reconstitution resulted in the generation of αβ and γδTCR IELs in a ratio of about 2:1 predominantly expressing the unusual CD8αα coreceptor. In addition, T cells within mesenteric lymph nodes (MLNs) were found, whereas no B cells were regenerated. The group concluded that CPs serve as a "gut thymus" and might be the side of extraintestinal lymphocyte development that has controversially been proposed over decades. Similar data were found in a second approach made by Lambolez et al.: flow cytometric isolation of "wall lymphocytes" (WLs) from the complete lamina propria characterized by the expression of c-kit, IL7-R, and CD25+ in the absence of lineage markers resulted in a population that phenotypically resembled CP cells.[6] It should be noted that CP cells are included in the WL population, whereas WLs are not necessarily restricted to CPs. The transfer of this cell population into thymectomized RAG-2/γ-chain-deficient mice again reconstituted the development of unusual CD8αα intraepithelial lymphocytes (IELs) as observed by the Japanese group. However, when compared to their thymic counterparts, CP cells showed only a limited amount of CD3-ε, RAG-1 and pre-Tα expression, suggesting that only a low proportion of the precursor cells show T cell commitment.

CONTROVERSIES IN CP FUNCTION

The hypothesis of CPs being the primary side of extrathymic T cell lymphopoiesis was challenged by observations in a transgenic mouse model that expresses GFP under the control of the RAG promoter. In this construct, Guy-Grand et al.[7] found that MLNs are the side of extrathymic T cell lymphopoesis in nude mice and—to a significant lesser extent—Peyer's patches, whereas no RAG activity was seen in CPs as well as in IELs. The developmental steps of MLN T cells found in this setting were similar to conventional thymic T cell development, but biased toward γδ chain synthesis. In euthymic mice the extrathymic developmental pathway was completely shut off and could only be unmasked in severe lymphocytotic depletion (e.g., after radiation), suggesting that IELs are more likely to be of thymic origin under normal conditions and that CPs are likely to possess a different function.

However, Nonaka *et al.* recently could show that CPs actually are able to generate extrathymic T cells by generating two mouse systems that lacked all lymph nodes, Peyer's patches, and isolated lymphoid follicles (ILFs) (nu/nu aly/aly double mutant mice; timed treated nu/+ mice [lymphotoxin-beta receptor-Ig and TNF receptor 55-Ig fusion protein]), whereas the development of CPs remained intact.[8] In this setting, the population size of a major γδ TCR CD8αα-IEL subset was maintained and the use of TCR-gamma-chain variable gene segments by these γδ-IELs was unaltered. In conclusion, the data suggest that CPs might harbor immature lymphocyte precursor cells, that are capable of differentiating into IELs. However, this process can only be unmasked under distinct settings and, therefore, is unlikely to be the primary role of these aggregates found throughout the murine gut. It also remains an open question whether "CPs-cells" constitute a single cell population and if they differentiate into other lymphocyte subsets under natural conditions.

RETINOIC ACID–RELATED ORPHAN RECEPTOR-γT

A significant input into the evaluation of CPs function came from genetic fate mapping experiments made by Eberl *et al.*[9,10] Firstly, the group found that both double-positive (DP) thymocytes and WLs are unique in their expression of the retinoic acid–related orphan receptor-γt (RORγt). The receptor is a splice variant of the widely expressed RORγ and is specifically expressed by lymphoid tissue–inducer cells (LTi) and is crucial for their generation and survival. RORγt is basically expressed by all lineage- c-kit+ lamina propria lymphocytes (corresponding to WL). RORγt-deficient mice have an impaired thymic lymphopoesis and strikingly have no CPs and no ILFs, whereas they show normal numbers of intestinal γδTCR IELs, suggesting that γδTCR IELs are not the progeny of DP thymocytes nor are these cells developing from WLs (including CP cells). Additionally, the rescue of RORγt cells by transgenic expression of the antiapoptotic protein Bcl-xL was able to restore DP thymocytes and the generation of αβTCR CD8αα IELs, but did not rescue WLs or CPs demonstrating that αβTCR CD8αα IELs are the progeny of DP thymocytes. These data strongly favor a different perspective of CP: CP might serve as organizers of inducible tertiary lymphoid tissue. WLs found aggregated within CPs phenotypically appear similar to fetal LTi cells that are among the first hematopoetic cells to colonize developing lymphoid tissue, such as Peyer's patch anlagen. LTi cells also express the heterotrimer lymphotoxin α1β2 crucially involved in the activation of local mesenchymal cells, suggesting that CP cells are involved in initiating immune responses inside the gut rather than being precursors of IELs.

CCR6 EXPRESSION INSIDE CP

The chemokine receptor CCR6 is the only receptor of the chemokine ligand CCL20 (Mip3α) that is specifically expressed by the follicle-associated epithelia of Peyer's patches.[11,12] CCR6 is expressed by B cells and subsets of T and dendritic cells.[13] Initial observations in CCR6-deficient mouse models suggested that the deletion of this receptor primarily affects the migration of myeloid DCs found within the follicle-associated dome region,[14,15] but extensive studies by Zhao et al. could not repeat these observations when comparing several different CCR6 knockout mouse models.[16] Recently, we could show by using an EGFP knockin mouse model that CCR6 seems not to affect cellular migration within PPs as receptor-deficient cells were correctly positioned.[17] However, a significant reduction of the size of PPs could be found in the absence of CCR6 paralleled with a loss of CD4 regulatory T cells. In addition, we found a significant reduction of M cells within the FAE. In summary, the deletion of CCR6 does influence the formation of PPs, but the effect seems not to be mediated by influencing the cellular migration inside PPs.

The influence of CCR6 on the development of IELs was appreciated by all knockout mouse models published so far. In order to specify the underlying mechanism we analyzed their phenotype in CCR6-deficient mice and found that unconventional CD8αα IELs are specifically affected by the deletion although no IEL expresses the receptor. These observations suggested that CCR6 might influence extrathymic T cell differentiation. In this context, we were able to show that CCR6 is not only highly expressed in PPs, but also in a second organized structure of the GALT[18]: CCR6 is expressed by 70–75% of cells found in CPs. Whereas the dendritic cells present in CPs do not express the receptor, it seems to be highly specific for the precursor cell type (lineage-marker-, c-kit+). In contrast, no CCR6 expression was found in bone marrow or thymic lin- c-kit+ cells, suggesting that this phenotype is restricted to the gut. However, the formation of CPs was not influenced by the deletion of the receptor. Although the expansion of CD8αα IELs in the absence of CCR6 intriguingly suggests that this might be related to the specific expression of this receptor inside CPs, it cannot be excluded that this phenomenon occurs as a secondary result of CCR6 deletion.

Preliminary data published by McDonald et al.[19] recently linked the expression of CCR6 inside CPs to the observations made by Eberl and colleagues: while characterizing the third organized component of the GALT the group found that CCR6-deficient mice specifically lack ILF. The data suggest that CCR6 is highly relevant for the progression of CPs to ILFs proposed by Eberl

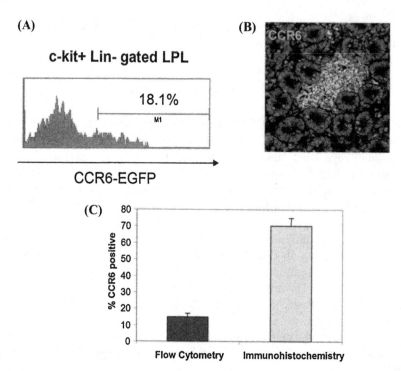

FIGURE 1. **(A)** FACS analysis of c-kit+ lin- lamina propria cells revealed a significant proportion of CCR6-expressing cells within the WL fraction (~15–20%; analysis of heterozygous EGFP-CCR6 knockin mice). However, when analyzed by immunohistochemistry **(B)**, a significant higher number of CP cells express this receptor (~ 70%, C), suggesting than within the lamina propria c-kit+ lin- cells must be found outside CPs and CCR6 is a marker for localization of these cells within CPs.

et al. In addition, it could be shown that immature and mature ILF formation are dependent upon CCR6-sufficient B lymphocytes, but it cannot be ruled out that CCR6 expression by other cellular subsets (e.g., CP cells) is also influencing ILF formation. Interestingly, CCL20 is not affecting lymphotoxin expression in B lymphocytes known to drive the progression of immature ILFs to mature ILFs, suggesting that the CCL20–CCR6 interaction drives a distinct early event in the progression of CPs to ILFs.

In conclusion, it seems likely that CPs are precursors of ILFs under natural conditions and that CCR6 is a factor that is specifically necessary for the early progression. However, if the development of ILFs is blocked by, for example, inhibition of CCR6 or lymphotoxin signaling, or if CP cells are transferred into an immunocompromised host, other developmental steps might favor a differentiation into IELs.

It is also noteworthy that CP cells have to be differentiated from WLs. Whereas CP cells are lymphocytes expressing c-kit and CD44 in the absence of lineage markers within CPs the term *wall lymphocyte* reflects lymphocytes prepared from the lamina propria also expressing c-kit and CD44 in the absence of lineage markers that are, however, anatomically not restricted to CPs. Whereas the overall expression of CCR6 within the WL cell population is between 15–20%, CP cells are expressing this receptor at a much higher level (70–80%; unpublished observations). In contrast, there is no major difference of RORγt expression in both populations, suggesting that LTi cells might also be present outside the organized lymphoid tissue. If CCR6-negative LTi cells found outside CPs constitute a different cell population when compared to CCR6-positive LTi-cells found inside CPs remains to be elucidated.

CPs IN HUMANS

The initial description of CPs in mice was followed by the search for similar structures in the human gut. Moghaddami et al.[20] identified a new lymphoid structure with an epithelium resembling follicle-associated epithelium that was termed *lymphocyte-filled villus*. These structures contain major histocompatibility complex class II-positive dendritic cells, memory T cells, and a variable amount of B cells. However, no evidence of aggregates of immature lymphocytes that express c-kit was found. The authors concluded that the human gut does not contain CPs. However, ILFs have already been appreciated in humans as tertiary lymphoid structures that are formed in autoimmune diseases, as well as in several inflammatory pathologies of the gastrointestinal tract. If CPs constitute the precursor structure for ILFs the presence of CP in the human gut has to be postulated, even though no clusters of c-kit-positive cells have been identified. In contrast, staining of the human gut for CCR6-expressing cells clearly identified lymphoid structures highly positive for CCR6 in the absence of c-kit, suggesting that similar mechanisms of tertiary lymphoid organ formation are present in the murine and human gut.

Recent work by Kaiserling et al.[21] as well as by Yeung et al.[22] also suggests that colonic ILF hyperplasia is observed in Crohn's disease and ulcerative colitis, and that the size of ILFs may correlate with the activity of the disease. In animal models, the induction of tertiary lymphoid structures in the colon has also been demonstrated after DSS as well as TNBS administration. These observations suggest that induction of ILF formation might not only be a consequence of intestinal inflammation, but also initiates or contributes to the disease perpetuation and that CCR6 might be a reasonable target for inhibiting this process.

REFERENCES

1. KANAMORI, Y., K. ISHIMARU, M. NANNO, et al. 1996. Identification of novel lymphoid tissues in murine intestinal mucosa where clusters of c-kit+ IL-7R+ Thy1+ lympho-hemopoietic progenitors develop. J. Exp. Med. **184**: 1449–1459.

2. TAYLOR, R.T., A. LUGERING, K.A. NEWELL & I.R. WILLIAMS. 2004. Intestinal cryptopatch formation in mice requires lymphotoxin alpha and the lymphotoxin beta receptor. J. Immunol. **173**: 7183–7189.

3. SAITO, H., Y. KANAMORI, T. TAKEMORI, et al. 1998. Generation of intestinal T cells from progenitors residing in gut cryptopatches. Science **280**: 275–278.

4. ISHIKAWA, H., H. SAITO, K. SUZUKI, et al. 1999. New gut associated lymphoid tissue "cryptopatches" breed murine intestinal intraepithelial T cell precursors. Immunol. Res. **20**: 243–250.

5. SUZUKI, K., T. OIDA, H. HAMADA, et al. 2000. Gut cryptopatches: direct evidence of extrathymic anatomical sites for intestinal T lymphopoiesis. Immunity **13**: 691–702.

6. LAMBOLEZ, F., O. AZOGUI, A.M. JORET, et al. 2002. Characterization of T cell differentiation in the murine gut. J. Exp. Med. **195**: 437–449.

7. GUY-GRAND, D., O. AZOGUI, S. CELLI, et al. 2003. Extrathymic T cell lymphopoiesis: ontogeny and contribution to gut intraepithelial lymphocytes in athymic and euthymic mice. J. Exp. Med. **197**: 333–341.

8. NONAKA, S., T. NAITO, H. CHEN, et al. 2005. Intestinal gamma delta T cells develop in mice lacking thymus, all lymph nodes, Peyer's patches, and isolated lymphoid follicles. J. Immunol. **174**: 1906–1912.

9. EBERL, G. & D.R. LITTMAN. 2004. Thymic origin of intestinal alphabeta T cells revealed by fate mapping of RORgammat+ cells. Science **305**: 248–251.

10. EBERL, G., S. MARMON, M.J. SUNSHINE, et al. 2004. An essential function for the nuclear receptor RORgamma(t) in the generation of fetal lymphoid tissue inducer cells. Nat. Immunol. **5**: 64–73.

11. BABA, M., T. IMAI, M. NISHIMURA, et al. 1997. Identification of CCR6, the specific receptor for a novel lymphocyte-directed CC chemokine LARC. J. Biol.Chem. **272**: 14893–14898.

12. GREAVES, D.R., W. WANG, D.J. DAIRAGHI, et al. 1997. CCR6, a CC chemokine receptor that interacts with macrophage inflammatory protein 3alpha and is highly expressed in human dendritic cells. J. Exp. Med. **186**: 837–844.

13. KUCHARZIK, T., J.T. HUDSON, III, R.L. WAIKEL, et al. 2002. CCR6 expression distinguishes mouse myeloid and lymphoid dendritic cell subsets: demonstration using a CCR6 EGFP knock-in mouse. Eur. J. Immunol. **32**: 104–112.

14. VARONA, R., R. VILLARES, L. CARRAMOLINO, et al. 2001. CCR6-deficient mice have impaired leukocyte homeostasis and altered contact hypersensitivity and delayed-type hypersensitivity responses. J. Clin. Invest. **107**: R37–R45.

15. COOK, D.N., D.M. PROSSER, R. FORSTER, et al. 2000. CCR6 mediates dendritic cell localization, lymphocyte homeostasis, and immune responses in mucosal tissue. Immunity **12**: 495–503.

16. ZHAO, X., A. SATO, C.S. DELA CRUZ, et al. 2003. CCL9 is secreted by the follicle-associated epithelium and recruits dome region Peyer's patch CD11b+ dendritic cells. J. Immunol. **171**: 2797–2803.

17. LUGERING, A., M. FLOER, S. WESTPHAL, et al. 2005. Absence of CCR6 inhibits CD4+ regulatory T-cell development and M-cell formation inside Peyer's patches. Am. J. Pathol. **166**: 1647–1654.

18. LUGERING, A., T. KUCHARZIK, D. SOLER, et al. 2003. Lymphoid precursors in intestinal cryptopatches express CCR6 and undergo dysregulated development in the absence of CCR6. J. Immunol. **171**: 2208–2215.

19. MCDONALD KG, M.J., I. WILLIAMS, T. KUCHARZIK & R. NEWBERRY. 2005. Cc chemokine receptor 6 is essential for isolated lymphoid follicle formation. Gastroenterology **128**: A21–A21.

20. MOGHADDAMI, M., A. CUMMINS & G. MAYRHOFER. 1998. Lymphocyte-filled villi: comparison with other lymphoid aggregations in the mucosa of the human small intestine. Gastroenterology **115**: 1414–1425.

21. KAISERLING, E. 2001. Newly-formed lymph nodes in the submucosa in chronic inflammatory bowel disease. Lymphology **34**: 22–29.

22. YEUNG, M.M., S. MELGAR, V. BARANOV, *et al.* 2000. Characterisation of mucosal lymphoid aggregates in ulcerative colitis: immune cell phenotype and TcR-gammadelta expression. Gut **47**: 215–227.

Peyer's Patches and M Cells as Potential Sites of the Inflammatory Onset in Crohn's Disease

ELISABET GULLBERG AND JOHAN D. SÖDERHOLM

Colorectal Surgery Unit, Department of Surgery, University Hospital,
SE-581 85 Linköping, Sweden

ABSTRACT: Clinical observations suggest that the sites of initial inflammation in ileal Crohn's disease (CD) are the lymphoid follicles, where the aphtoid lesions originate from small erosions of the follicle-associated epithelium (FAE). Lymphoid follicles and Peyer's patches (PPs) consist of a number of B-cell follicles with intervening T cell areas. The T cell follicular area is also populated by dendritic cells (DCs) and macrophages. A single layer of epithelial cells covering each follicle forms a dome between the surrounding villi. This FAE differs from normal villus epithelium in several ways that make the epithelial cells of the FAE more exposed to the luminal contents, more accessible to antigens, and in closer contact with the immune system. The most prominent feature is the presence of specialized M cells, which are optimized for antigen adherence and transport. M cells play an important role in the surveillance of the intestinal lumen, but also provide a route of entry for various pathogens. In this article we review the current knowledge on the epithelial phenotype of the human FAE, and changes of the FAE and M cells in intestinal inflammation, leading to a hypothesis of the role of the FAE and M cells in the pathogenesis of CD.

KEYWORDS: aphtoid lesion; follicle-associated epithelium; inflammatory bowel disease; lymphoid follicle

APHTHOID LESIONS AT LYMPHOID FOLLICLES—WHERE IT ALL STARTS?

The minute mucosal manifestations of Crohn's disease (CD) called aphtoid lesions are well recognized by every endoscopist. Rutgeerts et al. found that these aphtoid lesions are early endoscopic signs of recurrence in the neoterminal ileum following ileocolonic anastomosis,[1] and repeat colonoscopies

Address for correspondence: Johan D. Söderholm, M.D., Ph.D., Colorectal Surgery Unit, Department of Surgery, University Hospital, SE-581 85 Linköping, Sweden. Voice: +46-13-22-35-41; fax: +46-13-22-35-70.
e-mail: johda@ibk.liu.se

Ann. N.Y. Acad. Sci. 1072: 218–232 (2006). © 2006 New York Academy of Sciences.
doi: 10.1196/annals.1326.028

showed progression over time to more advanced lesions, such as larger, serpiginous ulcerations and stricturing of the lumen. The progression from aphtoid lesions to overt ulcers in the small intestine was subsequently confirmed in endoscopic and radiographic studies,[2,3] but was less obvious in colonic CD.[4]

Morson initially recognized that aphtoid lesions mainly occur at accumulations of lymphocytes and immune cells in the intestinal mucosa, the so-called lymphoid follicles.[5] Subsequently, Rickert found that aphtoid lesions can be found in 70% of CD patients.[6] The typical lesion varied in size from barely visible to up to 3 mm in diameter, with the characteristic light-microscopic appearance consisting of focal ulceration overlying an aggregate of lymphoid tissue. The aphtoid lesions were more common in the Peyer's patches (PP) of the distal small intestine,[1,2,6] where the lymphoid follicles collect into larger formations.[7] In carefully performed correlative studies with magnifying endoscopy and scanning electron microscopy, Fujimura and coworkers demonstrated that the aphtoid lesions of CD are preceded by ultra-structural erosions (150–200 microns in size) in the follicle-associated epithelium (FAE) of hyperemic lymphoid follicles.[8,9] The connection between the lymphoid tissue and CD pathogenesis is also corroborated by a similar peak for CD and number of PP as a function of age.[10] Taken together, these clinical observations suggest that the sites of initial inflammation in ileal CD are the lymphoid follicles, where the ulcerations originate from small erosions of the FAE. Which are the characteristics of the lymphoid follicles and the FAE that would make them predisposed to inflammation?

THE LYMPHOID FOLLICLE REGIONS AND PEYER'S PATCHES

Isolated lymphoid follicles (ILFs) or aggregates of these, the so-called PPs, can be found along the length of the small intestine and are particular abundant in the distal part of the ileum.[7,11] Both of these structures are today believed to be of great importance for the induction and regulation of gut mucosal immune responses.[12,13] ILFs and PPs develop before birth, although the full development of the PPs as inductive sites requires acquired antigenic challenge.[14] In mice, it has been shown that the development of PPs and ILFs is induced by the production of lymphotoxin (LT).[15,16] In the case of PPs, LT is produced by bone marrow progenitor cells as a response to local intestinal IL-7 production, whereas ILF formation seems dependent on LT-secreting B lymphocytes.[15] Interestingly, ILFs may develop in response to LT signaling also in adult age and do not require antigen-primed B cells for their maturation.[13,17] In adolescence, hundreds of patches can be found along the intestine.[11] The number of patches, the size, and the distribution of PPs and ILFs vary considerably in different individuals.[7,11,12]

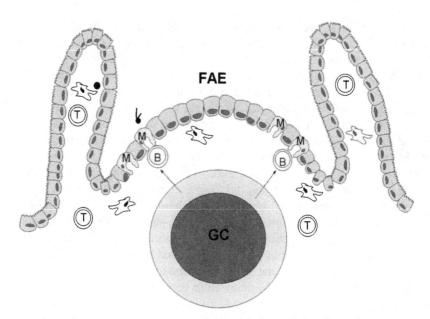

FIGURE 1. Structure of a lymphoid follicle and the FAE. See text for details. B, B cells; GC, germinal center; M, M cells; T, T cells.

Mature PPs consist of a number of B-cell follicles with intervening T cell areas. The follicular area is also populated by dendritic cells (DCs) and macrophages, which play an important role in the mucosal defense against ingested pathogens.[18] ILFs consist of a B-cell germinal center and scattered DCs, macrophages, and occasional T cells.[12] A single layer of epithelial cells covering each follicle forms a dome between the surrounding villi (FIG. 1). This FAE has been well studied in the PPs of animals and differs from normal villus epithelium in several ways that make the epithelial cells of the FAE more exposed to the luminal contents, more accessible to antigens, and in closer contact with the immune system.

SPECIALIZED EPITHELIAL PHENOTYPES IN THE FAE

Compared with regular entero- and colonocytes, the FAE has less production of mucus, expresses lower amounts of membrane-bound digestive enzymes, and has different glycosylation patterns in the brush border glycocalyx of the enterocytes.[19–22] The FAE also lacks the subepithelial myofibroblast sheath, and the basal lamina is more porous compared with regular epithelium.[23,24] However, the most prominent feature of this epithelium is the presence of specialized microfold cells, or M cells. These cells transport protein antigens, as well as viruses and bacteria, across the epithelial cell layer to underlying lymphocytes and DCs.[25] This sampling from the lumen is crucial for induction of protective mucosal immune responses, known as oral tolerance, but also provides a route of entry into the mucosa for various pathogens.[26] The M cells of the PPs and ILFs play an important role in this surveillance and sampling of the intestinal lumen, and the M-cell apical membrane is optimized for antigen adherence. It typically has microfolds, or ruffles, rather than microvilli, and the glycocalyx is thinner than that of absorptive cells.[27] Lymphocytes reside in a pocket, or invagination, of the basal plasma membrane, which results in close contact between lymphocytes and antigens transported across the thin apical membrane.[28] In addition, M cells do not express MHC class II molecules[29] and have few lysosomes.[30] It is therefore believed that most antigens cross M cells without being degraded.[31] Unfortunately, this increased capacity for presentation of intact antigens also provides a route of entry for pathogens into the mucosa. Thus, the human M cell is of utmost interest in trying to understand how the complex interplay between host and bacterial flora is regulated in health and in disease.

The FAE cell layer of the ILFs is not as well characterized as that of the PPs, but M cells have been identified also in the epithelium covering mouse and human ILFs.[32,33] Moreover, isolated lymphoid structures, called lymphocyte-filled villi, with epithelium-resembling FAE have been identified in the human small intestine,[34] and recently Jang et al. reported that M cells could be found in villus epithelium of the murine gut.[35] The exact pathways leading to changes in epithelial phenotype to the development of FAE and M cells are not known, but it was recently shown that FAE development is not B cell–dependent,[36] whereas CCR6 seems to play a role in the expansion of M cells, as reduced M-cell numbers are seen in CCR6$^{-/-}$ mice.[37] Recent studies have also characterized the tight-junction protein expression in the FAE of mice[38]: whereas claudin-3 and occludin were expressed throughout the dome, claudin-4 expression was stronger in the apex region of the dome, preferentially associated with apoptotic epithelial cells. Claudin-2 showed higher expression in the villus epithelium. Moreover, Clark and Hirst[39] found that the adherens junctions of murine M cells could be recognized by enhanced expression of beta-catenin, alpha-actinin, and polymerized actin. These findings may suggest that the paracellular pathway is also differentially regulated in the FAE and M cells.

Whereas the M-cell phenotype is quite well characterized in the mouse and rabbit PPs, human M cells remain poorly characterized and are thus difficult to study. In particular, the progress is hampered by lack of appropriate markers. TABLE 1 lists markers that have been identified as specific for M cells in various species.[39–50] UEA-1 is currently employed as an M-cell marker in the mouse intestine,[41,42] and vimentin and cytokeratin 18 are used as M-cell markers in the rabbit and pig intestine, respectively,[43,44] but these markers are not specific for human M cells.[51] During the past years, several attempts have been made to identify proteins or glycoconjugates specific to human M cells,[50–56] but so far, only markers with a reliable specificity for the entire FAE

TABLE 1. Markers of M cells in various species[a]

Type of marker	Human	Mouse	Rat	Rabbit	Pig
Lectin	SLAA[50,b]	UEA-1[41,42] EEA[48]			
Intermediate filaments			CK8[47]	Vimentin[43]	CK18[44]
Cytoskeletal proteins		F-actin[49] α-actinin[49] β1-integrin[49,c]			
Surface receptors	ICAM-1[32,c]				
Enzymes	Low AP[46]	Low AP[20]	Low AP[20]	Low AP[45]	
Others		IgA/IgG-adherence[40]	IgA/IgG-adherence[40]	IgA/IgG-adherence[40]	

ABBREVIATIONS: AP, alkaline phosphatase; ICAM, intracelluler adhesion molecule; SLAA, sialyl Lewis antigen A; EEA, *Euonymus europaeus* agglutinan; CK, cytokeratin.

[a]Lectins that only stain M cell in the caecal patch have been omitted.
[b]Negative results also obtained.[51]
[c]Colon.

TABLE 2. Markers of human FAE

Marker	Function	Reference
Cathepsin E	Protease	53
Sialyl Lewis antigen A	Lectin	50
CPE-R	*Clostridium perfringens* enterotoxin (CPE) receptor	54
TM4SF3	Tetraspan protein	54
β1-integrin	Surface receptor	57,59
TNFAIP3 (A20)	Antiapoptotic factor	58
CCL23	Putative DCs chemokine (human homologue of murine CCL9)	58
CD9	Tetraspan protein	59
Galectin 9	Lectin	60

have been found[50,53,54,57–60] (TABLE 2). Attempts to isolate FAE and M cells for subsequent culture *in vitro* have not been successful to date. However, in a seminal paper by Kerneís *et al.*, it was shown that coculture of PP lymphocytes and intestinal epithelial cells may trigger conversion of the epithelial cells to M cells.[61] This model and variants of it have been used to study M-cell function,[62–68] and as mentioned above, to discover novel FAE markers. Thus, the coculture model presents new possibilities to study the influence of genetic predisposition and proinflammatory cytokines on the interplay between FAE and luminal bacteria. However, the key question will still be how results obtained in the reductionistic coculture model correlate with the complex situation *in vivo*. The lack of specific M-cell markers in human intestine makes studies of the human FAE and M cells technically difficult and demanding. The obvious species differences in FAE surface markers do, however, call for studies of human intestine despite the difficulties. In our laboratory we have recently established techniques for reproducible sampling of human FAE at surgery and endoscopy, which makes functional and histochemical studies of human FAE possible.[111]

FAE AND M CELLS IN INTESTINAL INFECTION AND INFLAMMATION

Specific Route of Entry for Pathogens

As previously described, the FAE and M-cell phenotypes are optimized for antigen uptake. This sampling from the lumen is crucial for induction of protective mucosal immune responses, but also provides a route of entry into the mucosa for various microorganisms: bacteria, viruses, as well as protozoa. Many pathogens have developed strategies to survive M-cell transcytosis and go on to infect cells of the mucosa or the epithelium itself. For example, *Salmonella typhimurium* and *Shigella flexneri* are more or less specific colonizers of FAE and M cells.[69] The *Escherichia coli* strains EHEC and EPEC also show specific adherence to FAE when cultured *in vitro* together with human intestinal biopsies.[70,71] Whereas restricted adhesion of EPEC to FAE seems to be regulated by factors unrelated to intimin, EHEC adhesion to FAE in human intestinal *in vitro* culture is determined by bacterial expression of intimin gamma.[72] *Yersinia* spp. also bind to and invade FAE/M cells using specific binding of invasin to beta-1-integrin on the epithelial cell surface.[49,59,62] Moreover, reovirus and HIV use specific receptors to target and cross the FAE.[73-75] Prion proteins have also been suggested to be taken up via the FAE following oral ingestion.[76]

Induction of M Cells by Exposure to Bacteria

In 1987, Smith *et al.* reported that the number of M cells in mouse FAE increased after transfer of pathogen-free mice to normal housing conditions.[77] Since then, there have been several reports of *de novo* M-cell formation and increased uptake of particles after inoculation of mouse or rabbit intestinal loops with bacteria.[78-81] In some cases, the new M cells were observed as early as 1 h after the inoculation.[81] Gebert *et al.* recently challenged this, however, showing that increased uptake of particles after inoculation with bacteria depended on increased transport capacity in M cells already present in the FAE.[82] Considering the changes in epithelial morphology that must take place during the transition from absorptive cell to M cell, this explanation for the increased particle uptake maybe seems more conceivable. Either way, bacterial stimulation does lead to increased transcytosis, the mechanism remaining unknown.

In general, bacterial binding to and infection of the intestinal epithelium always leads to production of a cascade of proinflammatory cytokines, which recruits mononuclear cells to the site of infection.[83] Proinflammatory cytokine production by these cells, in turn, is likely to result in increased transcellular and paracellular permeability to macromolecules and particles. For instance, tumor necrosis factor (TNF)-α has been reported to induce transcytosis and bacterial translocation in intestinal epithelial cells in culture.[84,85] Moreover, it was recently shown that increased transcytosis of protein antigens in the human ileum could be correlated to TNF-α mRNA levels in the underlying mucosal tissue.[85]

FAE and M-Cell Changes in Animal Models of Inflammation

As initially described by Matsumoto *et al.*,[86] the senescence accelerated mouse P1 (SAMP1)/Yit mouse strain spontaneously develops a CD-like inflammation of the small intestine. At 30 weeks of age, a 100% penetrance of transmural intestinal inflammation was seen, which was most severe in the terminal ileum.[87] The majority of the inflammatory lesions were associated with PPs, and early inflammatory lesions with epithelial damage were commonly seen overlying these preexisting lymphoid aggregates, similar to aphtoid lesions in humans. Results suggesting that the FAE is more reactive or vulnerable than villus epithelium were shown by Velin et al.[88] In a model of chronic stress in rats an increase in transmucosal bacterial and antigen uptake was considerably more pronounced in the FAE compared with villus epithelium.

Studies using chemically induced models of intestinal inflammation also affect the FAE region. Kucharzik et al. showed increased M-cell formation, and expansion of mononuclear cells in the M-cell pockets, in indomethacin-induced enteritis in rats.[89] M-cell numbers already expanded 12 h after a single injection and returned to normal within 7 days. In inflamed tissue, M cells underwent apoptosis at an increased rate, and mononuclear cells were seen to pass into the intestinal lumen at these sites. Thus, M cells may be converted from intestinal epithelial cells inside the FAE by lympho-epithelial interaction under inflammatory conditions.[89,90] Also in the lambda-carrageenan colitis model in rats, the FAE was affected at an early stage, with pin-point ulcerations associated with the PPs.[91] Using the dextran sodium sulphate (DSS) colitis model in LT-α-deficient mice, Spahn et al.[92] found increased disease severity in mice lacking PPs and lymph nodes, whereas mice lacking only PPs had the same severity scores as DSS-treated control animals, suggesting an immunoregulatory role of the GALT (gut-associated lymphoid tissue).

FAE and M Cells in Intestinal Inflammation in Humans

In patients with spondylarthropathy, Cuvelier et al. found that the ileal mucosa had increased numbers of M cells (12–24% of epithelial cells in FAE compared with 0–6% in controls).[93] Occasionally, disruption of M-cell cytoplasm was seen, with lymphocytes entering the gut lumen at these sites, suggesting a possible mechanism for the development of aphtoid lesions.

In inflamed colonic specimens of human inflammatory bowel disease (IBD), expression of CCL20, a chemokine mediating recruitment of immature DCs and memory T cells, was increased several-fold in the epithelial cells of the FAE.[94] Accordingly, other groups have found increased numbers of DCs in colonic mucosa of CD,[95,96] as well as expression of M-DC8(+)DCs and Th1-type T cells in inflamed mucosa-associated lymphoid tissue of CD,[97,98] which may contribute to the high level of TNF-α production in CD.

THE FAE AND M CELLS IN CD—A WORKING HYPOTHESIS

The studies reviewed here indicate that the earliest observable lesions in ileal CD may be minute ulcers in the FAE, and that the FAE is reactive both to bacterial and inflammatory stimuli. The gut has several ways to survey and prepare the mucosa for antigen encounter. Both epithelial cells and antigen-sampling DCs recognize microbe-associated molecular patterns (MAMPs) expressed on bacteria,[99] which may trigger an inflammatory response. One example is the engagement of lipopolysaccahride (LPS) or microbial adhesins with toll-like receptors on epithelial cells. This stimulates chemokine production for recruitment of DCs to the intestinal epithelium.[100,101] It is presently not understood why there is a difference in the response to commensal and pathogen MAMPs. However, mechanisms may include the ability of commensals to specifically downregulate proinflammatory responses in epithelial cells[102] and the vast production of IgA to commensal antigens in the gut.[29] The importance of MAMP recognition is illustrated by the fact that dysregulation of MAMP signaling through mutations in the cytosolic receptor Nod2/CARD15 is associated with the susceptibility to develop CD.[103,104] Thus, the interaction between luminal antigens/microorganisms, epithelial cells, and DCs that takes place at the FAE may be a crucial step in the initiation of inflammation in CD.

Increased intestinal permeability has for many years been recognized as a pathogenic factor of possible etiologic importance in CD.[105,106] However, recent studies suggest the gut barrier defect in CD to be TNF-α-dependent.[85,107,108] One possibility is that the universal barrier dysfunction seen in CD is generated by signals initiated by immune–antigen interactions in the FAE. As antigens and bacteria that penetrate the FAE and M cells at a high rate are more prone to induce inflammatory responses,[109] our current working hypothesis is therefore that a reduced barrier function in the FAE initiates and/or perpetuates mucosal inflammation. Preliminary findings from our laboratory demonstrate increased transmucosal passage of nonpathogenic E. coli in the FAE of noninflamed ileum of CD, despite a normal permeability to protein antigens.[110] These findings suggest a previously unrecognized specific defect in the barrier to commensal bacteria in these specialized regions. Thereby an increased cross-talk between luminal bacteria and the inductive sites of the mucosal immune system could take place in CD. Unravelling the mechanisms involved in the FAE barrier defect may have important implications for the understanding of the pathogenesis of ileal CD.

REFERENCES

1. RUTGEERTS, P. et al. 1984. Natural history of recurrent Crohn's disease at the ileocolonic anastomosis after curative surgery. Gut 25: 665–672.
2. OLAISON, G., K. SMEDH & R. SJÖDAHL. 1992. Natural course of Crohn's disease after ileocolic resection: endoscopically visualised ileal ulcers preceding symptoms. Gut 33: 331–335.
3. MATSUMOTO, T. et al. 2000. Crohn's disease of aphthous type: serial changes in intestinal lesions. Br. J. Radiol. 73: 1046–1051.

4. Ni, X.Y. & H.I. Goldberg. 1986. Aphthoid ulcers in Crohn disease: radiographic course and relationship to bowel appearance. Radiology **158**: 589–596.
5. Morson, B.C. 1972. The early histological lesion of Crohn's disease. Proc. R. Soc. Med. **65**: 71–72.
6. Rickert, R.R. & H.W. Carter. 1980. The "early" ulcerative lesion of Crohn's disease: correlative light- and scanning electron-microscopic studies. J. Clin. Gastroenterol. **2**: 11–19.
7. Van Kruiningen, H.J. et al. 2002. Distribution of Peyer's patches in the distal ileum. Inflamm. Bowel Dis. **8**: 180–185.
8. Fujimura, Y., M. Hosobe & T. Kihara. 1992. Ultrastructural study of M cells from colonic lymphoid nodules obtained by colonoscopic biopsy. Dig. Dis. Sci. **37**: 1089–1098.
9. Fujimura, Y., R. Kamoi & M. Iida. 1996. Pathogenesis of aphthoid ulcers in Crohn's disease: correlative findings by magnifying colonoscopy, electron microscopy, and immunohistochemistry. Gut **38**: 724–732.
10. Van Kruiningen, H.J., L.M. Ganley & B.J. Freda. 1997. The role of Peyer's patches in the age-related incidence of Crohn's disease. J. Clin. Gastroenterol. **25**: 470–475.
11. Cornes, J.S. 1965. Peyer's patches in the human gut. Proc. R. Soc. Med. **58**: 716.
12. Velázquez, P., B. Wei & J. Braun. 2005. Surveillance B lymphocytes and mucosal immunoregulation. Spring. Sem. Immunopath. **26**: 453–462.
13. McDonald, K.G., J.S. McDonough & R.D. Newberry. 2005. Adaptive immune responses are dispensable for isolated lymphoid follicle formation: antigen-naïve, lymphotoxin-sufficient B lymphocytes drive the formation of mature isolated lymphoid follicles. J. Immunol. **174**: 5720–5728.
14. Yamanaka, T. et al. 2003. Microbial colonization drives lymphocyte accumulation and differentiation in the follicle-associated epithelium of Peyer's patches. J. Immunol. **170**: 816–822.
15. Koni, P.A. et al. 1997. Distinct roles in lymphoid organogenesis for lymphotoxins alpha and beta revealed in lymphotoxin beta-deficient mice. Immunity **6**: 491–500.
16. Debard, N. et al. 2001. Effect of mature lymphocytes and lymphotoxin on the development of the follicle-associated epithelium and M cells in mouse Peyer's patches. Gastroenterology **120**: 1173–1182.
17. Lorenz, R.G. et al. 2003. Isolated lymphoid follicle formation is inducible and dependent upon lymphotoxin-sufficient B lymphocytes, lymphotoxin beta receptor, and TNF receptor I function. J. Immunol. **170**: 5475–5482.
18. MacDonald, T.T. 2003. The mucosal immune system. Parasite Immunol. **25**: 235–246.
19. Owen, R.L. & A.L. Jones. 1974. Epithelial cell specialization within human Peyer's patches: an ultrastructural study of intestinal lymphoid follicles. Gastroenterology **66**: 189–203.
20. Owen, R.L. & D.K. Bhalla. 1983. Cytochemical analysis of alkaline phosphatase and esterase activities and of lectin-binding and anionic sites in rat and mouse Peyer's patch M cells. Am. J. Anat. **168**: 199–212.
21. Owen, R.L. 1999. Uptake and transport of intestinal macromolecules and microorganisms by M cells in Peyer's patches—a personal and historical perspective. Semin. Immunol. **11**: 157–163.
22. Clark, M.A., B.H. Hirst & M.A. Jepson. 2000. Lectin-mediated mucosal delivery of drugs and microparticles. Adv. Drug Deliv. Rev. **43**: 207–223.

23. SIERRO, F. *et al.* 2000. Transient expression of M-cell phenotype by enterocyte-like cells of the follicle-associated epithelium of mouse Peyer's patches. Gastroenterology **119:** 734–743.
24. TAKEUCHI, T. & T. GONDA. 2004. Distribution of the pores of epithelial basement membrane in the rat small intestine. J. Vet. Med. Sci. **66:** 695–700.
25. NEUTRA, M.R. 1999. M cells in antigen sampling in mucosal tissues. Curr. Top Microbiol. Immunol. **236:** 17–32.
26. SIEBERS, A. & B.B. FINLAY. 1996. M cells and the pathogenesis of mucosal and systemic infections. Trends Microbiol. **4:** 22–29.
27. GEBERT, A. 1996. M-cells in the rabbit tonsil exhibit distinctive glycoconjugates in their apical membranes. J. Histochem. Cytochem. **44:** 1033–1042.
28. KRAEHENBUHL, J.P. & M.R. NEUTRA. 2000. Epithelial M cells: differentiation and function. Annu. Rev. Cell Dev. Biol. **16:** 301–332.
29. MOWAT, A.M. 2005. Dendritic cells and immune responses to orally administered antigens. Vaccine **23:** 1797–1799.
30. OWEN, R.L., R.T. APPLE & D.K. BHALLA. 1986. Morphometric and cytochemical analysis of lysosomes in rat Peyer's patch follicle epithelium: their reduction in volume fraction and acid phosphatase content in M cells compared to adjacent enterocytes. Anat. Rec. **216:** 521–527.
31. NEUTRA, M.R. *et al.* 1987. Transport of membrane-bound macromolecules by M cells in follicle-associated epithelium of rabbit Peyer's patch. Cell Tissue Res. **247:** 537–546.
32. UEKI, T. *et al.* 1995. Expression of ICAM-I on M cells covering isolated lymphoid follicles of the human colon. Acta Med. Okayama **49:** 145–151.
33. ROSNER, A.J. & D.F. KEREN. 1984. Demonstration of M cells in the specialized follicle-associated epithelium overlying isolated lymphoid follicles in the gut. J. Leukoc. Biol. **35:** 397–404.
34. MOGHADDAMI, M., A. CUMMINS & G. MAYRHOFER. 1998. Lymphocyte-filled villi: comparison with other lymphoid aggregations in the mucosa of the human small intestine. Gastroenterology **115:** 1414–1425.
35. JANG, M.H. *et al.* 2004. Intestinal villous M cells: an antigen entry site in the mucosal epithelium. Proc. Natl. Acad. Sci. USA **101:** 6110–6115.
36. TUMANOV, A.V. *et al.* 2004. Lymphotoxin and TNF produced by B cells are dispensable for maintenance of the follicle-associated epithelium but are required for development of lymphoid follicles in the Peyer's patches. J. Immunol. **173:** 86–91.
37. LUGERING, A. *et al.* 2005. Absence of CCR6 inhibits CD4+ regulatory T-cell development and M-cell formation inside Peyer's patches. Am. J. Pathol. **166:** 1647–1654.
38. TAMAGAWA, H. *et al.* 2003. Characteristics of claudin expression in follicle-associated epithelium of Peyer's patches: preferential localization of claudin-4 at the apex of the dome region. Lab. Invest. **83:** 1045–1053.
39. CLARK, M.A. & B.H. HIRST. 2002. Expression of junction-associated proteins differentiates mouse intestinal M cells from enterocytes. Histochem. Cell Biol. **118:** 137–147.
40. WELTZIN, R. *et al.* 1989. Binding and transepithelial transport of immunoglobulins by intestinal M cells: demonstration using monoclonal IgA antibodies against enteric viral proteins. J. Cell Biol. **108:** 1673–1685.
41. CLARK, M.A. *et al.* 1993. Differential expression of lectin-binding sites defines mouse intestinal M-cells. J. Histochem. Cytochem. **41:** 1679–1687.

42. GIANNASCA, P.J. *et al.* 1994. Regional differences in glycoconjugates of intestinal M cells in mice: potential targets for mucosal vaccines. Am. J. Physiol. **267:** G1108–G1121.

43. JEPSON, M.A. *et al.* 1992. Co-expresion of vimentin and cytokeratins in M-cells of rabbit intestinal lymphoid follicle-associated epithelium. Histochem. J. **24:** 33–39.

44. GEBERT, A., H.J. ROTHKOTTER & R. PABST. 1994. Cytokeratin 18 is an M-cell marker in porcine Peyer's patches. Cell Tissue Res. **276:** 213–221.

45. SCHMEDTJE, J.F. 1965. Some histochemical characteristics of lymphoepithelial cells of the rabbit appendix. Anat. Rec. **151:** 412–413.

46. FARSTAD, I.N. *et al.* 1994. Heterogenity of M-cell-associated B and T cells in human Peyer's patches. Immunology **83:** 457–464.

47. RAUTENBERG, K., C. CICHON & M.A. SCHMIDT. 1996. Immunocytochemical characterization of the follicle-associated epithelium of Peyer's patches: anti-cytokeratin 8 antibody (Clone 4.1.18) as a molecular marker for rat M-cells. Eur. J. Cell Biol. **71:** 361–375.

48. SHARMA, R. *et al.* 1996. Lectin binding reveals divergent carbohydrate expression in human and mouse Peyer's patches. Histochem. Cell Biol. **105:** 459–465.

49. CLARK, M.A., B.H. HIRST & M.A. JEPSON. 1998. M-cell surface beta1 integrin expression and invasin-mediated targeting of *Yersinia pseudotuberculosis* to mouse Peyer's patch M cells. Infect. Immun. **66:** 1237–1243.

50. GIANNASCA, P. *et al.* 1999. Human intestinal M cells display the sialyl Lewis A antigen. Infect. Immun. **67:** 946–953.

51. WONG, N.A., M. HERRIOT & F. RAE. 2003. An immunohistochemical study and review of potential markers of human intestinal M cells. Eur. J. Histochem. **47:** 143–150.

52. UEKI, T. *et al.* 1995. Expression of ICAM-1 on M-cells covering isolated lymphoid follicles of the human colon. Acta Med. Okayama. **49:** 145–151.

53. FINZI, G. *et al.* 1993. Cathepsin E in follicle associated epithelium of intestine and tonsils: localization to M cells and possible role in antigen processing. Histochemistry **99:** 201–211.

54. LO, D. *et al.* 2004. Cell culture modeling of specialized tissue: identification of genes expressed specifically by follicle-associated epithelium of Peyer's patch by expression profiling of Caco-2/Raji co-cultures. Int. Immunol. **16:** 91–99.

55. ROTH-WALTER, F. *et al.* 2004. M cell targeting with *Aleuria aurantia* lectin as a novel approach for oral allergen immunotherapy. J. Allergy Clin. Immunol. **114:** 1362–1368.

56. JEPSON, M.A. *et al.* 1996. Targeting to intestinal M-cells. J. Anat. **189:** 507–516.

57. HAMZAOUI, N. *et al.* 2004. Expression and distribution of beta1 integrins in in vitro-induced M cells: implications for *Yersinia* adhesion to Peyer's patch epithelium. Cell Microbiol. **6:** 817–828.

58. ANDERLE, P. *et al.* 2005. Novel markers of the human follicle-associated epithelium identified by genomic profiling and microdissection. Gastroenterology **129:** 321–327.

59. GULLBERG, E. *et al.* 2005. Human follicle associated epithelium demonstrates increased CD9 and b1-integrin expression that is linked with selective transport into human Peyer's patches. Gastroenterology **128 (suppl. 4):** A128.

60. CICHON, C., L. GREUNE & M.A. SCHMIDT. 2005. Identification of Galectin 9 as a new marker molecule for "M-cell-like cells" and human "follicle-associated

epithelia": novel perspectives for mucosal vaccine development. Presented as poster #101 at "Inflammatory Bowel Disease: Research Drives Clinics," Muenster, Germany, September 2005.

61. KERNEÍS, S. *et al.* 1997. Conversion by Peyer's patch lymphocytes of human enterocytes into M cells that transport bacteria. Science **277:** 949–952.

62. SCHULTE, R. *et al.* 2000. Translocation of *Yersinia entrocolitica* across reconstituted intestinal epithelial monolayers is triggered by *Yersinia* invasin binding to beta1 integrins apically expressed on M-like cells. Cell. Microbiol. **2:** 173–185.

63. HEPPNER, F.L. *et al.* 2001. Transepithelial prion transport by M cells. Nat. Med. **7:** 976–977.

64. LIANG, E. *et al.* 2001. Permeability measurement of macromolecules and assessment of mucosal antigen sampling using in vitro converted M cells. J. Pharmacol. Toxicol. Methods **46:** 93–101.

65. El BAHI, S. *et al.* 2002. Lymphoepithelial interactions trigger specific regulation of gene expression in the M cell-containing follicle-associated epithelium of Peyer's patches. J. Immunol. **168:** 3713–3720.

66. FOTOPOULOS, G. *et al.* 2002. Transepithelial transport of HIV-1 by M cells is receptor-mediated. Proc. Natl. Acad. Sci. USA **99:** 9410–9414.

67. GULLBERG, E. *et al.* 2000. Expression of specific markers and particle transport in a new human intestinal M-cell model. Biochem. Biophys. Res. Commun. **279:** 808–813.

68. ROTH-WALTER, F. *et al.* 2005. Targeting antigens to murine and human M-cells with *Aleuria aurantia* lectin-functionalized microparticles. Immunol. Lett. **100:** 182–188.

69. JENSEN, V.B., J.T. HARTY & B.D. JONES. 1998. Interactions of the invasive pathogens *Salmonella typhimurium*, *Listeria monocytogenes*, and *Shigella flexneri* with M cells and murine Peyer's patches. Infect. Immun. **66:** 3758–3766.

70. PHILLIPS, A.D. *et al.* 2000. Enterohaemorrhagic *Escherichia coli* O157:H7 target Peyer's patches in humans and cause attaching/effacing lesions in both human and bovine intestine. Gut **47:** 377–381.

71. FITZHENRY, R.J. *et al.* 2002. Tissue tropism of enteropathogenic *Escherichia coli* strains belonging to the O55 serogroup. Infect. Immun. **70:** 4362–4368.

72. FITZHENRY, R.J. *et al.* 2002. Intimin type influences the site of human intestinal mucosal colonisation by enterohaemorrhagic *Escherichia coli* O157:H7. Gut **50:** 180–185.

73. HELANDER, A. *et al.* 2003. The viral sigma1 protein and glycoconjugates containing alpha2-3-linked sialic acid are involved in type 1 reovirus adherence to M cell apical surfaces. J. Virol. **77:** 7964–7977.

74. HUTCHINGS, A.B. *et al.* 2004. Secretory immunoglobulin A antibodies against the sigma1 outer capsid protein of reovirus type 1 Lang prevent infection of mouse Peyer's patches. J. Virol. **78:** 947–957.

75. FOTOPOULOS, G. *et al.* 2002. Transepithelial transport of HIV-1 by M cells is receptor-mediated. Proc. Natl. Acad. Sci. USA **99:** 9410–9414.

76. PRINZ, M. *et al.* 2003. Oral prion infection requires normal numbers of Peyer's patches but not of enteric lymphocytes. Am. J. Pathol. **162:** 1103–1111.

77. SMITH, M.W., P.S. JAMES & D.R. TIVEY. 1987. M cell numbers increase after transfer of SPF mice to a normal house enviroment. Am. J. Pathol. **128:** 385–389.

78. MEYNELL, H.M. *et al.* 1999. Up-regulation of microsphere transport across the follicle-associated epithelium of Peyer's patch by exposure to *Streptococcus pneumoniae R36a*. FASEB J. **13:** 611–619.
79. SAVIDGE, T.C., M.W. SMITH & P.S. JAMES. 1991. *Salmonella*-induced M-cell formation in germ-free Peyer's patch tissue. Am. J. Pathol. **139:** 177–184.
80. BORGHESI, C. *et al.* 1996. Modifications of the follicle-associated epithelium by short-term exposure to a non-intestinal bacterium. J. Pathol. **180:** 326–332.
81. BORGHESI, C., M.J. TAUSSIG & C. NICOLETTI. 1999. Rapid appearance of M cells after microbial challenge is restricted at the periphery of the follicle-associated epithelium of Peyer's patch. Lab. Invest. **79:** 1393–1401.
82. GEBERT, A. *et al.* 2004. Antigen transport into Peyer's patches: increased uptake by constant numbers of M cells. Am. J. Pathol. **164:** 65–72.
83. VISWANATHAN, V.K., R. SHARMA & G. HECHT. 2004. Microbes and their products: physiological effects upon mammalian mucosa. Adv. Drug Deliv. Rev. **56:** 727–762.
84. CLARK, E.C. *et al.* 2003. Glutamine deprivation facilitates tumour necrosis factor induced bacterial translocation in Caco-2 cells by depletion of enterocyte fuel substrate. Gut **52:** 224–230.
85. SÖDERHOLM, J.D. *et al.* 2004. Increased epithelial uptake of protein antigens in the ileum of Crohn's disease mediated by tumour necrosis factor alpha. Gut **53:** 1817–1824.
86. MATSUMOTO, S. *et al.* 1998. Inflammatory bowel disease-like enteritis and caecitis in a senescence accelerated mouse P1/Yit strain. Gut **43:** 71–78.
87. KOSIEWICZ, M.M. *et al.* 2001. Th1-type responses mediate spontaneous ileitis in a novel murine model of Crohn's disease. J. Clin. Invest. **107:** 695–702.
88. VELIN, A.K. *et al.* 2004. Increased antigen and bacterial uptake in follicle associated epithelium induced by chronic psychological stress in rats. Gut **53:** 494–500.
89. KUCHARZIK, T. *et al.* 2000. Characterization of M cell development during indomethacin-induced ileitis in rats. Aliment. Pharmacol. Ther. **14:** 247–256.
90. LUGERING, A. *et al.* 2004. Characterization of M cell formation and associated mononuclear cells during indomethacin-induced intestinal inflammation. Clin. Exp. Immunol. **136:** 232–238.
91. MOYANA, T.N. *et al.* 1994. Development of the early mucosal lesions in experimental inflammatory bowel disease—implications for pathogenesis. Exp. Mol. Pathol. **60:** 119–129.
92. SPAHN, T.W. *et al.* 2002. Induction of colitis in mice deficient of Peyer's patches and mesenteric lymph nodes is associated with increased disease severity and formation of colonic lymphoid patches. Am. J. Pathol. **161:** 2273–2282.
93. CUVELIER, C.A. *et al.* 1993. M cells are damaged and increased in number in inflamed human ileal mucosa. Eur. J. Morphol. **31:** 87–91.
94. KASER, A. *et al.* 2004. Increased expression of CCL20 in human inflammatory bowel disease. J. Clin. Immunol. **24:** 74–85.
95. SILVA, M.A. *et al.* 2004. Characterization and distribution of colonic dendritic cells in Crohn's disease. Inflamm. Bowel Dis. **10:** 504–512.
96. TE VELDE, A.A. *et al.* 2003. Increased expression of DC-SIGN+IL-12+IL-18+ and CD83+IL-12-IL-18- dendritic cell populations in the colonic mucosa of patients with Crohn's disease. Eur. J. Immunol. **33:** 143–151.

97. DE BAEY, A. *et al.* 2003. A subset of human dendritic cells in the T cell area of mucosa-associated lymphoid tissue with a high potential to produce TNF-alpha. J. Immunol. **170:** 5089–5094.
98. KUDO, T. *et al.* 2004. Polarized production of T-helper cell type 1 cells in Peyer's patches in Crohn's disease. Digestion **70:** 214–225.
99. DIDIERLAURENT, A. *et al.* 2002. How the gut senses its content. Cell. Microbiol. **4:** 61–72.
100. SIERRO, F. *et al.* 2001. Flagellin stimulation of intestinal epithelial cells triggers CCL20-mediated migration of dendritic cells. Proc. Natl. Acad. Sci. USA. **98:** 13722–13727.
101. COOK, D.N. *et al.* 2000. CCR6 mediates dendritic cell localization, lymphocyte homeostasis, and immune responses in mucosal tissue. Immunity **12:** 495–503.
102. NEISH, A.S. *et al.* 2000. Prokaryotic regulation of epithelial responses by inhibition of IkappaB-alpha ubiquitination. Science **289:** 1560–1563.
103. HUGOT, J.P. *et al.* 2001. Association of NOD2 leucine-rich repeat variants with susceptibility to Crohn's disease. Nature **411:** 599–603.
104. OGURA, Y. *et al.* 2001. A frameshift mutation in NOD2 associated with susceptibility to Crohn's disease. Nature **411:** 603–606.
105. MEDDINGS, J.B. 1997. Review article: intestinal permeability in Crohn's disease. Aliment. Pharmacol. Ther. **11** (Suppl 3): 47–53.
106. BJARNASON, I., A. MACPHERSON & D. HOLLANDER. 1995. Intestinal permeability: an overview. Gastroenterology **108:** 1566–1581.
107. SUENAERT, P. *et al.* 2002. Anti-tumor necrosis factor treatment restores the gut barrier in Crohn's disease. Am. J. Gastroenterol. **97:** 2000–2004.
108. ZEISSIG, S. *et al.* 2004. Downregulation of epithelial apoptosis and barrier repair in active Crohn's disease by tumour necrosis factor alpha antibody treatment. Gut **53:** 1295–1302.
109. NEUTRA, M.R., N.J. MANTIS & J.P. KRAEHENBUHL. 2001. Collaboration of epithelial cells with organized mucosal lymphoid tissues. Nat. Immunol. **2:** 1004–1009.
110. VELIN KEITA, A. *et al.* 2005. Disrupted barrier to non-pathogenic *E. coli* in the follicle-associated epithelium of non-inflamed ileum of patients with Crohn's disease. Gastroenterology **128 (suppl. 2):** A214.
111. KEITA, A.V., E. GULLBERG, A.C. ERICSON, *et al.* 2006. Characterization of antigen and bacterial transport in the follicle-associated epithelium of human ileum. Lab. Invest. **86:** 504–516.

Synergistic Costimulation by Both B7 Molecules Regulates Colitis Pathogenesis

GISEN KIM,[a] STEPHEN P. SCHOENBERGER,[b] ARLENE SHARPE,[c] AND MITCHELL KRONENBERG[a]

[a]Division of Developmental Immunology, La Jolla Institute for Allergy and Immunology, La Jolla, California 92037, USA

[b]Division of Cellular Immunology, La Jolla Institute for Allergy and Immunology, La Jolla, California 92037, USA

[c]Department of Pathology, Harvard Medical School, Boston, Massachusetts 02115, USA

ABSTRACT: It has been reported that B7-1 and B7-2 play different roles in the pathogenesis of autoimmunity, but this issue is controversial. Here we analyzed colitis induced by transfer of CD45RB^{high} CD4$^+$ T cells to immune-deficient recipients that lack expression of either B7-1 or B7-2. Surprisingly, disease was greatly accelerated in Rag$^{-/-}$ recipients deficient for either B7 molecule. Antigen presenting cells (APCs) lacking B7-1 or B7-2 stimulated T cell proliferation *in vitro*, but caused suboptimal IL-2 production, leading to decreased induction of CTLA-4. The data suggest that regulatory T cells function relatively normally in B7 single-deficient recipients, but they cannot restrain the increased pathogenesis by naïve cells primed in B7 single-deficient mice. Therefore, the inhibitory effect of CTLA-4 on pathogenic T cells likely slows colitis, even in the absence of regulatory T cells. While a full block of costimulation may prevent autoimmunity, our data indicate, surprisingly, that a partial block may in some cases augment disease.

KEYWORDS: costimulation; colitis; B7; CTLA-4; IL-2

INTRODUCTION

The B7-1 (CD80) and B7-2 (CD86) costimulatory molecules play critical roles in activation and regulation of T cells by binding to two counter receptors CD28 and CTLA-4. Constitutively expressed CD28 mediates a positive signal to T cells during priming that is indispensable for survival, proliferation, and IL-2 production.[1-5] On the contrary, CTLA-4 is upregulated upon T cell activation and mediates an inhibitory signal to activated T cells.[6,7] The critical role

Address for correspondence: M. Kronenberg, La Jolla Institute for Allergy and Immunology, 9420 Athena Circle, La Jolla, CA 92037, USA. Voice: 858-752-6540; fax: 858-225-0730.
e-mail: mitch@liai.org

Ann. N.Y. Acad. Sci. 1072: 233–241 (2006). © 2006 New York Academy of Sciences.
doi: 10.1196/annals.1326.012

of CTLA-4 in downregulating the immune response has been demonstrated in CTLA-4-deficient mice that develop lethal lymphoproliferative disease characterized by systemic accumulation of activated $CD4^+$ T cells.[8,9,10] Additionally, a series of studies have suggested an *in vivo* role for CTLA-4 in peripheral tolerance and anergy induction.[11,12] Doyle *et al.* reported on the role of CTLA-4 in restricting T cell clonal expansion,[13] which could be a major mechanism for the intrinsic restriction of T cell proliferation and cell cycle–driven differentiation of activated T cells. B7/CD28 costimulation enhances production of the potent T cell growth factor IL-2.[2] Besides driving proliferation or sensitizing activated T cells to cell death, IL-2 has been reported to be important for the induction of CTLA-4.[14] Therefore optimal $CD4^+$ T cell activation and IL-2 production might be key elements for the effective regulation of T cell responses through CTLA-4.

Two B7 molecules, B7-1 and B7-2 have overlapping functions in eliciting T cell effector functions but have distinct expression kinetics.[15] While B7-2 is constitutively expressed by mainly bone marrow–derived cells, B7-1 is induced after the activation and also is expressed by nonhematopoietic cells in the local tissues. Later upregulation and extralymph node expression of B7-1 suggest that the interaction of two inducible molecules, B7-1 and CTLA-4, might contribute to a feedback inhibition to avoid overstimulation of T cells.

Here we studied the role of B7 costimulation in an experimental mouse model of colitis induced by T cell transfer. In this model, injection of syngeneic $CD4^+$ T cells with a naïve phenotype ($CD45RB^{high}$) into immune-deficient $Rag^{-/-}$ or SCID mice results in the induction of chronic colitis that bears some features in common with human Crohn's disease, as differentiated Th1 cells are required for pathogenesis.[16,17,18] Surprisingly, transfer of the same donor cells into recipients that bear altered B7 expression revealed that the absence of only one B7 molecule, either B7-1 or B7-2, greatly accelerated disease. Our data further suggest that this acceleration may be mediated by decreased IL-2 synthesis, leading to decreased induction of CTLA-4 expression.

INSUFFICIENT COSTIMULATION DRAMATICALLY ACCELERATED COLITIS

To investigate the role of B7 molecules in the pathogenesis of experimental colitis in mice, we transferred 5×10^5 $CD4^+CD45RB^{high}$ T cells FACS-sorted from wild-type C57BL/6 (B6) spleens into B7 wild-type Rag-deficient mice (B6 $Rag1^{-/-}$) or two different single B7-deficient Rag-deficient mice ($B7\text{-}1^{-/-}Rag1^{-/-}$ or $B7\text{-}2^{-/-}Rag1^{-/-}$). Surprisingly, compared to B6 $Rag1^{-/-}$ recipients that developed chronic colitis by 6 to 10 weeks after the transfer, recipients lacking either B7-1 or B7-2 only developed the symptoms of wasting disease as early as 10–14 days after T cell transfer (TABLE 1). Histological analyses of the large intestines 14 days after transfer demonstrated

TABLE 1. Relative body weight change and histological scores of the large intestine

Donor cells	Recipients	Days post transfer	Body weight change (%)	Histological scores (1–14)
5×10^5 CD4$^+$CD45RB^{high}	B6 Rag1$^{-/-}$	14	+ 4.4 ±	4.2
5×10^5 CD4$^+$CD45RB^{high}	B7-1/2$^{-/-}$ Rag1$^{-/-}$	14	+ 1.9 ±	1.0
5×10^5 CD4$^+$CD45RB^{high}	B7-1$^{-/-}$ Rag1$^{-/-}$	14	−5.1 ±	8.4
5×10^5 CD4$^+$CD45RB^{high}	B7-2$^{-/-}$ Rag1$^{-/-}$	14	−10.9 ±	8.7
5×10^5 CD4$^+$CD45RB^{high} + 5×10^4 CD4$^+$CD25$^+$	B6 Rag1$^{-/-}$	28	+ 7.3 ±	1.0
5×10^5 CD4$^+$CD45RB^{high} + 5×10^4 CD4$^+$CD25$^+$	B7-2$^{-/-}$ Rag1$^{-/-}$	28	−19.0 ±	8.7

Recipients were injected with 5×10^5 of CD4$^+$CD45RB^{high} cells from B6 spleens in the absence or presence of 5×10^4 CD4$^+$CD25$^+$ cells from CD45.1 mice (The Jackson Laboratory, Bar Harbor, ME). Histological score for each recipient was averaged from three specimens obtained from proximal, middle, and distal parts of the large intestine.

massive cell infiltration and mucosal hyperplasia in both B7-1$^{-/-}$Rag1$^{-/-}$ and B7-2$^{-/-}$Rag1$^{-/-}$ mice, while only focal cell infiltration was seen at this relatively early time point in B6 Rag1$^{-/-}$ recipients. Inflammation was restricted to the large intestine, although mild T cell migration was seen in other organs, such as stomach, pancreas, and skin.

As has been reported, a cotransfer of CD4$^+$CD25$^+$ cells (5×10^4) with CD4$^+$CD45RB^{high} cells prevented disease induction in B6 Rag1$^{-/-}$ recipients. On the contrary, the same number of CD4$^+$CD25$^+$ cells failed to prevent disease in B7-2$^{-/-}$Rag1$^{-/-}$ recipients, which developed severe colitis by 28 days after the transfer (TABLE 1). To test the possibility that deficiency of a single B7 molecule might affect the expansion and/or the regulatory function of CD4$^+$CD25$^+$ cells, we carried out an *in vitro* coculture experiment. In this experiment, naïve CD4$^+$CD45RB^{high} cells from CD45.2 (B6) mice and CD4$^+$CD25$^+$ cells from congenic CD45.1 mice were cultured at a 4:1 ratio with gamma-irradiated T cell–depleted spleen cells from B7 wild-type (B6) or B7 single-deficient mice as antigen presenting cells (APCs). Cells were stimulated with 1.0 μg/mL of anti-CD3 monoclonal antibody (mAb). As shown in the FIGURE 1B, CD45.1$^+$ regulatory T cells proliferated comparably with B7 single-deficient APCs, compared to the same population that was cultured with B6 APCs. In addition, CD4$^+$CD25$^+$ cells suppressed the proliferation of CD4$^+$CD45RB^{high} cells comparably, even with B7 single-deficient APCs. This is evident in FIGURE 1C, as a decreased number of cell divisions was assessed by CFSE dye dilution. These data suggest that the failure in preventing disease in B7-2$^{-/-}$Rag1$^{-/-}$ recipients might be caused by an enhanced or dysregulated effector function of CD4$^+$CD45RB^{high} cells, not because of impaired functions of CD4$^+$CD25$^+$ cells.

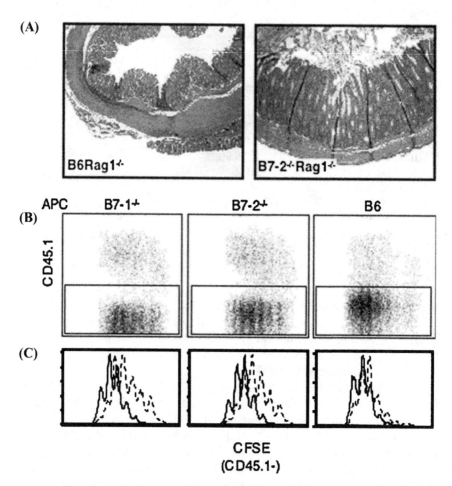

FIGURE 1. (A) Severe colitis in B7-2$^{-/-}$Rag1$^{-/-}$ recipients induced by a cotransfer of CD4$^+$CD25$^+$ cells with CD4$^+$CD45RB^{high} cells. 10^5 CD4$^+$CD45RB^{high} cells from B6 spleens and 5 × 10^4 CD4$^+$CD25$^+$ cells from spleens of CD45.1 mice (see TABLE 1) were coinjected in B6 Rag1$^{-/-}$ (left) and B7-2$^{-/-}$Rag1$^{-/-}$ mice (right). Four weeks later, specimens were obtained from large intestine and fixed in the 10% buffered formalin. **(B)** CD4$^+$CD25$^+$ cells exhibited a comparable proliferation with B7 single-deficient or wild-type APCs. 1 × 10^5 CD4$^+$CD45RB^{high} cells and 2.5 × 10^4 CD4$^+$CD25$^+$ cells (both labeled with CFSE) were stimulated with 1.0 μg/mL anti-CD3 mAb for 4 days in 96-well plates in the presence of irradiated CD90.2$^+$ cell-depleted spleen cells obtained from B7-1$^{-/-}$, B7-2$^{-/-}$, or B6 mice. CFSE dilution of CD45.1$^+$ (initially CD4$^+$CD25$^+$) or CD45.1$^-$ (initially CD4$^+$CD45RB^{high}) CD90.2$^+$ cells is shown. **(C)** CD4$^+$CD25$^+$ cells regulated proliferation of CD4$^+$CD45RB^{high} cells in the culture with B7 single-deficient APC. CFSE dilution of CD45.1$^-$ cells (initially CD4$^+$CD45RB^{high}) in the presence (dotted lines) or absence (solid lines) of CD4$^+$CD25$^+$ cells is shown. Suppressive function of CD4$^+$CD25$^+$ cells was maintained with B7 single-deficient APC, which is demonstrated as reduced CFSE dilution in the presence of CD4$^+$CD25$^+$ cells.

B7-1 AND B7-2 ARE REQUIRED FOR OPTIMAL IL-2 AND IL-2-DEPENDENT CTLA-4 EXPRESSION

We hypothesized that insufficient costimulation with either B7-1 or B7-2 might fail to fully induce CTLA-4, which could be responsible for the postulated regulation. Consistent with this, CD28 cross-linking, along with TCR stimulation, has been reported to play a role in upregulating CTLA-4.[19] To investigate the effect of B7 molecules on the upregulation of CTLA-4 by activated T cells, we used a similar culture system to that used in FIGURE 1. Sorted CD4$^+$CD45RB^{high} cells were cultured with B7 wild-type or B7-deficient APCs, as mentioned in FIGURE 1. Cells were cultured with anti-CD3 mAb for 3 or 4 days before staining total (intracellular and surface) CTLA-4 expression. T cells cultured with B7 single-deficient APCs expressed reduced levels of CTLA-4. Especially with B7-2$^{-/-}$ APCs, even high concentrations of anti-CD3 mAb (5.0 μg/mL) totally failed to induce CTLA4. Interestingly, T cell proliferation in the culture with B7-2$^{-/-}$ APCs was almost comparable to those with B6 APCs, despite a failure to induce CTLA-4. CTLA-4 expression in the culture was totally abrogated with addition of anti-IL-2 or anti-IL-2Rα (CD25) mAb, consistent with a previous report.[14] Because IL-2 production is highly enhanced by B7/CD28 costimulation,[2–14,20] we expected that lack of a single B7 molecule could influence the optimal induction of IL-2. In fact, IL-2 secretion by activated T cells was dramatically reduced in the culture with B7 single-deficient APCs compared to the culture with B6 APCs. Taken together, we conclude that optimal IL-2 production and subsequent IL-2-dependent CTLA-4 expression requires synergistic costimulation by both B7-1 and B7-2, although proliferation is essentially normal during priming with single B7-deficient APCs. Therefore, *in vivo* B7 single-deficient recipients could allow the activated donor T cells to proliferate in the absence of an optimal regulation by CTLA-4.

INCREASED T CELL CYTOKINES IN SINGLE B7-DEFICIENT RAG1$^{-/-}$ RECIPIENTS

In the majority of B7 single-deficient Rag1$^{-/-}$ recipients that received naïve CD4$^+$ T cells, thickening of the large intestine was found by 10 days after T cell transfer. At the same time, a characteristic feature that correlated with the rapid induction of colitis was an enlarged spleen and mesenteric lymph nodes as early as 7–10 days after transfer. Intracellular cytokine staining of spleen cells that were recovered 7 days post transfer and restimulated briefly demonstrated that the expanded spleen T cells from B7 single-deficient Rag1$^{-/-}$ recipients exhibited increased percentages of Th1 cytokine-producing cells, especially TNF-α and IL-2, compared to those from B6 Rag1$^{-/-}$ recipients (B7-1$^{-/-}$Rag1$^{-/-}$

and B7-2$^{-/-}$Rag1$^{-/-}$ to B6 Rag1$^{-/-}$, respectively: TNF-α, 36.0% and 49% to 14.9%; IL-2, 49% and 27.5% to 19.8%). In both types of recipients, many of the TNF-α highly positive CD4$^+$ T cells also were IL-2-positive. Furthermore, DNA content analysis using propidium iodide demonstrated that twofold and sixfold more of the TCR β^+ cells in B7-2$^{-/-}$ Rag1$^{-/-}$ recipients were in the S-G2-M phases of the cell cycle in the spleen and MLN, respectively. These data indicate that T cells primed in B7-2$^{-/-}$ Rag1$^{-/-}$ recipients were capable of more active proliferation upon restimulation compared to those in B6 Rag1$^{-/-}$ mice.

The increased *in vivo* T cell activation in B7-deficient Rag1$^{-/-}$ recipients could be due to the reduced induction of CTLA-4, as we observed *in vitro*. To determine whether the induction of CTLA-4 by activated CD4$^+$ T cells is affected by the absence of one B7 molecule *in vivo*, we analyzed TCRβ^+ donor cells that were recovered from lymph nodes at an early time point during priming, at 2 days post transfer. Donor T cells in peripheral and mesenteric lymph nodes of B7-2$^{-/-}$ Rag1$^{-/-}$ recipients expressed significantly lower levels of CTLA-4 than those in B6 Rag1$^{-/-}$ recipients.

BLOCKING IL-2-ACCELERATED COLITIS

To support our hypothesis that insufficient production of IL-2 during priming, because of reduced CD28 costimulation, causes a subsequent uncontrolled IL-2 synthesis and acceleration of pathogenesis, we blocked IL-2 signaling by injecting anti-IL-2 mAb immediately after the transfer of CD4$^+$CD45RB^{high} cells. After a single injection of a limiting amount (3 μg/mouse) of anti-IL-2 mAb, B6 Rag1$^{-/-}$ recipients developed accelerated colitis, demonstrated by an accumulation of cells, including TCRβ^+ donor cells, in the spleen and the large intestinal lamina propria at 2 weeks. Histological scores of the colon confirmed the induction of accelerated colitis with injection of anti-IL-2 mAb. Injection of a higher amount of anti-IL-2 mAb (100 μg/mouse) or later anti-IL-2 mAb injections did not accelerate colitis induction. This suggests that blocking IL-2 during priming is important for disease acceleration, and a possible later requirement for IL-2 in disease acceleration.

DISCUSSION

In the present study, we have demonstrated the indispensable roles of costimulation by both B7-1 and B7-2 in the regulation of activation-induced T lymphocyte proliferation. Reduced costimulation in either B7-1- or B7-2-deficient recipients resulted in a dramatic acceleration of colitis induction following transfer of CD4$^+$CD45RB^{high} cells.

We considered that CTLA-4, whose induction is dependent upon B7-CD28-mediated signals,[19] might provide one means to regulate T cell expansion and

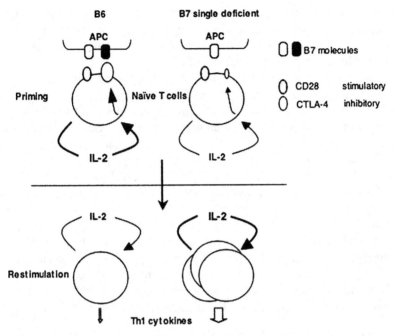

FIGURE 2. A model illustrating how priming with both B7 molecules (*left*) induces optimal IL-2 (thick arrows) and increased CTLA-4 (larger open symbol) compared priming with APCs expressing a single B7 molecule (*right*). Cells primed with APCs expressing a single type of B7 molecule proliferate more and secrete more IL-2 upon restimulation (*bottom*).

delay the onset of disease. In accord with a role for CTLA-4 in limiting the progression of pathogenesis, even in the absence of CD25$^+$ regulatory T cells, naïve CD4$^+$ T cells proliferated but did not fully increase their expression of CTLA-4 when cultured with APCs that lacked either B7-1 or B7-2.

In the present study, costimulation by the single B7-deficient APCs was sufficient for near-normal proliferation and survival of the primed T cells *in vitro*, but IL-2 production was seriously compromised. Our data indicate that IL-2 is likely to be a critical factor in the upregulation of CTLA-4 expression, allowing the activated T cells to escape regulation. The connections we propose between synergistic costimulation by both B7 molecules, optimal IL-2 synthesis, and CTLA-4 induction are diagrammed in FIGURE 2.

IL-2 has complex effects, some of which are independent of CTLA-4, as it influences both T lymphocyte growth and activation-induced cell death. Despite decreased IL-2 production following priming by B7 single-deficient APCs, activated T lymphocytes that accumulated in the spleen of B7 single-deficient Rag1$^{-/-}$ recipients 7 days post transfer were actively proliferating and capable of producing increased levels of IL-2, in addition to TNF-α, which is associated with colitis induction in this model. Consistent with a critical role for IL-2 during priming in limiting pathogenesis through CTLA-4 induction, and perhaps through other pathways as well, blocking of IL-2 signaling during the priming phase with a limiting amount of anti-IL-2 mAb dramatically accelerated the induction of colitis.

Regulating autoreactive CD4$^+$ T cells is critical for the maintenance of peripheral tolerance. Apart from regulatory T cells, activation-induced regulation of CD4$^+$ T lymphocytes is an additional important system for the maintenance of peripheral tolerance. IL-2 production by activated T cells could play a role as a sensor for the host to trigger multiple activation-induced regulatory systems, including activation-induced cell death and negative regulation through CTLA-4. Consistent with its important role, CTLA-4 polymorphisms have been linked to several human autoimmune diseases,[21] although such a linkage has not yet been reported for inflammatory bowel disease. Insufficient costimulation allows activated T lymphocytes to escape from this system because of impaired secretion of IL-2 by primed T cells, however, which could be a critical mechanism for the pathogenesis of autoimmune diseases, such as inflammatory bowel disease. Therefore, this study provided a good example showing that inappropriate T cell stimulation could cause a dysregulated immune reaction, which even overcomes the regulation by CD4$^+$CD25$^+$ regulatory T cells.

REFERENCES

1. BOISE, L.H. et al. 1995. CD28 costimulation can promote T cell survival by enhancing the expression of Bcl-XL. Immunity 3: 87–98.
2. FRASER, J.D. et al. 1991. Regulation of interleukin-2 gene enhancer activity by the T cell accessory molecule CD28. Science 251: 313–316.
3. JENKINS, M.K. et al. 1991. CD28 delivers a costimulatory signal involved in antigen-specific IL-2 production by human T cells. J. Immunol. 147: 2461–2466.
4. NORTON, S.D. et al. 1992. The CD28 ligand, B7, enhances IL-2 production by providing a costimulatory signal to T cells. J. Immunol. 149: 1556–1561.
5. GREEN, J.M. et al. 1994. Absence of B7-dependent responses in CD28-deficient mice. Immunity 1: 501–508.
6. VAN DER MERWE, P.A. et al. 1997. CD80 (B7-1) binds both CD28 and CTLA-4 with a low affinity and very fast kinetics. J. Exp. Med. 185: 393–403.
7. WALUNAS, T.L. et al. 1994. CTLA-4 can function as a negative regulator of T cell activation. Immunity 1: 405–413.
8. TIVOL, E.A. et al. 1995. Loss of CTLA-4 leads to massive lymphoproliferation and fatal multiorgan tissue destruction, revealing a critical negative regulatory role of CTLA-4. Immunity 3: 541–547.
9. WATERHOUSE, P. et al. 1995. Lymphoproliferative disorders with early lethality in mice deficient in Ctla-4. Science 270: 985–988.
10. CHAMBERS, C.A., T.J. SULLIVAN & J.P. ALLISON. 1997. Lymphoproliferation in CTLA-4-deficient mice is mediated by costimulation-dependent activation of CD4$^+$ T cells. Immunity 7: 885–895.

11. PEREZ, V.L. *et al.* 1997. Induction of peripheral T cell tolerance *in vivo* requires CTLA-4 engagement. Immunity **6:** 411–417.
12. GREENWALD, R.J. *et al.* 2001. CTLA-4 regulates induction of anergy *in vivo*. Immunity **14:** 145–155.
13. DOYLE, A.M. *et al.* 2001. Induction of cytotoxic T lymphocyte antigen 4 (CTLA-4) restricts clonal expansion of helper T cells. J. Exp. Med. **194:** 893–902.
14. ALEGRE, M.L. *et al.* 1996. Regulation of surface and intracellular expression of CTLA4 on mouse T cells. J. Immunol. **157:** 4762–4770.
15. BORRIELLO, F. *et al.* 1997. B7-1 and B7-2 have overlapping, critical roles in immunoglobulin class switching and germinal center formation. Immunity **6:** 303–313.
16. MORRISSEY, P.J. *et al.* 1993. CD4$^+$ T cells that express high levels of CD45RB induce wasting disease when transferred into congenic severe combined immunodeficient mice: disease development is prevented by cotransfer of purified CD4$^+$ T cells. J. Exp. Med. **178:** 237–244.
17. POWRIE, F. *et al.* 1993. Phenotypically distinct subsets of CD4$^+$ T cells induce or protect from chronic intestinal inflammation in C. B-17 scid mice. Int. Immunol. **5:** 1461–1471.
18. POWRIE, F. *et al.* 1994. Inhibition of Th1 responses prevents inflammatory bowel disease in scid mice reconstituted with CD45RBhi CD4$^+$ T cells. Immunity **1:** 553–562.
19. FINN, P.W. *et al.* 1997. Synergistic induction of CTLA-4 expression by costimulation with TCR plus CD28 signals mediated by increased transcription and messenger ribonucleic acid stability. J. Immunol. **158:** 4074–4081.
20. LINDSTEIN, T. *et al.* 1989. Regulation of lymphokine messenger RNA stability by a surface-mediated T cell activation pathway. Science **244:** 339–343.
21. UEDA, H. *et al.* 2003. Association of the T-cell regulatory gene CTLA4 with susceptibility to autoimmune disease. Nature **423:** 506–511.

Inflammatory Bowel Disease and the Apical Junctional Complex

MATTHIAS BRUEWER,[a] STANISLAV SAMARIN,[b] AND ASMA NUSRAT[b]

[a]Department of General Surgery, University of Muenster, Muenster 48149, Germany

[b]Epithelial Pathobiology Research Unit, Department of Pathology and Laboratory Medicine, Emory University, Atlanta, Georgia 30322, USA

ABSTRACT: A critical function of the intestinal mucosa is to form a barrier that separates luminal contents from the underlying interstitium. This intestinal barrier is primarily regulated by the apical junctional complex (AJC) consisting of tight junctions (TJs) and adherens junctions (AJs) and is compromised in a number of intestinal diseases, including inflammatory bowel disease (IBD). *In vitro* studies have demonstrated that proinflammatory cytokines, such as interferon-gamma (IFN-γ) and tumor necrosis factor-alpha (TNF-α), that are increased in the intestinal mucosa of patients with IBD can induce a leaky mucosal barrier. There is a growing evidence that the increased permeability and altered AJC structure observed in IBD are mediated by internalization of junctional proteins. This review summarizes barrier defects observed in IBD and addresses mechanisms by which proinflammatory cytokines, such as IFN-γ and TNF-α, modulate AJC structure and epithelial barrier function.

KEYWORDS: apical junctional complex; tight junctions; adherens junctions; cytokines; inflammatory bowel disease; endocytosis

INTRODUCTION

Idiopathic inflammatory bowel disease (IBD) encompassing Crohn's disease (CD) and ulcerative colitis (UC) is associated with intestinal inflammation and chronic-relapsing diarrhea. Although significant advances have been made in understanding the pathophysiology of IBD, we are far from understanding the etiologic pathways that lead to this chronic debilitating disorder. Etiologic factors for the disease appears to be multifactorial and contributions from genetic, environmental, and immune dysregulation have been proposed.

Address for correspondence: Asma Nusrat, Department of Pathology and Laboratory Medicine, Emory University, Whitehead Research Building, Room 105E, 615 Michael Street, Atlanta, GA 30322. Voice: 404-727-8543; fax: 404-727-3321.
e-mail: anusrat@emory.edu

Ann. N.Y. Acad. Sci. 1072: 242–252 (2006). © 2006 New York Academy of Sciences.
doi: 10.1196/annals.1326.017

The epithelial lining of the gastrointestinal tract functions as an important barrier that protects underlying tissue compartments from antigens and bacterial products in the lumen. A compromise in integrity of this barrier has been observed in patients with inflammatory bowel disease (IBD).[1–8] In UC the perturbations in permeability have been documented in inflamed intestinal segments, whereas in CD discrete intestinal permeability alterations have been noted not only in gut tissue with evident intestinal lesions, but also in areas lacking any sign of macroscopic injury.[9,10] However, the causes and consequences of the "leaky gut" in IBD are still incompletely understood. The leading concept assumes that the barrier dysfunction in CD reflects a very early event in the disease process that might be genetically driven and triggered by environmental factors, such as luminal antigens or bacteria.[11,12] The role of impaired barrier function in the causality of IBD has been proposed in a report documenting changes in intestinal permeability 8 years before the onset of CD.[13]

A familial link has been observed in both UC and CD and several IBD-related genes have been identified.[14–16] Interestingly, a number of studies have reported that 10–54% of first-degree relatives of CD patients had increased intestinal permeability in the absence of clinical symptoms.[3–6] The involvement of genetic factors is further supported by a study, in which, healthy first-degree relatives, increased mucosal permeability was associated with the presence of a NOD2/CARD15 mutation.[17] Furthermore, several studies have reported a high prevalence of increased intestinal permeability in spouses of CD patients,[6,7,18] suggesting that environmental factors may also play a role. It can therefore be envisioned that the altered mucosal barrier influences the physiologic immune response by increased exposure of immune cells to bacteria and luminal antigens, which in turn can contribute to the unsuppressed immune response that initiates and worsens disease outcome. In this regard, it is well established that the lesions and clinical symptoms of IBD are associated with the overproduction of proinflammatory cytokines, such as interferon-gamma (IFN-γ) and tumor necrosis factor-alpha (TNF-α).[19] This inflammatory process contributes to the further compromise in the epithelial barrier function.

Epithelial Paracellular Permeability and Barrier Function Are Regulated by the Apical Junctional Complex

The epithelial lining of the gastrointestinal tract forms a regulated, selectively permeable barrier permitting the passive entry of luminal nutrients, ions, and water while restricting pathogen access to underlying tissue compartments. The barrier function of epithelial cell monolayer is influenced by numerous physiological and pathological stimuli and is dynamically regulated by an apical intercellular junctional protein complex referred to as the apical junctional complex (AJC). The apical tight junction (TJ) and its subjacent adherens junction (AJ) constitute the AJC. The TJs function as a semipermeable gate permitting the passive entry of luminal nutrients, ions, and water, and at the same time preventing lateral diffusion of proteins and lipids between the outer leaflet of the apical and basolateral plasma membrane domains, thereby establishing distinctive microenvironments on both sides of polarized cells.[20,21] By freeze-fracture electron microscopy, TJs are visualized as a series of anastomosing intramembranous strands in which strand complexity correlates with the tightness of the epithelial barrier.[22]

In contrast with TJs, which are crucial for maintaining the barrier function, AJs are responsible for cell–cell recognition, initiating and maintaining cell–cell contacts.[23] The overall paradigm of protein organization in the AJC is the presence of a series of transmembrane proteins that affiliate with the underlying actin cytoskeleton via cytoplasmic plaque proteins (FIG. 1). Such affiliation with the actin cytoskeleton is important in regulating AJC function and epithelial barrier properties. Transmembrane proteins in the TJ include occludin, the claudin family of proteins, coxsackie adenovirus receptor (CAR), and junctional adhesion molecule-A (JAM-A), while cytoplasmic plaque proteins consist of a number of scaffolding and signaling molecules, such as zonula occludens (ZO) family proteins and cingulin.[20] In the AJs, the transmembrane protein E-cadherin associates with the catenin family of cytoplasmic proteins.[23] Numerous signaling molecules regulate AJC function in response to diverse physiologic and pathologic stimuli.[24–28] The AJC is now viewed as a dynamic signaling center in epithelial cells, which regulates epithelial cell polarization, differentiation, and paracellular permeability.

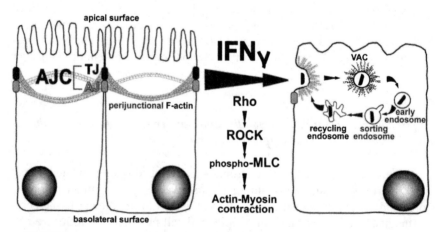

FIGURE 1. IFN-γ modulates TJ structure and induces endocytosis of TJ transmembrane proteins by Rho/ROCK signaling pathway.

Altered Structure of AJC Proteins Contributes to Impaired Barrier Function in IBD

As mentioned above, it is now evident that an important underlying mechanism of IBD is altered permeability across the intestinal epithelium.[29,30] This notion is further supported by findings in animal models of IBD[31–33] that have documented increased epithelial permeability prior to the inflammatory process. In contrast to CD, where altered epithelial barrier function may be a primary factor in the development of the disease,[4] it is presumed that in UC the increased peracellular permeability is secondary to the array of inflammatory signals.[34]

Because the integrity of the AJC determines normal barrier function in epithelia, it has been hypothesized that defects in AJC structure may underlie the increased mucosal permeability observed in patients with IBD.[31] Indeed, initial studies showed a reduced expression of the AJ molecules E-cadherin and α-catenin in the inflamed epithelium in both CD and UC.[35,36] Subsequent studies of Jankowski and co-workers have shown a strong correlation between the deregulation of two classic cadherin molecules, E- and P-cadherin, and the progression of the inflammation in the colon of both CD and UC patients. Morphologic analyses revealed that E-cadherin was focally absent from intercellular junctions and was detected in the cytoplasm.[37] These observations were supported by Gassler *et al.*,[38] showing that in an inactive–inflamed IBD specimen E-cadherin and α-catenin were affected, whereas no changes were observed in the noninflamed tissue. Similar findings were reported by Kucharzik *et al.*,[39] where downregulation of E-cadherin and β-catenin was limited to the areas of active inflammation.

Ultrastructural investigations using freeze-fracture electron microscopy provide information about morphological and structural alterations of the intestinal barrier system in patients with IBD. It was documented that TJs appeared to be abnormal, with an increased distance between enterocytes and a decrease in the number and complexity of TJ strands in both CD[40,41] and UC[34] patients. Moreover, by means of electrophysiological techniques, TJ alterations were found to contribute to the barrier defects in UC.[42] Using both immunohistochemical and protein analyses, Kucharzik *et al.*[39] described a substantial loss of occludin from TJs in the colonic mucosa of patients with UC and CD. Although other TJ proteins, such as ZO-1, JAM-A, and claudin-1 were also found to be decreased, downregulation of occludin was not limited to the areas of active inflammation. In contrast, using similar methods, Gassler *et al.* found a substantial loss of occludin from epithelial junctions exclusively in actively inflamed mucosal tissues from UC and CD patients. Interestingly, AJ molecules E-cadherin and α-catenin were affected in IBD tissues with active inflammation as well as in non-inflamed tissues.[38] The pathophysiological relevance of occludin downregulation for barrier function is incompletely understood since no permeability defects in the intestine were observed in the occludin-deficient mice.[43] This discrepancy could be related to redundancy of proteins that function similarly to occludin and can participate in regulation of epithelial barrier function in these mice.

While numerous mouse models have been generated to investigate the pathogenesis of IBD, intestinal permeability was studied in only a select number of those models and was found to be increased. These include TNBS (trinitrobenzene sulfonic acid)- and DSS (dextran sulfate sodium)-induced colitis, mice with deficient Il-10 gene, and MDR1a knockout mice.[44–48] More interestingly, in MDR1a knockout mice enhanced intestinal permeability was observed before the onset of inflammation. Nevertheless, the role of AJC proteins in this event has not yet been completely elucidated. Although protein levels of occludin, ZO-1, and claudin-1 were essentially similar to those of their respective controls, increased paracellular permeability was associated with decreased phosphorylation of occludin and ZO-1.[48] Moreover one mouse model was described in which the selective disruption of the AJ protein E-cadherin by tissue-specific expression of dominant-negative cadherin construct in small intestinal epithelial cells was associated with dissociation of the AJs and subsequently an inflammatory response similar to that observed in IBD.[31]

Proinflammatory Cytokines and Increased Paracellular Permeability

A growing body of evidence suggests that the immune system plays an important role in modulating intestinal permeability. While a number of proinflammatory cytokines have been proposed to contribute to the pathogenesis of IBD, the influence of two cytokines, IFN-γ and TNF-α, on epithelial permeability has been extensively investigated since the increased synthesis of these cytokines has been observed in the IBD mucosa.[49–51] Both IFN-γ and TNF-α have been shown to decrease epithelial barrier function across model epithelial cell lines, such as T84, Caco-2, and HT-29 intestinal epithelial cells.[52–56] We have observed that IFN-γ induces redistribution of TJ transmembrane proteins JAM-A, occludin, claudin-1, and claudin-4 away from the apical lateral membrane of T84 cells with minimal effect on AJC cytoplasmic plaque proteins.[56] Interestingly, variable effects of TNF-α have been observed in diverse epithelial cell lines.[52,54–56] It is, however, evident that TNF-α significantly potentiates the influence of INF-γ on epithelial barrier function.[56–58]

Endocytosis of AJC Proteins

As described above, we observed that the epithelial barrier defect in cells exposed to the proinflammatory cytokines IFN-γ and TNF-α was associated with redistribution of TJ transmembrane proteins. To further examine the barrier defect mediated by these cytokines we analyzed mechanisms by which

IFN-γ induces internalization of TJ proteins. Expressional downregulation of junctional proteins is unlikely to account for the rapid disassembly of epithelial junctions. Rapid disassembly of the AJC can, however, be achieved by endocytosis of AJC proteins.[59] Three major endocytic pathways[60] have been characterized in different cellular models of IBD. The first endocytic pathway involves polymerization of a specific coat protein, clathrin, on the intracellular face of the plasma membrane, resulting in formation of clathrin-coated pits. This mechanism was found to be important for internalization of AJC proteins in calcium-depleted T84 cells.[61] The second pathway involves invagination of cholesterol-enriched microdomains within the plasma membrane; these are referred to as membrane rafts. The raft pathway has been implicated in internalization of TJ proteins in T84 intestinal epithelial cells treated with *Clostridium botulinum* and *Escherichia coli* toxins.[62,63] The third pathway is the formation of large actin-coated vacuoles that are responsible for uptake of either solid particles (phagosomes) or liquids (macropinosomes) from the cell exterior. Our recent results revealed that exposure of T84 cells to IFN-γ results in internalization of TJ proteins into a subapical cytosolic compartment by macropinocytosis.[64] These observations support the role of all the three internalization pathways in mediating endocytosis of AJC proteins, that are differentially activated by diverse physiologic and pathologic stimuli.

The mechanism by which IFN-γ induces the endocytosis of epithelial TJ proteins has been extensively examined by our laboratory. Our studies suggest that IFN-γ-induced macropinosomes fuse with early endosomes, following which the internalized TJ transmembrane proteins are temporarily stored in a recycling endosomal compartment, from where they can be recycled back to the plasma membrane after withdrawal of IFN-γ (FIG. 1). This could be of clinical importance, as substantial fractions of TJ transmembrane proteins were observed in subapical vesicle-like structures in mucosal biopsies from patients with actively inflamed UC, supporting our *in vitro* observations.[64]

IFN-γ-induced macropinocytosis of TJ transmembrane proteins involves the reorganization of cortical actin cytoskeleton resulting in the formation of large F-actin-coated subapical vacuoles referred to as vacuolar apical compartments (VACs) (FIG. 1). The vacuolar apical compartments, containing internalized TJ proteins, were originated from the apical plasma membrane and their formation was not dependent on the rapid turnover of actin microfilaments. In contrast, the pharmacological inhibition of mammalian nonmuscle myosin II (MNMM II) prevented the formation of VACs, suggesting that the formation of VACs is driven by the myosin-II-mediated contraction.[65] Since the activity of myosin II requires phosphorylation of its light chain,[66,67] and our localization studies revealed the co-localization of MNMM II and phosphorylated myosin light chain (MLC) with VACs containing TJ proteins,[65] we further analyzed different signaling pathways that eventuate in the phosphorylation of MLC. Two serine-threonine protein kinases have been shown to phosphorylate MLC in cells: myosin light chain kinase (MLCK) and Rho-associated protein kinase

(ROCK).[68,69] It was previously shown that the alterations in the epithelial barrier function induced by both IFN-γ and TNF-α in Caco-2 cells can be reversed by a specific pharmacological inhibition of MLCK.[70] Nevertheless, our studies failed to demonstrate a role of MLCK in mediating IFN-γ-induced endocytosis of TJ proteins and consequent barrier defects. In contrast, we observed the direct phosphorylation of MLC by ROCK and found that pharmacological inhibition of ROCK completely prevented IFN-γ-induced formation of VACs. Additionally, IFN-γ upregulated the expression of ROCK in T84 cells, and, at the same time, activated its upstream effector Rho GTPase.[65] Thus our data support a role of IFN-γ induced Rho/ROCK signaling in development of VACs and endocytosis of TJ proteins (FIG. 1). These *in vitro* observations are supported by previous studies that have documented increased RhoA expression in mucosa of CD patients, and where pharmacological inhibition of ROCK prevented the inflammatory response.[71] Given these observations, a promising approach for treatment of barrier defects in patients with IBD will include the use of inhibitors for the Rho/ROCK signaling pathway.

CONCLUSION

Recent analyses of IBD tissues, mouse models of IBD, and *in vitro* cell culture studies have provided new insights into mechanisms of epithelial barrier disruption in IBD. From these studies, it is clear that the disassembly of AJC is triggered by inflammatory stimuli and selective TJ proteins are endocytosed at aberrant rates, thereby influencing AJC structure and permeability across the epithelium. Given the central role of AJC in regulating epithelial barrier function it is important in further understanding the intracellular and cell surface dynamics of AJC proteins and their modulation by pathologic stimuli. Such studies will facilitate development of therapeutic strategies to inhibit barrier defects observed in IBD.

ACKNOWLEDGMENTS

Studies from the authors' laboratories were funded by an NIH grant (DK59888) and the German Research Foundation (DFG) Br 2093/4-1.

REFERENCES

1. KATZ, K.D. *et al.* 1989. Intestinal permeability in patients with Crohn's disease and their healthy relatives. Gastroenterology **97:** 927–931.
2. TEAHON, K. *et al.* 1992. Intestinal permeability in patients with Crohn's disease and their first degree relatives. Gut **33:** 320–323.

3. HOLLANDER, D. 1993. Permeability in Crohn's disease: altered barrier functions in healthy relatives? Gastroenterology **104**: 1848–1851.
4. MAY, G.R., L.R. SUTHERLAND & J.B. MEDDINGS. 1993. Is small intestinal permeability really increased in relatives of patients with Crohn's disease? Gastroenterology **104**: 1627–1632.
5. YACYSHYN, B.R. & J.B. MEDDINGS. 1995. CD45RO expression on circulating CD19+ B cells in Crohn's disease correlates with intestinal permeability. Gastroenterology **108**: 132–137.
6. PEETERS, M. *et al.* 1997. Clustering of increased small intestinal permeability in families with Crohn's disease. Gastroenterology **113**: 802–807.
7. SODERHOLM, J.D. *et al.* 1999. Different intestinal permeability patterns in relatives and spouses of patients with Crohn's disease: an inherited defect in mucosal defence? Gut **44**: 96–100.
8. WYATT, J. *et al.* 1993. Intestinal permeability and the prediction of relapse in Crohn's disease. Lancet **341**: 1437–1439.
9. PEETERS, M. *et al.* 1994. Increased permeability of macroscopically normal small bowel in Crohn's disease. Dig. Dis. Sci. **39**: 2170–2176.
10. MARIN, M.L. *et al.* 1983. A freeze fracture study of Crohn's disease of the terminal ileum: changes in epithelial tight junction organization. Am. J. Gastroenterol. **78**: 537–547.
11. DeMEO, M.T. *et al.* 2002. Intestinal permeation and gastrointestinal disease. J. Clin. Gastroenterol. **34**: 385–396.
12. PODOLSKY, D.K. 2002. Inflammatory bowel disease. N. Engl. J. Med. **347**: 417–429.
13. IRVINE, E.J. & J.K. MARSHALL. 2000. Increased intestinal permeability precedes the onset of Crohn's disease in a subject with familial risk. Gastroenterology **119**: 1740–1744.
14. HUGOT, J.P. *et al.* 2001. Association of NOD2 leucine-rich repeat variants with susceptibility to Crohn's disease. Nature **411**: 599–603.
15. BRANT, S.R. *et al.* 2003. MDR1 Ala893 polymorphism is associated with inflammatory bowel disease. Am. J. Hum. Genet. **73**: 1282–1292.
16. OGURA, Y. *et al.* 2001. A frameshift mutation in NOD2 associated with susceptibility to Crohn's disease. Nature **411**: 603–606.
17. BUHNER, S. *et al.* 2006. Genetic basis for increased intestinal permeability in families with Crohn's disease: role of CARD15 3020insC mutation? Gut **55**: 342–347.
18. BRESLIN, N.P. *et al.* 2001. Intestinal permeability is increased in a proportion of spouses of patients with Crohn's disease. Am. J. Gastroenterol. **96**: 2934–2938.
19. FIOCCHI, C. 1998. Inflammatory bowel disease: etiology and pathogenesis. Gastroenterology **115**: 182–205.
20. TSUKITA, S., M. FURUSE & M. ITOH. 2001. Multifunctional strands in tight junctions. Nat. Rev. Mol. Cell. Biol. **2**: 285–293.
21. MADARA, J.L. 1998. Regulation of the movement of solutes across tight junctions. Annu. Rev. Physiol. **60**: 143–159.
22. CLAYBURGH, D.R., L. SHEN & J.R. TURNER. 2004. A porous defense: the leaky epithelial barrier in intestinal disease. Lab. Invest. **84**: 282–291.
23. YAP, A.S., W.M. BRIEHER & B.M. GUMBINER. 1997. Molecular and functional analysis of cadherin-based adherens junctions. Annu. Rev. Cell. Dev. Biol. **13**: 119–146.

24. FANNING, A.S. *et al.* 1998. The tight junction protein ZO-1 establishes a link between the transmembrane protein occludin and the actin cytoskeleton. J. Biol. Chem. **273:** 29745–29753.
25. CORDENONSI, M. *et al.* 1999. Cingulin contains globular and coiled-coil domains and interacts with ZO-1, ZO-2, ZO-3, and myosin. J. Cell. Biol. **147:** 1569–1582.
26. HASKINS, J. *et al.* 1998. ZO-3, a novel member of the MAGUK protein family found at the tight junction, interacts with ZO-1 and occludin. J. Cell. Biol. **141:** 199–208.
27. MA, T.Y. *et al.* 2000. Cytochalasin B modulation of Caco-2 tight junction barrier: role of myosin light chain kinase. Am. J. Physiol. Gastrointest. Liver Physiol. **279:** G875–G885.
28. TURNER, J.R. 2000. "Putting the squeeze" on the tight junction: understanding cytoskeletal regulation. Semin. Cell. Dev. Biol. **11:** 301–308.
29. TIBBLE, J.A. & I. BJARNASON. 2001. Non-invasive investigation of inflammatory bowel disease. World J. Gastroenterol. **7:** 460–465.
30. MEDDINGS, J.B. 1997. Review article: intestinal permeability in Crohn's disease. Aliment. Pharmacol. Ther. **11(Suppl 3):** 47–53; discussion 53–56.
31. HERMISTON, M.L. & J.I. GORDON. 1995. Inflammatory bowel disease and adenomas in mice expressing a dominant negative N-cadherin. Science **270:** 1203–1207.
32. HERMISTON, M.L. & J.I. GORDON. 1995. In vivo analysis of cadherin function in the mouse intestinal epithelium: essential roles in adhesion, maintenance of differentiation, and regulation of programmed cell death. J. Cell. Biol. **129:** 489–506.
33. PANWALA, C.M., J.C. JONES & J.L. VINEY. 1998. A novel model of inflammatory bowel disease: mice deficient for the multiple drug resistance gene, mdr1a, spontaneously develop colitis. J. Immunol. **161:** 5733–5744.
34. SCHMITZ, H. *et al.* 1999. Altered tight junction structure contributes to the impaired epithelial barrier function in ulcerative colitis. Gastroenterology **116:** 301–309.
35. KARAYIANNAKIS, A.J. *et al.* 1998. Expression of catenins and E-cadherin during epithelial restitution in inflammatory bowel disease. J. Pathol. **185:** 413–418.
36. DOGAN, A., Z.D. WANG & J. SPENCER. 1995. E-cadherin expression in intestinal epithelium. J. Clin. Pathol. **48:** 143–146.
37. JANKOWSKI, J.A. *et al.* 1998. Alterations in classical cadherins associated with progression in ulcerative and Crohn's colitis. Lab. Invest. **78:** 1155–1167.
38. GASSLER, N. *et al.* 2001. Inflammatory bowel disease is associated with changes of enterocytic junctions. Am. J. Physiol. Gastrointest. Liver Physiol. **281:** G216–G228.
39. KUCHARZIK, T. *et al.* 2001. Neutrophil transmigration in inflammatory bowel disease is associated with differential expression of epithelial intercellular junction proteins. Am. J. Pathol. **159:** 2001–2009.
40. MARIN, M.L. *et al.* 1983. Ultrastructural pathology of Crohn's disease: correlated transmission electron microscopy, scanning electron microscopy, and freeze fracture studies. Am. J. Gastroenterol. **78:** 355–364.
41. D'INCA, R. *et al.* 1995. Functional and morphological changes in small bowel of Crohn's disease patients: influence of site of disease. Dig. Dis. Sci. **40:** 1388–1393.
42. GITTER, A.H. *et al.* 2001. Epithelial barrier defects in ulcerative colitis: characterization and quantification by electrophysiological imaging. Gastroenterology **121:** 1320–1328.

43. SCHULZKE, J.D. *et al.* 2005. Epithelial transport and barrier function in occludin-deficient mice. Biochim. Biophys. Acta **1669:** 34–42.

44. KENNEDY, R.J. *et al.* 2000. Interleukin 10-deficient colitis: new similarities to human inflammatory bowel disease. Br. J. Surg. **87:** 1346–1351.

45. JIJON, H.B. *et al.* 2000. Inhibition of poly(ADP-ribose) polymerase attenuates inflammation in a model of chronic colitis. Am. J. Physiol. Gastrointest. Liver Physiol. **279:** G641–G651.

46. PARK, J.H. *et al.* 2002. Polynitroxylated starch/TPL attenuates cachexia and increased epithelial permeability associated with TNBS colitis. Inflammation **26:** 1–11.

47. VENKATRAMAN, A. *et al.* 2003. Amelioration of dextran sulfate colitis by butyrate: role of heat shock protein 70 and NF-kappaB. Am. J. Physiol. Gastrointest. Liver Physiol. **285:** G177–G184.

48. RESTA-LENERT, S., J. SMITHAM & K.E. BARRETT. 2005. Epithelial dysfunction associated with the development of colitis in conventionally housed mdr1a$^{-/-}$ mice. Am. J. Physiol. Gastrointest. Liver Physiol. **289:** G153–G162.

49. STALLMACH, A., T. GIESE & C. SCHMIDT. 2004. Cytokine/chemokine transcript profiles reflect mucosal inflammation in Crohn's disease. Int. J. Colorectal Dis. **19:** 308–315.

50. NIESSNER, M. & B.A. VOLK. 1995. Phenotypic and immunoregulatory analysis of intestinal T-cells in patients with inflammatory bowel disease: evaluation of an in vitro model. Eur. J. Clin. Invest. **25:** 155–164.

51. NIESSNER, M. & B.A. VOLK. 1995. Altered Th1/Th2 cytokine profiles in the intestinal mucosa of patients with inflammatory bowel disease as assessed by quantitative reversed transcribed polymerase chain reaction (RT-PCR). Clin. Exp. Immunol. **101:** 428–435.

52. MADARA, J.L. & J. STAFFORD. 1989. Interferon-gamma directly affects barrier function of cultured intestinal epithelial monolayers. J. Clin. Invest. **83:** 724–727.

53. YOUAKIM, A. & M. AHDIEH. 1999. Interferon-gamma decreases barrier function in T84 cells by reducing ZO-1 levels and disrupting apical actin. Am. J. Physiol. **276:** G1279–G1288.

54. SCHMITZ, H. *et al.* 1999. Tumor necrosis factor-alpha (TNFalpha) regulates the epithelial barrier in the human intestinal cell line HT-29/B6. J. Cell. Sci. **112 (Pt 1):** 137–146.

55. MARANO, C.W. *et al.* 1998. Tumor necrosis factor-alpha increases sodium and chloride conductance across the tight junction of CACO-2 BBE, a human intestinal epithelial cell line. J. Membr. Biol. **161:** 263–274.

56. BRUEWER, M. *et al.* 2003. Proinflammatory cytokines disrupt epithelial barrier function by apoptosis-independent mechanisms. J. Immunol. **171:** 6164–6172.

57. MANKERTZ, J. *et al.* 2000. Expression from the human occludin promoter is affected by tumor necrosis factor alpha and interferon gamma. J. Cell. Sci. **113 (Pt 11):** 2085–2090.

58. GITTER, A.H. *et al.* 2000. Epithelial barrier defects in HT-29/B6 colonic cell monolayers induced by tumor necrosis factor-alpha. Ann. N. Y. Acad. Sci. **915:** 193–203.

59. IVANOV, A.I., A. NUSRAT & C.A. PARKOS. 2004. The epithelium in inflammatory bowel disease: potential role of endocytosis of junctional proteins in barrier disruption. Novartis Found. Symp. **263:** 115–124; discussion 124–132, 211–218.

60. MUKHERJEE, S., R.N. GHOSH & F.R. MAXFIELD. 1997. Endocytosis Physiol. Rev. 77: 759–803.
61. IVANOV, A.I., A. NUSRAT & C.A. PARKOS. 2004. Endocytosis of epithelial apical junctional proteins by a clathrin-mediated pathway into a unique storage compartment. Mol. Biol. Cell. 15: 176–188.
62. HOPKINS, A.M. et al. 2003. Constitutive activation of Rho proteins by CNF-1 influences tight junction structure and epithelial barrier function. J. Cell. Sci. 116: 725–742.
63. NUSRAT, A. et al. 2001. Clostridium difficile toxins disrupt epithelial barrier function by altering membrane microdomain localization of tight junction proteins. Infect. Immun. 69: 1329–1336.
64. BRUEWER, M. et al. 2005. Interferon-gamma induces internalization of epithelial tight junction proteins via a macropinocytosis-like process. FASEB J. 19: 923–933.
65. UTECH, M. et al. 2005. Mechanism of IFN-γ induced endocytosis of tight junction proteins: myosin II-dependent vacuolarization of the apical plasma membrane. Mol. Biol. Cell.
66. BRESNICK, A.R. 1999. Molecular mechanisms of nonmuscle myosin-II regulation. Curr. Opin. Cell. Biol. 11: 26–33.
67. TAN, J.L., S. RAVID & J.A. SPUDICH. 1992. Control of nonmuscle myosins by phosphorylation. Annu. Rev. Biochem. 61: 721–759.
68. AMANO, M. et al. 1996. Phosphorylation and activation of myosin by Rho-associated kinase (Rho-kinase). J. Biol. Chem. 271: 20246–20249.
69. ADELSTEIN, R.S. 1982. Calmodulin and the regulation of the actin-myosin interaction in smooth muscle and nonmuscle cells. Cell 30: 349–350.
70. ZOLOTAREVSKY, Y. et al. 2002. A membrane-permeant peptide that inhibits MLC kinase restores barrier function in in vitro models of intestinal disease. Gastroenterology 123: 163–172.
71. SEGAIN, J.P. et al. 2003. Rho kinase blockade prevents inflammation via nuclear factor kappa B inhibition: evidence in Crohn's disease and experimental colitis. Gastroenterology 124: 1180–1187.

Antibody-Mediated Antigen Sampling across Intestinal Epithelial Barriers

M. CECILIA BERIN,[a] HONGXING LI,[b] AND KIRK SPERBER[b]

[a]Department of Pediatrics, Jaffe Food Allergy Institute, Mount Sinai School of Medicine, New York, New York, USA

[b]Department of Clinical Immunology and Immunobiology, Mount Sinai School of Medicine, New York, New York, USA

ABSTRACT: The epithelium of the gastrointestinal tract is the interface between luminal contents and the mucosal immune system. It must function as a selective barrier to limit penetration of antigens yet keep the mucosal immune system "informed" for the purpose of generating oral tolerance responses to food antigens or commensal organisms and host defense responses against pathogens. Alterations in epithelial barrier function have been proposed to play a significant role in gastrointestinal disease. In this review, we will discuss mechanisms of regulation of epithelial barrier function, and we will focus on the emerging understanding of how secreted immunoglobulins play a role in antigen-specific antigen sampling across the gastrointestinal epithelium.

KEYWORDS: antigen uptake; transcytosis; IgE; CD23

INTRODUCTION

A single layer of columnar epithelial cells comprises the interface between the external environment and the mucosal immune system. On the luminal side is found an abundance of antigenic dietary proteins, bacterial products, and commensal and occasionally pathogenic micro-organisms. On the mucosal side an array of resident immune cells including macrophages, dendritic cells, and B and T lymphocytes stand at the ready to defend the body against pathogenic micro-organisms, yet remain tolerant to the constant luminal presence of commensal micro-organisms. The epithelium has been shown to be

Address for correspondence: Cecilia Berin, Ph.D., Pediatric Allergy and Immunology, Box 1198, Mount Sinai School of Medicine, One Gustave L. Levy Place, New York, NY 10029, USA. Voice: 1-212-241-4986; fax: 1-212-426-1902.

e-mail: cecilia.berin@mssm.edu

Ann. N.Y. Acad. Sci. 1072: 253–261 (2006). © 2006 New York Academy of Sciences.

doi: 10.1196/annals.1326.002

a critical mediator of communication between the lumen and the mucosal immune system via the release of cytokines and chemokines that signal the presence of pathogens.[1] Another critical line of communication facilitated by the epithelium is the bidirectional transport of immunoglobulins that not only can neutralize antigens or pathogens in the lumen, but also provides information on the contents of the lumen to the mucosal immune system. This concept expands our current understanding of how the intestinal epithelium can function as a selective barrier that can be regulated during inflammatory conditions.

REGULATION OF EPITHELIAL BARRIER FUNCTION

Epithelial cells lining the gastrointestinal tract are held together at the apical pole by tight junctions that form intimate contacts to restrict the passive flow of molecules between cells. The tight junction is a major site of regulation of epithelial barrier function and, although under normal conditions they exclude the passage of macromolecules, under proinflammatory conditions the tight junctions can open to the extent that macromolecules can pass intact along this paracellular pathway. Studies on intestinal epithelial cell monolayers *in vitro* have shown that proinflammatory stimuli (IFN-γ, TNF-α, pathogenic bacteria) can induce an increase in epithelial permeability by regulation of the tight junction.[2,3] This increased permeability to macromolecules has also been documented in human inflammatory bowel disease.[4,5]

Although macromolecules such as protein antigens are normally restricted from traveling across tight junctions between cells, small amounts of intact protein antigen gain access to the systemic circulation after a meal. Transport of macromolecules in the normal epithelium has been shown to occur by the endocytic route, with a small amount of antigen taken up by fluid-phase endocytosis and delivered intact below the tight junction into the paracellular space.[6–8] Recent publications have made it increasingly clear that this pathway is also subject to regulation. Cytokines such as IL-4, TNF-α, and IFN-γ, which have been shown to regulate tight junction permeability, have also been shown to upregulate transcellular transport of macromolecules.[9–11] Transcellular transport of macromolecules is also elevated across epithelial cells in biopsies from patients with Crohn's disease, and this was observed to correlate with expression levels of the proinflammatory cytokine TNF-α.[10] Transepithelial transport of a nonpathogenic *Escherichia coli* (*E. coli*) strain across intestinal epithelial cell monolayers is also regulated by IFN-γ at doses not affecting the tight junctions, and via a lipid-raft-mediated transcellular uptake mechanism.[12] These studies highlight the concept that regulation of epithelial barrier function by proinflammatory factors can occur by parallel mechanisms, affecting both tight junctions and transcellular pathways.

EFFECT OF IMMUNIZATION ON EPITHELIAL BARRIER FUNCTION

There are differing reports on the impact of prior immunization on the uptake of antigens from the gastrointestinal lumen. Walker and colleagues have shown that oral or parenteral immunization leads to suppressed uptake of the immunizing antigen across the intestinal epithelium of rats.[13,14] This suppression was shown to be due to the formation of IgG–antigen complexes in the lumen that were taken up at a decreased rate compared to antigen alone.[15] Bockman and Cooper obtained different results and demonstrated that hamsters sensitized to ferritin had enhanced uptake of ferritin in intestinal epithelial cells.[16] These differing results could potentially be due to strain differences (perhaps including differences in IgG receptor expression) or due to differences in the techniques used to assess macromolecular uptake.

Studies in rodent models of food allergy support the hypothesis that prior immunization can enhance transcellular uptake of the sensitizing antigen. Small intestinal segments taken from rodents sensitized to an antigen by intraperitoneal injection with alum respond to administration of antigen on the luminal side with a rapid hypersensitivity response characterized by the induction of active chloride secretion, a driving force for diarrhea. Electron microscopy was used to track antigen uptake at various time points after addition to the luminal surface, showing that there are two distinct phases of antigen uptake in sensitized rats.[17] Very rapidly (2–3 min) after addition of antigen to the luminal surface, the antigen could be observed in vesicles throughout the epithelial cell and in the lamina propria. In contrast, when antigen was applied to the lumen of intestine from an unsensitized rat a slow transcytotic process was observed, leading to delivery of antigen to the lamina propria within 20–30 min. A greater amount of antigen was taken up into the epithelial cells in sensitized rats compared to unsensitized rats. This was found to be specific for the sensitizing antigen. After the initial rapid transcytotic event in sensitized animals, there was antigen-specific activation of subepithelial mast cells by cross-linking surface IgE, an event known to drive the allergen-induced secretory events in the intestine. Subsequent to mast cell activation, a slow opening of the tight junctions was observed, leading to nonspecific passage of macromolecules from the luminal to the serosal side of the epithelium.[17] The initial rapid transcytotic event was mast cell–independent, but the prolonged paracellular barrier defect [18] and subsequent late-phase inflammation [19] was mast cell–dependent. These studies highlight how regulation of both transcellular and paracellular epithelial barrier function can contribute to intestinal pathophysiology.

The initial phase of antigen uptake in sensitized rats was antigen-specific, such that enhanced uptake of the sensitizing antigen, but not a bystander antigen, was observed.[17] This antigen specificity suggested the involvement of a receptor-mediated uptake system. It had previously been reported that the low-affinity IgE receptor CD23 is expressed on human intestinal epithelial cells, and is upregulated in cow milk–induced enteropathy.[20] Subsequent studies in animal models showed that CD23 expression on intestinal epithelial cells was increased by sensitization, and that IgE and CD23 were involved in the enhanced antigen uptake and subsequent local hypersensitivity reactions in the intestinal mucosa.[21,22] This brings up an additional level of regulation of epithelial barrier function by antigen-specific sampling of luminal contents by mucosal immunoglobulins.

ANTIBODY-MEDIATED ANTIGEN SAMPLING ACROSS INTESTINAL EPITHELIAL BARRIERS

The best-studied system of immunoglobulin–epithelial interaction is the secretion of dimeric IgA by the polymeric immunoglobulin receptor (pIgR). This is a unidirectional transport system that delivers IgA to the lumen. IgA is not only active in the lumen, but can also neutralize intracellular viruses [23] and lipopolysaccharide (LPS) [24] on its way through the epithelial cell. The function of IgA as a major secretory immunoglobulin suggests that the general function of secreted antibodies is to prevent penetration of luminal antigens into the mucosa. A series of studies on the neonatal Fc receptor (FcRn) and its role in IgG transport has identified an additional function for secreted immunoglobulins.

FcRn and Antigen Sampling

FcRn was first described as a transporter of maternal immunoglobulins from the lumen of suckling rats.[25,26] FcRn is dramatically downregulated in rodent intestinal epithelial cells at the time of weaning, and was therefore assumed to be of relevance only during the neonatal period. FcRn is also expressed on human fetal intestine, yet the intestine is not a major site of transfer of passive immunity in humans. Further studies demonstrated that FcRn was expressed on human intestinal epithelial cells, as well as other cells in the gastrointestinal tract, into adulthood.[27] The known function of FcRn in transporting IgG from the lumen suggested that FcRn could potentially play a role in immune surveillance by capturing antibody and antigen from the lumen. Dickinson et al. showed that T84 human colonic epithelial cells expressed FcRn constitutively, and that this receptor could act as a bidirectional transporter of IgG.[28] Conclusive evidence that FcRn could contribute to antigen sampling and immune surveillance across the epithelial barrier was provided by Yoshida et al.[29] who showed that polarized cells transfected with human (h)FcRn could transcytose antigen in an IgG-dependent manner. In addition, transgenic mice expressing hFcRn and β2microglobulin could sample antigen from the intestinal lumen in an IgG-dependent manner and then deliver this antigen to

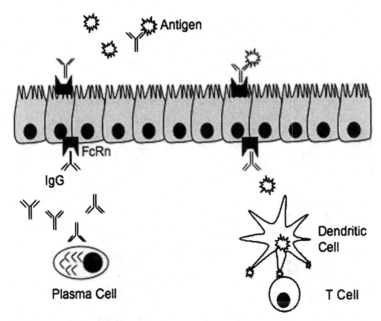

FIGURE 1. Antigen sampling by IgG/FcRn in mucosal immunity. IgG produced by mucosal plasma cells or in the lamina propria environment can be bound and transported to the intestinal lumen by FcRn. Once in the lumen, IgG can capture antigen and be transported in the apical to basal direction across intestinal epithelial cells by FcRn. One fate of antigen transported by IgG/FcRn is internalization by dendritic cells and migration to sites of presentation, that is, the mesenteric lymph node. Dendritic cells can present the captured antigen to T cells, resulting in an adaptive immune response. The figure summarizes data from Yoshida *et al.*[29]

lamina propria dendritic cells. This process was then shown to result in activation of antigen-specific T cells.[29] These studies show that the production of antigen-specific IgG within the gastrointestinal mucosa can be an initial step in allowing specific antigens enhanced access to the lamina propria via a FcRn-dependent transport pathway. FIGURE 1 summarizes this newly identified antigen-sampling pathway.

CD23 (FcεRII) and Antigen Sampling

Initial studies in rodent models of food allergy demonstrated that CD23 and IgE were necessary for enhanced antigen uptake by epithelial cells in sensitized rats and mice.[21,22] CD23 is a C-type lectin that is constitutively expressed on B cells, and is upregulated on a wider range of cells (monocytes, macrophages, keratinocytes) in response to stimulation with IL-4.[30] Two isoforms of CD23 have been described: the CD23a splice variant is expressed constitutively in B cells and the CD23b splice variant is upregulated in B cells and other cells.[30]

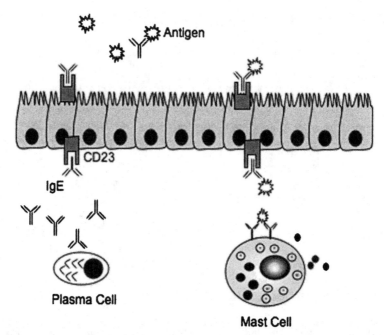

FIGURE 2. Antigen sampling by IgE/CD23 in allergic disease. IgE produced locally in the intestinal mucosa (e.g., in food-allergic individuals or in response to parasitic infection) is captured by CD23 and exported to the luminal aspect of the epithelial layer. IgE/antigen complexes formed in the lumen are retransported to the lamina propria, where the antigen complex can trigger mast cell activation and degranulation, and therefore initiate a local hypersensitivity reaction.

CD23a and CD23b have been shown to be functionally different, with only CD23a reported to be capable of facilitating endocytic uptake of IgE in humans,[31] although CD23b splice variants have been shown to endocytose IgE in a murine intestinal epithelial system.[32,33] Administration of antigen in the presence of antigen-specific IgE can enhance T cell and B cell responses to that antigen in a CD23- and B cell-dependent manner, presumably through IgE-mediated enhanced uptake and presentation of antigen by B cells bearing CD23.[34]

Recent studies are providing evidence that CD23, like FcRn, can function as an antigen-sampling mechanism across human epithelium when IgE is present on the apical side of the epithelium. Human CD23 transfected into HeLa cells undergoes constitutive endocytosis.[35] In addition, T84 human intestinal epithelial cells that constitutively express CD23 transcytose IgE in a bidirectional manner.[36] This transcytosis is inhibited when CD23 is suppressed by antisense oligonucleotides.[36] In recent experiments, we overexpressed CD23 in T84 cells by retroviral transfection and observed not only an increase in bidirectional transcytosis of IgE, but also a preferential apical-to-basal transport of antigen-IgE complexes[37] Antigen-IgE complexes captured from the luminal face of the epithelium were subsequently shown to degranulate mast cells. In order for CD23 to facilitate the uptake of antigen from the intestinal lumen, IgE must be present in the intestinal lumen. Although IgE is not classically considered to be a secretory immunoglobulin, transport of IgE into the intestinal lumen can reach high levels under conditions such as parasitic infection.[38] It has also been reported that IgE can be measured in intestinal lavage fluids of patients with food allergy.[39] We examined stool samples from patients undergoing graded oral food challenges, and detected allergen-specific IgE in stool samples from 6 of 10 food-allergic patients with IgE-mediated food allergies.[32] Therefore the presence of IgE in the lumen combined with constitutive expression of CD23 on the intestinal epithelium provides the components for an antigen-specific sampling mechanism across the intestinal epithelial barrier in allergic disease. FIGURE 2 illustrates the mechanism of CD23-mediated antigen sampling across the intestinal epithelial barrier. Although we have shown that one consequence of CD23-mediated IgE-antigen complex sampling is the degranulation of mast cells, the potential role of this trafficking pathway in the delivery of antigen to lamina propria antigen-presenting cells remains to be explored.

It has been recognized for many years that epithelial barrier function (as considered to be regulation at the level of the tight junction) can be regulated during inflammatory conditions. Recent findings that transcellular antigen transport pathways can also be regulated by inflammatory mediators, and that uptake can be antigen-selective on account of the contribution of secreted immunoglobulins extends not only our current concept of epithelial barrier function, but also the potential function of secreted immunoglobulins in health and disease.

REFERENCES

1. CARIO, E. 2005. Bacterial interactions with cells of the intestinal mucosa: toll-like receptors and NOD2. Gut **54:** 1182–1193.
2. BERKES, J. *et al.* 2003. Intestinal epithelial responses to enteric pathogens: effects on the tight junction barrier, ion transport, and inflammation. Gut **52:** 439–451.
3. NUSRAT, A., J.R. TURNER & J.L. MADARA. 2000. Molecular physiology and pathophysiology of tight junctions. IV. Regulation of tight junctions by extracellular stimuli: nutrients, cytokines, and immune cells. Am. J. Physiol. Gastrointest. Liver Physiol. **279:** G851–G857.
4. GITTER, A.H. *et al.* 2001. Epithelial barrier defects in ulcerative colitis: characterization and quantification by electrophysiological imaging. Gastroenterology **121:** 1320–1328.
5. SODERHOLM, J.D. *et al.* 2002. Augmented increase in tight junction permeability by luminal stimuli in the non-inflamed ileum of Crohn's disease. Gut **50:** 307–313.
6. CORNELL, R., W.A. WALKER & K.J. ISSELBACHER. 1971. Small intestinal absorption of horseradish peroxidase: a cytochemical study. Lab. Invest. **25:** 42–48.

7. WALKER, W.A. *et al.* 1972. Macromolecular absorption: mechanism of horseradish peroxidase uptake and transport in adult and neonatal rat intestine. J. Cell. Biol. **54:** 195–205.

8. WARSHAW, A.L. *et al.* 1971. Small intestinal permeability to macromolecules: transmission of horseradish peroxidase into mesenteric lymph and portal blood. Lab. Invest. **25:** 675–684.

9. BERIN, M.C. *et al.* 1999. Role for IL-4 in macromolecular transport across human intestinal epithelium. Am. J. Physiol. **276:** C1046–C1052.

10. SODERHOLM, J.D. *et al.* 2004. Increased epithelial uptake of protein antigens in the ileum of Crohn's disease mediated by tumour necrosis factor alpha. Gut **53:** 1817–1824.

11. TERPEND, K. *et al.* 1998. Protein transport and processing by human HT29-19A intestinal cells: effect of interferon gamma. Gut **42:** 538–545.

12. CLARK, E. *et al.* 2005. Interferon gamma induces translocation of commensal *Escherichia coli* across gut epithelial cells via a lipid raft-mediated process. Gastroenterology **128:** 1258–1267.

13. WALKER, W.A. K.J. ISSELBACHER & K.J. BLOCH. 1972. Intestinal uptake of macromolecules: effect of oral immunization. Science **177:** 608–610.

14. WALKER, W.A. K.J. ISSELBACHER & K.J. BLOCH. 1973. Intestinal uptake of macromolecules. II. Effect of parenteral immunization. J. Immunol. **111:** 221–226.

15. WALKER, W.A. *et al.* 1975. Intestinal uptake of macromolecules. III. Studies on the mechanism by which immunization interferes with antigen uptake. J. Immunol. **115:** 854–861.

16. BOCKMAN, D.E. & M.D. COOPER. 1973. Pinocytosis by epithelium associated with lymphoid follicles in the bursa of Fabricius, appendix, and Peyer's patches: an electron microscopic study. Am. J. Anat. **136:** 455–477.

17. BERIN, M.C. *et al.* 1997. Rapid transepithelial antigen transport in rat jejunum: impact of sensitization and the hypersensitivity reaction. Gastroenterology **113:** 856–864.

18. BERIN, M.C. *et al.* 1998. The influence of mast cells on pathways of transepithelial antigen transport in rat intestine. J. Immunol. **161:** 2561–2566.

19. YANG, P.C. *et al.* 2001. Mucosal pathophysiology and inflammatory changes in the late phase of the intestinal allergic reaction in the rat. Am. J. Pathol. **158:** 681–690.

20. KAISERLIAN, D. *et al.* 1993. Intestinal epithelial cells express the CD23/Fc epsilon RII molecule: enhanced expression in enteropathies. Immunology **80:** 90–95.

21. YANG, P.C. *et al.* 2000. Enhanced intestinal transepithelial antigen transport in allergic rats is mediated by IgE and CD23 (FcepsilonRII). J. Clin. Invest. **106:** 879–886.

22. YU, L.C. *et al.* 2001. Enhanced transepithelial antigen transport in intestine of allergic mice is mediated by IgE/CD23 and regulated by interleukin-4. Gastroenterology **121:** 370–381.

23. LAMM, M.E. 1998. Current concepts in mucosal immunity. IV. How epithelial transport of IgA antibodies relates to host defense. Am. J. Physiol. **274:** G614–G617.

24. FERNANDEZ, M.I. *et al.* 2003. Anti-inflammatory role for intracellular dimeric immunoglobulin A by neutralization of lipopolysaccharide in epithelial cells. Immunity **18:** 739–749.

25. BRAMBELL, F.W. 1966. The transmission of immunity from mother to young and the catabolism of immunoglobulins. Lancet **2:** 1087–1093.

26. JONES, E.A. & T.A. WALDMANN. 1971. The mechanism of intestinal uptake and transcellular transport of IgG in the neonatal rat. Gut **12:** 855–856.
27. ISRAEL, E.J. *et al.* 1997. Expression of the neonatal Fc receptor, FcRn, on human intestinal epithelial cells. Immunology **92:** 69–74.
28. DICKINSON, B.L. *et al.* 1999. Bidirectional FcRn-dependent IgG transport in a polarized human intestinal epithelial cell line. J. Clin. Invest. **104:** 903–911.
29. YOSHIDA, M. *et al.* 2004. Human neonatal Fc receptor mediates transport of IgG into luminal secretions for delivery of antigens to mucosal dendritic cells. Immunity **20:** 769–783.
30. YOKOTA, A. *et al.* 1988. Two species of human Fc epsilon receptor II (Fc epsilon RII/CD23): tissue-specific and IL-4-specific regulation of gene expression. Cell **55:** 611–618.
31. YOKOTA, A. *et al.* 1992. Two forms of the low-affinity Fc receptor for IgE differentially mediate endocytosis and phagocytosis: identification of the critical cytoplasmic domains. Proc. Natl. Acad. Sci. USA **89:** 5030–5034.
32. YU, L.C. *et al.* 2003. Intestinal epithelial CD23 mediates enhanced antigen transport in allergy: evidence for novel splice forms. Am. J. Physiol. Gastrointest. Liver Physiol. **285:** G223–G234.
33. MONTAGNAC, G. *et al.* 2005. Differential role for CD23 splice forms in apical to basolateral transcytosis of IgE/allergen complexes. Traffic **6:** 230–242.
34. GETAHUN, A., F. HJELM & B. HEYMAN. 2005. IgE enhances antibody and T cell responses *in vivo* via CD23+ B cells. J. Immunol. **175:** 1473–1482.
35. MONTAGNAC, G. *et al.* 2005. Intracellular trafficking of CD23: differential regulation in humans and mice by both extracellular and intracellular exons. J. Immunol. **174:** 5562–5572.
36. TU, Y. *et al.* 2005. CD23-mediated IgE transport across human intestinal epithelium: inhibition by blocking sites of translation or binding. Gastroenterology **129:** 928–940.
37. LI X.M. *et al.* 2006. Transcytosis of IgE-antigen complexes by CD23a in human intestinal epithelial cells and its role in food allergy. Gastroenterology doi: 10.1053/J. gastro.#2006.03.044.
38. NEGRAO-CORREA, D., L.S. ADAMS & R.G. BELL. 1996. Intestinal transport and catabolism of IgE: a major blood-independent pathway of IgE dissemination during a *Trichinella spiralis* infection of rats. J. Immunol. **157:** 4037–4044.
39. BELUT, D. *et al.* 1980. IgE levels in intestinal juice. Dig. Dis. Sci. **25:** 323–332.

Molecular Mechanisms of Disturbed Electrolyte Transport in Intestinal Inflammation

URSULA SEIDLER,[a] HENRIKE LENZEN,[a] AYHAN CINAR,[a] TESFAYE TESSEMA,[a] ANDRÉ BLEICH,[b] AND BRIGITTE RIEDERER[a]

[a]Department of Gastroenterology, Hepatology, and Endocrinology, Hannover Medical School, Germany

[b]Institute of Animal Research, Hannover Medical School, Germany

ABSTRACT: Diarrhea is the hallmark of both ulcerative colitis (UC) and Crohn's disease. Loss of resorptive area, destruction of epithelial cells, leaky tight junctions, and release of inflammatory mediators and products from immune cells that stimulate fluid secretion all have been implicated in the pathogenesis of inflammatory diarrhea. Very early studies in patients, however, have pinpointed the overwhelming transport abnormality in inflamed intestinal mucosa: a virtually complete loss of sodium resorptive capacity. Recently, tools have become available to study the molecular basis of disturbances in the major electrolyte transport systems during intestinal inflammation. This review gives a brief overview of the historical development of research related to electrolyte transport in inflammatory bowel disorders, focusing on the studies performed in humans, and highlights recent understanding of the molecular mechanisms that may help explain the origin of diarrhea in intestinal inflammation.

KEYWORDS: ion transport; sodium absorption; anion secretion; Na^+/H^+ exchange; intestine; inflammation; NHE3; CFTR; pd3 proteins

EARLY STUDIES IN INTESTINAL ION TRANSPORT PROPERTIES IN PATIENTS

Diarrhea occurs in 50% of acute flare-ups of Crohns disease and virtually 100% in ulcerative colitis (UC), and is often the leading symptom causing distress to the patients. Therefore, clinician scientists applied methods that had been developed in animal research very early to the study of patients.

Hans Ussing developed an *in vitro* system in which the electrical behavior of an isolated mucosa during electrolyte transport could be studied—the

Address for correspondence: Ursula Seidler, Department of Gastroenterology, Hepatology, and Endocrinology, Hannover Medical School, Germany.
e-mail: seidler.ursula@mh-hannover.de

Ann. N.Y. Acad. Sci. 1072: 262–275 (2006). © 2006 New York Academy of Sciences.
doi: 10.1196/annals.1326.024

famous "Ussing chamber."[1] He found that frog skin *in vitro* generated a surface-negative potential difference (PD) due to the active absorption of Na^+ ions.[2,3] Transepithelial ion transport resulting in the generation of a PD is now called "electrogenic ion transport," and the current that is necessary to bring the PD continuosly to zero voltage is called "short circuit current" (Isc) and is a real-time measurement of net electrogenic transport across an epithelium.

Shortly afterwards, it was found that such a negative PD was also generated by the intestinal mucosa,[4,5] and devices were designed to measure the PD *in vivo* and in patients.[6] Edmonds *et al.* measured the rectal PD in UC patients sequentially and found that the rectal PD became positive during acute flare-ups, followed by recovery to negative values during the healing phase.[7] At the time, this was interpreted exclusively as a loss of active Na^+ resorption, because it was not widely recognized yet that the intestinal mucosa also secreted Cl^- in an electrogenic fashion.[8]

Similar experiments were repeated by others. Archampong *et al.*,[9] and later the group of Leslie Turnberg,[10] performed bilateral[22] Na^+ isotope flux studies in distal colonic mucosa (harvested during surgical resection in patients with UC and patients undergoing resection for other causes) in classical Ussing-chambers and noted a very strong reduction of sodium absorption, or even sodium "secretion," in untreated UC patients, whereas steroid-treated patients displayed a return to absorptive rates.

Allan *et al.* studied Na^+ absorption in proctocolectomized patients with either UC or Crohn's disease (CD) and a radiologically normal small bowel. They found that despite clinical and radiographic remission, Na^+ absorption was markedly diminished in the intestine of CD patients.[11] They interpreted this as an indication for CD being a generalized rather than a focal disease.

Sandle *et al.* studied the rectal PD in patients with active UC and healthy controls before and 5 h after a single i.v. dose of steroids.[12] They confirmed the strong reduction in PD in UC patients, but found that steroids increased the PD to the same degree in normal and UC patients. Obviously, enterocyte ion transport could be regulated despite severe inflammation.

EFFECT OF INFLAMMATORY MEDIATORS ON INTESTINAL ANION SECRETION

In the late '60s, investigators recognized that bacterial enterotoxins and other agents known for their diarrheal properties elicited an electrogenic Cl^- secretion in the isolated intestinal mucosa in Ussing chambers, and this could be measured by an increase in Isc.[13–16] In the '80s and '90s, scientific interest focused on the effects of inflammatory mediators on intestinal Cl^- secretion. A great number of inflammatory mediators were found to stimulate electrogenic Cl^- secretion when applied to isolated intestinal mucosa of various species in Ussing-chamber systems, or applied to intestinal cell lines which express apical

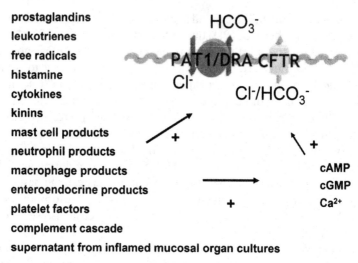

FIGURE 1. Many inflammatory mediators and products from cells involved in the inflammatory response have been found to elicit a Isc, indicative of electrogenic anion secretion, when applied to intestinal cell lines or intact intestinal epithelium from several species *in vitro*. PAT1: putative anion transport 1, also named SLC26A6; DRA: downregulated in adenoma, also named SLC26A3; CFTR: cystic fibrosis transmembrane regulator.

Cl^- channels, such as T84, HT29, or Caco-2 cells. Among those mediators were arachidonic acid metabolites,[17-19] cytokines,[20-23] tachykinins,[24] reactive oxygen metabolites,[25-27] as well as substances released from neutrophils,[28-30] macrophages,[31,32] mast cells,[33-35] and platelets[36,37] that were only partially characterized. In addition, the supernatant of inflamed human colonic mucosa in organ culture stimulated electrogenic Cl^- secretion when added to rat colonic mucosa in Ussing chambers.[37-39] Thus, is could be unequivocally demonstrated that a whole battery of substances released during intestinal inflammation elicited an anion secretory response in healthy intestinal mucosa. FIGURE 1 summarizes the findings. Some of the inflammatory mediators were found to elicit Cl^- secretion via activation of the classic second messenger systems cyclic adenosine 3′,5′-phosphate (cAMP), cyclic guanosine 5′-monophosphate (cGMP), or an elevation of intracellular Ca^{2+}, whereas the intracellular signal transduction pathway of others is still under debate.

INFLAMMATION RESULTS IN DISTURBANCES OF CL^- SECRETORY RESPONSE TO SECRETAGOGUES

Although such inflammatory secretagogues were being actively searched for, researchers noticed that the inflamed intestinal mucosa did not respond normally to stimulation. Hubel *et al.* reported that an increase in intracellular cAMP elicited a Cl^- secretory response in normal, but not in inflamed human

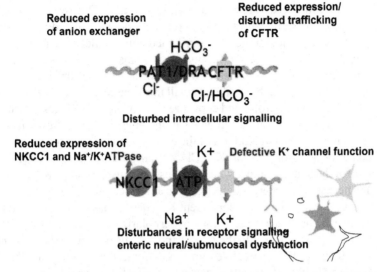

FIGURE 2. Potential molecular mechanisms for the hyporesponsiveness of inflamed intestinal mucosa to secretagogues of electrogenic anion secretion. The respective references are found in the text. NKCC1: $Na^+K^+2Cl^-$ Cotransporter Isoform 1.

jejunum.[40] Kachur *et al.* found that inflamed rat colonic tissue displayed a reduced response to a number of secretagogues whose effect was receptor-mediated, but not to theophyllin, which increases intracellular cAMP levels by phosphodiesterase inhibition.[41] They concluded that inflammation may result in an uncoupling of receptors to second-messenger systems or desensitization of receptor-linked secretory mechanisms. Another group also reported a reduction in Cl^- secretory responsiveness in experimentally inflamed rat colonic tissue and concluded that it reflected a defective cAMP production, possibly caused by disturbances within the enteric neural system.[42]

Studies of colonic mucosa from patients with UC confirmed the relative lack of electrogenic Cl^- secretion despite the obvious presence of high concentrations of inflammatory mediators whose secretory action in normal tissues was undisputed.[10,12,43] As the molecular transport mechanisms involved in electrogenic anion transport became evident, investigators searched for the reasons for this intrinsic unresponsiveness to secretory stimuli during inflammation.

FIGURE 2 summarizes the major transport pathways involved in electrogenic ion secretion, and the potential disturbances that were implicated in causing a reduced secretory responsiveness of inflamed mucosa. First, apical anion transporters could be downregulated or dysfunctional. Indeed, both a reduced,[44] an increased,[45] and no change in[42,46] expression of the cystic fibrosis transmembrane regulator (CFTR) anion channel has been described in enterocytes under the influence of inflammatory mediators or during intestinal inflammation. Recently, netric oxide (NO) release was reported to result in impaired trafficking of CFTR to the apical membrane.[47] One report described reduced expression of the apical anion exchanger downregulated in adenoma (DRA) in the apical membrane of the inflamed colon.[48] Second, downregulation or dysfunction of basolateral transport proteins could interfere with the uptake of anions destined for secretion or result in a lack of driving force. In an elegant study, in which human fetal small intestine was implanted into nude mice, it was shown that prolonged exposure to interferon-γ, a cytokine known to be present at high concentration levels in the mucosal tissue during inflammation, resulted in a dowregulation of the expression levels for the basolateral Cl^- uptake mechanism, the $Na^+K^+2Cl^-$ cotransporter isoform 1 (NKCC1), as well as for the sodium pump, which creates the transmembrane K^+ and Na^+ gradients necessary to energize electrogenic anion secretion.[46] Recently, a defect in the activation of a Ca^{2+}-dependent K^+ channel has been described that could reduce the basolateral membrane hyperpolarization and thus the driving force for apical Cl^- efflux. On the other hand, cAMP-dependent K^+ channels have been found to be hyperactive during inflammation, making the concept of defective K^+-channel activation controversial at the present time.[49]

A Spanish group of investigators performed elegant experiments in which they evoked inflammation of the distal colon in rats, and studied the proximal, noninflamed colon in Ussing chambers.[50] They found a decrease in the stimulatory effect of Ca^{2+}-dependent agonists, which was reverted by blockers of neural transmission. Direct activation of enterocyte cAMP-dependent signalling caused a normal secretory response. Thus, regional inflammation can result in widespread disturbance of intestinal secretory function.

Recently, the molecular mechanisms of reduced secretory function in intestinal tissue that had just recovered from a bout of experimental colitis was studied. Wallace and coworkers demonstrated that cyclooxygenase-2 expression was elevated as long as 6 weeks after induction of inflammation, and that this resulted in increased production of prostaglandin (PG) D2, an antiinflammatory prostaglandin that results in reduced epithelial responsiveness.[51] Similar mechanisms may well be operative in the chronic colitis of patients with inflammatory bowel disease.

In conclusion, experimental research in animal models as well as observations in clinical samples suggest that despite the ample presence of inflammatory mediators in inflamed intestinal tissues, multiple disturbances within the anion secretory pathways result in a diminished responsiveness to secretagogues.

CELLULAR BASIS FOR DEFECTIVE SODIUM ABSORPTION IN INFLAMED INTESTINE

As mentioned above, early studies had already uncovered the massive reduction in intestinal Na^+ absorption in inflamed colonic tissue from UC patients.

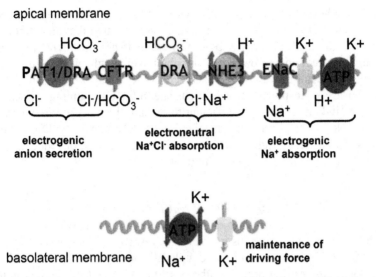

FIGURE 3. Major ion transport pathways involved in the regulation of fluid movement in the intestine. NHE3: Na^+/H^+ exchanger isoform 3; ENaC: epithelial Na^+ channel.

In 1990, Sandle *et al.* realized that this may be caused by a multicomponent change of the biophysical properties of the inflamed colonocytes, leading to a reduction in electrogenic Na^+ absorption, an increased paracellular leakiness, a relative predominance of anion secretion over sodium absorption, and a reduced basolateral sodium pump activity.[43] FIGURE 3 displays the major transport pathways that regulate intestinal fluid movements, as we understand them now. Clearly, this picture is not complete.

ENaC Channel Dysfunction

As tools became available to do so, Geoffrey Sandle's group, as well as others, tried to establish the molecular basis for these defects.[52,53] Immunohistochemical studies demonstrated a marked decrease in apical staining for the ß and γ subunit of the epithelial Na^+ channel (EnaC).[53] Expression of the α subunit is constitutive, but results in a low-conductive state of the channel, whereas the expression of the ß and γ subunit is aldosterone-dependent in the colon and results in a high-conductive state.[54]

It is known, however, that the expression of the ENaC is under the control of aldosterone and therefore not regularly expressed in the presence of a balanced electrolyte and fluid status and highly variable among individuals. Amasheh *et al.* performed an excellent study in which they placed biopsy specimens of patients with UC and of healthy controls into Ussing chambers and induced an electrogenic, amiloride-sensitive Na^+ current by the addition of aldosterone *in vitro* in the healthy but not the inflamed tissue.[55] They then extracted mRNA and protein from the biopsy samples and demonstrated that aldosterone had resulted in an ENaC ß- and γ-subunit expression in healthy but not in inflamed tissue. They went on to show that the incubation of healthy tissue with a combination of the cytokine tumor necrosis factor (TNF)-α and interferon-γ caused a similar loss of responsiveness of the tissue to EnaC-subunit upregulation.

These findings are *per se* sufficient to explain the markedly reduced electrogenic Na$^+$ absorption in the distal colon of UC patients. Additional disturbances such as leaky tight junctions, epithelial apoptosis, or reduced driving force for ion transport, may be additional features.

Electroneutral NaCl Absorption

The major salt and water absorptive mechanism in the intestine is electroneutral NaCl absorption, mediated by a coupled action of Na$^+$/H$^+$ and Cl$^-$/HCO$_3^-$ exchange in the brush border membrane of the enterocyte.[56,57] The ion transport proteins that mediate electroneutral salt absorption are largely, but not completely, identified.[58,59] The Na$^+$/H$^+$ exchanger isoform Na$^+$/H$^+$ Exchanger Isoform 3 (NHE3) and the Cl$^-$/HCO$_3^-$ exchanger SLC26A3 or DRA are the predominant transport pathways with particularly high expression in the ileum and proximal colon, segments most strongly affected by Crohn's disease.[60] Therefore, investigators wondered about the influence of inflammation on electroneutral NaCl absorption in the more proximal parts of the intestine. However, because these parts of the intestine are difficult to reach for study, few data are available.

Musch *et al.* investigated the effect of acute T cell activation by anti-CD3 antibody on intestinal fluid loss in mice, and also studied EIPA (an inhibiter of Na$^+$/H$^+$ exchange)-sensitive Na$^+$ absorption in the small intestine.[61] They observed an increase in enteropooling (fluid in the intestinal lumen), an increase in paracellular permeability, as well as a marked reduction in EIPA-sensitive Na$^+$ uptake, a reduced anion secretory response, and a decrease in Na$^+$/K$^+$ adenosine 5′-triphosphate (ATP)ase activity, as early as 3 h after acute T cell stimulation. The same group demonstrated that interferon-γ resulted in a decrease in expression and function of NHE3 and NHE2 in an intestinal cell line 6 h after exposure, and in rat intestine 48 h after injection.[62] Thus, acute release of high concentrations of inflammatory cytokines results in a generalized depression of enterocyte cellular transport function.

We studied the question of electroneutral salt absorption and NHE3 expression in the IL-2 knockout (KO) mouse, a murine model for chronic intestinal inflammation, in which the disease manifests itself predominantly in the proximal colon and distal ileum.[63] We also observed an extreme reduction of electroneutral salt absorption in the proximal colon, but the NHE3 mRNA and protein expression levels were only slightly reduced despite massive epithelial infiltration and thickening. Likewise, NHE3 mRNA expression in colonic biopsies of UC patients was found to be depressed only in those with severe inflammation, whereas increased NHE3 mRNA expression was found in mild inflammation.[45]

This suggested that lack of NHE3 expression cannot be the major explanation for the severely disturbed electroneutral salt absorptive function in chronic proximal colonic inflammation. To get further insight into the molecular mechanisms of disturbed electroneutral salt absorption, we studied the time course of inflammation and disturbed salt absorption in the IL-10 KO mouse model for chronic immune-mediated inflammation. We measured NHE3 activity fluorometrically in surface colonocytes, using the pH-sensitive dye BCECF, and NHE3 mRNA and protein expression by quantitative polymerase chain reaction (PCR) and immunohistochemistry. Surprisingly, we found a marked increase in NHE3 mRNA expression in the proximal colon and distal ileum of the IL-10 KO mice when kept in a normal animal housing environment. We speculate that this increased NHE3 mRNA expression reflects the proliferative stimulus that results in the crypt hyperplasia, but obviously also affects the surface-predominant NHE3. Immunohistochemical studies showed completely preserved apical NHE3 protein staining (FIG. 4A), which, in the IL-10 KO mouse, extended somewhat into the opening of the crypt mouths. However, acid-activated NHE3 function was severely depressed (FIG. 4B). This demonstrates that NHE3 function rather than expression is disturbed in chronically inflamed intestine. The potential molecular basis for this could be a reduction in the PDZ-adapter proteins that retain NHE3 in the plasma membrane and regulate its transport function by aiding in the formation of multiprotein signalling complexes.[64]

SUMMARY AND UNRESOLVED QUESTIONS FOR FUTURE RESEARCH

Patients with inflammatory bowel disease (IBD) often suffer from diarrhea. Ion transport studies *in vivo* and *in vitro* have uncovered the dramatic loss of sodium (and, as a consequence, fluid) absorptive capacity of the inflamed intestinal mucosa of IBD patients several decades ago. Despite the generation of numerous inflammatory mediators with anion (and fluid) secretagogue action during intestinal inflammation, the inflamed intestinal mucosa has a diminished ability to respond to them. The molecular mechanisms that cause this reduced anion secretory responsiveness are controversially discussed and may include disturbed expression and/or trafficking of apical anion exit and basolateral entry transporters, a reduction in the electrochemical gradient across the apical membrane, and disturbances in signal transduction within the enteric nervous system as well as the enterocyte itself.

The research tools to study the molecular basis for the sodium absorptive defect have only recently become available. In the distal colon, inflammation

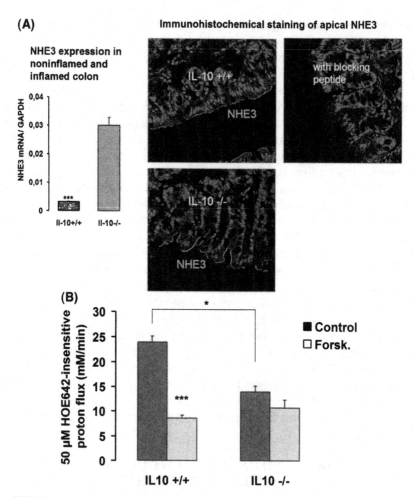

FIGURE 4. (A) Upregulation of NHE3 mRNA and correct apical NHE3 sorting in IL-10 -/- mice raised in normal laboratory housing conditions (with intestinal inflammation and cryptal hyperplasia). **(B)** Despite the apical presence of NHE3, its transport function, measured as the cariporide-insensitive proton efflux rate in the surface cells of the proximal colon of IL-10 +/+ and -/-mice by a fluorometric approach[65] is markedly disturbed. Both the acid-activated NHE3 transport activity was markedly reduced in the inflamed colon, and its inhibition by forskolin was reduced. This resembles the defect found in mice that lack PDZ-adapter proteins that regulate NHE3 function.

interferes with the ability of aldosterone to induce ENaC channel subunit ß- and γ-expression and thus upregulate electrogenic Na⁺ absorption. In the more proximal parts of the colon and the ileum, inflammation causes a functional disturbance of electroneutral salt absorption, whose molecular cause is not yet clear and may be different in acute and chronic inflammation. Cell culture experiments indicate that very high concentrations of inflammatory cytokines result in a downregulation of Na⁺/K⁺ ATPase activity, an increase

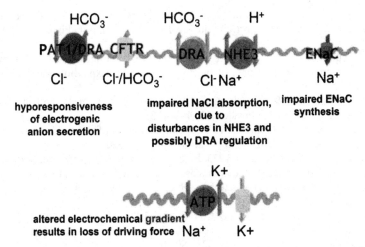

FIGURE 5. Summary of the major changes in intestinal electrolyte transport found to occw during intestinal inflammation.

in intracellular Na^+ concentration, and a decrease in NHE2 and NHE3 expression. Chronic inflammation of native intestine also results in a severe reduction of electroneutral Na^+ absorption, but the mechanism does not appear to be related to Na^+/K^+ ATPase inhibition and dowregulation of apical Na^+ transport protein expression, but rather to a regulatory defect whose molecular nature has yet to be clarified. Dysfunction or downregulation of PDZ-adapter proteins, which are mandatory for the organization of the multiprotein complexes that regulate NHE3 transport activity, may be one of these defects.

ACKNOWLEDGMENTS

The author thanks the many people whose encouragement, intellectual exchange, and practical help allowed her and her group to enter the field of epithelial dysfunction during intestinal inflammation. In particular, my thanks go to Jörg-Dieter Schulzke and Michael Fromm and their groups, Charité Berlin, Chris Lytle and coworkers, University of California at Riverside, and to the members of the Sonderforschungsbereich 621 "Pathobiology of the intestinal mucosa." The work was supported by a grant from the DFG SFB621/C9.

REFERENCES

1. USSING, H.H. 1965. Transport of electrolytes and water across epithelia. Harvey Lect. **59:** 1–30.
2. LEVI, H. & H.H. USSING. 1949. Resting potential and ion movements in the frog skin. Nature **164:** 928.

3. USSING, H.H. & K. ZEHRAN. 1951. Active transport of sodium as the source of electric current in the short-circuited isolated frog skin. Acta Physiol. Scand. **23:** 111–127.
4. CHALFIN, D., I.L. COOPERSTEIN & C.A. HOGBEN. 1958. Fluid and electrolyte movement across intestinal wall of bullfrog. Proc. Soc. Exp. Biol. Med. **99:** 746–748.
5. COOPERSTEIN, I.L. & C.A. HOGBEN. 1959. Ionic transfer across the isolated frog large intestine. J. Gen. Physiol. **42:** 461–473.
6. EDMONDS, C.J. & R. GODFREY. 1970. A simple method of measuring transmucosal P.D. in man and its clinical application. Clin. Sci. **38:** 11P.
7. EDMONDS, C.J. & D. PILCHER. 1973. Electrical potential difference and sodium and potassium fluxes across rectal mucosa in ulcerative colitis. Gut **14:** 784–789.
8. FIELD, M. 1993. Intestinal electrolyte secretion: history of a paradigm. Arch. Surg. **128:** 273–278.
9. ARCHAMPONG, E.Q., J. HARRIS & C.G. CLARK. 1972. The absorption and secretion of water and electrolytes across the healthy and the diseased human colonic mucosa measured in vitro. Gut **13:** 880–886.
10. HAWKER, P.C., J.S. MCKAY & L.A. TURNBERG. 1980. Electrolyte transport across colonic mucosa from patients with inflammatory bowel disease. Gastroenterology **79:** 508–511.
11. ALLAN, R., D.M. STEINBERG, K. DIXON & W.T. COOKE. 1975. Changes in the bidirectional sodium flux across the intestinal mucosa in Crohn's disease. Gut **16:** 201–204.
12. SANDLE, G.I., J.P. HAYSLETT & H.J. BINDER. 1986. Effect of glucocorticoids on rectal transport in normal subjects and patients with ulcerative colitis. Gut **27:** 309–316.
13. FIELD, M., G.R. PLOTKIN & W. SILEN. 1968. Effects of vasopressin, theophylline and cyclic adenosine monophosphate on short-circuit current across isolated rabbit ileal mucosa. Nature **217:** 469–471.
14. KIMBERG, D.V., M. FIELD, J. JOHNSON, *et al.* 1971. Stimulation of intestinal mucosal adenyl cyclase by cholera enterotoxin and prostaglandins. J. Clin. Invest. **50:** 1218–1230.
15. PIERCE, N.F., C.C. CARPENTER, JR., H.L. ELLIOTT & W.B. GREENOUGH, III. 1971. Effects of prostaglandins, theophylline, and cholera exotoxin upon transmucosal water and electrolyte movement in the canine jejunum. Gastroenterology **60:** 22–32.
16. FIELD, M., D. FROMM, Q. AL AWQATI & W.B. GREENOUGH, III. 1972. Effect of cholera enterotoxin on ion transport across isolated ileal mucosa. J. Clin. Invest. **51:** 796–804.
17. FIELD, M., M.W. MUSCH, R.L. MILLER & E.J. GOETZL. 1984. Regulation of epithelial electrolyte transport by metabolites of arachidonic acid. J. Allergy Clin. Immunol. **74:** 382–385.
18. GIANNELLA, R.A., R.E. GOTS, A.N. CHARNEY, *et al.* 1975. Pathogenesis of *Salmonella*-mediated intestinal fluid secretion: activation of adenylate cyclase and inhibition by indomethacin. Gastroenterology **69:** 1238–1245.
19. CALDERARO, V., A. GIOVANE, B. DE SIMONE, *et al.* 1991. Arachidonic acid metabolites and chloride secretion in rabbit distal colonic mucosa. Am. J. Physiol. **261:** G443–G450.
20. WARDLE, T.D. & L.A. TURNBERG. 1994. Potential role for interleukin-1 in the pathophysiology of ulcerative colitis. Clin. Sci. (London) **86:** 619–626.

21. McKAY, D.M. & P.K. SINGH. 1997. Superantigen activation of immune cells evokes epithelial (T84) transport and barrier abnormalities via IFN-gamma and TNF alpha: inhibition of increased permeability, but not diminished secretory responses by TGF-beta2. J. Immunol. **159:** 2382–2390.
22. OPRINS, J.C., C. VAN DER BURG, H.P. MEIJER, *et al.* 2002. Tumour necrosis factor alpha potentiates ion secretion induced by histamine in a human intestinal epithelial cell line and in mouse colon: involvement of the phospholipase D pathway. Gut **50:** 314–321.
23. DANAHAY, H., H. ATHERTON, G. JONES, *et al.* 2002. Interleukin-13 induces a hypersecretory ion transport phenotype in human bronchial epithelial cells. Am. J. Physiol. **282:** L226–L236.
24. GAGINELLA, T.S. & J.F. KACHUR. 1989. Kinins as mediators of intestinal secretion. Am. J. Physiol. **256:** G1–G15.
25. NGUYEN, T.D. & A.T. CANADA. 1994. Modulation of human colonic T84 cell secretion by hydrogen peroxide. Biochem. Pharmacol. **47:** 403–410.
26. GRISHAM, M.B., T.S. GAGINELLA, C. VON RITTER, *et al.* 1990. Effects of neutrophil-derived oxidants on intestinal permeability, electrolyte transport, and epithelial cell viability. Inflammation **14:** 531–542.
27. TAMAI, H., J.F. KACHUR, D.A. BARON, *et al.* 1991. Monochloramine, a neutrophil-derived oxidant, stimulates rat colonic secretion. J. Pharmacol. Exp. Ther. **257:** 887–894.
28. MADARA, J.L., C. PARKOS, S. COLGAN, *et al.* 1992. Cl- secretion in a model intestinal epithelium induced by a neutrophil-derived secretagogue. J. Clin. Invest. **89:** 1938–1944.
29. MADARA, J.L., T.W. PATAPOFF, B. GILLECE-CASTRO, *et al.* 1993. 5'-adenosine monophosphate is the neutrophil-derived paracrine factor that elicits chloride secretion from T84 intestinal epithelial cell monolayers. J. Clin. Invest. **91:** 2320–2325.
30. PARKOS, C.A., S.P. COLGAN & J.L. MADARA. 1994. Interactions of neutrophils with epithelial cells: lessons from the intestine. J. Am. Soc. Nephrol. **5:** 138–152.
31. ROCHA, M.F., J.J. SIDRIM, A.M. SOARES, *et al.* 2000. Supernatants from macrophages stimulated with microcystin-LR induce electrogenic intestinal response in rabbit ileum. Pharmacol. Toxicol. **87:** 46–51.
32. ROCHA, M.F., A.M. SOARES, C.A. FLORES, *et al.* 1998. Intestinal secretory factor released by macrophages stimulated with *Clostridium difficile* toxin A: role of interleukin 1beta. Infect. Immun. **66:** 4910–4916.
33. BARRETT, K.E. 1991. Immune-related intestinal chloride secretion. III. Acute and chronic effects of mast cell mediators on chloride secretion by a human colonic epithelial cell line. J. Immunol. **147:** 959–964.
34. ROCHA, M.F., J.E. AGUIAR, J.J. SIDRIM, *et al.* 2003. Role of mast cells and proinflammatory mediators on the intestinal secretion induced by cholera toxin. Toxicon **42:** 183–189.
35. CROWE, S.E., G.K. LUTHRA & M.H. PERDUE. 1997. Mast cell mediated ion transport in intestine from patients with and without inflammatory bowel disease. Gut **41:** 785–792.
36. MACNAUGHTON, W.K. & D.G. GALL. 1991. Mechanisms of platelet-activating factor-induced electrolyte transport in the rat jejunum. Eur. J. Pharmacol. **200:** 17–23.

37. WARDLE, T.D., L. HALL & L.A. TURNBERG. 1996. Platelet activating factor: release from colonic mucosa in patients with ulcerative colitis and its effect on colonic secretion. Gut **38:** 355–361.
38. WARDLE, T.D., L. HALL & L.A. TURNBERG. 1993. Inter-relationships between inflammatory mediators released from colonic mucosa in ulcerative colitis and their effects on colonic secretion. Gut **34:** 503–508.
39. WARDLE, T.D., L. HALL & L.A. TURNBERG. 1992. Use of coculture of colonic mucosal biopsies to investigate the release of eicosanoids by inflamed and uninflamed mucosa from patients with inflammatory bowel disease. Gut **33:** 1644–1651.
40. HUBEL, K.A. & K.S. RENQUIST. 1990. Ion transport in normal and inflamed human jejunum in vitro: changes with electric field stimulation and theophylline. Dig. Dis. Sci. **35:** 815–820.
41. KACHUR, J.F., A. KESHAVARZIAN, R. SUNDARESAN, *et al.* 1995. Colitis reduces short-circuit current response to inflammatory mediators in rat colonic mucosa. Inflammation **19:** 245–259.
42. SANCHEZ, D.M., R. PEREZ, O. MARTINEZ-AUGUSTIN, *et al.* 2002. Disturbances of colonic ion secretion in inflammation: role of the enteric nervous system and cAMP. Pflugers Arch. **444:** 378–388.
43. SANDLE, G.I., N. HIGGS, P. CROWE, *et al.* 1990. Cellular basis for defective electrolyte transport in inflamed human colon. Gastroenterology **99:** 97–105.
44. FISH, S.M., R. PROUJANSKY & W.W. REENSTRA. 1999. Synergistic effects of interferon gamma and tumour necrosis factor alpha on T84 cell function. Gut **45:** 191–198.
45. LOHI, H., S. MAKELA, K. PULKKINEN, *et al.* 2002. Upregulation of CFTR expression but not SLC26A3 and SLC9A3 in ulcerative colitis. Am. J. Physiol. **283:** G567–G575.
46. BERTELSEN, L.S., L. ECKMANN & K.E. BARRETT. 2004. Prolonged interferon-gamma exposure decreases ion transport, NKCC1, and Na+-K+-ATPase expression in human intestinal xenografts in vivo. Am. J. Physiol. **286:** G157–G165.
47. SKINN, A.C. & W.K. MACNAUGHTON. 2005. Nitric oxide inhibits cAMP-dependent CFTR trafficking in intestinal epithelial cells. Am. J. Physiol. **289:** G739–G744.
48. YANG, H.Y., W. JIANG, E.E. FURTH, *et al.* 1998. Intestinal inflammation reduces expression of DRA, a transporter responsible for congenital chloride diarrhea. Am. J. Physiol. **275:** G1445–G1453.
49. SANDLE, G.I. 2005. Pathogenesis of diarrhea in ulcerative colitis: new views on an old problem. J. Clin. Gastroenterol. **39:** S49–S52.
50. PEREZ-NAVARRO, R., O. MARTINEZ-AUGUSTIN, I. BALLESTER, *et al.* 2005. Experimental inflammation of the rat distal colon inhibits ion secretion in the proximal colon by affecting the enteric nervous system. Naunyn Schmiedebergs Arch. Pharmacol. **371:** 114–121.
51. ZAMUNER, S.R., N. WARRIER, A.G. BURET, *et al.* 2003. Cyclooxygenase 2 mediates post-inflammatory colonic secretory and barrier dysfunction. Gut 2003. **52:** 1714–1720.
52. GREIG, E. & G.I. SANDLE. 2000. Diarrhea in ulcerative colitis: the role of altered colonic sodium transport. Ann. N. Y. Acad. Sci. **915:** 327–332.
53. GREIG, E.R., R.P. BOOT-HANDFORD, V. MANI & G.I. SANDLE. 2004. Decreased expression of apical Na+ channels and basolateral Na+, K+-ATPase in ulcerative colitis. J. Pathol. **204:** 84–92.

54. CANESSA, C.M., L. SCHILD, G. BUELL, *et al.* 1994. Amiloride-sensitive epithelial Na+ channel is made of three homologous subunits. Nature **367:** 463–467.
55. AMASHEH, S., C. BARMEYER, C.S. KOCH, *et al.* 2004. Cytokine-dependent transcriptional down-regulation of epithelial sodium channel in ulcerative colitis. Gastroenterology **126:** 1711–1720.
56. SHULL, G.E., M.L. MILLER & P.J. SCHULTHEIS. 2000. Lessons from genetically engineered animal models VIII: absorption and secretion of ions in the gastrointestinal tract. A. J. Physiol **278:** G185–G190.
57. KERE, J. & P. HOGLUND. 2000. Inherited disorders of ion transport in the intestine. Curr. Opin. Genet. Dev. **10:** 306–309.
58. GAWENIS, L.R., X. STIEN, G.E. SHULL, *et al.* 2002. Intestinal NaCl transport in NHE2 and NHE3 knockout mice. Am. J. Physiol. **282:** G776–G784.
59. SCHULTHEIS, P.J., L.L. CLARKE, P. MENETON, *et al.* 1998. Renal and intestinal absorptive defects in mice lacking the NHE3 Na+/H+ exchanger. Nat. Genet. **19:** 282–285.
60. JACOB, P., H. ROSSMANN, G. LAMPRECHT, *et al.* 2002. Down-regulated in adenoma mediates apical Cl-/HCO3- exchange in rabbit, rat, and human duodenum. Gastroenterology **122:** 709–724.
61. MUSCH, M.W., L.L. CLARKE, D. MAMAH, *et al.* 2002. T cell activation causes diarrhea by increasing intestinal permeability and inhibiting epithelial Na+/K+-ATPase. J. Clin. Invest. **110:** 1739–1747.
62. ROCHA, F., M.W. MUSCH, L. LISHANSKIY, *et al.* 2001. IFN-gamma downregulates expression of Na(+)/H(+) exchangers NHE2 and NHE3 in rat intestine and human Caco-2/bbe cells. Am. J. Physiol. **280:** C1224–C1232.
63. BARMEYER, C., M. HARREN, H. SCHMITZ, *et al.* 2004. Mechanisms of diarrhea in the interleukin-2-deficient mouse model of colonic inflammation. Am. J. Physiol. **286:** G244–G252.
64. DONOWITZ, M., B. CHA, N.C. ZACHOS, *et al.* 2005. NHERF Family and NHE3 Regulation. J. Physiol. **567:** 3–18. Eprint May 19.
65. BACHMANN, O., B. RIEDERER, H. ROSSMANN, *et al.* 2004. The Na^+/H^+ Exchanger isoform 2 is the predomenant NHE isoform in murene colonic crypts NHE3 upregulation. Am. J. Physiol. Gastrointest. Liver Physiol. **287:** E125–133. E-publication Feb. 12, 2004.

Neutrophil Transepithelial Migration and Epithelial Barrier Function in IBD

Potential Targets for Inhibiting Neutrophil Trafficking

ALEX C. CHIN AND CHARLES A. PARKOS

Epithelial Pathobiology Unit, Department of Pathology and Laboratory Medicine, Emory University Atlanta, Georgia 30322, USA

ABSTRACT: Neutrophil (PMN) transmigration across mucosal epithelia is a hallmark of inflammatory conditions, such as ulcerative colitis and Crohn's disease. PMN accumulation within epithelial crypts and in the intestinal lumen directly correlates with clinical disease activity and epithelial injury. Currently, the mechanisms by which PMNs migrate across mucosal epithelia are incompletely understood and a better understanding of this process will likely provide new insights into novel treatment strategies for inflammatory bowel disease. In this article, we discuss current advances that define PMN transepithelial migration, specifically focusing on PMN–epithelial adhesive interactions and signaling events. We also describe how these interactions might be specifically targeted for the development of therapeutic strategies to manage mucosal inflammation.

KEYWORDS: meutrophil; transmigration; epithelium; apical junction complex; permeability; IBD

INTRODUCTION

Inflammatory bowel disease (IBD), including Crohn's disease and ulcerative colitis, is a multifactorial immunological disorder, commonly occurring in developed countries, with approximately 1.3 million and 1.9 million people affected in North America and Europe, respectively.[1] Although the pathogenesis of IBD remains obscure, advances in this field have shed more light on this debilitating and complex collection of diseases. Recent studies have postulated that the alteration in intestinal barrier function plays an important role in the

Address for correspondence: Charles A. Parkos, M.D., Ph.D., Department of Pathology and Laboratory Medicine, Emory University, 615 Michael Street, Atlanta, GA, USA 30322. Voice: 404-727-8533; fax: 404-727-8538.

e-mail: cparkos@emory.edu

Ann. N.Y. Acad. Sci. 1072: 276–287 (2006). © 2006 New York Academy of Sciences.
doi: 10.1196/annals.1326.018

pathogenesis of IBD.[2,3] Furthermore, epithelial injury, disease activity, and patients' symptoms have been shown to correlate with the histological finding of extensive polymorphonuclear leukocyte (neutrophil or PMN) migration across the epithelium in active cases of IBD.[4] Although it has been shown that high numbers of intraepithelial PMN (beneath the tight junction) do not correlate with an IBD-like syndrome *in vivo*,[5] it is postulated that high-density PMN migration across the epithelium and into the lumen is necessary to influence epithelial functions ranging from barrier maintenance to electrolyte secretion.[6–9] In this review, we will discuss the recent advances that define the multistep mechanism(s) by which PMNs migrate across epithelial surfaces and further discuss potential therapeutic targets aimed at fine-tuning PMN trafficking in inflammatory diseases.

EXPERIMENTAL MODELS

Much of the information obtained from PMN transepithelial migration has been derived from *in vitro* experiments using epithelial monolayers cultured on permeable supports, peripheral blood PMNs, and imposition of chemoattractant gradients. Traditionally, such transepithelial migration experiments have been performed such that PMNs transmigrate in an apical to basolateral direction across epithelial monolayers. For these assays, peripheral blood PMNs are added to epithelial monolayers that are grown on the upper or inner surface of permeable transwell supports. Although this method can prove to be useful in determining direct PMN–epithelial interactions, the direction of PMN migration is actually in the opposite direction of what occurs under physiologically relevant conditions. To model PMN migration across epithelial monolayers in the physiologically relevant basolateral-to-apical direction, years ago we developed an *in vitro* system whereby peripheral blood PMNs are added to the basal aspect of epithelial monolayers that are grown in inverted fashion on the underside of permeable transwell supports.[7] Given that epithelial cells grow in a polarized manner by virtue of a well-defined apical junctional complex, studies using these two methods have been successful in identifying appropriate apical and basolateral ligands for PMN at various stages of transepithelial migration.

PMN–Epithelial Interactions that Promote PMN Transmigration

PMN transepithelial migration is the integration of several distinct steps involving different cell surface receptors and their respective ligands (FIG. 1). Once the PMNs have emigrated from the bloodstream across the endothelium and migrated through the extracellular matrix, they initially contact the

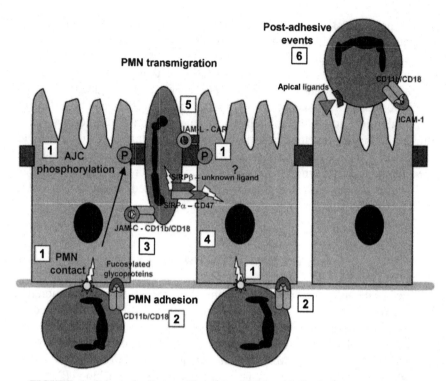

FIGURE 1. Schematic diagram illustrating PMN–epithelial interactions. (**1**) Initially, PMN contact with the epithelial basolateral surface induces signaling and subsequent apical junctional protein phosphorylation. This event is rapid and reversible, and may facilitate the passage of PMNs through the paracellular space. (**2**) Concurrent with contact, PMNs adhere to the basolateral surface via CD11b/CD18 interactions with epithelial fucosylated glycoproteins and other currently undefined ligands. (**3**) During transmigration, CD11b/CD18 is also used by PMNs to bind desmosomal JAM-C. This is the first indication that adhesive interactions between PMNs and epithelial intercellular junctions occur. (**4**) In addition, the rate of transmigration is modulated through PMN SIRPα and epithelial CD47 interactions. Since CD47 is also expressed on PMNs, there exists the possibility of *cis* interactions between PMN CD47 or SIRPα. Ligation of PMN SIRPβ with a yet to be identified ligand appears to enhance PMN transmigration. These interactions suggest that initialization of concomitant signaling plays a role in transmigration. (**5**) In addition to adhesive interactions at the desmosomes, PMNs also bind to epithelial CAR via JAML. Since CAR is expressed at the tight junctions, this suggests that PMNs may use intercellular junctional proteins as ligands to successively navigate epithelial surfaces to reach the site of injury. These observations indicate that epithelial intercellular junctions may be targeted to develop therapeutic agents specifically aimed at controlling mucosal inflammation. (**6**) Upon arrival in the lumen after migration across the epithelial intercellular junction, PMNs adhere to apical ICAM-1 that may facilitate the retention of PMNs at the site of injury. During some disease conditions, autoantibodies decorating epithelial luminal surfaces may also enhance PMN retention and activation via Fc-mediated events.

basolateral aspect of the mucosal epithelium and induce signaling events that ultimately result in rapid and reversible opening of the intercellular junctions to facilitate PMN transmigration.[10] The signaling mechanism of PMN contact-induced epithelial permeability remains incompletely understood, but studies have demonstrated that high PMN density is required and that this event is CD11b/CD18-independent.[10] Interestingly, others have reported that low-density PMN transepithelial migration can occur without the disruption of barrier function,[6,11] suggesting that mucosal damage is associated with high-density PMN infiltration into tissues. More studies are needed to determine the identity of the specific receptors and signaling events that are responsible for the PMN-induced epithelial barrier changes. The discovery of receptors that mediate such responses may provide therapeutic advantages to control the increase in intestinal permeability associated with IBD and other inflammatory disorders.

CD11b/CD18 Plays a Central Role in PMN Transmigration

The initial step of PMN transepithelial migration involves adhesion of PMNs to the basolateral aspect of the mucosal epithelium and is mediated by the leukocyte β2 integrin CD11b/CD18 (Mac-1, CR3).[7] This initial event is unlike leukocyte transendothelial migration, which relies on both CD11b/CD18 and another β2 integrin CD11a/CD18 (LFA-1) for firm adhesion. In the same line, CD62 (E-, L-, and P-selectins) and CD31 (platelet endothelial cell adhesion molecule, PECAM) play important roles in PMN–endothelial interactions, but do not mediate transepithelial migration.[12] It is likely that the differences between endothelial and epithelial microenvironments are accountable for some of the variations in the cell surface receptors necessary for mediating PMN transmigration in each milieu. While it is important to distinguish the transendothelial from transepithelial components associated with leukocyte migration, it is clear that CD11b/CD18 plays a crucial role in both microenvironments. Incubation with CD11b/CD18 inhibitory monoclonal antibodies has been shown to block approximately 90% of PMN migration across epithelial monolayers.[10] Given that CD11b/CD18 plays a crucial role during initial adhesion to both the endothelium and epithelium, inhibition of this integrin may provide therapeutic benefits by preventing PMN adhesion and transmigration from the vasculature to the mucosae. However, the mode of delivery of inhibitory therapeutics may induce nonspecific effects, given that CD11b/CD18 plays a role in both transendothelial and transepithelial leukocyte migration. In addition, since PMNs have been shown to increase epithelial permeability in a CD11b/CD18-independent fashion, inhibition of this step may not confer protection associated with alteration of epithelial function induced by PMN contact.

Role of JAMs and Other CTX Family Members
in Transepithelial Migration

Although CD11b/CD18 plays a pivotal role in PMN transmigration, the identity of the epithelial counterreceptors during initial adhesion remains elusive, but it is likely that they may include basally localized fucosylated glycoproteins.[13] Recently, members of a different class of proteins termed *junctional adhesion molecules* (JAMs) have been recently shown to play a role in leukocyte migration across endothelial[14-17] and epithelial[18,19] monolayers. JAMs are cell surface immunoglobulin superfamily members that share similarities to fellow members of the cortical thymocyte of *Xenopus* (CTX) family including nectins, coxsackie adenovirus receptor (CAR), and other related proteins involved in cell adhesion and migration. Some members of the JAM/CTX family of proteins that have been identified include JAM-A, JAM-B, JAM-C, JAM-D, and a JAM-like protein (JAML).[20,21]

JAM-A is abundantly expressed at the epithelial apical junctional complex that encompasses both the tight and adherens junctions. In addition to epithelial cells, JAM-A has also been shown to be expressed on PMNs[22] and endothelia, and studies have shown that it plays a role in murine leukocyte transendothelial migration.[14,17] Furthermore, JAM-A deficiency in mice results in enhanced spontaneous random endothelial cell motility,[23] while attenuating PMN transendothelial migration.[24] A more recent study has shown that JAM-A- deficient murine PMNs exhibited reduced diapedesis with high numbers adhering to the endothelium or suspended between endothelial cells and the basement membrane.[25] Conversely in humans, multiple inhibitory anti-JAM-A antibodies were unable to inhibit both transendothelial and transepithelial migration.[22,26] Given that studies have shown that JAM-A exhibits homophilic interactions between cells[27,28] and that PMNs also express JAM-A, these observations might be explained by homophilic adhesive interactions between PMNs and epithelial cells or perhaps heterophilic interactions between JAM proteins. Further studies have suggested that JAM-A regulates epithelial cell morphology through the small GTPase Rap1,[29] while others have shown that calcium/calmodulin-dependent serine protein kinase plays a role in epithelial signaling.[29,30] It is thus likely that JAM-A homo-/heterophilic interactions and subsequent induction of cell signaling pathways may mediate cell motility and shape in endothelial and epithelial cells. Indeed, the maintenance of cell shape through JAM-A may facilitate endothelial cell anchorage to the matrix[23] or may enhance $\beta 1$ integrin-mediated adhesion in epithelial cells.[29] Although it remains to be seen in humans, a recent study reported that JAM-A may enhance murine PMN detachment and directional movement.[25] Taken together, these observations suggest that effects of JAM-A on cellular morphology in leukocytes as well as endothelial and epithelial cells may thus affect leukocyte transmigration in indirect ways.

While JAM-A has been shown to be expressed at the tight junctions, recent studies have shown that another JAM family member termed *JAM-C* is abundantly expressed at epithelial desmosomes and specifically binds to CD11b/CD18 on the I domain.[18] This observation confirmed earlier studies demonstrating that CD11b/CD18 binds JAM-C on platelets.[31] It was also shown that anti-JAM-C monoclonal antibodies and soluble JAM-C fusion proteins partially inhibited the rate of PMN migration across epithelial monolayers.[18] These observations support the hypothesis that PMNs may use epithelial intercellular junctional components as counterreceptors to crawl across the epithelium. Although inhibition of JAM-C does not have an equivalently potent inhibitory effect as that of anti-CD11b/CD18 antibodies, blockade of JAM-C significantly decreases the rate of PMN migration across intestinal epithelial monolayers by approximately 50%. This suggests that there are other epithelial CD11b/CD18 receptor ligands and that inhibition of JAM-C as well as other epithelial intercellular junctional proteins may provide therapeutic advantages to specifically fine-tune PMN infiltration across mucosal epithelial surfaces. Indeed, a recent study reported that neutralizing antibodies to JAM-C significantly attenuated PMN infiltration into the bronchoalveolar space after intranasal instillation of lipopolysaccharide (LPS) in mice.[32]

The incomplete inhibition of PMN transmigration by anti-JAM-C antibodies suggests that other ligands must be involved in regulating PMN migration across epithelial barriers, particularly at the level of the tight junction. Another member of the JAM family termed *JAML* (JAM-like protein) was shown to be highly expressed on granulocytes and to enhance leukocyte adhesion to endothelial cells.[21] Subsequently, it was shown that JAML plays an important role in regulating PMN transepithelial migration.[19] From recombinant protein/cell-binding and cell-labeling screening experiments, the membrane proximal loop of JAML has been shown to bind to the distal loop of the coxsackie adenovirus receptor (CAR) expressed at epithelial tight junctions.[19] In addition, JAML and CAR fusion proteins specifically inhibited PMN transepithelial migration, although this effect was incomplete.[19] These findings with JAML and CAR again indicate that additional epithelial receptors for migrating PMN are likely to exist within the epithelial paracellular space. In support of this contention, addition of a mixture of both JAM-C and CAR inhibitory antibodies to PMN transepithelial migration assays resulted in more inhibition than either agent alone but failed to completely block PMN transepithelial migration.[19]

The recent findings with JAML and CAR may confer opportunities in specific targeting of PMN transmigration at the level of the epithelium. Indeed, studies have shown that CAR is highly expressed in epithelial tissues while being poorly expressed in endothelial cells.[33] Conceivably, epithelial CAR might be targeted to specifically inhibit mucosal inflammation while not affecting other leukocyte functions. However, given the wide distribution of JAM proteins in leukocytes and/or epithelial cells, more studies are needed to determine the binding interactions between JAM members or with other proteins, and whether their respective signaling pathways play a role in PMN transepithelial migration.

CD47 and SIRPs Mediate Signaling Events During PMN Transepithelial Migration

Regulation of PMN transepithelial migration has also been shown to involve a cell surface immunoglobulin superfamily member termed *CD47* (integrin-associated protein, IAP). CD47 is expressed in many cell types including both PMNs and epithelial cells[34] and has been shown to be upregulated in epithelial tissues in IBD. Studies have shown that CD47 mediates PMN transmigration across the vascular endothelium, extracellular matrix, and the intestinal epithelium.[35–37] Furthermore, CD47 regulates PMN transepithelial migration after initial CD11b/CD18-mediated adhesion has occurred.[36,37] Specifically, the rate of PMN transmigration is delayed upon incubation with inhibitory CD47 antibodies.[37] Other studies have shown that signal regulatory protein-α (SIRPα), a transmembrane Ig superfamily member also expressed on PMN but not epithelia, can act as a cellular receptor for CD47,[38] and this has raised the possibility of multidirectional signaling in *trans* between PMNs and epithelial cells and/or in *cis* within PMNs. Subsequent studies have shown that ligation of SIRPα with inhibitory antibodies or CD47 and is fusion proteins partially inhibited PMN transepithelial migration as opposed to the delayed effect achieved with anti-CD47 antibodies.[39] These observations suggest that different signaling pathways exist between CD47 and SIRPα, activation. Indeed, investigation into possible signaling pathways has implicated the role of tyrosine kinase(s) signaling in CD47 ligation and phosphatidylinositol-3-kinase activation upon SIRPα ligation.[39] Conversely, further studies have shown that antibody-mediated ligation of a closely related SIRP family member also expressed on PMN that does not bind CD47, and is termed *SIRP*β, enhances PMN transepithelial migration.[40] These observations indicate that different signaling cascades downstream of SIRP family members may play a role in regulating PMN transmigration. Given that CD47 expression is upregulated in IBD and is associated with enhanced PMN migration, further studies examining CD47 and SIRPs are necessary in order to develop pharmacological inhibitors to manipulate PMN transepithelial migration. Indeed, phage panning techniques have been used to develop a specific blocking peptide that mimics a CD47 epitope that binds SIRPα[41] and inhibits PMN transepithelial migration. Such approaches may be useful for designing a template for anti-inflammatory agents.

Postadhesive Interactions Between PMNs and Epithelial Cells Contribute to Pathophysiology

After PMNs have negotiated the apical junctional complex, they reach the apical epithelial plasma membrane and lumen of the intestine. In the event of microbial invasion, apical PMNs act to destroy luminal pathogens by activating an NADPH oxidase that leads to the release of toxic oxygen radicals. Consequently, excessive release of these free oxygen radicals associated with high-density PMN mucosal infiltration leads to extensive tissue damage observed in many inflammatory diseases including IBD. Furthermore, apical PMNs also release 5'-AMP, which is converted to adenosine by epithelial CD73.[42,43] Adenosine binds to epithelial A2b receptors, which, in turn, activates chloride secretion that acts to flush out offending agents.[42,43]

In active IBD, high numbers of PMNs are frequently observed to be associated with the apical surface of the epithelium, and it is hypothesized that the deposition of autoantibodies on the apical surfaces of the epithelium under inflammatory conditions may partly explain this phenomenon. In active episodes of ulcerative colitis, autoantibodies against epithelial cells and complement products have been observed to decorate the apical surfaces of epithelial cells.[44] To emulate this phenomenon, past studies have shown that a specific immunoglobulin G1 raised against T84 epithelial cell membranes retains PMNs at the apical surface through Fc-mediated interactions.[45] In addition, ICAM-1 is found to be expressed only at the apical surfaces of epithelial cells under inflammatory conditions and this may serve to retain PMNs via adhesive interactions with CD11b/CD18.[46,47] This adhesive mechanism may play a particularly important role since similar shear fluid forces seen in the vasculature come into effect again in the gut lumen. Eliminating the high numbers of PMNs retained at the apical surfaces of the epithelium in active cases of IBD appears to have therapeutic potential. However, more studies need to be done to test this hypothesis.

While apically expressed ICAM-1 may be involved in retention of PMNs, CD55 (decay-accelerating factor, DAF) has been implicated as an antiadhesive ligand that promotes release of PMNs from the apical surface of the epithelium.[48,49] Although CD97, expressed by a variety of leukocytes, has been shown to bind CD55,[50–52] this interaction does not seem to be the case between PMNs and epithelial cells.[49] Currently, the PMN counterreceptor to CD55 remains to be identified, and the PMN counterreceptor to CD55 may prove to be a ligand other than CD97. To date, several microbial antigens derived from RNA viruses and bacteria have been shown to bind CD55,[53] thus suggesting a possible role for targeting leukocytic and epithelial CD55 to prevent microbial infection. CD55 is also highly expressed in leukocytes including PMNs,[53] but the role of PMN-expressed CD55 during transepithelial migration has yet to be established. Nevertheless, mucosal epithelial surfaces are readily available for topical administration of therapeutic agents and this may prove to be beneficial for decreasing the numbers of apical PMNs that parallel the degree of patients' symptoms during acute inflammation. Indeed, delivery of peptide mimetics may help control pathophysiological changes by reducing epithelial-associated PMNs.[49]

CONCLUSIONS

In this review, we have highlighted features of PMN migration across mucosal epithelia and how each distinct step can be specifically targeted for the development of therapeutic agents. PMN transepithelial migration occurs in a polarized fashion that calls for specific events associated with its microenvironment. Initial contact with the basolateral aspect of the epithelium leads to a rapid and reversible opening of the apical junctional complex that is CD11b/CD18-independent. The temporary breakdown in epithelial barrier function may facilitate PMN transmigration and prevent irreversible damage to the epithelium. Concurrently, PMNs adhere to the basolateral membranes via interactions between CD11b/CD18 and yet unidentified epithelial fucosylated glycoproteins. Cell signaling events mediated by CD47-SIRPα and SIRPβ activation regulate PMN transmigration. Adhesive interactions with apical junctional components enable the PMNs to crawl across the epithelium. Migrating PMNs encounter the desmosomes, where they bind to JAM-C via CD11b/CD18. Then they traverse the tight junctions by binding to CAR via JAML. Transmigrated PMNs are retained at the apical surface by Fc- and ICAM-1-mediated adhesive events, where they undergo antimicrobial activities that may promote mucosal defense or result in detrimental tissue damage. More studies are warranted to further uncover the multifaceted process associated with PMN transepithelial migration. Small-compound inhibitors of these interactions may thus prove to have considerable therapeutic applications for IBD. The development of targeted therapy may serve to fine-tune PMN transepithelial migration and facilitate the management of inflammatory disorders.

ACKNOWLEDGMENTS

This work was supported, in part by NIH Grants DK61379, DK72564, HL72124 (to C. A. Parkos), a grant from the NIH Digestive Diseases Research Development Center (DK64399), and a fellowship from the Canadian Association of Gastroenterology, Canadian Institutes of Health Research, and Axcan Pharma Inc. (to A. C. Chin).

REFERENCES

1. LOFTUS, E.V. JR. & W.J. SANDBORN. 2002. Epidemiology of inflammatory bowel disease. Gastroenterol. Clin. North Am. **31:** 1–20.
2. IRVINE, E.J. & J.K. MARSHALL. 2000. Increased intestinal permeability precedes the onset of Crohn's disease in a subject with familial risk. Gastroenterology **119:** 1740–1744.
3. SCHMITZ, H. *et al.* 1999. Altered tight junction structure contributes to the impaired epithelial barrier function in ulcerative colitis. Gastroenterology **116:** 301–309.

4. KUMAR, N.B., T.T. NOSTRANT & H.D. APPELMAN. 1982. The histopathologic spectrum of acute self-limited colitis (acute infectious-type colitis). Am. J. Surg. Pathol. **6:** 523–529.
5. KUCHARZIK, T. *et al.* 2005. Acute induction of human IL-8 production by intestinal epithelium triggers neutrophil infiltration without mucosal injury. Gut **54:** 1565–1572.
6. NASH, S., J. STAFFORD & J.L. MADARA. 1987. Effects of polymorphonuclear leukocyte transmigration on barrier function of cultured intestinal epithelial monolayers. J. Clin. Invest. **80:** 1104–1113.
7. PARKOS, C.A. *et al.* 1991. Neutrophil migration across a cultured intestinal epithelium: dependence on a CD11b/CD18-mediated event and enhanced efficiency in the physiologic direction. J. Clin. Invest. **88:** 1605–1612.
8. PARKOS, C.A., S.P. COLGAN & J.L. MADARA. 1994. Interactions of neutrophils with epithelial cells: lessons from the intestine. J. Am. Soc. Nephrol. **5:** 138–152.
9. NUSRAT, A. *et al.* 1997. Neutrophil migration across model intestinal epithelia: monolayer disruption and subsequent events in epithelial repair. Gastroenterology **113:** 1489–1500.
10. EDENS, H.A. *et al.* 2002. Neutrophil transepithelial migration: evidence for sequential, contact-dependent signaling events and enhanced paracellular permeability independent of transjunctional migration. J. Immunol. **169:** 476–486.
11. PARSONS, P.E. *et al.* 1987. The effect of neutrophil migration and prolonged neutrophil contact on epithelial permeability. Am. J. Pathol. **129:** 302–312.
12. COLGAN, S.P. *et al.* 1995. Receptors involved in carbohydrate binding modulate intestinal epithelial-neutrophil interactions. J. Biol. Chem. **270:** 10531–10539.
13. ZEN, K. *et al.* 2002. CD11b/CD18-dependent interactions of neutrophils with intestinal epithelium are mediated by fucosylated proteoglycans. J. Immunol. **169:** 5270–5278.
14. MARTIN-PADURA, I. *et al.* 1998. Junctional adhesion molecule, a novel member of the immunoglobulin superfamily that distributes at intercellular junctions and modulates monocyte transmigration. J. Cell. Biol. **142:** 117–127.
15. DEL MASCHIO, A. *et al.* 1999. Leukocyte recruitment in the cerebrospinal fluid of mice with experimental meningitis is inhibited by an antibody to junctional adhesion molecule (JAM). J. Exp. Med. **190:** 1351–1356.
16. JOHNSON-LEGER, C.A. *et al.* 2002. Junctional adhesion molecule-2 (JAM-2) promotes lymphocyte transendothelial migration. Blood **100:** 2479–2486.
17. OSTERMANN, G. *et al.* 2002. JAM-1 is a ligand of the beta(2) integrin LFA-1 involved in transendothelial migration of leukocytes. Nat. Immunol. **3:** 151–158.
18. ZEN, K. *et al.* 2004. JAM-C is a component of desmosomes and a ligand for CD11b/CD18-mediated neutrophil transepithelial migration. Mol. Biol. Cell. **15:** 3926–3937.
19. ZEN, K. *et al.* 2005. Neutrophil migration across tight junctions is mediated by adhesive interactions between epithelial coxsackie and adenovirus receptor and a junctional adhesion molecule-like protein on neutrophils. Mol. Biol. Cell. **16:** 2694–2703.
20. BAZZONI, G. 2003. The JAM family of junctional adhesion molecules. Curr. Opin. Cell. Biol. **15:** 525–530.
21. MOOG-LUTZ, C. *et al.* 2003. JAML, a novel protein with characteristics of a junctional adhesion molecule, is induced during differentiation of myeloid leukemia cells. Blood **102:** 3371–3378.

22. LIU, Y. *et al.* 2000. Human junction adhesion molecule regulates tight junction resealing in epithelia. J. Cell. Sci. **113(Pt 13):** 2363–2374.
23. BAZZONI, G. *et al.* 2005. Expression of junctional adhesion molecule-A prevents spontaneous and random motility. J. Cell. Sci. **118:** 623–632.
24. KHANDOGA, A. *et al.* 2005. Junctional adhesion molecule-A deficiency increases hepatic ischemia-reperfusion injury despite reduction of neutrophil transendothelial migration. Blood **106:** 725–733.
25. CORADA, M. *et al.* 2005. Junctional adhesion molecule-A-deficient polymorphonuclear cells show reduced diapedesis in peritonitis and heart ischemia–reperfusion injury. Proc. Natl. Acad. Sci. USA **102:** 10634–10639.
26. SHAW, S.K. *et al.* 2001. Reduced expression of junctional adhesion molecule and platelet/endothelial cell adhesion molecule-1 (CD31) at human vascular endothelial junctions by cytokines tumor necrosis factor-alpha plus interferon-gamma does not reduce leukocyte transmigration under flow. Am. J. Pathol. **159:** 2281–2291.
27. BAZZONI, G. *et al.* 2000. Homophilic interaction of junctional adhesion molecule. J. Biol. Chem. **275:** 30970–30976.
28. MANDELL, K.J., I.C. MCCALL & C.A. PARKOS. 2004. Involvement of the junctional adhesion molecule-1 (JAM1) homodimer interface in regulation of epithelial barrier function. J. Biol. Chem. **279:** 16254–16262.
29. MANDELL, K.J. *et al.* 2005. Junctional adhesion molecule 1 regulates epithelial cell morphology through effects on beta1 integrins and Rap1 activity. J. Biol. Chem. **280:** 11665–11674.
30. MARTINEZ-ESTRADA, O.M. *et al.* 2001. Association of junctional adhesion molecule with calcium/calmodulin-dependent serine protein kinase (CASK/LIN-2) in human epithelial caco-2 cells. J. Biol. Chem. **276:** 9291–9296.
31. SANTOSO, S. *et al.* 2002. The junctional adhesion molecule 3 (JAM-3) on human platelets is a counterreceptor for the leukocyte integrin Mac-1. J. Exp. Med. **196:** 679–691.
32. AURRAND-LIONS, M. *et al.* 2005. Junctional adhesion molecule-C regulates the early influx of leukocytes into tissues during inflammation. J. Immunol. **174:** 6406–6415.
33. DORNER, A.A. *et al.* 2005. Coxsackievirus-adenovirus receptor (CAR) is essential for early embryonic cardiac development. J. Cell. Sci. **118:** 3509–3521.
34. REINHOLD, M.I. *et al.* 1995. In vivo expression of alternatively spliced forms of integrin-associated protein (CD47). J. Cell. Sci. **108(Pt 11):** 3419–3425.
35. COOPER, D. *et al.* 1995. Transendothelial migration of neutrophils involves integrin-associated protein (CD47). Proc. Natl. Acad. Sci. USA **92:** 3978–3982.
36. PARKOS, C.A. *et al.* 1996. CD47 mediates post-adhesive events required for neutrophil migration across polarized intestinal epithelia. J. Cell. Biol. **132:** 437–450.
37. LIU, Y. *et al.* 2001. The role of CD47 in neutrophil transmigration. Increased rate of migration correlates with increased cell surface expression of CD47. J. Biol. Chem. **276:** 40156–40166.
38. BROWN, E.J. & W.A. FRAZIER. 2001. Integrin-associated protein (CD47) and its ligands. Trends Cell. Biol. **11:** 130–135.
39. LIU, Y. *et al.* 2002. Signal regulatory protein (SIRPalpha), a cellular ligand for CD47, regulates neutrophil transmigration. J. Biol. Chem. **277:** 10028–10036.

40. LIU, Y. *et al.* 2005. SIRPbeta 1 is expressed as a disulfide-linked homodimer in leukocytes and positively regulates neutrophil transepithelial migration. J. Biol. Chem. **280:** 36132–36140.
41. LIU, Y. *et al.* 2004. Peptide-mediated inhibition of neutrophil transmigration by blocking CD47 interactions with signal regulatory protein alpha. J. Immunol. **172:** 2578–2585.
42. COLGAN, S.P. *et al.* 1993. Lipoxin A4 modulates transmigration of human neutrophils across intestinal epithelial monolayers. J. Clin. Invest. **92:** 75–82.
43. STROHMEIER, G.R. *et al.* 1997. Surface expression, polarization, and functional significance of CD73 in human intestinal epithelia. J. Clin. Invest. **99:** 2588–2601.
44. HALSTENSEN, T.S. *et al.* 1990. Epithelial deposition of immunoglobulin G1 and activated complement (C3b and terminal complement complex) in ulcerative colitis. Gastroenterology **98:** 1264–1271.
45. REAVES, T.A. *et al.* 2001. Neutrophil transepithelial migration: regulation at the apical epithelial surface by Fc-mediated events. Am. J. Physiol. Gastrointest. Liver Physiol. **280:** G746–G754.
46. PARKOS, C.A. *et al.* 1996. Expression and polarization of intercellular adhesion molecule-1 on human intestinal epithelia: consequences for CD11b/CD18-mediated interactions with neutrophils. Mol. Med. **2:** 489–505.
47. HUANG, G.T. *et al.* 1996. Infection of human intestinal epithelial cells with invasive bacteria upregulates apical intercellular adhesion molecule-1 (ICAM)-1 expression and neutrophil adhesion. J. Clin. Invest. **98:** 572–583.
48. KING, P.D. *et al.* 1990. The role of CD44, CD45, CD45RO, CD46 and CD55 as potential anti-adhesion molecules involved in the binding of human tonsillar T cells to phorbol 12-myristate 13-acetate-differentiated U-937 cells. Eur. J. Immunol. **20:** 363–368.
49. LAWRENCE, D.W. *et al.* 2003. Antiadhesive role of apical decay-accelerating factor (CD55) in human neutrophil transmigration across mucosal epithelia. J. Exp. Med. **198:** 999–1010.
50. HAMANN, J. *et al.* 1996. The seven-span transmembrane receptor CD97 has a cellular ligand (CD55, DAF). J. Exp. Med. **184:** 1185–1189.
51. HAMANN, J. *et al.* 1998. Characterization of the CD55 (DAF)-binding site on the seven-span transmembrane receptor CD97. Eur. J. Immunol. **28:** 1701–1707.
52. QIAN, Y.M. *et al.* 1999. Structural characterization of mouse CD97 and study of its specific interaction with the murine decay-accelerating factor (DAF, CD55). Immunology **98:** 303–311.
53. LEA, S. 2002. Interactions of CD55 with non-complement ligands. Biochem. Soc. Trans. **30:** 1014–1019.

Disrupted Barrier Function through Epithelial Cell Apoptosis

JOERG-DIETER SCHULZKE,[a] CHRISTIAN BOJARSKI,[a]
SEBASTIAN ZEISSIG,[a,b] FRANK HELLER,[a] ALFRED H. GITTER,[b]
AND MICHAEL FROMM[b]

[a]Department of Gastroenterology, Infectious Diseases and Rheumatology,
Campus Benjamin Franklin, Charité, Berlin, Germany

[b]Department of Clinical Physiology, Campus Benjamin Franklin, Charité,
Berlin, Germany

ABSTRACT: Epithelial barrier function is determined by trans- and paracellular permeabilities, the latter of which is mainly influenced by tight
junctions (TJs) and apoptotic leaks within the epithelium. The present
article aims to present experimental evidence for a functional role of
epithelial apoptoses by means of cell culture models as well as in tissues
from patients with inflammatory bowel disease. It is shown that epithelial
apoptoses are sites of elevated conductance within the intestinal epithelium and that proinflammatory cytokines like TNF-α upregulate both
the apoptotic rate and single apoptotic conductivity, making cytokine-
induced apoptosis functionally far more relevant than is spontaneous
apoptosis. In ulcerative colitis and Crohn's disease (CD), but not in collagenous colitis, apoptotic rates are increased to about 5%, in mild-to-
moderately inflamed colon specimens, where as the control apoptotic rate
is about 2%. Thus, epithelial apoptoses lead to a loss of ions and water into
the intestinal lumen, causing leak flux diarrhea and enabling small antigens of <4,000 Da in the intestinal lumen to enter the intestinal mucosa,
thereby perpetuating inflammatory responses. In addition to TNF-α, interleukin (IL)-13 is an important inductor of epithelial apoptosis in Th2
immune responses. Therapeutically, TNF-α-antibodies (infliximab) can
restore barrier function in Crohn's disease by downregulating epithelial
apoptoses, while epithelial TJs are unaffected.

KEYWORDS: apoptosis; barrier function; Crohn's disease; diarrhea;
interferon-γ; interleukin-13; tight junctions; TNF-α; ulcerative colitis

Address for correspondence: Dr. Joerg D. Schulzke, Charité, Campus Benjamin Franklin, Medizinische Klinik I, Gastroenterology, Infectious Diseases and Rheumatology, Department of Medical
Engineering, University of Applied Sciences, Jena, 12200 Berlin, Germany. Voice: +49-30-8445-2666;
fax: +49-30-8445-4239.
e-mail: Joerg.Schulzke@Charite.De

Ann. N.Y. Acad. Sci. 1072: 288–299 (2006). © 2006 New York Academy of Sciences.
doi: 10.1196/annals.1326.027

INTRODUCTION

The structure of the intestinal mucosa is maintained by a sensitive balance between the (apoptotic) loss of cells and cell regeneration. This balance is disturbed in the inflamed intestine where the epithelium is exposed to several toxins and proinflammatory cytokines with the potential to induce necrosis and apoptosis. In chronic inflammatory bowel disease (IBD), the frequency of epithelial apoptosis is considerably increased, which is thought to contribute to the impairment of intestinal barrier function.[12] Among the cytokines that have been identified to induce apoptosis in intestinal epithelia, tumor necrosis factor-α (TNF-α) has a central role, which was first described in renal LLC-PK1 cells by Mullin and coworkers.[8] Induction of apoptosis by TNF-α is accompanied by alteration of tight junction (TJ) structure.[10] Therefore, conventional measurements of the overall transmural, respectively, transepithelial, electrical resistance (R^t, "TEER"), or its reciprocal, overall transepithelial conductivity (G^t), alone cannot resolve whether barrier impairments are caused by apoptosis. However, by measuring the spatial distribution of transepithelial conductivity with the *conductance scanning technique* it is possible to get more insight into the functional meaning of epithelial apoptoses. As a selective tool to upregulate apoptotic rate, the topoisomerase I-inhibitor, camptothecin, can be used in intestinal cell culture models, which is a potent inductor of apoptosis in epithelial cell lines.[11]

METHODS

Colon Specimens

Inflamed colonic specimens were analyzed from patients with ulcerative colitis with mild-to-moderate macroscopic disease activity. Control specimens were taken from patients undergoing resection of sigmoidal or rectal cancer. Specimens were used after removal of the muscularis propria and were mounted in Ussing chambers as described earlier.[9]

HT-29/B6 Cells

Experiments were performed on HT-29/B6 monolayers,[7] which grow as highly differentiated polarized monolayers. They were routinely cultured in 25-cm^2 culture flasks in RPMI 1640 (Biochrom, Berlin, Germany) containing 2% stabilized L-glutamine and supplemented with 10% FCS at 37°C in an atmosphere of 95% O_2 and 5% CO_2. For electrophysiological measurements, cells were seeded on Millicell PCF filters (effective area 0.6 cm^2, Millipore) with an average concentration of 7×10^5 cells/cm^2. Three filters were placed together into one conventional culture dish (OD, 60 mm) filled with 10 mL of culture medium. Confluence of the monolayers was reached after 7 days.

Ussing Experiments

Ussing-type experiments on human colon specimens were performed using a computer-controlled voltage clamp device (CVC 6, Fiebig, Berlin, Germany) as described previously.[9] Short-circuit current (I_{SC}), open-circuit transepithelial voltage, and transepithelial resistance were recorded on hard disk. Exposed tissue area was 0.28 cm^2. I_{SC} values were corrected for bath resistance. All experiments were performed in the presence of amiloride (10^{-4} M) in order to block electrogenic Na$^+$ absorption, which could have been elicited during anesthesia by elevated plasma aldosterone levels.

In HT-29/B6 cell monolayers, as a measure of epithelial ion permeability, the overall electrical resistance (R^t, $\Omega \cdot cm^2$) of the monolayers was determined in Ussing chambers specially designed for the insertion of Millicell filters.[7] Unidirectional tracer flux measurements from mucosa-to-serosa were performed under short-circuit conditions with ^{3}H-lactulose or ^{3}H-polyethylene glycol (PEG) 4000. Here, the medium also contained nonlabeled tracer molecules, 20 mmol·L^{-1} lactulose or 1 mmol·L^{-1} PEG 4000, respectively. Four 15-min flux periods were analyzed after the addition of camptothecin. Samples were taken from the mucosal and serosal side, and radioactivity was counted by a Tri-Carb 2100TR Liquid Scintillation Analyzer (Packard, Meriden, CT, USA). Fluxes were calculated with the standard formula described previously.[1]

Alternating Current (AC) Impedance Analysis

Impedance analysis allows determination of epithelial (R^e) and subepithelial (R^{sub}) portion of the total wall resistance (R^t).[9] In brief: the voltage responses after transepithelial application of 35 μA/cm^2 eff. sine wave AC of 48 discrete frequencies in a range from 1 to 65 kHz were detected by phase-sensitive amplifiers (Model 1250 Frequency Response Analyzer and Model 1286 Electrochemical Interface; Solartron Schlumberger, Farnborough, Hampshire, UK). Complex impedance values were calculated after correction for the bath resistance and the frequency behavior of the measuring setup. Then, for each tissue the impedance locus was plotted in a Nyquist diagram and a circle segment was fitted by least-squares analysis. From this circle segment, three variables of an electrical equivalent circuit were obtained that consisted of a resistor and a capacitor in parallel representing the epithelium and a resistor in series to this unit representing the subepithelium. On account of the frequency-dependent electrical characteristics of the capacitor, total wall resistance (R^t) is obtained at low frequencies, whereas the subepithelial resistance (R^{sub}) is obtained by high frequencies. The epithelial resistance (R^e) was obtained from $R^e = R^t - R^{sub}$.

Conductance Scanning

This method allows determination of the spatial distribution of conductivity in flat epithelia.[4] The monolayers were mounted horizontally between the two half-chambers of the conductance scanning apparatus. The cells were viewed through a 40× water immersion object lens (Zeiss, Oberkochen, Germany). Alternating electric current (300 μAcm^2, 24 Hz) was clamped across the epithelium and the electrical field generated in the mucosal bath solution was measured with a probe at a constant distance of 25 m above the epithelial surface. The probe was positioned in the center of the microscope's visual field by means of a mechanical micromanipulator. The probe consisted of a pair of microelectrodes that were connected to a differential amplifier and an AC bridge system with synchronous demodulation. The position of the probe in relation to the cells was adjusted by moving the experimental chamber with a remote-controlled electrically driven micromanipulator (Model 5171, Eppendorf, Hamburg, Germany). The distance to the surface was determined by lifting the epithelium until it barely touched the probe, which induced characteristic disturbance in the electric signal. The local current density was calculated from the electrical field measured with the probe and the specific resistivity of the bath solution. The spatial distribution of current density was even above nonapoptotic areas far from apoptoses, but peaked above apoptoses. Nonapoptotic conductivity was determined from the division of current density above nonapoptotic areas by the transepithelial voltage. Since the current density rose toward apoptoses, the current associated with a single apoptosis was computed by spatial integration of the current density exceeding the nonapoptotic current density. From this current and the transepithelial voltage, apoptotic conductance was determined. The arithmetic mean of conductances associated with apoptosis, multiplied by the density of apoptoses, yielded apoptotic conductivity. In this manner, the overall epithelial conductivity was differentiated into the nonapoptotic epithelial conductivity, which is the conductivity of homogeneous nonapoptotic areas of the epithelium, and the apoptotic conductivity, which is the conductivity of all apoptoses in the area investigated. The corresponding density of apoptoses was counted using conventional light microscopy in four monolayers.

Statistical Analysis

Results are given as means ± SEM. Significance was tested by means of the two-tailed Student's *t*-test. $P < 0.05$ was considered significant.

RESULTS

Single-Cell Apoptosis

The apparent local conductivity, that is, local current density divided by transepithelial voltage, is shown in a typical recording along a line between the apoptotic cell and a nonapoptotic area (FIG. 1). Because the current density was measured 25 μm above the mucosal surface, the current associated with apoptosis was determined by integration of the bell-shaped distribution of the local transepithelial current. Thus, our recordings differentiated between (*a*) the current through areas of nonapoptotic cells, exhibiting a planar spatial distribution, and (*b*) the current associated with sites of apoptosis, exhibiting a bell-shaped distribution forming a maximum above the apoptotic cell. The

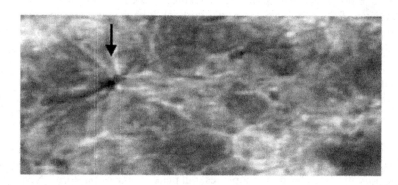

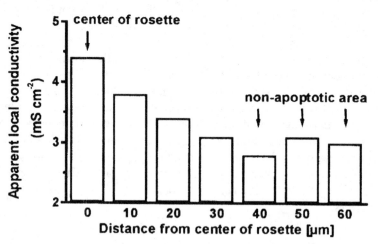

FIGURE 1. Apparent local conductivity (local current density measured with the mobile probe, divided by the transepithelial voltage) along a line between an apoptosis (*arrow*) and a nonapoptotic area with homogeneous conductivity. HT-29/B6 cells were treated for 48 h with 20 μg/ mL camptothecin.[1]

spatial distribution of epithelial conductivity away from apoptotic rosettes was even, but the conductivity rose to peaks of different magnitude in the rosettes' centers. As the first central finding, there was a large increase in local conductivity in an apoptotic site compared to nonapoptotic regions within the same epithelial layer.

Influence of TNF-α on Apoptosis

The overall basic epithelial conductivity, measured in the homogeneous nonapoptotic areas, was 3.1 0.1 mS cm^2, and it increased with TNF-α treatment to 8.1 0.1 mS/cm^2. The conductance associated with single apoptoses was determined by the measurement of the current density along a line between the rosette's center and the area with homogeneous conductivity, integration over the area, division by the transepithelial voltage, and subtraction of basic epithelial conductivity. The histogram (FIG. 2A) shows that under controlled conditions most apoptotic rosettes exhibited conductances below 200 nS. The mean conductance of single apoptoses was 48 nS (range 0–280 nS). With TNF-α, however, most apoptoses showed conductances between 200 and 600 nS and the mean conductance of single apoptoses had increased to 597 nS (range 67–1,542 nS). The contribution of apoptoses to the total epithelial conductivity (FIG. 2 B, shaded bars) was 0.18 mS/cm^2, or 5.5%, under controlled conditions. With TNF-α it increased to 6.57 mS/cm^2, or 45% of the total epithelial conductivity.[4]

Epithelial Apoptoses and Mucosal Barrier Function in Ulcerative Colitis Patients

The data are presented in TABLE 2. R^e as obtained by transmural AC impedance analysis was dramatically decreased, indicating impaired epithelial barrier function. This was, on the one hand, due to TJ alterations (data not shown) and, on the other hand, to an increase in the epithelial apoptotic rate as measured in terminal deoxynucleotidyl transferase-mediated deoxyuridine triphosphate nick-end labeling (TUNEL)- and DAPI-stained thin sections from mild-to-moderately inflamed ulcerative colitis specimens (data not shown). A similar increase in apoptotic rate to about 5% was also observed in mild-to-moderately inflamed Crohn's disease (CD) specimens (FIG. 3).

Functional Consequences of Epithelial Apoptoses as Indicated by Flux and Conductance Scanning Measurements after Exposure of HT-29/B6 Monolayers to Camptothecin

Camptothecin increased the mucosa-to-serosa fluxes of paracellular tracer molecules concomitant with the increase in ion permeability (TABLE 1). The

(A)

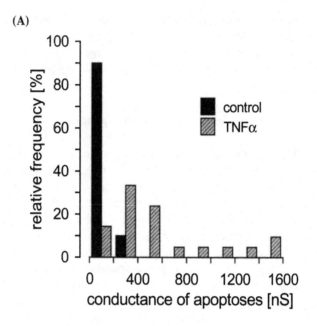

(B)

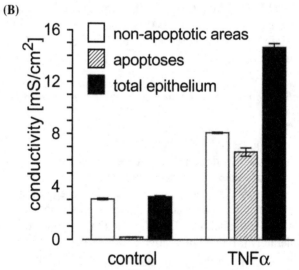

FIGURE 2. (A) Relative frequency of single apoptoses with different conductances as determined under controlled conditions and with TNF-α preincubation. The right shift of the histogram with TNF-α indicates the occurrence of apoptoses with high conductance. With TNF-α the apoptotic rate increased threefold (data not shown). **(B)** Contribution of apoptoses and of nonapoptotic area to the overall tissue conductivity. In controls, apoptoses contributed 5.5% to total conductivity. With TNF-α exposure basic epithelial conductivity of nonapoptotic areas increased 2.6-fold, while that of apoptoses increased by a factor of 37. Hence, with TNF-α exposure, apoptoses contributed 45% to the overall epithelial conductivity.[4]

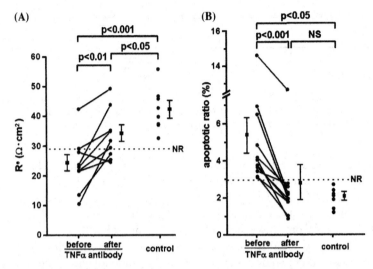

FIGURE 3. Effect of TNF-α-antibody therapy on epithelial barrier function and apoptoses in CD. **(A)** R^e obtained by transmural impedance analysis of control ($n = 8$) and CD ($n = 9$) before and 2 weeks after TNF-α antibody therapy. **(B)** Apoptotic ratio of controls ($n = 8$) and CD patients ($n = 11$) before and 2 weeks after infliximab (5 mg/kg body weight) treatment determined in TUNEL-stained sections. Individual data are given as means ± SEM. Upper limit of normal range (NR) as obtained from mean of control ± 2 SD is indicated by the *dotted line* (Zeissig *et al.*, 2004).

flux of ^{3}H-lactulose increased 2.6-fold in cells treated with 20 μg/mL^1 camptothecin for 48 h. This indicates an increased permeability in the paracellular route. By contrast, the flux of ^{3}H-PEG 4000 remained unchanged (TABLE 1). The I_{sc} was not changed by the addition of camptothecin (-4.67 ± 0.05 vs. -6.10 ± 2.08 μA/cm^2 in control, n. s., $n = 8$), militating against an increase in transcellular conductivity due to activation of active transport sites.

In these experiments, the overall epithelial conductivity doubled after treatment with 20 μg/mL^1 camptothecin. This was not due to an increase in non-apoptotic epithelial conductivity, which was not altered by the addition of

TABLE 1. Influence of epithelial apoptosis on barrier function

	R^t Ω/cm^2	$J_{lactulose}^{ms}$ nmol/h^1/cm^2	$J_{PEG4000}^{ms}$ nmol/h^1/cm^2
Control	457 ± 22	86 ± 4	10.8 ± 1.0
Camptothecin	210 ± 41	205 ± 4	10.5 ± 1.0
P	<0.001	<0.001	n.s.

Transmural electrical resistance (R^t) and unidirectional mucosa-to-serosa ^{3}H-labeled tracer fluxes in HT-29/B6 cell monolayers treated with 20 μg/mL camptothecin for 48 h versus controls. Data represent mean ± SEM.

TABLE 2. Epithelial barrier function in inflammatory bowel disease

	R^e	n
Control	$95 \pm 5 \ \Omega/cm^2$	10
Ulcerative colitis	$20 \pm 3 \ \Omega/cm^2$	11
P	<0.001	

R^e as obtained by transmural AC impedance analysis on mild-to-moderately inflamed ulcerative colitis specimens and controls. Data represent mean $\pm$ SEM.

camptothecin (2.53 ± 0.35 vs. 3.06 ± 0.07 mS/cm^2, n.s., $n = 11$), but was the result of an increase in apoptotic conductivity that increased 22-fold (from 0.17 ± 0.02 to 3.84 ± 1.03 mS/cm^2, $P < 0.01$, $n = 11$). This increase in apoptotic conductivity was caused, on the one hand, by a higher density of apoptoses, which increased from 24.4 ± 4.6 to 103.0 ± 9.2 mm^2 ($P < 0.01$, $n = 4$), and, on the other hand, by a higher single apoptosis conductance, which was dramatically increased compared to that in untreated cell monolayers (720 ± 230 nS vs. 48 ± 19 nS, $P < 0.01$, $n = 11$).[1]

Influence of TNF-α Antibody Therapy on the Mucosa in CD

The data are shown in FIGURE 3A. In control, R^e was 42 ± 3 Ω/cm^2 ($n = 8$). In CD before treatment, R^e was lower than in control (24 ± 3 Ω/cm^2; $n = 9$; $P < 0.001$ vs. control). TNF-α antibody therapy increased R^e to 34 ± 3 Ω/cm^2 ($P < 0.01$ when compared to R^e before therapy). Two weeks after TNF-α antibody therapy, six of nine patients (67%) achieved an R^e within the normal range (as defined by mean of control ± 2 SD to be 29 to 56 Ω/cm^2 ($n = 8$)).

Thin sections of sigmoid colon from 8 controls and from 11 CD patients before and 2 weeks after infliximab were stained with TUNEL. Apoptotic ratio was determined as a percentage of apoptotic enterocytes. Numerical results from TUNEL-stained sections are shown in FIGURE 3B. There was a higher apoptotic ratio in CD patients ($5.3 \pm 1.0\%$; $n = 11$) compared to controls ($2.1 \pm 0.2\%$; $n = 8$; $P < 0.05$). After therapy, apoptotic ratio was decreased to $2.9 \pm 1.0\%$ in CD ($n = 11$; $P < 0.001$). Thus, all CD patients had an apoptotic ratio above the normal range (as defined by mean of control ± 2 SD to be

TABLE 3. Effect of pro-inflammatory cytokines on epithelial apoptosis

	Control	Interferon-γ (100 U/L)	IL-13 (10 ng/mL)
Apoptotic rate	$1.0 \pm 0.5\%$ ($n = 6$)	$1.1 \pm 0.5\%$ ($n = 6$)	$5.6 \pm 0.9\%$ ($n = 6$)
P		n.s. versus control	< 0.001 versus control

Epithelial cell apoptosis is induced by IL-13. Apoptosis of HT-29/B6 monolayers stained with TUNEL. Apoptotic rate is the percentage of TUNEL-positive cells per total counted cells. Data represent mean $\pm$ SEM. Significance was tested versus untreated control monolayers.

1.2 to 3.0 ($n = 8$)) before therapy. Two weeks after TNF-α antibody therapy, 10 of 11 (91%) reached an apoptotic ratio within the normal range.[13]

Interleukin (IL)-13 Upregulates Epithelial Apoptoses

The effect of IL-13 on epithelial apoptosis was investigated in HT-29/B6 cell monolayers. The data are shown in TABLE 3. Apoptotic ratios were determined in control, IL-13, and interferon-γ-treated cells after 48-h incubation with either cytokine. The number of apoptotic cells was determined after TUNEL staining by manual counting in monolayers. We found that control monolayers exhibited a rate of $1.0 \pm 0.5\%$ ($n = 6$) apoptotic cells, whereas after IL-13 treatment with 10 ng/mL, apoptotic rate was increased to $5.6 \pm 0.9\%$ ($n = 6$). In comparison, interferon-γ did not induce apoptosis.[5]

DISCUSSION

There has been a long debate on the functional role of epithelial apoptosis. Many authors argue that single-cell apoptosis can be a rather regular and more or less sealed process that occurs without disruption of the epithelial permeability barrier.[6] This "perfect seal" dogma, based on circumstantial morphological evidence, is disproven by our own data[1,4]) and a recent careful study of Bruewer *et al.*[2] only seemingly supports it. Bruewer *et al.*[2] showed that caspase inhibition by ZVAD blocked apoptosis in interferon-γ/TNF-α–exposed T84 monolayers, but did not prevent the decrease in electrical resistance. However, the magnitude of the resistance reduction from 1,800 to about 200 Ω/cm^2 after 72 h of cytokine exposure indicates an almost complete breakdown of intestinal barrier function that could have superposed the change in apoptotic conductivity.

This means that other barrier features, such as induction of necrosis or TJ alterations, may have predominated in the functional response to caspase inhibition in T84 cells. Indeed, the interpretation of Bruewer and coworkers themselves in their article was that it cannot be ruled out that apoptoses represent conductive spots.

Thus, we address the question to what extent epithelial apoptoses are functionally relevant by raising four lines of arguments. As a first and undisputable finding, conductance scanning revealed that epithelial apoptoses represent "hot spots" of conductance. Second, single-cell apoptotic conductivity was much more pronounced when induced by the proinflammatory cytokine TNF-α than observed in case of spontaneous apoptotic events. Thus, TNF-α increased both, apoptotic frequency and the conductivity of single apoptoses. The contribution of apoptoses to the total epithelial conductivity was 5.5% under controlled conditions. With TNF-α it increased to 45% of the total epithelial conductivity.

Thus, the TNF-α-induced conductance increase was based on 44% degradation of TJs in nonapoptotic areas and on 56% apoptosis-related conductivity changes, the latter indicating pronounced local barrier defects.

As the third relevant set of data, the apoptotic rate was found to be induced to a level of about 4–5% in mild-to-moderately inflamed colon mucosa in ulcerative colitis as well as in CD. This had a significant effect on epithelial barrier function as indicated by induction of apoptosis in HT-29/B6 cell monolayers and the therapeutic effect of TNF-α antibodies in CD. In contrast to ulcerative colitis and CD, the apoptotic rate was not elevated in collagenous colitis.[3]

In order to investigate which size of molecule becomes permeant after apoptosis induction, epithelial apoptosis was upregulated by the topoisomerase-1 inhibitor, camptothecin. The increase in overall conductivity was caused by increases in the number as well as the mean conductance associated with single apoptoses.[1] Nonapoptotic conductivity did not change after addition of camptothecin. In contrast, TNF-α increased also the nonapoptotic conductivity.[4] This was explained by an effect of TNF-α on the TJs of nonapoptotic epithelium demonstrated by freeze-fracture electron microscopy.[9] Hence, unlike TNF-α, camptothecin is a selective tool for the induction of apoptosis. Our results showing that barrier defects at the site of apoptosis lead to an increase in epithelial conductivity corroborate the hypothesis that apoptosis causes barrier dysfunction in intestinal epithelia.

The present findings show camptothecin to affect apoptosis with a concomitant increase of both conductivity and mucosa-to-serosa fluxes of the paracellular marker ^{3}H-lactulose. In contrast, the flux of PEG 4000 was unchanged after camptothecin exposure. Thus, the size of potentially noxious agents penetrating apoptosis-related leaks in the mucosal barrier to molecules must be smaller than 1.2 nm. Neither bacteria nor viruses can penetrate the leaks caused by apoptosis induced by camptothecin. Because the permeability to molecules with 4,000 Da and more was unaltered, it is unlikely that molecules of a size sufficient to possess antigenic properties can pass through the damaged epithelium. By contrast, smaller molecules, for example, haptens, may penetrate through the apoptotic leaks.[1]

A fourth argument emerged from studies of the functional role of TNF-α-antibodies on the inflamed colonic mucosa of CD patients. A concomitant decrease in apoptotic rate and repair in epithelial barrier function as indicated by R^e measurements was obtained 14 days after TNF-α-antibody therapy. In contrast, epithelial TJ structure was not affected. Also, a similar degree of upregulation in apoptotic rate by camptothecin was necessary in HT-29/B6 cells, in order to achieve a similar relative resistance decrease. Camptothecin induced an increase in apoptotic rate from 2.6% to 5.4%, which caused a 40% reduction in transepithelial resistance in HT-29/B6. This resembles the situation in CD, where infliximab induced a decrease in apoptotic rate from 5.3% to 2.9% with a 43% lower transepithelial resistance before treatment.[13]

As the last important finding in this article, in addition to TNF-α, IL-13 was also identified to be a potent inductor of epithelial apoptosis. Thus, IL-13 has to be seen as the key Th2-effector cytokine in ulcerative colitis, which triggers apoptosis, while TNF-α is predominant in Th1-immune response as in CD.[5]

REFERENCES

1. BOJARSKI, C., A.H. GITTER, K. BENDFELDT, *et al.* 2001. Permeability of human HT-29/B6 colonic epithelium as a function of apoptosis. J. Physiol. **535:** 541–552.

2. BRUEWER, M., A. LUGERING, T. KUCHARZIK, *et al.* 2003. Proinflammatory cytokines disrupt epithelial barrier function by apoptosis-independent mechanisms. J. Immunol. **171:** 6164–6172.

3. BÜRGEL, N., C. BOJARSKI, J. MANKERTZ, *et al.* 2002. Mechanisms of diarrhea in collagenous colitis. Gastroenterology **123:** 433–443.

4. GITTER, A.H., K. BENDFELDT, J.D. SCHULZKE & M. FROMM. 2000. Leaks in the epithelial barrier caused by spontaneous and TNFα-induced single-cell apoptosis. FASEB J. **14:** 1749–1753.

5. HELLER, F., P. FLORIAN, C. BOJARSKI, *et al.* 2005. Interleukin-13 is the key effector Th2 cytokine in ulcerative colitis that affects epithelial tight junctions, apoptosis, and cell restitution. Gastroenterology **129:** 550–564.

6. JONES, B.A. & G.J. GORES. 1997. Physiology and pathophysiology of apoptosis in epithelial cells of the liver, pancreas, and intestine. Am. J. Physiol. **273:** G1176–G1188.

7. KREUSEL, K.M., M. FROMM, J.D. SCHULZKE & U. HEGEL. 1991. Cl-secretion in epithelial monolayers of mucus forming human colon cells (HT-29/B6). Am. J. Physiol. **261:** C574–C582.

8. MULLIN, J.M., K.V. LAUGHLIN, C.W. MARANO, *et al.* 1992. Modulation of tumor necrosis factor-induced increase in renal (LLC-PK1) transepithelial permeability. Am. J. Physiol. **263:** F915–F924.

9. SCHMITZ, H., C. BARMEYER, M. FROMM, *et al.* 1999a. A decrease in tight junction complexity contributes to the severely impaired epithelial barrier function in ulcerative colitis. Gastroenterology **116:** 301–309.

10. SCHMITZ, H., M. FROMM, C.J. BENTZEL, *et al.* 1999b. Tumor necrosis factor-alpha (TNFα) regulates the epithelial barrier in the human intestinal cell line HT-29/B6. J. Cell. Sci. **112:** 137–146.

11. SHIMIZU, T. & Y. POMMIER. 1997. Camptothecin-induced apoptosis in p53-null human leukemia HL60 cells and their isolated nuclei: effects of the protease inhibitors Z-VAD-fmk and dichloroisocoumarin suggest an involvement of both caspases and serine proteases. Leukemia **11:** 1238–1244.

12. STRATER, J., I. WELLISCH, S. RIEDL, *et al.* 1997. CD95 (APO-1/Fas)-mediated apoptosis in colon epithelial cells: a possible role in ulcerative colitis. Gastroenterology **113:** 160–167.

13. ZEISSIG, S., C. BOJARSKI, N. BUERGEL, *et al.* 2004. Downregulation of epithelial apoptosis and barrier repair in active Crohn's disease by tumour necrosis factor α antibody treatment. Gut **53:** 1295–1302.

Growth Factors as Treatment Options for Intestinal Inflammation

BRIAN K. DIECKGRAEFE,[a] JOSHUA R. KORZENIK,[b]
AND SHRIKANT ANANT[c]

[a]Division of Gastroenterology, Siteman Cancer Center, Washington University School of Medicine, St. Louis, Missouri, USA

[b]Inflammatory Bowel Disease Center, Gastrointestinal Unit, Massachusetts General Hospital, Harvard Medical School, Boston, Massachusetts, USA

[c]Department of Medicine, Molecular Biology and Pharmacology, Siteman Cancer Center, Washington University School of Medicine, Saint Louis, Missouri, USA

ABSTRACT: On the basis of several studies that have been completed to date, some growth factors appear promising for the treatment of inflammatory bowel disease: keratinocyte-like growth factor-2 (KGF-2), epidermal growth factor (EGF) enemas used in combination with oral mesalamine, somatropin (human growth hormone), and sargramostim (recombinant human GM–CSF). The results of these studies are highlighted and suggest that new insights into the regulation of intestinal immunity may provide effective synergistic or single-agent treatment alternatives to immunosuppression for inflammatory bowel disease. These data focus on the reparative components of mucosal homeostasis.

KEYWORDS: growth factors; Crohn's disease; inflammatory bowel disease; sargramostim

INTRODUCTION

Growth factors have recently emerged as potential targets for the modulation of intestinal inflammation and repair. At least 30 different growth factors are relevant for the maintenance of gut mucosal integrity, including transforming growth factor β (TGF-β), insulin-like growth factor (IGF), keratinocyte-like growth factor (KGF), epidermal growth factor (EGF), growth hormone (GH), and the colony-stimulating factors (granulocyte–macrophage colony-stimulating factor [GM–CSF], granulocyte colony-stimulating factor [G-CSF],

Address for correspondence: Brian K. Dieckgraefe, M.D., Ph.D., Gastroenterology, Campus Box 8124, 660 South Euclid Avenue, Washington University School of Medicine, St. Louis, MO 63110. Voice: 314-362-8940; fax: 314-362-8959.
e-mail: dieck@im.wustl.edu

Ann. N.Y. Acad. Sci. 1072: 300–306 (2006). © 2006 New York Academy of Sciences.
doi: 10.1196/annals.1326.007

and macrophage colony-stimulating factor [M-CSF]).[1,2] Each of these regulatory peptide families plays an important role in the modulation of cellular proliferation, differentiation, angiogenesis, and inflammation; moreover, they serve an important function as messengers between the intestinal mucosa, enteric nervous system, and immune system.[1] This article highlights a few of the most promising findings with these agents, including keratinocyte growth factor-2 (KGF-2), EGF, GH, and GM–CSF.

KERATINOCYTE GROWTH FACTOR

Han and colleagues investigated the use of subcutaneous (s.c.) and intravenously (i.v.) administered KGF-2 in a Lewis rat model of indomethacin-induced intestinal ulceration.[3] In this study, rats injected with indomethacin (7.5 mg/kg per day × 2 days) also received daily s.c. or i.v. injections of 1 or 5 mg/kg KGF-2 or human serum albumin (HSA) for 5 days beginning 1 day prior to indomethacin treatment. As shown in FIGURE 1, i.v. administration of KGF-2 nearly prevented the weight loss associated with indomethacin-induced intestinal ulceration.

EPIDERMAL GROWTH FACTOR

Sinha and colleagues evaluated the efficacy of EGF in a randomized, double-blind, placebo-controlled study of 24 patients with left-sided ulcerative colitis.[4] Patients were randomly assigned to receive daily enemas containing 5 μg of EGF in 100 mL of an inert carrier ($n = 12$) or placebo ($n = 12$) for 2 weeks; all patients received concomitant oral mesalamine treatment (median daily dose, 2.4 g) for a total of 12 weeks. As shown in FIGURE 2, median Ulcerative Colitis Disease Activity Index (UCDAI) scores were similar at base line for the EGF and placebo groups (9.5 and 9.0, respectively). After 2 weeks of treatment, significantly greater improvements were seen in mean UCDAI scores in the patients treated with EGF compared with those receiving placebo ($P < 0.001$). This pattern continued at the 4-week assessment, with 7 of 12 patients in the EGF-treated group and 1 of 12 patients in the placebo-treated group achieving remission, which was defined as a UCDAI score of 0 or 1 ($P = 0.03$).

GROWTH HORMONE

Slonim and colleagues conducted a randomized, double-blind, placebo-controlled study of recombinant human GH (somatropin) therapy in 37 patients with moderate-to-severe active Crohn's disease (CD).[5] Patients self-administered somatropin by s.c. injection, with a loading dose of 5 mg/day for

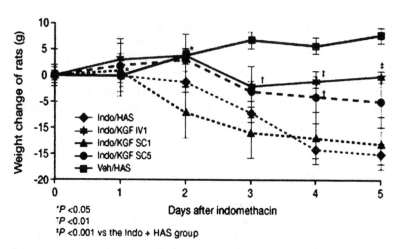

FIGURE 1. Keratinocyte growth factor-2 (KGF-2) reduces acute indomethacin-induced injury. Indo = indomethacin; HAS = human serum albumin; VEH = vehicle. (Reprinted from Han *et al.*,[2] with permission from The American Physiological Society.)

the first week, followed by a maintenance dose of 1.5 mg/kg per day for up to 4 months, and were instructed to increase their protein intake to 2 g/kg body weight per day; patients continued using other medications for CD as needed.

As shown in FIGURE 3, baseline mean Crohn's Disease Activity Index (CDAI) scores were somewhat higher in patients receiving somatropin than in the placebo group (287 vs. 213, $P = 0.09$). After the first month of treatment, however, patients who received somatropin demonstrated significantly lower mean CDAI scores compared with those patients in the placebo group ($P = 0.02$). Similar results were seen at subsequent monthly assessments, with mean

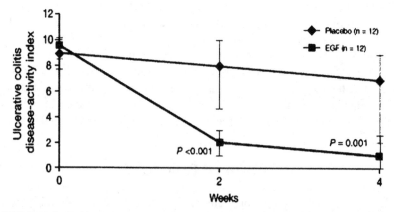

FIGURE 2. Epidermal growth factor enemas and oral mesalamine reduce disease activity in patients with ulcerative colitis. (From Sinha *et al.*[4] by permission of the Massachusetts Medical Society.)

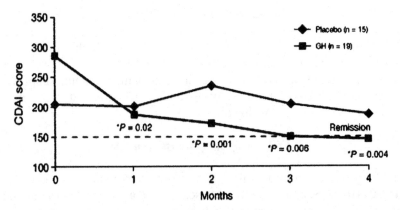

FIGURE 3. Human growth hormone (somatropin) in active CD: Change from base line in mean Crohn's Disease Activity Index (CDAI) scores. Note: only the 15 placebo-treated patients for whom follow-up data were available were included in the analysis. GH = growth hormone.

CDAI scores decreasing by a total of 143 ($\pm$144) points in the somatropin group and 19 ($\pm$63) points in the placebo group at the end of the study ($P=0.004$).

GRANULOCYTE–MACROPHAGE COLONY-STIMULATING FACTOR

Colony-stimulating factors are characterized by their ability to induce the formation of distinct hematopoietic cell lineages. Key members of this peptide family include GM–CSF, G-CSF, M-CSF, and interleukin-3 (IL-3). Although the hematopoietic tissues are the predominant site of action for these peptides, they are produced throughout the body, including the intestine, and are also produced by constituents of the lamina propria (primarily macrophages/monocytes).[1] GM–CSF is expressed by CD4+ T cells and Paneth cells in the intestine. Receptors for GM–CSF have been identified on intestinal epithelial cells, including Paneth cells.[6] GM–CSF increases proliferation of crypt epithelial cells.[7] Moreover, GM–CSF is expressed at high levels in those regions of the gastrointestinal tract that are associated with the greatest concentration of luminal microbial colonization. Taken together, these findings suggest a regulatory role for GM–CSF in maintaining mucosal homeostasis.

The greatest body of evidence supporting the use of colony-stimulating factors in intestinal inflammation comes from studies conducted with GM–CSF in patients with CD. Sargramostim (Leukine®, Berlex Inc., Seattle, WA, USA) is a recombinant version of the naturally occurring human growth factor GM–CSF, most commonly used for myeloid cell recovery after chemotherapy. Sargramostim was chosen for evaluation in patients with CD because of its ability to stimulate the innate immune system through direct effects on neutrophils, monocytes, macrophages, and dendritic cells.

Sargramostim in CD

An initial pilot study of sargramostim demonstrated a high rate of clinical response and remission with limited toxicity in 15 patients with moderately-to-severely active CD who were not receiving concomitant immunosuppressive therapy.[8] On the basis of these promising results, a phase II study was initiated to compare sargramostim with placebo.

Efficacy of Sargramostim in CD

In the phase II study, a total of 124 patients with moderately-to-severely active CD (defined as a baseline CDAI score >200 and <475, and a minimum 6-month history of CD) were randomly assigned to receive either 6 μg/kg per day of sargramostim ($n = 81$) or placebo ($n = 43$) s.c. for 8 weeks.[9] The use of corticosteroids and immunosuppressant therapies was prohibited throughout the study; however, patients were allowed to continue treatment with stable doses of antibiotics or aminosalicylates. Efficacy measures included changes from base line in disease severity (measured by CDAI score), mucosal healing (measured using the Crohn's Disease Endoscopic Index of Severity [CDEIS]), and health-related quality of life (measured by Inflammatory Bowel Disease Questionnaire [IBDQ] score), while safety was assessed according to the incidence of adverse events.

In patients treated with sargramostim, response and remission rates were significantly improved over the course of the study compared with placebo (FIG. 4). For example, significantly more patients treated with sargramostim demonstrated a ≥100-point decrease in CDAI score at the end of the 8-week treatment period than patients who received placebo (48% vs. 26%, $P = 0.013$). Similarly, a greater proportion of patients receiving sargramostim achieved a complete remission (CDAI score ≤150) compared with those receiving placebo (40% vs. 19%, $P = 0.014$). The time to response was significantly shorter in the sargramostim-treated group ($P = 0.018$), and the significant between-group differences in response and remission were maintained at the 30-day posttreatment follow-up visit (FIG. 4). Sargramostim therapy was also associated with improvements in mucosal healing and particularly, in quality of life. Although baseline IBDQ scores were comparable for both treatment groups, significantly greater improvements were seen in the sargramostim group throughout treatment, with scores ranging from 155 at day 29 ($P = 0.017$ vs. placebo), to 156 at day 57 ($P = 0.030$ vs. placebo), and to 153 at the end of the 30-day follow-up period ($P = 0.013$ vs. placebo).

Safety Experience with Sargramostim

Both the pilot and placebo-controlled studies indicated that sargramostim is generally safe and well tolerated in patients with CD. Mild-to-moderate

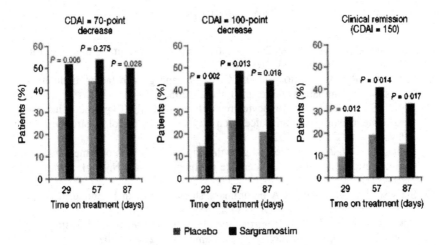

FIGURE 4. Sargramostim improves response and remission in patients with CD. (From Korzenik *et al.*[9] permission of the Massachusetts Medical Society.)

injection-site reactions and bone pain were more common in the sargramostim group; however, the incidence of injection-site reactions decreased after the second week of treatment, and bone pain was generally transient and manageable. Furthermore, the incidence of bone pain is substantially reduced with retreatment.

SUMMARY

On the basis of several studies that have been completed to date, some growth factors appear promising for the treatment of inflammatory bowel disease:

- KGF-2 was well tolerated in patients with ulcerative colitis, although there was no evidence of efficacy at doses of up to 50 μg/kg;
- EGF enemas were effective for the treatment of left-sided ulcerative colitis when used in combination with oral mesalamine;
- Somatropin (human GH) has shown benefit in a preliminary study of patients with CD; and
- Sargramostim (recombinant human GM–CSF) has demonstrated significant benefits in a randomized, double-blind, placebo-controlled, phase II study in patients with active CD. Additional trials are currently under way to determine the long-term efficacy and tolerability of sargramostim in this patient population.

Taken together, the results of these studies suggest that new insights into the reparative components of mucosal homeostasis may ultimately provide effective synergistic or single-agent treatment alternatives to immunosuppression for inflammatory bowel disease.

REFERENCES

1. DIGNASS, A.U. & A. STURM. 2001. Peptide growth factors in the intestine. Eur. J. Gastroenterol. Hepatol. **13:** 763–770.
2. PLAYFORD, R.J. & S. GHOSH. 2005. Cytokines and growth factor modulators in intestinal inflammation and repair. J. Pathol. **205:** 417–425.
3. HAN, D.S. *et al.* 2000. Keratinocyte growth factor-2 (FGF-10) promotes healing of experimental small intestinal ulceration in rats. Am. J. Physiol. Gastrointest. Liver Physiol. **279:** G1011–G1022.
4. SINHA, A. *et al.* 2003. Epidermal growth factor enemas with oral mesalamine for mild-to-moderate left-sided ulcerative colitis or proctitis. N. Engl. J. Med. **349:** 350–357.
5. SLONIM, A.E. *et al.* 2000. A preliminary study of growth hormone therapy for Crohn's disease. N. Engl. J. Med. **342:** 1633–1637.
6. FUKUZAWA, H. *et al.* 2003. Identification of GM-CSF in Paneth cells using single-cell RT-PCR. Biochem. Biophys. Res. Commun. **312:** 897–902.
7. RAMSAY, R.G. *et al.* 2004. Colony-stimulating factor-1 promotes clonogenic growth of normal murine colonic crypt epithelial cells in vitro. J. Interferon Cytokine Res. **24:** 416–427.
8. DIECKGRAEFE, B.K. & J.R. KORZENIK. 2002. Treatment of active Crohn's disease with recombinant human granulocyte-macrophage colony-stimulating factor. Lancet **360:** 1478–1480.
9. KORZENIK, J.R. *et al.* 2005. Sargramostim for active Crohn's disease. N. Engl. J. Med. **352:** 2193–2201.

The Bacterial Weaponry

Lessons from *Shigella*

PHILIPPE J. SANSONETTI

Unité de Pathogénie Microbienne Moléculaire, INSERM U389, and Howard Hughes Medical Institute, Institut Pasteur, 28 Rue du Docteur Roux, 75724 Paris Cedex 15, France

ABSTRACT: *Shigella*, a Gram-negative bacterial species of the family Enterobacteriaceae, causes bacillary dysentery in humans, an acute rectocolitis that reflects the capacity of the microorganism to disrupt, invade, and cause the inflammatory destruction of the intestinal epithelium. Here, the pathogenesis of *Shigella* infection is analyzed in the context of the disruption of the homeostatic balance that protects the gut against inflammation in the presence of its commensal flora. Thus a unified view by which enteroinvasive pathogens allow identification of key signalling molecules and pathways involved in the regulation of intestinal inflammation, thereby providing keys to understand inflammatory bowel diseases (IBDs) such as Crohn's disease and ulcerative colitis.

KEYWORDS: *Shigella*; invasion; epithelium; inflammation; Nod; peptidoglycan

INTRODUCTION

In addition to its functions of digestion, nutrient, water and electrolyte transport, and production of hormones, the intestinal epithelium plays a major role of barrier between the host and the external environment. The colon, for instance, is exposed to the huge bacterial load of its commensal microflora, and intestinal epithelial cells (IECs) are the primary cells to interact with luminal bacteria.[1] This barrier function is largely devoted to protection against invasion and systemic dissemination of the microorganisms of the commensal flora and against pathogenic microorganisms subverting its organization. The intestinal epithelium integrates three barriers,[2] physical, functional, and immunological. This barrier is in permanent cross-talk with the microorganisms, IECs being a major partner in this dialogue because of their strategic position of interface.[3] Microorganisms are constantly sampled from the intestinal lumen

Address for correspondence: Philippe J. Sansonetti, Unité de Pathogénie Microbienne Moléculaire, INSERM U389, and Howard Hughes Medical Institute, Institut Pasteur, 28 Rue du Docteur Roux, 75724 Paris cedex 15, France. Voice: 33-145-68-8342; fax: 33-145-68-8953.
e-mail: psanson@pasteur.fr

Ann. N.Y. Acad. Sci. 1072: 307–312 (2006). © 2006 New York Academy of Sciences.
doi: 10.1196/annals.1326.025

into the inductive sites of the intestinal immune system and the intestinal flora plays a role in gut maturation.[4] Coevolution of mammals with their intestinal flora has led to a situation of tolerance whose mechanisms have only recently started to be recognized.[5] The homeostatic balance that is shown to prevail represents a complex and fragile equilibrium because the exposed surface is large (i.e., 200 m^2), and the microbial density enormous (i.e., 10^{11-12} bacteria/gram of stool in the colon). Thus this fragile balance can, at any moment, be subverted by toxins or pathogenic microorganisms. The concept of innate immunity and its regulation is central to this homeostatic balance, leading to a status of controlled "physiological inflammation" whose disruption by pathogens, particularly enteroinvasive bacteria, causes the rupture, invasion, and inflammatory destruction of the barrier.[6,7] Identification of the receptors and signaling pathways with which enteroinvasive microorganisms interact and interfere is essential because tracking bacteria in their "proinflammatory journey" may allow us to identify key molecules in the regulation of intestinal inflammation. As a matter of fact, pathogenic microbes have been coevolving with mammals, particularly humans, for such a long period that, under selective pressure, particularly the host's innate immune response, they have accumulated genes encoding effectors that regulate the host response to allow successful colonization by the pathogen. Not surprisingly, recent discoveries regarding genetic determination of chronic inflammatory bowel diseases (IBDs) such as Crohn's disease reveal that common signaling pathways are affected, central to which is the Nod family of intracellular sensors of bacterial peptidoglycan (PGN).[8,9]

SHIGELLA AS A PARADIGM OF RUPTURE, INVASION, AND INFLAMMATORY DESTRUCTION OF THE EPITHELIAL BARRIER

Shigella, the causative agent of bacillary dysentery, is a Gram-negative bacterial species that represents an extraodinary tool to address the above questions.[10] It has been possible to identify a series of molecular mechanisms that reflect stepwise interactions mediated by bacterial effectors encoded by a virulence plasmid[11] and delivered to eukaryotic cells by a Type III secretory system (TTSS).[12] This series of cross-talk allows entry of the bacterium into epithelial cells by a macropinocytic event, reflecting massive reorganization of the host cell cytoskeleton, which is triggered by activation of small guanosine triphosphatases (GTPases) of the Rho family[13] and of a cascade involving src and its phosphorylated substrate cortactin,[14] both inducing actin nucleation and assembly via activation of the Arp2/3 complex. Following entry and lysis of the phagocytic vacuole, bacteria escape into the cytoplasm and move intracellularly in an actin-dependent process involving a plasmid-encoded outer membrane protein, IcsA,[15] the host-cell protein N-WASP (neural Wiskott-Aldrich protein) and the actin nucleating complex Arp2/3.[16] Bacteria then spread from cell to cell following engagement of adherence junction components.[17] Of major importance to this series of events is a paracrine regulation mediated through hemi-channels by which infected cells release adenosine 5'-triphosphate (ATP) and cause Ca^{2+} fluxes in yet uninfected cells of the epithelial lining, thus creating a highly permissive state of invasion.[18]

The whole process leads to massive intracellular colonization of the intestinal epithelium, which accounts for the development of mucosal inflammation because each invaded cell gets reprogrammed by intracellular microorganisms to express a proinflammatory program dominated by the expression of IL-8,[19] thus triggering massive recruitment of polymorphonuclear leukocytes (PMNs).[20] Acute recruitment of this mucosal infiltrate of PMNs is essential to eradicate shigellae because PMNs appear to be the major effectors of their killing,[21] but this occurs at the cost of massive epithelial destruction.[22] The role of antibacterial peptides expressed by IECs in the control of pathogens in the course of an acute infection remains to be definitely demonstrated, but even more interestingly, poor expression of cryptdins by Paneth cells may be related to the triggering of uncontrolled inflammation in Crohn's disease.[23] Intracellular sensing and proinflammatory programming is based upon recognition of the *Shigella* PGN by Nod proteins,[24] particularly Nod1, which is able to discriminate between PGN from Gram-negative and Gram-positive bacteria.[25,26] This has set a new paradigm of intracellular sensing of bacteria, leading to "inside-in" signaling that activates the NF-κB and c-Jun N-terminal kinase (JNK) pathways, and thus the transcription of numerous proinflammatory genes. Nod molecules are composed of three domains: a leucine-rich C-terminal domain (LRR), which is likely to participate in the recognition of the PGN fragments; a central nucleotide binding Site (NBS) domain; and one or two caspase-recruiting domains (CARDs). Nod1 recognizes a muropeptide characterized by the presence of a tripeptide with a molecule of meso-diaminopimelate in position 3, and Nod2 recognizes a simpler and generic muropeptide present in all PGNs, the muramyl-dipeptide (MDP).[27] This whole process accounts for the break in tolerance induced by invasive pathogens and promotes Nod molecules to the rank of an essential system for the perception of bacterial insults to the epithelium. Key questions now are (i) whether the Nod molecules also participate in the homeostatic balance that controls the commensal flora, and (ii) how bacterial pathogen-associated molecular patterns (PAMPs) are, in general presented to intracellular Nod molecules. In the case of intracellular shigellae, the answer is rather straightforward. Regarding extracellular pathogens, recent work on *Helicobacter pylori* interacting with gastric epithelial cells has shown that the Type IV secretory system encoded by the *cag* operon was able to introduce *H. pylori* PGN fragments into target cells along with the Cag protein effectors.[28] A new theme is now emerging, "cellular pampology," which should address the cell biology of capture and internalization of PAMPs, both in epithelial and phagocytic cells and their presentation to molecular sensors such as the Nod molecules.

Another emerging theme is how invasive shigellae cope with the strong innate response they elicit, and manage to survive and efficiently colonize the epithelial surface before proceeding to invasion. Accumulating evidence indicates that a group of effector proteins encoded by the Shigella virulence plasmid and secreted through the Type III secretion system are likely to be strong regulators of the innate and possibly adaptive immune response. These proteins (i.e., Osp[s] and IpaH[s] are expressed only during periods of activation of the secretory system, even though it is not yet clear whether the Type III system is constantly activated *in vivo* or simply turned on every time bacteria meet the eukaryotic cell surface, particularly the epithelium. In any event, one of these proteins, OspG, has recently been shown to downregulate activation of the NF-κB signaling pathway. It does so through a very original process in which it binds to ubiquitin-transfering enzymes Ubc5 and Ubc7, thus blocking the degradation of I-kB.[29] One may thus expect that a battery of anti-inflammatory proteins will soon be unraveled in *Shigella*.

CONCLUSION

Time has come to take a unifying approach to intestinal inflammation by developing in parallel (i) studies aimed at understanding the homeostatic mechanisms allowing tolerance of the intestinal flora; (ii) studies aimed at understanding how (enteroinvasive) pathogens cause intestinal inflammation and break this tolerance process; and, last but not least, (iii) studies aimed at understanding, mostly following identification of candidate genes, the molecular mechanisms of IBDs. These are clearly intertwined topics that will provide a deeper understanding of the basic mechanisms of physiology.

ACKNOWLEDGMENTS

I wish to thank the members of Unité de Pathogénie Microbienne Moléculaire and Group Immunité Innée et Signalisation for their contributions, which I have only briefly summarized here.

REFERENCES

1. KAGNOFF, M.F. & L. ECKMANN. 1997. Epithelial cells as sensors for microbial infection. J. Clin. Invest. **100:** 6–10.
2. MADARA, J.L., S. NASH, R. MOORE & K. ATISOOK. 1990. Structure and function of the intestinal epithelial barrier in health and disease. Monogr. Pathol. **31:** 306–324.

3. SANSONETTI, P.J. 2004. War and peace at mucosal surfaces.. Nat. Rev. Immunol. **4:** 953–964.
4. BACKHED, F., R.E. LEY, J.L. SONNENBURG, *et al.* 2005. Host-bacterial mutualism in the human intestine. Science **307:** 1915–1920.
5. MACDONALD, T.T. & G. MONTELEONE. 2005. Immunity, inflammation, and allergy in the gut. Science **307:** 1920–1925.
6. SANSONETTI, P.J. 2001. Rupture, invasion and inflammatory destruction of the intestinal barrier by *Shigella*, making sense of prokaryote-eukaryote cross-talk. FEMS Microbiol. Rev. **25:** 3–14.
7. COSSART, P. & P.J. SANSONETTI. 2004. Bacterial invasion: the paradigms of enteroinvasive pathogens. Science **304:** 242–248.
8. HUGOT, J.P., M. CHAMAILLARD, H. ZOUALI, *et al.* 2001. Association of NOD2 leucine-rich repeat variants with susceptibility to Crohn's disease. Nature **411:** 599–603.
9. OGURA, Y., D.K. BONEN, N. INOHARA, *et al.* 2001. A frameshift mutation in NOD2 associated with susceptibility to Crohn's disease. Nature **411:** 603–606.
10. FERNANDEZ, M.I. & P.J. SANSONETTI. 2003. *Shigella* interaction with intestinal epithelial cells determines the innate immune response in shigellosis. Int. J. Med. Microbiol. **293:** 55–67.
11. SANSONETTI, P.J., D.J. KOPECKO & S.B. FORMAL. 1982. Involvement of a large plasmid in the invasive ability of *Shigella flexneri*. Infect. Immun. **35:** 852–860.
12. BLOCKER, A., P. GOUNON, E. LARQUET, *et al.* 1999. Role of *Shigella*'s type III secretion system in insertion of IpaB and IpaC into the host membrane. J. Cell Biol. **147:** 683–693.
13. TRAN VAN NHIEU, G., E. CARON, A. HALL & P.J. SANSONETTI. 1998. IpaC determines filopodia formation during *Shigella* entry into epithelial cells. EMBO J. **18:** 3249–3262.
14. BOUGNÈRES, L., S. GIRARDIN, S.A. WEED, *et al.* 2004. Cortactin and Crk cooperate to trigger actin polymerization during *Shigella* invasion of epithelial cells. J. Cell Biol. **166:** 225–235.
15. BERNARDINI, M.L., J. MOUNIER, H. d'HAUTEVILLE, *et al.* 1989. Identification of *ics*A, a plasmid locus of *Shigella flexneri* which governs bacterial intra- and intercellular spread through interaction with F-actin. Proc. Natl. Acad. Sci. USA **86:** 3867–3871.
16. EGILE, C., T.P. LOISEL, V. LAURENT, *et al.* 1999. Activation of the CDC42 effector N-WASP by the *Shigella icsA* protein promotes actin nucleation by Arp2/3 complex and bacterial actin-ased motility. J. Cell Biol. **146:** 1319–1332.
17. SANSONETTI, P.J., J. MOUNIER, M.C. PRÉVOST & R.M. MEGE. 1994. Cadherin expression is required for the spread of *Shigella flexneri* between epithelial cells. Cell **76:** 829–839.
18. TRAN VAN NHIEU, G., C. CLAIR, R.R. BRUZZONE, *et al.* 2003. Connexin-dependent intercellular communication increases *Shigella* invasion and dissemination in epithelial cells. Nat. Cell Biol. **5:** 720–726.
19. PÉDRON, T., C. THIBAULT & P.J. SANSONETTI.The invasive phenotype of *Shigella flexneri* directs a distinct gene expression pattern in the human intestinal epithelial cell line Caco-2. J. Biol. Chem. **278:** 33878–33886.
20. PHILPOTT, D.J., S. YAMAOKA, S.A. ISRAËL & P.J. SANSONETTI. 2000. Invasive *Shigella flexneri* activates NF-κB through an LPS-dependent innate intracellular response and leads to IL-8 expression in epithelial cells. J. Immunol. **165:** 903–914.

21. WEINRAUCH, Y., D. DRUJAN, S.D. SHAPIRO, et al. 2002. Neutrophil elastase targets virulence factors of enterobacteria. Nature **417:** 91–94.
22. SANSONETTI, P.J., J. ARONDEL, M. HUERRE, et al. 1999. Interleukin-8 controls bacterial transepithelial translocation at the cost of epithelial destruction in experimental shigellosis. Infect. Immun. **67:** 1471–1480.
23. OGURA, Y., S. LALA, W. XIN, et al. 2003. Expression of Nod2 in Paneth cells: a possible link to Crohn's ileitis. Gut **52:** 1591–1597.
24. GIRARDIN, S.E., R. TOURNEBIZE, M. MAVRIS, et al. 2001. CARD4/Nod1 mediates NF-kB and JNK activation by invasive *Shigella flexneri.* EMBO Reports **2:** 736–742.
25. CHAMAILLARD, M., M. HASHIMOTO, Y. HORIE, et al. 2003. An essential role for Nod1 in host recognition of bacterial peptidoglycan containing diaminopimelic acid. Nat. Immunol. **4:** 702–707.
26. GIRARDIN, S.E., I. GOMPERTS-BONECA, L.A.M. CARNEIRO, et al. 2003. Nod1 detects specifically Gram-negative bacteria through GlcNAc-MurNAc tripeptide, a peptidoglycan motif. Science **300:** 1584–1587.
27. GIRARDIN, S., I. GOMPERTS-BONECA, J. VIALA, et al. 2003. Nod2 is a general sensor of peptidoglycan through muramyldipeptide (MDP) detection. J. Biol. Chem. **278:** 8869–8872.
28. VIALA, J., C. CHAPUT, I. GOMPERTS-BONECA, et al. 2004. Nod1 responds to peptidoglycan delivered by the *Helicobacter pylori* cag pathogenicity island. Nat. Immunol. **5:** 1166–1174.
29. KIM, D.W., G. LENZEN, A.L. PAGE, et al. 2006. The *Shigella flexneri* of effector OspG interfere with innate immune responses by targeting ubiquitin-conjugating enzymes. Proc. NatL. Acad. Sci. USA **102:** 14046–14051.

Microbial-Epithelial Cell Crosstalk during Inflammation

The Host Response

MARTIN F. KAGNOFF

Departments of Medicine and Pediatrics, Laboratory of Mucosal Immunology and the Wm. K. Warren Medical Research Center for Celiac Disease, University of California, San Diego, La Jolla, California 920393-0623, USA

ABSTRACT: The intestinal epithelium forms a single cell barrier that separates the host's internal milieu from luminal contents. This article examines the role of the intestinal epithelium as a critical component of a communications network that is essential for transmitting signals generated in response to infection with microbial pathogens to cells of the innate and acquired immune systems in the underlying intestinal mucosa. It further highlights the importance of intestinal epithelium in mediating host antimicrobial defense through the production of antimicrobial peptides of the defensin and cathelicidin families.

KEYWORDS: antimicrobial peptide; bacteria; cathelicidin; chemokine; CXCL8; CCL20; defensin; intestinal epithelial cell; innate immunity; mCRAMP

A single layer of polarized epithelium separates intestinal luminal contents that are in contact with the external environment from the host's internal milieu. Formerly viewed as a simple barrier, it is now known that this single layer of intestinal epithelial cells is a dynamic component of a communications network that conveys signals from environmental cues to cells in the underlying subepithelial region. Moreover, signals generated by the epithelium in response to a diversity of microbes and microbial products have a key role in the initiation of host innate mucosal immune responses that are critical for "homeland protection." Signals generated by intestinal epithelial cells can result in the chemoattraction and/or activation of subepithelial mononuclear cell populations including dendritic cells, neutrophils, monocytes/macrophages, T cells, B cells, mast cells, and eosinophils as well as other cell types. Those cells in turn can generate mediators that signal the paracrine activation of other

Address for correspondence: Martin F. Kagnoff, M.D., Professor of Medicine and Pediatrics, University of California at San Diego, La Jolla, CA 92093. Voice: 858-534-4633; fax: 858-534-5691.
e-mail: mkagnoff@ucsd.edu

Ann. N.Y. Acad. Sci. 1072: 313–320 (2006). © 2006 New York Academy of Sciences.
doi: 10.1196/annals.1326.038

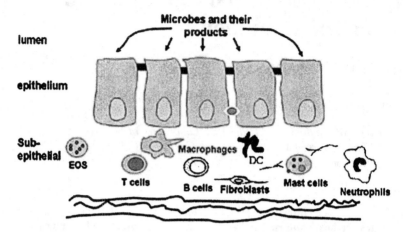

FIGURE 1. The epithelium as a part of a communications network: Pathogenic microbes and their products activate signaling pathways in intestinal epithelial cells. Mediators produced by intestinal epithelial cells are released and can chemoattract and act on target cells of the innate and acquired immune system (e.g., dendritic cells DC, neutrophils, T cells) in the underlying subepithelial region. Cells in the subepithelial region, in turn, produce proinflammatory mediators that can act on neighboring subepithelial mononuclear cells and other cell types, as well as activate basolaterally expressed receptors on epithelial cells and alter epithelial cell functions.

subepithelial cells. Further, some of these mediators feed back to the intestinal epithelium and alter epithelial cell functions (FIG. 1).

Important host strategies are involved in the interaction of the epithelium with enteric pathogens and their products. We have used enteric pathogens and their products to probe the repertoire of host intestinal epithelial responses to enteric pathogens that employ a variety of strategies to infect the host. We do not address the influence of the commensal microflora herein, but do note that commensal bacteria have a key role in the normal development and maturation of the intestinal mucosa, and in activating the production of products that can be viewed as mucosal-protective,[1-3] as discussed by others in this volume.

Some enteric pathogens adhere to the apical epithelial membrane. Pathogens, such as enteropathogenic *Escherichia coli* (EPEC) and enterohemorrhagic *E. coli* (EHEC), are generally noninvasive, yet develop an intimate association with the apical epithelial cell membrane, where they form a characteristic attaching and effacing lesion and, through a type III secretion system, inject bacterial proteins into host intestinal epithelial cells. These bacterial products alter epithelial cell signaling pathways and epithelial cell functions, and can result in the activation of host proinflammatory signals that are important for signaling the onset of mucosal inflammation. Still other epithelial cell–adherent but noninvasive pathogens, such as the protozoan parasite

Giardia lamblia, are not proinflammatory. Nonetheless, they can engage in intimate crosstalk with the host's intestinal epithelium and alter the epithelial cell's production of host defense molecules that otherwise could detrimentally alter the parasite's life cycle.[4] Still other enteric pathogens invade the epithelium but not deeper layers of the mucosa. Such pathogens (e.g., *Cryptosporidium parvum*, *Chlamydia trachomatis*) undergo key parts of their life cycle within the intestinal epithelium and, although they may activate low levels of inflammatory signals, for the most part this appears to be a byproduct of activating the NF-κB pathway, whose major role under these circumstances appears to be its anti-apoptotic function.[5,6] Thus, such pathogens activate NF-κB and anti-apoptotic pathways in order to keep the epithelial cell alive for a sufficient duration of time to allow the pathogen to undergo critical phases in its reproductive cycle. Thereafter, the epithelial cell undergoes lysis and releases infective life stages of the parasite that can go on to infect additional epithelial cells. Finally, a group of systemically invasive microorganisms (e.g., *Salmonella* sp., *Shigella* sp., *Listeria monocytogenes*, enteroinvasive *E. coli*) invades epithelial cells and deeper layers of the intestinal mucosa. Such organisms and their products can be potent activators of host epithelial cell proinflammatory signals.

This article highlights two aspects of the host epithelial response. The first is the role of the intestinal epithelium and host epithelial cells as a defense "early warning system" following an encounter with microbial pathogens. The second is the role of the intestinal epithelium in mediating antimicrobial defense through the production of antimicrobial peptides.

ROLE OF INTESTINAL EPITHELIUM AS A MUCOSAL DEFENSE EARLY WARNING SYSTEM

It is now known that intestinal epithelial cells can sense enteric microbes and microbial products and, in response to that interaction, signal the onset of epithelial cell and mucosal innate defense mechanisms. Sensing is accomplished through arrays of membrane-associated pattern-recognition molecules, such as the toll-like receptors and intracellular pattern-recognition molecules, such as the Nod proteins.[7,8] Signaling through those pathways culminates in the generation of chemoattractant cytokines that variably function to chemoattract acute inflammatory cells (e.g., neutrophils and monocytes), cells that can link innate and acquired immunity (e.g., dendritic cell populations), and cells that are key in mediating acquired immunity, including T and B lymphocyte populations.

CXCL8 (IL-8) is a prototypic chemokine produced by the intestinal epithelium that can chemoattract and activate neutrophils. In response to microbial infection, there is increased gene transcription of CXCL8, which is accompanied by increased levels of CXCL8 mRNA transcripts and ensuing increased production and release of CXCL8 from the basolateral surface of intestinal epithelial cells.[9–11] Moreover, relative to other neutrophil chemoattractants (e.g., CXCL5, also known as ENA-78), CXCL8 is produced more rapidly, is more potent, and is produced in larger quantities.[12] This led to the concept of spatial and temporal gradients of epithelial chemokine production wherein chemokines, such as CXCL8, that were produced more rapidly and in larger quantities, and that predictably would imprint a chemokine gradient at a greater distance from epithelial cells, but whose production was relative short-lived, may have a more prominent role in the early chemoattraction of neutrophils to and within the intestinal mucosa. In contract chemokines like CXCL5 which are produced in lesser amounts and are less potent, but whose upregulation is longer-lived, may be more important in bringing neutrophils in closer proximity to the epithelium, where they subsequently rely on other mediators and receptors to cross between intestinal epithelial cells and enter the crypt lumen.

Another example of a prototypic chemokine produced by intestinal epithelium is CCL20 (MIP3α). CCL20 uses CCR6 expressed on some populations of dendritic cells and T cells and by the apical membrane of intestinal epithelium, as its cognate receptor. In the intestinal tract of mice, CCL20 is constitutively expressed by the epithelium overlying Peyer's patches. However, CCL20, which functions as an NF-κB target gene, can be markedly upregulated throughout the intestinal epithelium during inflammatory responses, such as those seen in mice systemically injected with bacterial lipopolysaccharide or in human epithelium.[13] The latter has been shown both in a human intestinal xenograft model after challenge with bacterial products like flagellin[14] or exposure to proinflammatory mediators and in the epithelium of patients with ulcerative colitis.[15] Of note, the key functional targets of CCL20 in the gut mucosa, outside of Peyer's patches, require further study. Although CCL20 can signal through apical expressed CCR6 on intestinal epithelial cells in cell culture models,[16] whether or not this is important *in vivo* and whether CCL20 is the major natural ligand for CCR6 expressed by intestinal epithelium remains to be determined.

The discussion above highlights two epithelial chemokines. However, the intestinal epithelium can produce, in addition to those that mainly function as neutrophil or dendritic cell chemoattractants, chemokines that function as monocyte/macrophage chemoattractants (e.g., MCP-1),[17] CCL22 (MDC), which can chemoattract CD4 T-cell populations that produce TH2 type cytokines,[18] and CCL9 and CCL10 (Mig and IP-10), which chemoattract TH1 type CD4 cytokine-producing cells.[19] Moreover, chemokine production can be relatively compartmentalized within different regions of the intestine, with small intestinal epithelium producing, for example, CCL25, a chemoattractant for gut homing T cells that express CCR9,[20] and the colon epithelium producing CCL28, which chemoattracts IgA plasmablasts expressing the receptor CCR10.[21]

HOST INTESTINAL EPITHELIAL CELLS AS AN ANTIMICROBIAL DEFENSE SYSTEM

Intestinal epithelial cells produce antimicrobial peptides both constitutively and under regulated conditions. For example, intestinal epithelial cells in the small intestine and colon constitutively produce human β-defensin (HBD) 1 and Paneth cells in the small intestine produce the α-defensins HD5 and HD6.[22] In contrast, the sole human cathelicidin LL37/hCAP18 is constitutively produced largely by epithelial cells that line the surface of the crypts in the colon, with little production by small intestinal epithelium.[23] Unlike HBD-1, another human β-defensin, HBD-2, is a NF-κB target gene that is produced mainly under inflammatory conditions and predominately in the colon.[22] HBD-3, in contrast, is a γ-interferon–regulated gene reported to be expressed in the colon and small intestine, mainly in the crypt region, and has been noted to be upregulated to some extent in ulcerative colitis.[24]

Cathelicidins expressed by intestinal epithelium have been studied recently by our laboratory.[23,25,26] Cathelicidins are multifunctional antimicrobial peptides that are present in all mammalian species. They can mediate antimicrobial activities, as well as chemoattract populations on mononuclear cells, and have LPS-binding activity. In humans and mice, cathelicidins are produced as propeptides with a conserved signal sequence, a cathelin domain, and a C-terminal domain which, when proteolytically cleaved, has antimicrobial activity.[27] The sole human cathelicidin is LL37/hCAP18, whereas mCRAMP is the orthologue in mice. Both LL37/hCAP18 and mCRAMP are relatively restricted in their distribution in the intestinal tract to the surface epithelial cells of colon crypts.[25,26] Using a mutant mouse model in which the mCRAMP gene (*cnlp*) was genetically knocked out, we showed recently that mCRAMP can play an important role in abrogating surface colonization of the colon epithelium with an apical surface-adherent pathogen that has many virulence properties in common with EPEC and EHEC.[26] Whereas epithelial antimicrobial peptides often appear to be functionally more potent as antimicrobials when different classes of those peptides are combined, we showed that early in the course of infection *in vivo* mCRAMP, by itself, was sufficient to prevent surface colonization with this pathogen. On the basis of studies from our group and others, it is clear that the distribution of different antimicrobial defense molecules is regionally restricted in the intestine, and within a given region, restricted to cell types that differ in either lineage or differentiation state. Such differences favor the notion that different antimicrobial defense molecules are host-adapted to mediate different functional roles in various intestinal sites.

In summary, in this brief article we have focused on the production of two prototypic chemokines and a selected few antimicrobial defense molecules produced by intestinal epithelium that were highlighted in this symposium. Nonetheless, it is important to remember that intestinal epithelial cells are an

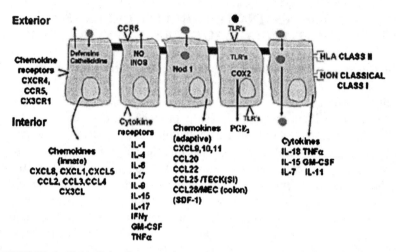

FIGURE 2. Epithelial cells are an integral component of a communications network important in host mucosal defense. Intestinal epithelial cells produce mediators and express receptors important in innate and adapative mucosal immunity. Examples of such mediators are a selected group of chemokines, cytokines, and prostaglandins (e.g., PGE_2). Epithelial cells also express receptors for cytokines and chemokines. Microbial products activate epithelial cell signaling pathways through pattern-recognition receptors that are located on the cell surface (e.g., some TLRs) and cytoplasmic (e.g., Nod proteins). Another arm of host antimicrobial defense is mediated by antimicrobial peptides (e.g., defensins, cathelicidin).

essential component of a rather complex communications network that can convey multiple signals from luminal contents to the underlying subepithelial region. Several of the receptors and products expressed by the intestinal epithelium that play a key role in innate mucosal defense are depicted in FIGURE 2. Although pathogens and their products are powerful tools to probe host intestinal epithelial responses and the role of the epithelium in innate and acquired immune networks, we note that the epithelium also produces products that function to maintain the balance between physiologic inflammation and pathologic mucosal inflammation. In this regard, a number of anti-inflammatory strategies are essential for normal host mucosal function. Further, when the intestinal epithelium is injured, the host employs remarkable strategies to restore essential epithelial integrity, and these also are tightly integrated with the host's epithelial cell pro- and anti-inflammatory functions.[28–30]

ACKNOWLEDGMENTS

This work was supported by NIH Grants DK35108, DK 58960, and a grant from the Wm. K. Warren Foundation.

REFERENCES

1. RAKOFF-NAHOUM, S., J. PAGLINO, F. ESLAMI-VARZANEH, *et al.* 2004. Recognition of commensal microflora by toll-like receptors is required for intestinal homeostasis. Cell **118:** 229–241.

2. MAZMANIAN, S.K., C.H. LIU, A.O. TZIANABOS & D.L. KASPER. 2005. An immunomodulatory molecule of symbiotic bacteria directs maturation of the host immune system. Cell **122:** 107–118.

3. KELLY, D., J.I. CAMPBELL, T.P. KING, *et al.* 2004. Commensal anaerobic gut bacteria attenuate inflammation by regulating nuclear-cytoplasmic shuttling of PPAR-γ and RelA. Nat. Immunol. **5:** 104–112.

4. ECKMANN, L., F. LAURENT, T.D. LANGFORD, *et al.* 2000. Nitric oxide production by human intestinal epithelial cells and competition for arginine as potential determinants of host defense against the lumen-dwelling pathogen *Giardia lamblia.* J. Immunol. **164:** 1478–1487.

5. MCCOLE, D.F., L. ECKMANN, F. LAURENT & M.F. KAGNOFF. 2000. Intestinal epithelial cell apoptosis following *Cryptosporidium parvum* infection. Infect. Immun. **68:** 1710–1713.

6. KARIN, M. & A. LIN. 2002. NF-κB at the crossroads of life and death. Nat. Immunol. **3:** 221–227.

7. GIRARDIN, S.E., R. TOURNEBIZE, M. MAVRIS, *et al.* 2001. CARD4/Nod1 mediates NF-κB and JNK activation by invasive *Shigella flexneri.* EMBO Rep. **2:** 736–742.

8. KIM, J.G., S.J. LEE & M.F. KAGNOFF. 2004. Nod1 is an essential signal transducer in intestinal epithelial cells infected with bacteria that avoid recognition by toll-like receptors. Infect. Immun. **72:** 1487–1495.

9. ECKMANN, L., H.C. JUNG, C. SCHURER-MALY, *et al.* 1993. Differential cytokine expression by human intestinal epithelial cell lines: regulated expression of interleukin 8. Gastroenterology **105:** 1689–1697.

10. ECKMANN, L., M.F. KAGNOFF & J. FIERER. 1993. Epithelial cells secrete the chemokine interleukin-8 in response to bacterial entry. Infect. Immun. **61:** 4569–4574.

11. KAGNOFF, M.F. & L. ECKMANN. 1997. Epithelial cells as sensors for microbial infection. J. Clin. Invest. **100:** 6–10.

12. YANG, S.K., L. ECKMANN, A. PANJA & M.F. KAGNOFF. 1997. Differential and regulated expression of C-X-C, C-C, and C-chemokines by human colon epithelial cells. Gastroenterology **113:** 1214–1223.

13. IZADPANAH, A., M.B. DWINELL, L. ECKMANN, *et al.* 2001. Regulated MIP-3α/CCL20 production by human intestinal epithelium: mechanism for modulating mucosal immunity. Am. J. Physiol. Gastrointest. Liver Physiol. **280:** G710–G719.

14. MIYAMOTO, Y., M. IIMURA, J.B. KAPER, *et al.* 2006. Role of Shiga toxin versus H7 flagellin in enterohaemorrhagic *Escherichia coli* signaling of human colon epithelium *in vivo.* Cell. Microbiol. **8:** 869–879.

15. KEATES, S., A.C. KEATES, E. MIZOGUCHI, *et al.* 1997. Enterocytes are the primary source of the chemokine ENA-78 in normal colon and ulcerative colitis. Am. J. Physiol. **273:** G75–G82.

16. YANG, C.C., H. OGAWA, M.B. DWINELL, *et al.* 2005. Chemokine receptor CCR6 transduces signals that activate p130Cas and alter cAMP-stimulated ion trans-

port in human intestinal epithelial cells. Am. J. Physiol. Cell Physiol. **288:** C321–C328.

17. REINECKER, H.C., E.Y. LOH, D.J. RINGLER, *et al.* 1995. Monocyte-chemoattractant protein 1 gene expression in intestinal epithelial cells and inflammatory bowel disease mucosa. Gastroenterology **108:** 40–50.

18. BERIN, M.C., M.B. DWINELL, L. ECKMANN & M.F. KAGNOFF. 2001. Production of MDC/CCL22 by human intestinal epithelial cells. Am. J. Physiol. Gastrointest. Liver Physiol. **280:** G1217–G1226.

19. DWINELL, M.B., N. LUGERING, L. ECKMANN & M.F. KAGNOFF. 2001. Regulated production of interferon-inducible T-cell chemoattractants by human intestinal epithelial cells. Gastroenterology **120:** 49–59.

20. KUNKEL, E.J., J.J. CAMPBELL, G. HARALDSEN, *et al.* 2000. Lymphocyte CC chemokine receptor 9 and epithelial thymus-expressed chemokine (TECK) expression distinguish the small intestinal immune compartment: epithelial expression of tissue-specific chemokines as an organizing principle in regional immunity. J. Exp. Med. **192:** 761–768.

21. OGAWA, H., M. IIMURA, L. ECKMANN & M.F. KAGNOFF. 2004. Regulated production of the chemokine CCL28 in human colon epithelium. Am. J. Physiol. Gastrointest. Liver Physiol. **287:** G1062–G1069.

22. O'NEIL, D.A., E.M. PORTER, D. ELEWAUT, *et al.* 1999. Expression and regulation of the human β-defensins hBD-1 and hBD-2 in intestinal epithelium. J. Immunol. **163:** 6718–6724.

23. HASE, K., L. ECKMANN, J.D. LEOPARD, *et al.* 2002. Cell differentiation is a key determinant of cathelicidin LL-37/human cationic antimicrobial protein 18 expression by human colon epithelium. Infect. Immun. **70:** 953–963.

24. FAHLGREN, A., S. HAMMARSTROM, A. DANIELSSON & M.L. HAMMARSTROM. 2004. β-Defensin-3 and -4 in intestinal epithelial cells display increased mRNA expression in ulcerative colitis. Clin. Exp. Immunol. **137:** 379–385.

25. HASE, K., M. MURAKAMI, M. IIMURA, *et al.* 2003. Expression of LL-37 by human gastric epithelial cells as a potential host defense mechanism against *Helicobacter pylori.* Gastroenterology **125:** 1613–1625.

26. IIMURA, M., R.L. GALLO, K. HASE, *et al.* 2005. Cathelicidin mediates innate intestinal defense against colonization with epithelial adherent bacterial pathogens. J. Immunol. **174:** 4901–4907.

27. ZAIOU, M. & R.L. GALLO. 2002. Cathelicidins, essential gene-encoded mammalian antibiotics. J. Mol. Med. **80:** 549–561.

28. GRETEN, F.R., L. ECKMANN, T.F. GRETEN, *et al.* 2004. IKKβ links inflammation and tumorigenesis in a mouse model of colitis-associated cancer. Cell **118:** 285–296.

29. EGAN, L.J., A. DE LECEA, E.D. LEHRMAN, *et al.* 2003. Nuclear factor-κB activation promotes restitution of wounded intestinal epithelial monolayers. Am. J. Physiol. Cell Physiol. **285:** C1028–C1035.

30. CHEN, L.W., L. EGAN, Z.W. LI, *et al.* 2003. The two faces of IKK and NF-κB inhibition: prevention of systemic inflammation but increased local injury following intestinal ischemia-reperfusion. Nat. Med. **9:** 575–581.

A New Look at Crohn's Disease

Breakdown of the Mucosal Antibacterial Defense

JAN WEHKAMP AND EDUARD F. STANGE

Robert Bosch Hospital and Dr. Margarete Fischer Bosch Institute of Clinical Pharmacology, Auerbachstr. 112, D-70376 Stuttgart, Germany

ABSTRACT: Crohn's disease (CD), a chronic inflammatory disease of the intestinal mucosa is usually located in the small intestine (ileum) and or in the colon. Ileal CD has been linked to a mutation in the *NOD2* gene, a bacterial recognition protein. A disturbed antimicrobial defense as provided by an arsenal of different epithelial defensins seems to be a critical factor in disease pathogenesis. Defensins are antimicrobial peptides and in the ileum are mainly expressed in Paneth cells (PCs), epithelial cells that also express *NOD2*. In the colon, defensins are expressed by enterocytes or metaplastic PCs. Ileal CD patients are characterized by a reduced antibacterial activity and a specific reduction of ileal PC defensins. In ileal Crohn's patients displaying a *NOD2* mutation, this decrease is even more pronounced. In contrast, CD of the colon is characterized by an impaired induction of beta defensins in enterocytes. In conclusion, the regional localizations of CD, either ileal or colonic disease, can be linked to different defects in defensin expression. In line with these new findings, we predict that future therapeutic strategies aimed at restoring the host–microbe balance at the intestinal mucosa may prove superior to those that broadly suppress inflammation and adaptive immunity.

KEYWORDS: intestinal bacteria; defensins; gastrointestinal infection; ileal Crohn's disease; colonic Crohn's disease; *NOD2*

INTRODUCTION

On the basis of its clinical features and histopathology, inflammatory bowel disease (IBD) is often grouped into two major entities, ulcerative colitis and Crohn's disease (CD). In both forms of IBD, intestinal microbiota are thought to trigger the disease in genetically susceptible individuals. Although the inflammation seen in patients with ulcerative colitis is typically restricted to the

Address for correspondence: Jan Wehkamp, M.D., Robert Bosch Hospital, Internal Medicine I, and Dr. Margarete Fischer Bosch Institute for Clinical Pharmacology, Auerbachst., 112, D-70376 Stuttgart, Germany. Voice: +49-0-711/8101-3753; fax: +49-0-711/85-92-95.
e-mail: jan.wehkamp@ikp-stuttgart.de

Ann. N.Y. Acad. Sci. 1072: 321–331 (2006). © 2006 New York Academy of Sciences.
doi: 10.1196/annals.1326.030

colon, that of CD occurs at many sites, most commonly in the ileum of the small intestine and in the colon.[1] About a third of patients with CD have a mutation in the *NOD2* gene, which encodes an intracellular bacterial pattern-recognition receptor.[2,3] Furthermore, clinical analyses have revealed that this mutation is associated with the clinical phenotype of ileal CD, whereas no clear genetic association is known so far for the colonic type of CD (for a recent review see Ref. 4). The possible role of diminished defensin levels in CD has been the focus of recent investigation and the overview provided by this meeting aims to summarize some of these new findings.

PATHOPHYSIOLOGY: THE ROLE OF LUMINAL AND MUCOSAL BACTERIA

In health, the normal host relationship with the commensal luminal micro-biota is beneficial, but the same commensal bacteria may have a pathogenic role in inflammatory diseases. For many years, there has been an ongoing discussion that IBDs are caused by a specific, hitherto unrecognized infection. The potential role of several pathogenic microbes like M*ycobacterium*, *Listeria*, rubella (measles) infection, and *Saccharomyces* has been discussed recently.[5,6] In summary, the multitude of identified mucosal pathogens or an-tibodies does not seem to be restricted to a single microorganism and suggests that the mucosa in CD is more susceptible in general to harbor commensal as well as potentially pathogenic bacteria. There is a tremendous increase in the mucosa-associated bacterial counts in the neoterminal ileum after ileocecal re-section for CD, and this colonization may be related to postoperative relapse.[7] Different groups have convincingly and repeatedly demonstrated that the mu-cosa in IBD is characterized by adherent and sometimes invading *Escherichia coli* strains from the lumen.[8–11] In contrast, normal mucosa is virtually ster-ile when washed a few times in saline. Although the causal link has not yet been proven, a breakdown in the expression or function of the antimicrobial mucosal barrier may well explain these findings. A very interesting study by Darfeuille-Michaud and colleagues in France has described adherent invasive *E. coli* strains specifically in the ileal mucosa of CD patients, but not in ul-cerative colitis.[11] Another recent study has found increased levels of adherent *E. coli* in CD colonic mucosa as well as in colon cancer.[10] All these findings fit well with the hypothesis of a break in mucosal tolerance towards various luminal bacteria in IBDs.[12] These findings indicate that Crohn's mucosa may often be the target of various infections but there is no proof that the disease is caused by these agents. In further support of this idea, the immune response in the gut mucosa is not specific for any of these suspicious agents, but rather a general response to a multitude of organisms. Moreover, it is conceivable that there may be a primary defect in the peptide barrier of intestinal antibiotic defensins, which protect the normal mucosa extremely efficiently against ad-herent or invasive microbes. We are convinced that a thorough understanding of these functionally relevant peptides is crucial for the understanding of mucosal biology and that an impaired balance of these effector molecules might explain many aspects of pathogenesis in IBDs, especially CD.[13]

DEFENSIN EXPRESSION AND REGULATION IN THE INTESTINAL TRACT

Although the gastrointestinal tract is colonized by and exposed to a multitude of different bacteria, intestinal infection or translocation of bacterial agents is the exception, not the rule, and is mostly limited to highly pathogenic bacteria or predisposing disease states. The constitutive production of defensins in the intestinal tract helps to limit invasion and adherence of pathogenic and commensal bacteria. The most abundant, constitutively expressed defensins are found in Paneth cells (PCs) of the small intestine.[14] PC antimicrobials, which are stored in secretory granules, are released into the intestinal lumen on stimulation with bacterial products including lipopolysaccharide (LPS) and muramyl dipeptide (MDP).[15] All types of defensins—α, β, and θ—characteristically have microbicidal activity against bacteria, and some also have activity against fungi, viruses, and protozoa.[6, 16, 17] Like other cationic antimicrobial peptides, defensins are thought to kill target microbes by disrupting their membrane integrity via a mechanism known as the "Shai-Matsuzaki-Huang model."[18] Many important studies in the field of defensins have focused on the human and nonvertebrate skin as another barrier of the body exposed to a multitude of bacteria. These studies resulted in the isolation of various peptides exhibiting potent antibiotic activity towards both Gram-positive and -negative bacteria, as well as enveloped viruses and fungi.[19–21] A similar system of antibiotic peptides is apparently synthesized and secreted by the intestinal mucosa as part of innate immunity, but has received little attention, at least in the field of clinical gastroenterology. With more knowledge about defensins in the gastrointestinal tract, especially over the last 5 years, we start to better appreciate the enormous complexity of expression and regulation of these peptides. A total of six α-defensins and four epithelial β-defensins have been identified in the different parts of human intestinal mucosa so far. The α-defensins include human neutrophil peptides 1–4, produced by granulocytes, and human defensin 5 and 6, synthesized in PCs.[22]

REGULATION AND EXPRESSION OF β-DEFENSINS

The β-defensins are of epithelial origin and are abundant in skin, urogenital tract, intestine, and lung.[23] Defensins can be divided into constitutive forms, for example, HBD-1 with its widespread stable distribution,[24] and inducible peptides like HBD-2.[19] The mechanisms of activation are still under investigation and are very complex. Induction by cytokines, such as IL-1β and tumor necrosis factor (TNF)-α, has been shown in addition to a direct response to bacterial components, such as lipopolysaccharides and lipoproteins.[25,26] Signaling pathways include toll-like receptors (TLRs), especially TLR2 and 4,[27,28] and recent work has also focused on various intestinal epithelial cells.[29] Intestinal epithelial cells express various pattern-recognition receptors recognizing microbial "pathogen-associated molecular patterns" as "non-self" to rapidly initiate innate immune responses of survival and to activate defence strategies against luminal pathogens.[30,31] This system of several functional TLRs appears to be a key regulator of the innate response system. Different TLRs are responding to different pathogens and bacterial components, including lipopolysaccharide, flagellin, and others. In the context of pathogen recognition receptors, *NOD2*/CARD15 is an intracellular receptor for peptidoglycan that induces NFκB,[3] which in turn is known to trigger HBD-2 transcription. In colonic epithelial cells *in vitro*, a recent study has shown a specific, NFκB– and AP1– dependent, induction of HBD2 by probiotic bacteria such as *E. coli* (Nissle, 1917) and *Lactobacillus*.[32] In the same study normal LPS., probiotic *E. coli* Nissle LPS, as well as 50 other *E. coli* strains tested did not induce HBD2.[32] The induction of HBD2 by LPS has been described for the airway epithelia[26] and by indirect IL-1 signaling in skin.[33] The lack of response to LPS in the colon is consistent with the lack of HBD2 expression in the uninflamed state.[34,35] Although *in vitro* studies of HBD2 suggest an activation by inflammatory agents or inflammation itself,[33,36,37] the induction of HBD2 does not necessarily correlate with proinflammatory cytokines like IL-8 or TNF-α *in vivo*.[34] Consistent with these findings in the colon, the upregulation of HBD2 in gastritis, was restricted to that triggered by *Helicobacter pylori* infection.[38] Future studies will hopefully be able to address these complicated interactions and their regulation *in vivo*.

GUARDIANS OF THE SMALL INTESTINE: PC α-DEFENSINS

An illustration and HE staining of PCs in the small intestine are shown in FIGURE 1. Human defensin 5 is released as a propeptide from PC and, at least in man, is activated by trypsin in the lumen of the intestinal crypts.[39] The functional importance of PC α-defensins is illustrated by two mouse models. First, mice rendered deficient in their PC α-defensin-processing enzyme do not produce mature homologues of the human α-defensins and are highly susceptible to orally administered challenges with bacterial pathogens.[40] Second, and conversely, HD5 transgenic mice are protected against infection, which demonstrates a potent *in vivo* activity of this peptide against pathogenic bacteria in the lumen.[41] These investigators showed that HD5 expression in these mice is specific to PCs and is similar to endogenous defensin gene expression. The storage and processing of transgenic HD5 also matches that observed in

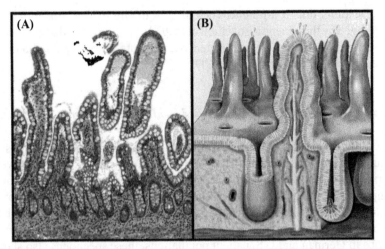

FIGURE 1. Hematoxylin–eosin staining **(A)** as well as schematic demonstration **(B)** of the small intestine. PCs are expressed at the base of the crypts. These cells seem to play a critical role in the pathogenesis of CD. PCs are the only source of α-defensins HD5 and HD6, which are the major antibacterial factors in the ileum. In mice small intestinal PC defensins contribute to 70% of antibiotic activity.[15] This antimicrobial activity is reduced in patients with ileal CD, which corresponds with a specific decrease in PC-defensin expression[43] (Figures published with the permission of *Nature Immunology*).

humans. HD5 transgenic mice were markedly resistant to orally administered challenges with virulent *Salmonella typhimurium* compared with controls.[41] Together these studies of transgenic mice provide support for a critical *in vivo* role of PC α-defensins in innate immunity of the small intestinal mucosa. It has been shown in mice that bacteria such as *Salmonella*, are able to downregulate PC defensin expression.[42] Mice PC defensins contribute to 70% of total ileal antimicrobial activity and these ileal peptides are released after stimulation with LPS and other bacterial products.[15] The extremely abundant expression of PC and PC defensins correlates with the different milieu of colonic and ileal bacterial flora: In the presence of PCs in the small intestine, the bacterial counts are low. In contrast, in the absence of significant numbers of PCs in the colon, intestinal bacteria are a significant proportion of the luminal content and are found into numbers that exceed the total number of eukaryotic cells in the human body.

DEFENSIN EXPRESSION IN DIFFERENT CLINICAL PHENOTYPES OF CD

The separation of CD into different clinical phenotypes is based on the concept that CD is not a single disease, but rather different disorders with common clinical features. On the basis of different clinical observations and classifications, drastic differences in innate immunity and bacterial milieu, and encouraged by the genetic association of *NOD2* mutations with disease location in the small intestine, we segregated our patients according to anatomical disease location, ileal and colonic CD.

Ileal CD and Diminished Ileal PC α-Defensins

PCs are the major source of antimicrobial peptides in the small intestine, including human α-defensins HD5 and HD6. Over the last couple of years, we rigorously tested the hypothesis that reduced expression of PC α-defensins compromises mucosal host defenses and predisposes patients to CD of the ileum. We recently reported that patients with CD of the ileum have reduced antibacterial activity in their intestinal mucosal extracts.[43] In two independent studies in German and U.S. patient populations, these specimens also showed decreased expression of PC α-defensins (mRNA and protein), whereas the expression of other PC products either remained unchanged or increased when compared with controls.[43,44] The specific decrease of α-defensins was independent of the degree of inflammation in the specimens and was not observed in either CD of the colon, ulcerative colitis, or pouchitis. The functional consequence of α-defensin-expression levels was examined by using a transgenic mouse model, where we found that changes in HD5-expression levels, comparable to those observed in CD, had a pronounced impact on the luminal microbiota.[43]

PCs also express *NOD2*,[45] which further supports the idea of a possible role for PC antimicrobials in CD. The human studies mentioned above, as well as independent studies in a rodent model, further substantiate a link between *NOD2* mutations and PC α-defensins.[43,44,46] Interestingly, even though all patients with ileal CD have diminished HD5 and HD6 levels, this decrease is most pronounced in patients with a *NOD2* mutation.[43,44] In the study using a rodent model, Kobayashi and colleagues reported a decrease of PC α-defensin (cryptidin) mRNA expression in mice lacking the *NOD2* gene.[46] The *NOD2* knockout mice were unable to detect muramyl dipeptide, the ligand for *NOD2*. Most interestingly, these mice were more susceptible to an oral, but not systemic, infection with the pathogenic bacterium *Listeria monocytogenes*, supporting the importance of *NOD2* in epithelial antimicrobial function.[46] Even though there seems to be a clear link between *NOD2* function and α-defensin expression, the mechanistic details are still obscure. The studies of different patient populations with ileal CD suggest that reduced PC defensins are ultimately linked to disease and the specific deficiency of PC defensins that characterizes ileal CD may compromise innate immune defenses of the ileal mucosa and initiate and/or perpetuate this disease. A model for the role of defensins and intestinal bacteria in the pathogenesis and disease progression of CD is proposed in FIGURE 2.

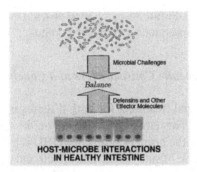

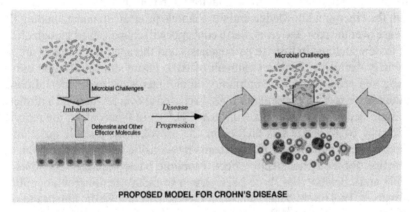

FIGURE 2. Proposed model for the role of intestinal bacteria and host defensins in the pathogenesis and disease progression of CD. The healthy intestinal tract is characterized by a sensitive balance of host antimicrobial peptides and intestinal microbes (*top*). In CD this balance is disturbed. Because of insufficient expression and function of antimicrobial defensin molecules, intestinal microbes are able to invade the mucosa. With further progression of disease the bacterial influx provokes an inflammatory response. (Source: Wehkamp *et al.* Nature *Clinical* Practice, September 2005.[13] Also available at www.nature.com/clinicalpractice/gastrohep).

Colonic CD and Attenuated Induction of β-Defensins

Two studies have investigated the expression of HBD2 in ulcerative colitis finding a strong induction in case of inflammation.[36,47] When comparing colonic HBD2 expression among patients with CD and ulcerative colitis there is a striking difference: Whereas in ulcerative colitis patients strong HBD2 induction is observed, this induction seems to be attenuated in the inflamed tissue of CD patients.[34,35,37] Two β-defensins with a different antimicrobial spectrum, HBD3 and HBD4, seem to follow this distribution pattern, although their mRNA-expression levels are lower.[34,48] In summary, except for HBD1, defensins are almost absent in normal colonic tissue. In ulcerative colitis patients there is an increased defensin synthesis, but a lack of (or weakened) response is noted in CD. Future research may provide mechanistic details and reveal the functional consequences of these findings.

Therapeutic Consequences and Conclusion

Currently, the principal treatment for both diseases is a suppression of the inflammatory process. This strategy was based on the former belief of most experts in the field that the primary problem in IBD is a disregulated adaptive immune system. Because of substantial side effects and uncontrolled relapses, this therapy remains far from satisfactory for both patients and physicians. With the emerging knowledge and tremendous progress in understanding this disease over the past few years, these concepts will change, even though different understandings in disease pathogenesis and therapeutic strategies are not mutually exclusive. For the treatment of IBD, future strategies might aim to strengthen protective innate immunity. Some interesting experimental observations leave room for speculation. As discussed above, PC-derived antimicrobials are decreased in patients with ileal CD.[43,44] In this context, the reported efficiency of *Trichuris suis* therapy in CD provokes the testable question of whether the stimulation of PC defensins by parasitic worms might be an explanation for their therapeutic effect. Probiotic bacteria like *E. coli* (Nissle, 1917) and *Lactobacillus*, have been shown to induce antimicrobial peptides strongly.[32] This might be an important mechanism to help the mucosa to prevent bacterial invasion.[32] Probiotic bacteria are the first therapeutic agents for IBD that we know bolster the production of antimicrobial peptides,[32] but it is likely that other therapeutic agents could have similar effects. In summary, this new view of disease pathophysiology suggests that therapeutic strategies aimed at restoring the host–microbe balance at the intestinal mucosa may prove superior to those that broadly suppress inflammation and adaptive immunity.

ACKNOWLEDGMENTS

Jan Wehkamp and Eduard F. Stange are supported by the Robert Bosch Foundation, Stuttgart, Germany. Jan Wehkamp was also supported in part by the NIH (AI 32738 and AI 50843). The authors thank many scientists in the field for valuable discussion, and apologize to those colleagues who we were unable to reference owing to space constraints.

REFERENCES

1. PODOLSKY, D.K. 2002. Inflammatory bowel disease. N. Engl. J Med. **347:** 417–429.
2. HUGOT, J.-P., C. CHAMAILLARD, *et al.* 2001. Association of NOD2 leucine-rich repeat variants with susceptibility to Crohn's disease. Nature **411:** 599–603.

3. OGURA, Y., D.K. BONEN, *et al.* 2001. A frameshift mutation in NOD2 associated with susceptibility to Crohn's diease. Nature **411**: 603–606.
4. GASCHE, C. & P. GRUNDTNER. 2005. Genotypes and phenotypes in Crohn's disease: do they help in clinical management? Gut **54**: 162–167.
5. FELLERMANN, K., J. WEHKAMP, *et al.* 2003. Crohn's disease: a defensin deficiency syndrome ? Eur. J. Gastroenterol. Hepatol. **15**: 627–634.
6. WEHKAMP, J., M. SCHMID, *et al.* 2005. Defensin deficiency, intestinal microbes and clinical phenotypes of Crohn's disease. J. Leukoc. Biol. **77**: 460–465.
7. NEUT, C., P. BULOIS, *et al.* 2002. Changes in the bacterial flora of the neoterminal ileum after ileocolonic resection for Crohn's disease. Am. J. Gastroenterol. **97**: 939–946.
8. DARFEUILLE-MICHAUD, A., C. NEUT, *et al.* 1998. Presence of adherent *Escherichia coli* strains in ileal mucosa of patients with Crohn's disease. Gastroenterology **115**: 1405–1413.
9. SWIDSINSKI, A., A. LADHOFF, *et al.* 2002. Mucosal flora in inflammatory bowel disease. Gastroenterology **122**: 44–54.
10. MARTIN, H.M., B.J. CAMPBELL, *et al.* 2004. Enhanced *Escherichia coli* adherence and invasion in Crohn's disease and colon cancer. Gastroenterology **127**: 80–93.
11. DARFEUILLE-MICHAUD, A., J. BOUDEAU, *et al.* 2004. High prevalence of adherent-invasive *Escherichia coli* associated with ileal mucosa in Crohn's disease. Gastroenterology **127**: 412–421.
12. DUCHMANN, R., E. MAY, *et al.* 1999. T cell specifity and cross reactivity towards enterobacteria, *Bacteroides*, *Bifidobacterium*, and antigens from resident intestinal flora in humans. Gut **44**: 812–818.
13. WEHKAMP, J., K. FELLERMANN, *et al.* 2005. Mechanisms of disease: defensins in gastrointestinal diseases. Nat. Clin. Pract. **2**: 406–415.
14. BEVINS, C.L. 2004. The Paneth cell and the innate immune response. Curr. Opin. Gastroenterol. **20**: 572–580.
15. AYABE, T., D.P. SATCHELL, *et al.* 2000. Secretion of microbicidal alpha-defensins by intestinal Paneth cell response to bacteria. Nat. Immunol. **1**: 113–118.
16. LEHRER, R.I., A.K. LICHTENSTEIN, *et al.* 1993. Defensins: antimicrobial and cytotoxic peptides of mammalian cells. Ann. Rev. Immunol. **11**: 105–128.
17. LEHRER, R.I. & C.L. BEVINS. 2004. Defensins and other antimicrobial peptides. *In* Mucosal Immunology. Mestecky J., Bienenstock J., Lammet M.E., W. Strober, *et al.* Eds.: 95–110. Academic Press. New York
18. ZASLOFF, M. 2002. Antimicrobial peptides of multicellular organisms. Nature **415**: 389–395.
19. HARDER, J., J. BARTELS, *et al.* 1997. A peptide antibiotic from human skin [letter] [see comments]. Nature **387**: 861.
20. HARDER, J., J. BARTELS, *et al.* 2001. Isolation and characterization of human - defensin-3, a novel human inducible peptide antibiotic. J. Biol. Chem. **276**: 5707–5713.
21. ZASLOFF, M. 1992. Antibiotic peptides as mediators of innate immunity. Curr. Opin. Immunol. **4**: 3–7.
22. JONES, D.E. & C.L. BEVINS. 1992. Paneth cells of the human small intestine express an antimicrobial peptide gene. J. Biol. Chem. **267**: 23216–23225.
23. GANZ, T. 2003. Defensins: antimicrobial peptides of innate immunity. Nat. Rev. Immunol. **3**: 710–720.
24. ZHAO, C., I. WANG, *et al.* 1996. Widespread expression of beta-defensin hBD-1 in human secretory glands and epithelial cells. FEBS Lett. **396**: 319–322.

25. BECKER, M.N., G. DIAMOND, et al. 2000. CD14-dependent lipopolysaccharide-induced beta-defensin-2 expression in human tracheobronchial epithelium. J. Biol. Chem. 275: 29731–29736.
26. DIAMOND, G., J.P. RUSSELL, et al. 1996. Inducible expression of an antibiotic peptide gene in lipopolysaccharide-challenged tracheal epithelial cells. Proc. Natl. Acad. Sci. USA 93: 5156–5160.
27. WANG, X., Z. ZHANG, et al. 2003. Airway epithelia regulate expression of human beta-defensin 2 through Toll-like receptor 2. FASEB J. 17: 1727–1729.
28. BIRAGYN, A., P.A. RUFFINI, et al. 2002. Toll-like receptor 4-dependent activation of dendritic cells by beta-defensin 2. Science 298: 1025–1029.
29. VORA, P., A. YOUDIM, et al. 2004. {beta}-defensin-2 expression is regulated by TLR signaling in intestinal epithelial cells. J. Immunol. 173: 5398–5405.
30. OTTE, J.M., K. KIEHNE, et al. 2003. Antimicrobial peptides in innate immunity of the human intestine. J. Gastroenterol. 38: 717–726.
31. CARIO, E., G. GERKEN, et al. 2002. "For whom the bell tolls!"—innate defense mechanisms and survival strategies of the intestinal epithelium against luminal pathogens. Z. Gastroenterol. 40: 983–990.
32. WEHKAMP, J., J. HARDER, et al. 2004. NF-kB and AP-1 mediated induction of human beta defensin-2 in intestinal epithelial cells by E. coli Nissle 1917: a novel effect of a probiotic bacterium. Infect. Immun. 72: 5750–5758.
33. LIU, L., A.A. ROBERTS, et al. 2003. By IL-1 signaling, monocyte-derived cells dramatically enhance the epidermal antimicrobial response to lipopolysaccharide. J. Immunol. 170: 575–580.
34. WEHKAMP, J., J. HARDER, et al. 2003. Inducible and constitutive beta-defensins are differentially expressed in Crohn's disease and ulcerative colitis. Inflamm. Bowel Dis. 9: 215–223.
35. FAHLGREN, A., S. HAMMARSTROM, et al. 2003. Increased expression of antimicrobial peptides and lysozyme in colonic epithelial cells of patients with ulcerative colitis. Clin. Exp. Immunol. 131: 90–101.
36. O'NEIL, D.A., E.M. PORTER, et al. 1999. Expression and regulation of the human β-defensins hBD-1 and hBD-2 in intestinal epithelium. J. Immunol. 163: 6718–6724.
37. WEHKAMP, J., K. FELLERMANN, et al. 2002. Human beta-defensin 2 but not beta-defensin 1 is expressed preferentially in colonic mucosa of inflammatory bowel disease. Eur. J. Gastroenterol. Hepatol. 14: 745–752.
38. WEHKAMP, J., K. SCHMIDT, et al. 2003. Defensin pattern in chronic gastritis: HBD-2 is differentially expressed with respect to Helicobacter pylori status. J. Clin. Pathol. 56: 352–357.
39. GHOSH, D., E. PORTER, et al. 2002. Paneth cell trypsin is the processing enzyme for human defensin-5. Nat. Immunol. 3: 583–590.
40. WILSON, C.L., A.J. OUELLETTE, et al. 1999. Regulation of intestinal alpha-defensin activation by the metalloproteinase matrilysin in innate host defense. Science 286: 113–117.
41. SALZMAN, N.H., D. GHOSH, et al. 2003. Protection against enteric salmonellosis in transgenic mice expressing a human intestinal defensin. Nature 422: 522–526.
42. SALZMAN, N.H., M.M. CHOU, et al. 2003. Enteric salmonella infection inhibits Paneth cell antimicrobial peptide expression. Infect. Immun. 71: 1109–1115.
43. WEHKAMP, J., N.H. SALZMAN, et al. 2005. Reduced Paneth cell {alpha}-defensins in ileal Crohn's disease. Proc. Natl.: Acad. Sci. USA 102: 18129–18134.

44. WEHKAMP, J., J. HARDER, *et al.* 2004. NOD2 (CARD15) mutations in Crohn's disease are associated with diminished mucosal α-defensin expression. Gut **53:** 1658–1664.
45. LALA, S., Y. OGURA, *et al.* 2003. Crohn's disease and the NOD2 gene: a role for Paneth cells. Gastroenterology **125:** 47–57.
46. KOBAYASHI, K.S., M. CHAMAILLARD, *et al.* 2005. Nod2-dependent regulation of innate and adaptive immunity in the intestinal tract. Science **307:** 731–734.
47. FURRIE, E., S. MACFARLANE, *et al.* 2005. Synbiotic therapy (*Bifidobacterium longum*/synergy 1) initiates resolution of inflammation in patients with active ulcerative colitis: a randomised controlled pilot trial. Gut **54:** 242–249.
48. FAHLGREN, A., S. HAMMARSTROM, *et al.* 2004. beta-defensin-3 and -4 in intestinal epithelial cells display increased mRNA expression in ulcerative colitis. Clin. Exp. Immunol. **137:** 379–385.

Toll-Like Receptor Signaling and its Relevance to Intestinal Inflammation

ELKE CARIO[a] AND DANIEL K. PODOLSKY[b]

[a]Division of Gastroenterology and Hepatology, University Hospital of Essen, Essen, Germany

[b]Gastrointestinal Unit, Massachusetts General Hospital, Center for the Study of Inflammatory Bowel Disease, Harvard Medical School, Boston Massachusetts 02114, USA

ABSTRACT: This review discusses the current progress in the understanding of how commensal-mediated activation of toll-like receptors (TLRs) may be involved in the regulation of physiological and pathophysiological processes of the intestinal mucosa including tissue regeneration and inflammation. While regulation of TLRs and their downstream signaling mediators might be used to prevent and treat inflammatory bowel diseases, paradoxically, at this time, it remains uncertain whether this would be more effectively accomplished by enhancing or inhibiting these pathways.

KEYWORDS: Innate immunity; inflammatory bowel diseases; resident microflora; host defense; intestinal epithelium; therapy

The intestinal mucosa must rapidly recognize luminal pathogens to initiate controlled immune responses, but maintain hyporesponsiveness to omnipresent harmless commensals. In order to be able to continuously screen the microbial composition of luminal contents, readily recognize potential imbalances, and rapidly initiate innate immune responses, immune cells of the intestinal mucosa are equipped with a diverse set of pattern-recognition receptors (PRRs), including toll-like receptors (TLRs). An important role of TLRs in microbial recognition, induction of antimicrobial genes, and the control of adaptive immune responses has begun to emerge from recent studies.

Eleven mammalian TLRs have been identified. They are characterized by three common structural features: a divergent ligand-binding extracellular domain with leucine-rich repeats, a short transmembrane region, and a highly homologous cytoplasmic toll/IL-1 receptor domain--similar to that of the

Address for correspondence: Elke Cario, M.D., University Hospital of Essen, Division of Gastroenterology & Hepatology, Institutsgruppe I, Virchowstr. 171, D-45147 Essen, Germany. Voice: +49-201-723-4527; fax: +49-211-495-7035.

e-mail: elke.cario@uni-due.de

Ann. N.Y. Acad. Sci. 1072: 332–338 (2006). © 2006 New York Academy of Sciences.
doi: 10.1196/annals.1326.006

interleukin-1 receptor family and essential for initiation of downstream signaling cascades. TLRs are inducibly or constitutively expressed in varying combinations by many different cell types throughout the whole gastrointestinal tract, including intestinal epithelial cells,[1] monocytes/macrophages,[2] myofibroblasts,[3] endothelial cells,[4] and dendritic cells.[5]

Different so-called pathogen-associated molecular patterns (PAMPs) selectively activate different TLRs, that is, each TLR binds specific "molecular signatures" of different classes of micro-organisms or individual features present on diverse commensals or pathogens; for example, TLR2, lipopeptide; TLR4, lipopolysaccharide; TLR5, flagellin, and TLR9, CpG DNA. Subcellular compartmentalization of TLRs appears to be a critical determinant of immune responsiveness.[6] Individual TLRs differentially activate distinct, but also partially overlapping, signaling events via diverse cofactors and adaptor proteins mediating specific immune responses. To date, at least five different adaptor proteins have been identified in humans: MyD88, Mal/TIRAP, TRIF/TICAM-1, TRAM/Tirp/TICAM-2, and SARM. Downstream, different signaling modules and partially interacting complexes result in the activation of several transcription factors, including NF-κB, AP-1, Elk-1, CREB, and STATs. These result in the subsequent transcriptional activation of unique and common genes encoding pro- and anti-inflammatory cytokines and chemokines as well as the induction of costimulatory molecules that control the activation of antigen-specific and non-specific adaptive immune responses by lamina propria cells. Several proteins that negatively modulate immune responses by interference with the TLR signaling complex have recently been identified including Tollip,[7,8] PPARγ,[9] SIGIRR (or TIR8),[10,11] and A20.[12] These proteins may block exaggerated inflammatory responses to omnipresent harmless commensals and their products in the healthy intestine.

Accumulating evidence underscores the important role that basal activation of TLRs plays in innate host defense in the healthy intestinal mucosa, maintaining mucosal as well as commensal homeostasis. Commensals not only suppress[13,14] but also actively induce expression of a variety of host genes that participate in important physiological functions, including barrier protection and defense strategies.[15] Recent observations imply that the continuous recognition of selective commensals by TLR2/4 under steady-state conditions is essential in mucosal protection against exogenous injury.[16] Moreover, TLR2 can directly confer intestinal epithelial barrier function.[17] Commensal-derived signals also protect the host via TLR4 by inhibiting allergic responses to food antigens.[18] Finally, TLR signaling pathways may critically be involved in commensal-induced antimicrobial peptide production, such as defensins,[19] thus helping to prevent pathogenic bacteria from crossing the mucosal barrier. However, the full spectrum of host-beneficial signaling pathways activated by commensal-derived TLR ligands, which may balance responsiveness and survival and confer integrity of the healthy, intestinal mucosa, remains to be identified in depth.

The pathogenesis of chronic recurrent intestinal inflammation in IBD is thought to involve broken epithelial barrier function and diverse environmental triggers including, most importantly, the luminal flora, with subsequent aberrant stimulation of the underlying mucosal immune system in genetically susceptible individuals.[20] "Healthy" intestinal mucosa expresses low concentrations of TLR2 or TLR4 protein *in vivo*.[21] However, TLR4 expression is significantly increased in intestinal epithelial cells (IECs) and lamina propria mononuclear cells (LPMNCs) throughout the lower gastrointestinal tract in association with acute IBD[5,21,22] and murine colitis.[23,24] Th1 cytokines, such as IFN-γ and TNF-α, strongly upregulate TLR4 expression in IECs, possibly acting in an autocrine loop, which may lead to perpetuation of intestinal inflammation by altering TLR4 responsiveness to commensals.[25,26]

The most common variant of TLR4 (D299G polymorphism) has been associated with IBD in some populations,[27] but the functional phenotypic significance remains unresolved in IBD. Several studies have recently demonstrated that TLR4-mutant (C3H/HeJBir) and TLR4-deficient mice show increased susceptibility to DSS colitis.[16,28–31] Observed differences between studies in susceptibility may be caused by different degrees of genetic back-crosses.[32] Toxic effects on colonic epithelium with loss of commensal-mediated cytoprotection of the intestinal epithelial barrier due to TLR4/MyD88 dysfunction and subsequent bacterial translocation have been suggested as possible mechanisms by which DSS induces increased morbidity and mortality in TLR4/MyD88-deficient mice. Furthermore, activated macrophages in the colonic epithelial progenitor niche promote proliferation and survival of epithelial progenitors, which may be severely impaired in the absence of MyD88 in DSS injury.[33]

The outcome of TLR-specific signaling effects may show considerable variation between cell types and different stages of disease, but the precise molecular mechanisms of pathophysiology are not yet understood. While basal TLR4 activation may be protective against *acute* injury through its beneficial effects in the intestinal epithelium, other data imply that aberrant TLR4/MyD88 signaling may favor *chronic* intestinal inflammation through its detrimental proinflammatory effects in the underlying lamina propria. A recent study demonstrated that myeloid cell–specific deletion of Stat3 results in development of chronic enterocolitis with enhanced Th1 responses in mice. Crossing Stat3 knockout with TLR4 knockout mice dramatically reduced intestinal inflammation, suggesting that commensal-mediated TLR4 dysfunction of mucosal T cells contributes to the development of intestinal inflammation through the Th1 pathway.[34] This hypothesis is supported by the recent observation that blocking TLR4 with a specific antagonist inhibited development of Th1-mediated colitis in MDR1-α-deficient mice.[35] Interestingly, spontaneous development of enterocolitis also appears to be significantly lessened in IL10 null mice in the absence of MyD88 (R. Medzhitov, personal communication), suggesting that commensal-mediated signaling via the adaptor molecule MyD88 may be involved in aberrant generation of IFNγ-producing Th1-type cells that drive disease in this colitis model.

Signaling through different TLRs may result in considerable qualitative differences in Th1-mediated immune responses.[36] Different commensal bacterial species selectively initiate intestinal inflammation with distinctly different kinetics and anatomic distribution in IL10 null mice,[37] implying variation of agonist recognition and engagement with cell signaling between individual TLRs and other PRRs. Moreover, when back-crossed onto several genetic backgrounds, IL10 knockout mice demonstrate significant differences in the severity of colitis activity,[38] TLR4-deficient C3H/HeJ mice are resistant to endotoxin shock, but paradoxically predisposed to gram-negative bacteria, such as *Salmonella typhimurium*.[39,40] Thus, D299G mutation could confer hypersensitivity to *E. coli* and other gram-negative commensal or pathogenic ligand causing unwanted inflammation in IBD. Interestingly, dominant antigens in sera from colitic C3H/HeJBir mice, and also from subsets of IBD patients, seem to be flagellins.[41-43] Flagellin-specific CD4(+) T cells induce severe colitis when adoptively transferred into immunodeficient SCID mice,[42] implying aberrant TLR5 (and/or other TLR)-mediated T regulatory immune response in colitis. Further studies are needed to dissect the complex interplay of environmental and microbial factors as well as distinct pattern-recognition molecules with functional variations in distinct cell types (and also organs) that may modify disease expression, leading to diverse IBD phenotypes in the genetically susceptible host.

Further characterization of the physiologic and pathophysiologic mechanisms within this network of possible cell–cell, ligand–ligand, and PRR–PRR signaling interactions could lead to promising, novel approaches that differentially exploit the TLR pathways as means to induce salutary immune responses for treatment of IBD. Administration of bacterial DNA derived from the normal gut flora ameliorates acute DSS colitis and inhibits induction of proinflammatory cytokines,[29,44,45] Prophylactic application of selective TLR ligands could enhance commensal-mediated tissue-protective processes in order to prevent acute flare-ups in IBD. Once an acute inflammatory episode has been initiated, some of the untoward effects of intestinal inflammation could be abrogated by blocking uncontrolled signal transduction by specific TLR inhibitors, such as the lipid A-mimetic, CRX-526, which has antagonistic activity for TLR4,[35] thus dampening tissue-destructive effects.

ACKNOWLEDGMENTS

This work was supported by grants from the Deutsche Forschungsgemeinschaft (to E.C.) and the NIH (to D.K.P.).

REFERENCES

1. CARIO, E. *et al.* 2000. Lipopolysaccharide activates distinct signaling pathways in intestinal epithelial cell lines expressing toll-like receptors. J. Immunol. **164:** 966–972.

2. SMITH, P.D. *et al.* 2001. Intestinal macrophages lack CD14 and CD89 and consequently are down-regulated for LPS- and IgA-mediated activities. J. Immunol. **167:** 2651–2656.

3. OTTE, J.M., I.M. ROSENBERG & D. K. PODOLSKY. 2003. Intestinal myofibroblasts in innate immune responses of the intestine. Gastroenterology **124:** 1866–1878.

4. MAASER, C. *et al.* 2004. Human intestinal microvascular endothelial cells express toll-like receptor 5: a binding partner for bacterial flagellin. J. Immunol. **172:** 5056–5062.

5. HART, A.L. *et al.* 2005. Characteristics of intestinal dendritic cells in inflammatory bowel diseases. Gastroenterology **129:** 50–65.

6. CARIO, E. *et al.* 2002. Commensal-associated molecular patterns induce selective toll-like receptor-trafficking from apical membrane to cytoplasmic compartments in polarized intestinal epithelium. Am. J. Pathol. **160:** 165–173.

7. MELMED, G. *et al.* 2003. Human intestinal epithelial cells are broadly unresponsive to toll-like receptor 2-dependent bacterial ligands: implications for host-microbial interactions in the gut. J. Immunol. **170:** 1406–1415.

8. OTTE, J. M., E. CARIO & D. K. PODOLSKY. 2004. Mechanisms of cross hyporesponsiveness to toll-like receptor bacterial ligands in intestinal epithelial cells. Gastroenterology **126:** 1054–1070.

9. DUBUQUOY, L. *et al.* 2003. Impaired expression of peroxisome proliferator-activated receptor gamma in ulcerative colitis. Gastroenterology **124:** 1265–1276.

10. GARLANDA, C. *et al.* 2004. Intestinal inflammation in mice deficient in Tir8, an inhibitory member of the IL-1 receptor family. Proc. Natl. Acad. Sci. USA **101:** 3522–3526.

11. QIN, J. *et al.* 2005. SIGIRR inhibits interleukin-1 receptor- and toll-like receptor 4-mediated signaling through different mechanisms. J. Biol. Chem. **280:** 25233–25241.

12. BOONE, D.L. *et al.* 2004. The ubiquitin-modifying enzyme A20 is required for termination of toll-like receptor responses. Nat. Immunol. **5:** 1052–1060.

13. NEISH, A.S. *et al.* 2000. Prokaryotic regulation of epithelial responses by inhibition of IkappaB-alpha ubiquitination. Science **289:** 1560–1563.

14. KELLY, D. *et al.* 2004. Commensal anaerobic gut bacteria attenuate inflammation by regulating nuclear-cytoplasmic shuttling of PPAR-gamma and RelA. Nat. Immunol. **5:** 104–112.

15. HOOPER, L.V. & J.I. GORDON. 2001. Commensal host-bacterial relationships in the gut. Science **292:** 1115–1118.

16. RAKOFF-NAHOUM, S. *et al.* 2004. Recognition of commensal microflora by toll-like receptors is required for intestinal homeostasis. Cell **118:** 229–241.

17. CARIO, E., G. GERKEN & D.K. PODOLSKY. 2004. Toll-like receptor 2 enhances ZO-1-associated intestinal epithelial barrier integrity via protein kinase C. Gastroenterology **127:** 224–238.

18. BASHIR, M.E. *et al.* 2004. Toll-like receptor 4 signaling by intestinal microbes influences susceptibility to food allergy. J. Immunol. **172:** 6978–6987.

19. VORA, P. *et al.* 2004. Beta-defensin-2 expression is regulated by TLR signaling in intestinal epithelial cells. J. Immunol. **173:** 5398–5405.
20. PODOLSKY, D.K. 2002. Inflammatory bowel disease. N. Engl. J. Med. **347:** 417–429.
21. CARIO, E. & D.K. PODOLSKY. 2000. Differential alteration in intestinal epithelial cell expression of toll-like receptor 3 (TLR3) and TLR4 in inflammatory bowel disease. Infect. Immun. **68:** 7010–7017.
22. HAUSMANN, M. *et al.* 2002. Toll-like receptors 2 and 4 are up-regulated during intestinal inflammation. Gastroenterology **122:** 1987–2000.
23. ORTEGA-CAVA, C.F. *et al.* 2003. Strategic compartmentalization of toll-like receptor 4 in the mouse gut. J. Immunol. **170:** 3977–3985.
24. SINGH, J. C. *et al.* 2005. Toll-like receptor-mediated responses of primary intestinal epithelial cells during the development of colitis. Am. J. Physiol. Gastrointest. Liver Physiol. **288:** G514–G524.
25. ABREU, M.T. *et al.* 2002. TLR4 and MD-2 expression is regulated by immune-mediated signals in human intestinal epithelial cells. J. Biol. Chem. **277:** 20431–20437.
26. SUZUKI, M., T. HISAMATSU & D. K. PODOLSKY. 2003. Gamma interferon augments the intracellular pathway for lipopolysaccharide (LPS) recognition in human intestinal epithelial cells through coordinated up-regulation of LPS uptake and expression of the intracellular toll-like receptor 4-MD-2 complex. Infect. Immun. **71:** 3503–3511.
27. FRANCHIMONT, D. *et al.* 2004. Deficient host-bacteria interactions in inflammatory bowel disease? The toll-like receptor (TLR)-4 Asp299gly polymorphism is associated with Crohn's disease and ulcerative colitis. Gut **53:** 987–992.
28. ELSON, C.O., Y. CONG & J. SUNDBERG. 2000. The C3H/HeJBir mouse model: a high susceptibility phenotype for colitis. Int. Rev. Immunol. **19:** 63–75.
29. RACHMILEWITZ, D. *et al.* 2004. Toll-like receptor 9 signaling mediates the anti-inflammatory effects of probiotics in murine experimental colitis. Gastroenterology **126:** 520–528.
30. FUKATA, M. *et al.* 2005. Toll-like receptor-4 is required for intestinal response to epithelial injury and limiting bacterial translocation in a murine model of acute colitis. Am. J. Physiol. Gastrointest. Liver Physiol. **288:** G1055–G1065.
31. OHKAWARA, T. *et al.* 2005. Macrophage migration inhibitory factor contributes to the development of acute dextran sulphate sodium-induced colitis in toll-like receptor 4 knockout mice. Clin. Exp. Immunol. **141:** 412–421.
32. MAHLER, M. *et al.* 1998. Differential susceptibility of inbred mouse strains to dextran sulfate sodium-induced colitis. Am. J. Physiol. **274:** G544–G551.
33. PULL, S.L. *et al.* 2005. Activated macrophages are an adaptive element of the colonic epithelial progenitor niche necessary for regenerative responses to injury. Proc. Natl. Acad. Sci. USA **102:** 99–104.
34. KOBAYASHI, M. *et al.* 2003. Toll-like receptor-dependent production of IL-12p40 causes chronic enterocolitis in myeloid cell-specific Stat3-deficient mice. J. Clin. Invest. **111:** 1297–1308.
35. FORT, M.M. *et al.* 2005. A synthetic TLR4 antagonist has anti-inflammatory effects in two murine models of inflammatory bowel disease. J. Immunol. **174:** 6416–6423.
36. AGRAWAL, S. *et al.* 2003. Cutting edge: different toll-like receptor agonists instruct dendritic cells to induce distinct Th responses via differential modulation of

extracellular signal-regulated kinase-mitogen-activated protein kinase and c-Fos. J. Immunol. **171:** 4984–4989.

37. KIM, S.C. *et al.* 2005. Variable phenotypes of enterocolitis in interleukin 10-deficient mice monoassociated with two different commensal bacteria. Gastroenterology **128:** 891–906.

38. BERG, D.J. *et al.* 1996. Enterocolitis and colon cancer in interleukin-10-deficient mice are associated with aberrant cytokine production and CD4(+) TH1-like responses. J. Clin. Invest. **98:** 1010–1020.

39. O'BRIEN, A.D. *et al.* 1980. Genetic control of susceptibility to *Salmonella typhimurium* in mice: role of the LPS gene. J. Immunol. **124:** 20–24.

40. BIHL, F. *et al.* 2003. Overexpression of toll-like receptor 4 amplifies the host response to lipopolysaccharide and provides a survival advantage in transgenic mice. J. Immunol. **170:** 6141–6150.

41. TARGAN, S.R. *et al.* 2005. Antibodies to CBir1 flagellin define a unique response that is associated independently with complicated Crohn's disease. Gastroenterology **128:** 2020–2028.

42. LODES, M.J. *et al.* 2004. Bacterial flagellin is a dominant antigen in Crohn disease. J. Clin. Invest. **113:** 1296–1306.

43. SITARAMAN, S.V. *et al.* 2005. Elevated flagellin-specific immunoglobulins in Crohn's disease. Am. J. Physiol. Gastrointest. Liver Physiol. **288:** G403–G406.

44. OBERMEIER, F. *et al.* 2005. In vivo CpG DNA/ TLR9 interaction induces regulatory properties in CD4+CD62L+-T-cells which prevent intestinal inflammation in the SCID-transfer model of colitis. Gut **54:** 1428–1436.

45. JIJON, H. *et al.* 2004. DNA from probiotic bacteria modulates murine and human epithelial and immune function. Gastroenterology **126:** 1358–1373.

Probiotics

Do They Help to Control Intestinal Inflammation?

S.K. BÖHM AND W. KRUIS

ABSTRACT: There is currently a growing appreciation for the role of the enteric flora in health and disease. In the past years overwhelming evidence has accumulated for the role of commensal gut bacteria in the inflammatory bowel diseases Crohn's disease and ulcerative colitis. Both entities are mainly located in areas with high bacterial concentrations. Reduction of the enteric bacterial concentration by antibiotics, lavage, or surgical bypass results in a mitigation of symptoms, while experimental colitis models depend on the presence of the bacterial flora and the NOD2/CARD15-mutation results in inefficient clearance of invasive bacteria. Those findings helped to bring the concept of probiotic therapy to the forefront, a therapy that had been known for millennia, but had been disregarded by the scientific world. Probiotics are meanwhile established in the maintenance therapy of ulcerative colitis and chronic recurrent or refractory pouchitis. Promising data exist for the primary prevention of pouchitis. Probiotic research at the intersection of gastroenterology, immunology and microbiology is highly dynamic in both the basic and the clinical field. Further understanding of the complex molecular mechanisms leading to the effectiveness of probiotics will also spur the development of more successful probiotic formulations.

KEYWORDS: inflammatory bowel disease (IBD); Crohn's disease; ulcerative colitis; pouchitis; probiotics; Escherichia coli; Bifidobacterium; lactobacillus

INTRODUCTION

The current hypothesis in the pathogenesis of the chronic idiopathic inflammatory bowel diseases (IBD), Crohn's disease and ulcerative colitis, suggests that these are caused by an overly aggressive cell-mediated immune response to luminal commensal bacteria in genetically susceptible hosts.[1,2] Most therapeutic approaches currently aim at modulating the immune response; another rational strategy, however, is to modify the intestinal flora. This intended modification may follow different aims according to the understanding of the role

Address for correspondence: S.K. Böhm, Evangelisches Krankenhaus Kalk, Abteilung für Innere Medzin, Universität Zu Köln, Buchforststr. 2, Köln, Germany.
e-mail: boehm@evkk.de

Ann. N.Y. Acad. Sci. 1072: 339–350 (2006). © 2006 New York Academy of Sciences.
doi: 10.1196/annals.1326.005

of the intestinal flora in health and disease. Following the dysbiosis theory[3] one goal may be to shift the intestinal ecosystem from a pro- to a more anti-inflammatory state. Another facet may be to try to eliminate bacterial antigens that constantly drive the pathogenic immune response. A different concept is to consider probiotic therapy in terms of specific molecules modulating defined targets in the gut mucosal and systemic immune system.[4]

Although the therapeutic use of food fermented with micro-organisms has already been described in the classical Roman literature,[5] the term *probiotics* was only coined in 1965 by Lilly and Stillwell.[6] They described a growth-promoting effect on the ciliate *Tetrahymena* by a factor produced by protozoan micro-organisms. Parker extended the definition of probiotics in 1974 as "organisms and substances which contribute to intestinal microbial balance" and described thereby a dietary supplement for animals.[7] Fuller in 1989 put more emphasis on the importance of the living cells in probiotics and defines them as "a live microbial food supplement which beneficially affects the host animal by improving its intestinal microbalance.[8] A beneficial effect in man was emphasized in the definition of probiotics by von Havenaar and Huis in't Veld:[9] "A viable mono- or mixed-culture of micro-organisms, which applied to animal or man, beneficially affects the host by improving the properties of the indigenous microflora." The Joint Food and Agriculture Organization (FAO) of the United Nations and the World Health Organization currently gives the following definition: "Probiotics are life micro-organisms which, when administered in adequate amounts, confer a health benefit on the host. The FAO further demands that probiotics are well characterized regarding genus, species, strain, minimum viable number of organisms at the end of shelf-life, and effective dose related to the health claim."

The history of the term "probiotics" mirrors the rapid development the understanding and use of micro-organisms in human conditions and diseases has taken over the last decade. The definition will surely have to be further adapted as we learn even more about actions of probiotic micro-organisms and their interaction with the host. For example, it is becoming clear from animal models that probiotics mediate some of their anti-inflammatory effects through nonviable components. Nonmethylated DNA (CpG) from VSL3 and a randomly selected *Escherichia coli* (*E. coli*) strain suppresses experimental colitis in several models through toll-like receptor 9 (TLR 9).[10]

The ancient concept of a beneficial effect of certain bacteria in fermented milk was scientifically investigated by the Russian Nobel Price winner Elie Metchnikoff, who proposed in 1907 that the lactic acid producing strain *Lactobacillus bulgaricus* contained in yoghurt is able to displace pathological intestinal flora.[11] Alfred Nissle was the first to treat a patient with inflammatory bowel disease with a newly identified and isolated probiotic bacterial strain. He studied soldiers during World War I and isolated bacteria from the stool of soldiers who remained healthy despite the fact that most of their comrades suffered from diarrhea. He used one isolate, *E. coli* strain Nissle 1917 (DSM

6601, serotype O6:K5:H1), to treat a 20-year-old female with chronic active ulcerative colitis. She was treated for 7 weeks with up to 200 mg/day of the strain and achieved remission after 5 weeks.[12] Probiotic therapy remained in the academic back room and was ridiculed until major advances were made in two different fields: firstly in the understanding of the importance of the human intestinal microbiota for a healthy mucosal immunity[13-17] and secondly in the understanding of the importance of the commensal flora in the pathogenesis of experimental and human inflammatory bowel conditions.[1, 18] Now the body of literature on probiotic organisms used in human therapeutic studies is rapidly increasing.[19] We review the evidence for a beneficial effect of probiotics in inflammatory bowel disease. The first controlled studies on this topic started to be published in 1997.

ULCERATIVE COLITIS

Maintenance of Remission

One of those early studies was performed by Kruis and colleagues.[20] They recruited 120 patients with ulcerative colitis in remission in a randomized, double-blind study comparing mesalamine (500 mg tid) with *E. coli* Nissle 1917 (200 mg; 5 × 10^{10} living bacteria). The end point of the study was the relapse rate after 3 months using the clinical activity index of Rachmilewitz as outcome measure for disease activity. Relapse rates were not different between groups, with 11.3% in the mesalamine group and 16% in the *E. coli* Nissle 1917 group.[20]

A slightly more complex study design was used by Rembacken *et al.*, [21] who enrolled 116 patients with active ulcerative colitis. All patients received a 1-week course of gentamicin (80 mg tid) to suppress the native *E. coli* flora and tapering prednisolone systemically plus rectal hydrocortisone enemas for 3 months to induce remission. From the outset of the study patients were randomized to receive either mesalamine (800 mg tid) or *E. coli* Nissle 1917 (200 mg bid) in addition. Patients not reaching remission after 3 months under this regimen were excluded from the study. After reaching remission patients received a reduced dose of mesalamine (400 mg tid) or *E. coli* Nissle 1917 (200 mg qd) and were followed up for up to 12 months. Time to remission and the numbers of patients achieving remission were not different whether mesalamine (75%) or *E. coli* Nissle 1917 (68%) was added to the prednisolone treatment. The number of patients relapsing was also not different between treatment groups. However, the reported 1-year relapse rate of 73% for the mesalamine group is uncharacteristically high and comparable to historical placebo rates. This may have been due to recruitment of patients soon after exacerbation instead of patients during a long-standing remission. In addition, the criteria for relapse were a more rigorous variation of the colitis-activity index (CAI) described by Rachmilewitz.

The scientific community had reservations about the latter studies regarding the short observation period of 3 months,[20] the nonstandardized criteria for relapse,[21] and the lack of statistical power for equivalence testing.[20,21] Kruis and colleagues therefore undertook a second study to investigate the efficacy of *E. coli* Nissle 1917 in maintenance therapy of ulcerative colitis.[22] Three hundred twenty-seven patients were randomized in a double-dummy, double-blind trial to *E. coli* Nissle 1917 (200 mg qd) or mesalamine (500 mg tid) and observed for 12 months. All 327 patients underwent the intent-to-treat analysis, 222 patients were available for the per-protocol analysis. Definitions for remission and relapse were based on the clinical activity index and the endoscopic index described by Rachmilewitz. Analysis of the per-protocol group after 12 months demonstrated a relapse rates that was 33.9% in the *E. coli* Nissle 1917 group and 36.4% in the mesalamine group, statistically equivalent ($P = 0.003$). In addition, there was no difference in number and kind of adverse events between groups. *E. coli* Nissle 1917 therefore is a safe alternative for prevention of relapse in ulcerative colitis. This is mirrored in the German guidelines for treatment of ulcerative colitis and acknowledged in recent reviews.[23,24]

In smaller, less well-designed studies the effect of other probiotics in maintaining remission in ulcerative colitis was evaluated. The probiotic preparation VSL3, containing four strains of *Lactobacilli*, three strains of *Bifidobacteria*, and *Streptococcus salivarius* ssp. thermophilus (5×10^{11} cells/g), was evaluated in an open-label uncontrolled trial.[25] Twenty patients received the preparation (3 g bid) for 1 year. Fifteen of 20 patients remained in remission.

Ishikawa and colleagues divided 21 patients into a group receiving fermented milk containing *Bifidobacteria* strains and *Lactobacillus acidophilus* (BFM) in numbers of 1×10^{10} per 100 mL milk (100 mL per day) and a group receiving no further treatment.[26] After 1 year symptoms were exacerbated in 3 of 11 subjects in the group receiving the fermented milk and in 9 of 10 in the control group. Colonoscopic findings were not different between the groups.[26]

Another small study examined the effect of an ill-defined mixture of three strains of bacteria including *Bifidobacteria* on maintaining remission in ulcerative colitis.[27] This publication omits crucial data about the patient characteristics as well as definitions for active disease and remission. Thirty patients were recruited, remission was induced with sulfasalazine and glucocorticoids, and patients were then randomized to receive "bifico" or placebo for 2 months. Relapses occurred in 3 of 15 patients (20%) of the probiotics group compared to 14 of 15 (93%) in the placebo group. In accompanying studies in tissue biopsies it was determined that the expression of the proinflammatory factors NF-κB, IL-1β and TNF-α was lower after probiotic treatment and that expression of the anti-inflammatory cytokine IL-10 was increased compared to placebo treatment.[27]

Active Ulcerative Colitis

The successful use of probiotic preparations in maintenance therapy of ulcerative colitis encouraged investigators to evaluate this approach in recent years in few pilot studies for active disease.

First Guslandi and colleagues studied 25 patients with a mild-to-moderate clinical flare-up of ulcerative colitis while being on maintenance treatment with 1g mesalamine tid for at least 3 months.[28] The patients had a history of poorly tolerating steroids in earlier flare-ups and were therefore treated in an open-label trial with *Saccharomyces boulardii* (250 mg tid) in addition to mesalamine for 4 weeks. Twenty-four patients completed the study, a significant reduction in the disease activity index according to Rachmilewitz was observed, and 17 of 24 patients (68%) achieved remission confirmed endoscopically.

A Japanese group performed a randomized, double-blind, placebo-controlled trial [29] examining the effectiveness of the fermented milk containing *Bifidobacteria* strains and *Lactobacillus acidophilus* (BFM) already used in the maintenance therapy of ulcerative colitis.[26] Twenty patients with mild-to-moderate active ulcerative colitis randomly received BFM or placebo for 12 weeks in addition to their standard treatment with sulfasalazine or mesalamine. Remission was achieved in 4 of 10 patients (40%) in the verum group and 3 of 9 patients (33%) in the placebo group. However, the clinical activity index at 12 weeks was significantly reduced by BFM compared with the control group. The endoscopic activity score and histological score also decreased significantly in the BFM group, while the improvement was not statistically significant in the control group. In contrast, the values for the endoscopic and the histological score at the 12 weeks end point did not differ between groups.

Finally, Bibiloni and colleagues performed an open-label trial evaluating the efficacy of VSL#3 in 34 patients with mildly to moderately active ulcerative colitis who had not responded to mesalamine therapy.[30] Patients were allowed to stay on steady medication with oral or rectal mesalamine, corticosteroids, and 6-mercaptopurine and azazathioprine. They received 1.8×10^{12} viable bacteria bid for 6 weeks. Intent-to-treat analysis demonstrated that remission defined by reaching a disease activity index ≤ 2 was achieved in 18 of 34 patients (53%) and response defined by a decrease in the disease activity index of ≥ 3 in 8 of 34 patients (24%).

Borody *et al.*[31] extended the case reported by Bennet and Brinkman[32] 14 years earlier about the successful treatment of ulcerative colitis with the unconventional approach of exogeneous bacteria by retention enema. Borody now reported favorable responses to fecal bacteriotherapy in a series of six difficult-to-treat patients with long-standing ulcerative colitis. The patients had been treated with moderate- to high-dose steroids and four patients had received azathioprine, 6-mercaptopurine, or cyclosporin. Five of six patients had responded to these drugs, although marked symptoms recurred when the medication was reduced or discontinued. The patients were eager to avoid the use of long-term anti-inflammatory and immunosuppressive therapy. Patients were conditioned with a 7- to 10- day course of antibiotics including van-comycin, metronidazole, and rifampicin to suppress clostridia followed by an orthostatic lavage with 3 liters of a PEG-based oral solution. The patients were asked to name suitable donors for feces samples, donors were required to be healthy and to have normal bowel function. Feces were screened for a wide panel of pathogens. Donor feces (200–300 g) were diluted in 200 to 300 mL normal saline solution and administered to the patient via enema; the process was repeated daily for 5 days. Anti-inflammatory therapy was withdrawn immediately or after 4 to 6 weeks. A complete reversal of symptoms was reported in all patients by 4 months after the fecal bacteriotherapy and patients remained free of clinical, colonoscopic, or histological evidence of ulcerative colitis in any patient with observation times ranging from 1 to 13 years.[31] These astonishing results are provoking and warrant further investigation because an intervention most different from a standardized probiotic therapy seems to produce the most dramatic success.

In conclusion there are some promising leads for a beneficial effect of probiotic preparations in acute ulcerative colitis, but more data from well-designed, larger studies are needed to further support the idea that probiotics are not only able to prevent reinflammation of ulcerative colitis in remission, but also to suppress inflammation of acute colitis.

POUCHITIS

Ileal pouch anal anastomosis (IPAA) is performed in patients undergoing proctocolectomy for ulcerative colitis. Pouchitis is a nonspecific inflammation of the ileal reservoir, which occurs in up to 50% of patients after a mean follow-up of 40 months. The fact that pouchitis occurs in only 5% of patients undergoing IPAA following proctocolectomy for FAP suggests that pouchitis is a re-manifestation of IBD under new conditions. Its cause is largely unknown, but some studies have found reduced numbers of lactobacilli and *Bifidobacteria* within the pouch, suggesting a contribution of dysbiosis to the development of the syndrome. Although most patients respond to a short course of antibiotics (metronidazole, ciprofloxacin), approximately 10% of patients develop recurrent or refractory disease.[23,33,34]

Gionchetti and colleagues were the first to report the ability of VSL#3 to prevent recurrence of chronically relapsing pouchitis.[35] They studied the secondary prevention of pouchitis in 40 patients in whom acute pouchitis had been treated successfully with ciprofloxacin plus rifaximin. In a double-blinded, placebo-controlled design, patients were randomized to receive orally either placebo or 6 g VSL#3 once daily for 9 months. Of the 20 patients who received placebo all (100%) relapsed within the study period, while 17 of

20 (85%) patients who received verum remained in remission ($P < 0.001$). In the group receiving VSL#3, disease activity gauged by the pouchitis disease activity index was zero, the presence of viable VSL#3-derived micro-organisms could be demonstrated at the end of the study period, discontinuation of VSL#3 resulted in recurrent pouchitis within 3 months, and no adverse effects were noted. These results were confirmed by Mimura and colleagues in another randomized, placebo-controlled study.[36] Remission had been induced in 36 patients by a combination of metronidazole and ciprofloxacin. Seventeen of 20 patients (85%) receiving 6 g VSL#3 once daily for 1 year remained in remission compared with only 1 of 16 patients (6%) in the placebo group ($P < 0.001$). Furthermore, patients in the VSL#3 group reported an enhanced quality of life.

An even wider and more intriguing indication for VSL#3 was suggested by another study made by Gionchetti and colleagues. They demonstrated that this probiotic is effective in primary prevention of pouchitis when therapy is started immediately after IPAA surgery.[37] Forty patients undergoing colectomy were randomized to receive 3 g VSL#3 or placebo once daily for 1 year. Acute pouchitis developed in 40% of patients receiving placebo but only in 10% of patients receiving VSL#3 ($P < 0.05$). VSL#3-treated patients had better quality of life, with two fewer stools per day on average than the placebo group. Another well-designed randomized controlled study to confirm these results is still missing. In a study with a historical control group, daily treatment with *Lactobacillus rhamnosus* GG resulted in occurrence of the first episode of symptomatic pouchitis in 7% at 3 years postoperatively, whereas 29% of placebo-treated patients developed pouchitis ($P = 0.01$).[38]

In contrast to their efficiency in primary and secondary prevention of pouchitis, probiotics up to this point have failed to demonstrate efficiency in the induction of remission in acute pouchitis. *Lactobacillus rhamnosus* GG administered orally for 3 months colonized only 40% of study participants and did not reverse symptoms of acute pouchitis.[39] Similarly, a combination of *Lactobacillus acidophilus* and *Bifidobacterium lactis* in fermented milk (Cultura) failed to demonstrate a therapeutic benefit in acute pouchitis.[40]

Current guidelines developed by gastroenterological societies of various countries recommend the probiotic formulation VSL#3 in the treatment of chronic recurrent or refractory pouchitis. The currently available data were deemed too preliminary to recommend VSL#3 in the primary prevention of pouchitis.[23,33]

CROHN'S DISEASE

Although one of the two pioneer studies in modern probiotic therapy published in 1997 examined the efficacy of *E. coli* Nissle 1917 in maintaining remission in Crohn's disease,[41] the use of probiotics in this entity of inflammatory bowel disease is still the least substantiated.

Malchow performed a randomized, double-blind study in 75 patients with active Crohn's disease (CDAI > 150) located either in the large bowel only or in both large and small bowel.[41] The patients received a tapering dose of prednisolone starting with 60 mg and 200 mg *E. coli* Nissle 1917 or placebo for 1 year. *E. coli* Nissle and placebo groups did not differ in the rate of remission regardless of disease location. However, the time before onset of remission was considerably shorter in patients receiving the probiotic preparation with a mean of 30 days versus 51 days in the control group. The relapse rate was not different between treatment groups in patients suffering from ileocolitis. In contrast, in patients with Crohn's colitis the relapse rate was only 30% in the verum group compared to 70% in the placebo group. None of the results in this study reached statistical significance.

Guslandi and colleagues performed to this date the only other study examining the effect of probiotics on medically induced remission.[42] Thirty-two patients with predominantly ileocolic disease were randomized to a regimen of 3 g mesalamine or 2 g mesalamine and 1g *Saccharomyces boulardii* per day for 6 months. Relapse occurred statistically significantly more often in 10 of 16 patients (38%) in the mesalamine-only group compared to only 1 of 16 patients (6%) in the mesalamine plus *Saccharomyces boulardii* group.

Prantera *et al.* [43] undertook a randomized, double-blind trial in 45 patients to determine the effect of *Lactobacillus* GG in surgically induced remission in Crohn's disease. Patients received *Lactobacillus* GG or placebo within 10 days following resection of the affected segment for 52 weeks. The unexpected difference of 60% relapses in the *Lactobacillus* GG group compared to 35% in the placebo group was not statistically significant.

A more successful outcome of a probiotic maintenance therapy in surgically induced remission in Crohn's disease was reported by Campieri and colleagues, who compared[44] a combination of rifixamin plus VSL#3 or mesalamine. The study has still not been published as full paper.

A small randomized, double-blind, placebo-controlled study with 11 patients failed to demonstrate a positive effect of *Lactobacillus* GG in inducing or maintaining remission in moderate-to-active Crohn's disease (CDAI 150–300).[45] McCarthy and colleagues demonstrated in an open-label uncontrolled trial that *Lactobacillus salivarius* UCC118 resulted in a significant reduction of the CDAI in 25 patients with mild to moderately active Crohn's disease; the paper is only published in abstract form.[46] *Lactobacillus* GG was also reported to improve clinical status and gut barrier function in four children with mildly to moderately active, stable Crohn's disease in a 6-month open-label pilot evaluation.[47]

CONCLUSION

Currently available data demonstrate that probiotics are more effective in preventing relapse of inflammatory processes than suppressing active disease.

This is illustrated by the solid evidence for activity of *E. coli* Nissle 1917 in maintaining remission in ulcerative colitis and of VSL#3 in preventing relapse of chronic pouchitis. These indications have found entry into guidelines. There is also preliminary evidence that VSL#3 may prevent pouchitis when administered immediately after surgery. Use of probiotics in active inflammation is intriguing, but sufficient data are missing. Therefore additional large-scale, high-quality trials need to be performed to clarify the efficacy of probiotic preparations for these and other indications.

Studies with probiotics are complex in that individual probiotic preparations have individual properties and individual patients may respond differently to one and the same probiotic. With ongoing research elucidating more and more individual molecular mechanisms of probiotic bacteria targeting the host immune system, probiotic interventions will move more and more away from the simplistic concept of repopulating the intestinal flora with "friendly" bacteria.[4] Following this path, we soon may see genetically engineered bacteria delivering anti-inflammatory cytokines or other biologically active molecules to the gut in human studies. Proof of principle and efficacy have been demonstrated with *Lactococcus lactis* engineered to secrete IL-10 [48] or trefoil factor [49] within the gut of murine IBD models. This rapidly evolving field at the intersection of immunology, microbiology, and gastroenterology holds a lot of promise for IBD patients.

REFERENCES

1. SARTOR, R.B. 2004. Therapeutic manipulation of the enteric microflora in inflammatory bowel diseases: antibiotics, probiotics and prebiotics. Gastroenterology **126:** 1620–1633.
2. SHANAHAN, F. 2005. Physiological basis for novel drug therapies used to treat the inflammatory bowel diseases. I. Pathophysiological basis and prospects for probiotic therapy in inflammatory bowel disease. Am. J. Physiol. Gastrointest. Liver Physiol. **288:** G417–G421.
3. TAMBOLI, C.P., C. NEUT, P. DESREUMAUX, *et al.* 2004. Dysbiosis in inflammatory bowel disease. Gut **53:** 1–4.
4. GHOSH, S., D. VAN HEEL & R.J. PLAYFORD. 2004. Probiotics in inflammatory bowel disease: is it all gut flora modulation? Gut **53:** 620–622.
5. C. PLINIUS SECUNDUS (23/24–79). Naturalis historiae. **XXVIII: 36,** 135.
6. LILLY, D.M. & R.H. STILLWELL. 1965. Probiotics: growth promoting factors produced by microorganisms. Science **147:** 747–748.
7. PARKER, R.B. 1974. Probiotics, the other half of the antibiotic story. Anim. Nutr. Health **29:** 4–8.
8. FULLER, R. 1989. Probiotics in man and animals. J. Appl. Bacteriol. **66:** 365–378.
9. HAVENAAR, R. & J.H.J. HUISIN'T VELD. 1992. Probiotics: a general view. *In* B.J.B. Wood, Ed.: The Lactic Acid Bacteria, Vol.1: The Lactic Acid Bacteria in Health and Disease. 151–170. Elsevier Applied SciencesLondon.

10. RACHMILEWITZ, D., K. KATAKARA, F. KARMELI, *et al.* 2004. Toll-like receptor 9 signaling mediates the anti-inflammatory effects of probiotics in murine experimental colitis. Gastroenterology **126:** 520–528.
11. METCHNIKOFF, E. 1907. The prolongation of life: optimistic studies. *In* M. Chalmers, Ed.: 161–183. Butterworth-Heinemann, London.
12. NISSLE, A. 1918. Die antagonistische Behandlung chronischer Darmstörungen mit Colibakterien. Med. Klein. **2:** 29–33.
13. TLASKALOVA-HOGENOVA, H., R. STEPANKOVA, T. HUDCOVIC, *et al.* 2004. Commensal bacteria (normal microflora), mucosal immunity and chronic inflammatory and autoimmune diseases. Immunol. Lett. **93:** 97–108.
14. SHANAHAN, F. 2004. Host-flora interactions in inflammatory bowel disease. Inflamm. Bowel Dis. **10:** S16–S24.
15. ISOLAURI, E., S. SALMINEN & A.C. OUWEHAND. 2004. Probiotics. Best Pract. Res. Clin. Gastroenterol. **18:** 299–313.
16. BÄCKHED, F., R.E. LEY, J.L. SONNENBURG, *et al.* 2005. Host-bacterial mutualism in the human intestine. Science **307:** 1915–1920.
17. TANNOCK, G.W. 2005. Commentary: remembrance of microbes past. Int. J. Epidemiol. **34:** 13–15.
18. SCHULTZ, M., J. SCHÖLMERICH & H.C. RATH. 2003. Rationale for probiotic and antibiotic treatment strategies in inflammatory bowel diseases. Dig. Dis. **21:** 105–128.
19. MONTROSE, D.C. & M.H. FLOCH. 2005. Probiotics used in human studies. J. Clin. Gastroenterol. **39:** 469–484.
20. KRUIS, W., E. SCHÜTZ, P. FRIC, *et al.* 1997. Double-blind comparison of an oral *Escherichia coli* preparation and mesalazine in maintaining remission of ulcerative colitis. Aliment. Pharmacol. Ther. **11:** 853–858.
21. REMBACKEN, B.J., A.M. SNELLING, P.M. HAWKEY, *et al.* 1999. Non-pathogenic *Escherichia coli* versus mesalazine for the treatment of ulcerative colitis: a randomised trial. Lancet **354:** 635–639.
22. KRUIS, W., P. FRIC, J. POKROTNIEKS, *et al.* 2004. Maintaining remission of ulcerative colitis with the probiotic *Escherichia coli* is as effective as with standard mesalazine. Gut **53:** 1617–1623.
23. HOFFMANN, J.C., M. ZEITZ, S.C. BISCHOFF, *et al.* 2004. Diagnostik und Therapie der Colitis ulcerosa: Ergebnisse einer evidenzbasierten Konsensuskonferenz der Deutschen Gesellschaft für Verdauungs- und Stoffwechselerkrankungen zusammen mit dem Kompetenznetz chronisch entzündliche Darmerkrankungen. Z. Gastroenterol. **42:** 984–1032.
24. SARTOR, R.B. 2005. Probiotic therapy of intestinal inflammation and infections. Curr. Opin. Gastroenterol. **21:** 44–50.
25. VENTURI, A., P. GIONCHETTI, F. RIZZELLO, *et al.* 1999. Impact on the composition of the faecal flora by a new probiotic preparation: preliminary data on maintenance treatment of patients with ulcerative colitis. Aliment. Pharmacol. Ther. **13:** 1103–1108.
26. ISHIKAWA, H., I. AKEDO, Y. UMESAKI, *et al.* 2003. Randomized controlled trial of the effect of bifidobacteria-fermented milk on ulcerative colitis. J. Am. Coll. Nutr. **22:** 56–63.
27. CUI, H.-H., C.-L. CHEN, J.-D. WANG, *et al.* 2004. Effects of probiotic on intestinal mucosa of patients with ulcerative colitis. World J. Gastroenterol. **10:** 1521–1525.
28. GUSLANDI, M., P. GIOLLI & P.A. TESTONI. 2003. A pilot trial of *Saccharomyces boulardii* in ulcerative colitis. Eur. J. Gastroenterol. Hepatol. **15:** 697–698.

29. KATO, K., S. MIZUNO, Y. UMESAKI, et al. 2005. Randomized placebo-controlled trial assessing the effect of bifidobacteria-fermented milk on active ulcerative colitis. Aliment. Pharmacol. Ther. **20:** 1133–1141.

30. BIBILONI, R., R.N. FEDORAK, G.W. TANNOCK, et al. 2005. VSL3 probiotic-mixture induces remission in patients with active ulcerative colitis. Am. J. Gastroenterol. **100:** 1539–1546.

31. BORODY, T.J., E.F. WARREN, S. LEIS, et al. 2003. Treatment of ulcerative colitis using fecal bacteriotherapy. J. Clin. Gastroenterol. **37:** 42–47.

32. BENNET, J.D. & M. BRINKMAN. 1989. Treatment of ulcerative colitis by implantation of normal colonic flora. Lancet **333:** 164.

33. KORNBLUTH, A. & D.B. SACHAR. 2004. Ulcerative colitis practice guidelines in adults (update): American College of Gastroenterology, Practice Parameters Committee. Am. J. Gastroenterol. **99:** 1371–1385.

34. RIOUX, K.P., K.L. MADSEN & R.N. FEDORAK. 2005. The role of enteric microflora in inflammatory bowel disease: human and animal studies with probiotics and prebiotics. Gastroenterol. Clin. N. Am. **34:** 465–482.

35. GIONCHETTI, P., F. RIZZELLO, A. VENTURI, et al. 2000. Oral bacteriotherapy as maintenance treatment in patients with chronic pouchitis: a double-blind, placebo-controlled trial. Gastroenterology **119:** 305–309.

36. MIMURA, T., F. RIZZELLO, U. HELWIG, et al. 2004. Once-daily high-dose probiotic therapy (VSL3) for maintaining remission in recurrent or refractory pouchitis. Gut **53:** 108–114.

37. GIONCHETTI, P., F. RIZZELLO, U. HELWIG, et al. 2003. Prophylaxis of pouchitis onset with probiotic therapy: a double-blind, placebo-controlled trial. Gastroenterology **124:** 1202–1209.

38. GOSSELINK, M.P., W.R. SCHOUTEN, L.M. VAN LIESHOUT, et al. 2004. Delay of the first onset of pouchitis by oral intake of the probiotic strain *Lactobacillus rhamnosus* GG. Dis. Colon Rectum **47:** 876–884.

39. KUISMA, J., S. MENTULA, H. JARVINEN, et al. 2003. Effect of *Lactobacillus rhamnosus* GG on ileal pouch inflammation and microbial flora. Dis. Colon Rectum **46:** 1476–1483.

40. LAAKE, K.O., P.D. LINE, L. AABAKKEN, et al. 2003. Assessment of mucosal inflammation and circulation in response to probiotics in patients operated with ileal pouch anal anastomosis for ulcerative colitis. Scand. J. Gastroenterol. **38:** 409–414.

41. MALCHOW, H. 1997. Crohn's disease and *Escherichia coli*: a new approach in therapy to maintain remission of colonic Crohn's disease? J. Clin. Gastroenterol. **25:** 653–658.

42. GUSLANDI, M., G. MEZZI, M. SORGHI, et al. 2000. *Saccharomyces boulardii* in maintenance treatment of Crohn's disease. Dig. Dis. Sci. **45:** 1462–1464.

43. PRANTERA, C., M.L. Scribano, G. FALASCO, et al. 2002. Ineffectiveness of probiotics in preventing recurrence after curative resection for Crohn's disease: a randomised controlled trial with *Lactobacillus* GG. Gut **51:** 405–409.

44. CAMPIERI, M., F. RIZZELLO, A. VENTURI, et al. 2000. Combination of antibiotic and probiotic treatment is efficacious in prophylaxis of postoperative recurrence of Crohn's disease: a randomised controlled study versus mesalamine. Gastroenterology **118:** A781.

45. SCHULTZ, M., A. TIMMER, H.H. HERFARTH, et al. 2004. *Lactobacillus* GG in inducing and maintaining remission of Crohn's disease. BMC Gastroenterology **4:** 5–8.

46. McCarthy, J., L. O'Mahony, C. Dunne, *et al.* 2001. An open trial of a novel probiotic as an alternative to steroids in mild/moderately active Crohn's disease. Gut **49:** A2447.
47. Gupta, P., H. Andrew, B.S. Kirschner, *et al.* 2000. Is lactobacillus GG helpful in children with Crohn's disease? Results of a preliminary open-label study. J. Pediatr. Gastroenterol. Nutr. **31:** 453–457.
48. Steidler, L., W. Hans, L. Schotte, *et al.* 2000. Treatment of murine colitis by *Lactococcus lactis* secreting interleukin-10. Science **289:** 1352–1355.
49. Vandenbroucke, K., W. Hans, J. van Huysse, *et al.* 2004. Active delivery of trefoil factors by genetically modified *Lactococcus lactis* prevents and heals acute colitis in mice. Gastroenterology **127:** 502–513.

Homeostatic Effects of TLR9 Signaling in Experimental Colitis

JONGDAE LEE,[a] DANIEL RACHMILEWITZ,[b] AND EYAL RAZ[a]

[a]Department of Medicine, University of California, San Diego, La Jolla, California 92093–0663, USA

[b]Division of Medicine, Shaare Zedek Medical Center, Jerusalem, Israel

ABSTRACT: The commensal microflora of the intestinal tract confer multiple health benefits to the host, including amelioration of inflammatory bowel disease (IBD). Yet, the exact mechanisms by which it ameliorates experimental colitis in animals and human IBD are largely unknown. We tested whether the attenuation of experimental colitis by probiotic bacteria is mediated by toll-like receptor (TLR) signaling. The severity of colitis was attenuated by delivery of nonviable, γ-irradiated, or by viable probiotics, but not by heat-killed probiotics, in wild-type mice in mice deficient in TLR2 or TLR4. In contrast we did not observe any inhibition of experimental colitis by probiotics, in mice deficient in MyD88 or TLR9. Furthermore, administration of probiotic DNA ameliorated the severity of experimental colitis, whereas methylated probiotic DNA, calf thymus DNA, and Dnase-treated probiotics had no effect. In subsequent studies, we identified that TLR9-induced type 1 IFN mediates the anti-inflammatory effects in experimental colitis. The addition of neutralization antibodies to type 1 IFN abolished the anti-inflammatory effects, whereas the administration of recombinant IFN-β mimicked the anti-inflammatory effects induced by TLR9 agonists. Taken together, these results indicate that the protective effects of probiotics are mainly mediated by their own DNA rather than by their metabolites or their ability to colonize the colon. These findings underscore the diverse effects of indigenous microbial TLR ligands in intestinal homeostasis and intestinal inflammation and suggest that strategies, that modulate type 1 IFN may be of therapeutic value for intestinal inflammatory conditions.

KEYWORDS: TLR; toll-like receptor; type 1 interferon; homeostasis; commensal bacteria

INTRODUCTION

Inflammatory bowel disease (IBD) includes Crohn's disease and ulcerative colitis, both of which are characterized by flare-up periods and possible

Address for correspondence: Eyal Raz, M.D., Department of Medicine, University of California, San Diego, La Jolla, California 92093-0663, USA. Voice: 858-534-5444; fax: 858-534-5399.
e-mail: eraz@ucsd.edu

Ann. N.Y. Acad. Sci. 1072: 351–355 (2006). © 2006 New York Academy of Sciences.
doi: 10.1196/annals.1326.022

life-long relapses. Clinical and experimental evidence suggests that the etiology of IBD is multifactorial, involving susceptibility genes and environmental factors, such as intestinal microflora or their products, and it is the interaction of these factors with the immune system that leads to dysregulated mucosal immunity and chronic intestinal inflammation.[1]

Probiotics are live commensal micro-organisms of the intestinal tract. It is believed that they confer health benefits to the host by one or more of the following mechanisms: (1) production of various antimicrobial metabolites, (2) competitive exclusion of enteric pathogens, and (3) neutralization of dietary carcinogens and modulation of mucosal immune responses. Current probiotic therapy is mainly advocated for its immunomodulatory properties and anti-inflammatory activities at mucosal sites.[1,2] The rationale for using probiotics in IBD is based on evidence implicating enteric bacteria in the pathogenesis of various models of murine colitis and IBD in humans.[3] Indeed, probiotic therapy has been effective for the attenuation of experimental colitis,[4] prevention of pouchitis, and maintenance of remission of pouchitis, Crohn's disease, and ulcerative colitis.[5] Despite these beneficial effects, the exact mechanisms and the molecular pathways by which probiotics ameliorate experimental colitis and IBD are largely unknown.

Toll-like receptors function as sentinels of innate immunity. By recognizing signature microbial compounds they trigger the transcriptional activation of proinflammatory cytokines (e.g., IL-12, TNF-α) and chemokines (e.g., RANTES), as well as costimulatory molecules (e.g., CD40). The activation of this proinflammatory program initiates defense mechanisms that are vital for host survival.[6] Therefore, various TLR$^{-/-}$ mice as well as mice deficient in TLR-related adaptor proteins (e.g., MyD88) fail to mount protective responses and succumb to various microbial infections.[7] Bacterial DNA and its synthetically derived immunostimulatory DNA sequence oligonucleotides (ISS–ODN, also known as CpG–ODN) contain unmethylated CpG dinucleotide motifs within consensus sequences and are ligands of TLR9. Like other TLR ligands, such as LPS, ISS–ODN has a broad range of activities on the mammalian innate immune system. In particular, ISS–ODN induces the secretion of Th1-type cytokines and upregulates the expression of costimulatory molecules on antigen-presenting cells.[8] These immunostimulatory characteristics of ISS–ODN have been used to elicit Th1-dependent immune responses[9] and mucosal immunity,[10] leading to an enhanced host defense against invading pathogens.

Since ISS–ODN mimics the immunomodulatory activities of bacterial DNA, we hypothesized a role for probiotic DNA in the inhibition of colonic inflammation and therefore conducted studies that explored the mechanisms by which probiotics ameliorate experimental colitis.

RESULTS AND DISCUSSION

Persuasive evidence indicates that intestinal microflora play an important role in the initiation and the perpetuation of murine experimental colitis and human IBD.[3] However, the molecular mechanisms by which probiotics exert their therapeutic effects have not been identified. The impact of probiotics on intestinal barrier function, their diverse metabolic activities, their competitive exclusion of intestinal indigenous microflora, and their interaction with the mucosal immune system have all been implicated in mediating their therapeutic effects.[1,2]

In a recent study, we provided biochemical, immunologic, and genetic evidence that implicated TLR signaling, especially TLR9, in mediating the protective effect of probiotics (VSL-3) on various models of experimental colitis.[11] The administration of γ-irradiated probiotics effectively ameliorated experimental colitis, as did the administration of viable probiotics. Since the irradiated probiotics were unable to grow in culture, it is unlikely that either their metabolites or their competitive inhibition with indigenous microflora were responsible for the protective effects on the colonic mucosa. Therefore, we reasoned that the anti-inflammatory activities could be the product of the activation of innate immunity (e.g., via TLR) by structural microbial probiotic components.[11]

To further verify the role of TLR signaling in the probiotic-induced amelioration of experimental colitis, mice deficient in TLR2, TLR4, TLR9, or MyD88 were treated with dextran sodium sulfate (DSS) and irradiated probiotics. The administration of γ-irradiated probiotics ameliorated the clinical, biochemical, and histological parameters of colitis in TLR2- or TLR4-deficient mice but not in TLR9- or MyD88-deficient mice, indicating the involvement of the TLR9 signaling pathway in the observed amelioration of colonic inflammation.[11] The inhibition of colonic inflammation by probiotic DNA or by ISS–ODN was reproduced in DSS- and TNBS-induced colitis as well as in spontaneous colitis in IL-10-deficient mice.[11,12] Thus, in contrast to the current paradigm related to the proinflammatory role of TLR-activated innate immunity, our data indicated that TLR9 signaling results in the activation of an anti-inflammatory program that attenuates inflammation in different models of experimental colitis.

Subsequent studies addressed the molecular basis for the anti-inflammatory effects induced by TLR9 signaling in models of experimental colitis. We found that two genetically distinct, but phenotypically similar animals responded differently to ISS–ODN (i.e., TLR9 ligand) administration.[13] While DSS-induced colitis in RAG$^{-/-}$ mice was inhibited by ISS–ODN, colitis in SCID mice was not. We used these ISS-responsive and ISS-resistant phenotypes to dissect the anti-inflammatory role of TLR9 signaling in colonic inflammation.[13] Analysis of the response to ISS–ODN of these two mouse strains revealed defective TLR9-induced type 1 IFN production in SCID mice. Furthermore, we observed that IFN-α/βR$^{-/-}$ mice are extremely sensitive to colitis inflicted by DSS and that the administration of ISS–ODN to these mice increased their mortality. In addition, the lack of inhibition of DSS-induced colitis in ISS-treated wild-type mice adoptively transferred with bone marrow–derived macrophages (BMDM) from IFN-α/βR$^{-/-}$, but not with BMDM from wild-type mice, also suggests that TLR9-induced type 1 IFN inhibits the inflammatory response of activated macrophages. Finally, the administration of recombinant IFNβ to DSS-treated mice mimicked the anti-inflammatory effects on colonic inflammation induced by ISS–ODN.[13] Collectively, this set of data indicates that type 1 IFN has a physiological and protective role on colonic injury and that it also cross-regulates the other proinflammatory activities induced by TLR9 triggering.[13] Indeed, in subsequent preliminary studies we observed that basolateral administration of IFN-α to polarized monolayers of intestinal epithelial cells protected the cells against apoptosis and disruption of the epithelial tight junctions induced by DSS (E. Raz, unpublished material). Thus, type 1 IFN may protect against colonic inflammation by preventing epithelial barrier dysfunction.

Recent study documented the protective effect of other TLR ligands on colonic injury.[14] Our previous studies identified the anti-inflammatory effects of TLR9 agonists on experimental colitis and identified that TLR-induced type 1 IFN mediates these protective effects on colonic inflammation. These findings and the hypersensitivity to DSS observed in IFN-α/βR$^{-/-}$ mice expand the already known activities of type 1 IFN and indicate an important role for type 1 IFN in intestinal homeostasis. Taken together, these results suggest that strategies designed to trigger the production of type 1 IFN in the intestinal tract by the administration of certain TLR ligands (e.g., ISS–ODN, probiotic DNA) or probiotics are of therapeutic value for intestinal inflammatory conditions.

ACKNOWLEDGMENTS

This work was supported by NIH grants AI40682 and DK35108.

REFERENCES

1. SHANAHAN, F. 2001. Inflammatory bowel disease: immunodiagnostics, immunotherapeutics, and ecotherapeutics. Gastroenterology **120:** 622–635.
2. HOOPER, L.V. & J.I. GORDON. 2001. Commensal host-bacterial relationships in the gut. Science **292:** 1115–1118.
3. PODOLSKY, D.K. 2002. Inflammatory bowel disease. N. Engl. J. Med. **347:** 417–429.
4. MADSEN, K., A. CORNISH, P. SOPER, et al. 2001. Probiotic bacteria enhance murine and human intestinal epithelial barrier function. Gastroenterology **121:** 580–591.
5. HART, A.L., A.J. STAGG & M.A. KAMM. 2003. Use of probiotics in the treatment of inflammatory bowel disease. J. Clin. Gastroenterol. **36:** 111–119.
6. TAKEDA, K., T. KAISHO & S. AKIRA. 2003. Toll-like receptors. Annu. Rev. Immunol. **21:** 335–376.
7. KOPP, E. & R. MEDZHITOV. 2003. Recognition of microbial infection by toll-like receptors. Curr. Opin. Immunol. **15:** 396–401.

8. KRIEG, A.M. 2002. CpG motifs in bacterial DNA and their immune effects. Annu. Rev. Immunol. **20:** 709–760.
9. ROMAN, M., E. MARTIN-OROZCO, J.S. GOODMAN, *et al.* 1997. Immunostimulatory DNA sequences function as T helper-1-promoting adjuvants. Nat. Med. **3:** 849–854.
10. HORNER, A. A., A. RONAGHY, P.M. CHENG, *et al.* 1998. Immunostimulatory DNA is a potent mucosal adjuvant. Cell. Immunol. **190:** 77–82.
11. RACHMILEWITZ, D., K. KATAKURA, F. KARMELI, *et al.* 2004. Toll-like receptor 9 signaling mediates the anti-inflammatory effects of probiotics in murine experimental colitis. Gastroenterology **126:** 520–528.
12. RACHMILEWITZ, D., F. KARMELI, K. TAKABAYASHI, *et al.* 2002. Immunostimulatory DNA ameliorates experimental and spontaneous murine colitis. Gastroenterology **122:** 1428–1441.
13. KATAKURA, K., J. LEE, D. RACHMILEWITZ, *et al.* 2005. TLR9-induced type-1 IFN protects mice from experimental colitis. J. Clin. Invest. **115:** 695–702.
14. RAKOFF-NAHOUM, S., J. PAGLINO, F. ESLAMI-VARZANEH, *et al.* 2004. Recognition of commensal microflora by toll-like receptors is required for intestinal homeostasis. Cell **118:** 229–241.

Helminths and Mucosal Immune Modulation

JOEL V. WEINSTOCK

Division of Gastroenterology-Hepatology, Department of Internal Medicine, Tufts New England Medical Center, Boston, Massachusetts 02111, USA

ABSTRACT: Geographic and ethnic variations in ulcerative colitis and Crohn's disease frequency suggest that environmental factors affect disease risk. Prevention of parasitic worms (helminths) through improved hygiene may be one factor leading to the increased disease prevalence. Helminths alter host mucosal and systemic immunity. Animals exposed to helminths are protected from experimental colitis and other immunological diseases, and helminthic colonization can be used to treat ongoing murine and human disease. Helminths induce mucosal T cells to make Th2 and regulatory cytokines. Helminth-induced mucosal IL4, TGFβ, and IL10 likely are part of the protective process. Helminths affect pathways of innate immunity like TLR4 expression and function. Worms also induce various regulatory-type T-cell subsets in the gut that limit effector T-cell growth and function. These effects of once ever-present helminths may have protected people from immune-mediated illnesses like inflammatory bowel disease.

KEYWORDS: Crohn's disease; immune regulation; T cells; helminths; ulcerative colitis

INTRODUCTION

Inflammatory bowel disease (IBD) may result from loss of immune tolerance to normal commensal enteric bacteria. Geographic and ethnic variations in IBD frequency suggest that environmental factors affect the risk of disease.[1] In industrialized countries and in countries undergoing the process of industrialization, there has been an increase in the frequency of IBD and other immunological diseases like multiple sclerosis and asthma.[2]

Helminths are worm-like parasitic animals. Humans and helminths have coexisted throughout our evolution. They strongly modulate the host's immune system to allow their own survival. Prevention of helminthic colonization and

Address for correspondence: Joel V. Weinstock, M.D., Division of Gastroenterology, Tufts New England Medical Center, 750 Washington Street, P.O. Box 233, Boston, MA 02111. Voice: 617-636-8387; fax: 617-636-4505.

e-mail: jweinstock2@Tufts-NEMC.org

Ann. N.Y. Acad. Sci. 1072: 356–364 (2006). © 2006 New York Academy of Sciences.
doi: 10.1196/annals.1326.033

loss of the influence of these organisms on immune function, particularly during childhood development, may be one of the factors promoting the rise in IBD frequency. Moreover, exposure to helminths has therapeutic potential for people with IBD[3-5] and other immunologic disorders. This article reviews the possible mechanisms through which helminths control immunologic diseases like IBD.

ENVIRONMENTAL INFLUENCES ON IBD FREQUENCY

Genetic traits influence the risk of IBD, but are not the etiologic cause of these diseases. Monozygotic opposed to dizygotic twin pairs separated at birth have a higher concordance rate for Crohn's disease (CD), and to a lesser extent ulcerative colitis (UC), suggesting a role for genes in disease susceptibility.[6,7] People with selective defects in the NOD2 (CARD 15) gene are more likely to get CD,[8-10] but most patients with this genetic defect do not get CD and only 10% of CD patients have this defect. While there are other genes that modestly influence disease susceptibility, no single gene has a predominant role in disease etiology, and gene variation does not explain the rapid worldwide rise in IBD frequency.

Environmental factors affect the risk of disease.[1] Cigarette smoking increases the chance for CD,[11] while appendicitis followed by appendectomy lowers the incidence of UC.[12-14] In a small subset of patients, disease onset is provoked by an immune response to pathogenic organisms like *Entamoeba histolytica* or cytomegalovirus.

IBD has a striking geographic variation in disease frequency. In the United States and Europe, IBD is more common in the North than South.[15,16] The prevalence of IBD, and particularly CD, has steadily increased in Western Europe and North America in the 20th century,[17] now affecting one in 250 people in some affluent regions.[18,19] CD and UC remain rare in South America,[20] Central America, the Mediterranean region,[21,22] Africa,[23,24] and Asia.[25,26] Migration studies suggest that children born to individuals who relocate from regions of low CD or UC frequency to areas of high disease prevalence acquire greater disease risk.[27-29]

In the United States, CD originally was mostly restricted to the Jewish population, but now is routinely diagnosed in non-Jewish whites, and in people of African-American and Hispanic origin. Jewish populations living in countries near the equator have lower rates of disease, except for those residing in South Africa.[30,31] Jewish immigrants to Israel from Mediterranean and Middle Eastern countries have a lower frequency of IBD compared to people from Western Europe and North America.[32] IBD is rare in the Arab community of Israeli.[33]

Patients with CD are likely to live in more hygienic environments and have houses with indoor plumbing and hot water.[34,35] IBD is more common in urban versus rural areas,[36] and less common in people having jobs exposing them to dirt.[37] Prior prisoner-of-war status or combat in tropical regions lowers the risk of disease.[38] The clinical spectrum of IBD is still changing, as suggested by IBD demographic and clinical data from Wisconsin, northern Stockholm,[39] and northern France.[40]

ANIMAL MODELS OF HELMINTHIC MODULATION OF IMMUNOLOGIC DISEASE

Epidemiological data suggest that very hygienic life styles and underexposure to organisms like helminths predispose to IBD. Animal models support this concept by showing that helminths can prevent IBD onset and reverse developed disease. Trinitrobenzene sulfonic acid (TNBS) in alcohol placed in the colon of a rodent induces Th1-type colitis. Infection with the intestinal roundworm *T. muris* or *H. polygyrus* or the vascular fluke *S. mansoni*[41] or treatment with schistosome ova[42] protects rodents from TNBS-induced colitis. The intestinal roundworm *Trichinella spiralis*[43] or the rat intestinal tapeworm *Hymenolepis diminuta* also protects. Mice deficient in IL-10 develop a chronic Th1-type colitis that is prevented or reversed by colonization with *T. muris* or *H. polygyrus*,[17,44] or by exposure to non-viable schistosome ova. Helminths also protect in other rodent models of immunological disease like experimental autoimmune encephalomyelitis,[45,46] type 1 diabetes,[47] rheumatoid arthritis,[48] Graves' hyperthyroidism,[49] and food allergy (peanut extract).[50]

HELMINTHIC INTERACTIONS WITH THE HOST AND PROTECTIVE IMMUNITY

Helminths exert a strong influence on the host immune system. They usually stimulate production of Th2 cytokines (IL-4, IL-5, IL-9, and IL-13).[51–55] A Th2, opposed to Th1, cytokine response[56] is host-protective against intestinal worms. The immune response to helminths also alters host immunity to immunologic stimuli unrelated to the parasite. Studies in humans suggest that exposure to various helminths decreases T-cell signal transduction, lowers expression of CD28 with increased expression of CTLA4, reduces proliferation to recall antigens/mitogens, decreases DTH responses,[57] and raises IL10 levels.[58] In mice, the Th2 response to helminths can deviate Th1 antigenic immunity toward Th2.[59–61] People carrying helminths can show immune bias away from the Th1 response normally elicited with tetanus vaccination[62] or *in vitro* mitogen stimulation.[58] Even maternal helminth infection during pregnancy skews normal Th1 immune reactivity of newborn children.[63]

The Th1 pathway of inflammation (IL-12, IL-18, and IFN-γ) is active in CD,[64] and activated Th1 cells probably have a role in this disease. Mice treated with rectal TNBS develop severe colitis driven by Th1 cytokines. Intestinal helminths restrain the intestinal mucosa from mounting a Th1-type cytokine response (IFN-γ, IL-12 p40-related cytokines) in the distal regions of the bowel and protect mice from TNBS colitis.

The process of helminth regulation of Th1 function could be mediated through several mechanisms. Mucosal lamina propria mononuclear cells (LPMCs) produce large amounts of Th2 cytokines (e.g., IL-4, IL-13) and regulatory factors (e.g., IL-10, TGF-β, PGE$_2$) after worm exposure, suggesting cytokine regulation as an important mechanism. In TNBS colitis, abrogation of the Th2 pathway blocks worm protection, attesting to the importance of these cytokines for worm protection, at least in this animal model of IBD. Enhancement of mucosal production of IL-10, TGF-β, and PGE$_2$ also is noteworthy since the absence of any of these cytokines can lead to Th1-type murine colitis.[65-67] In worm-infected mice, blocking the IL-10 receptor restores IFN-γ and IL-12 production in LPMCs cultured *in vitro*. This suggests that IL-10 is also important in this local regulatory process (paper submitted). IL-10 KO mice get colitis. *H. polygyrus* reverses this colitis after it is established and curtails mucosal IFN-γ secretion.[44] Colonization also decreases LPMC production of IL-12p40. This reduction in established colitis occurs without IL-10, suggesting that IL-10 is not essential for control of inflammation or suppression of Th1-type cytokine production. Anti-IL-12p40 mAb treatment, but not IFN-γ mAbs, also mitigates this colitis. This suggests that only IL-12p40, which is a component of IL-12 and IL-23, is essential for the inflammation.

However, during worm infestation, there can be concomitant dampening of Th2-type reactivity[50,68,69] and decreased lymphocyte responsiveness to various antigens and mitogens. This suggests that worms trigger additional regulatory pathways beyond those that limit Th1 cytokine production.

Regulatory T cells can induce peripheral tolerance and constrain mucosal reactivity.[70-72] Such regulatory cells can control self-reactive T cells and are functionally important in limiting inflammation in various animal models of IBD.[73] There are several regulatory T-cell phenotypes. For instance, some express CD4, while others CD8.[74] There are naturally occurring CD4+ CD25+ regulatory T cells that develop in the thymus. Also described are CD4+ regulatory T cells that produce high levels of IL-10 and/or TGF-β (Tr1, Th3).[75]

Helminths may induce production of regulatory T cells in their host. T cells from the mesenteric lymph node (MLN) of *H. polygyrus*-colonized IL-10-deficient mice, unlike MLN cells from their worm-free IL-10 littermates, abrogate established colitis when transferred into IL-10-deficient recipients.[44] Also, lamina propria (LP) T cells from distal bowel segments of healthy wild-type (WT) mice can make large amounts of IL-10 and TGF-β after *H. polygyrus* infection. These T cells acquired after worm infection limit IFN-γ production from stimulated effector T cells *in vitro* (paper submitted). They express CD4, function without the need of cell contact, and act partially through production of IL-10.

Also, LP T cells from *H. polygyrus*-infected mice, in contrast to LP T cells from uninfected controls, strongly suppress proliferation of both CD4+ and

CD8+ splenic T cells coming from uninfected animals. This regulatory activity lies exclusively within the LP CD8+ T-cell subset and needs direct interactions between the CD8 regulatory T cell and the activated responder T cell. Regulatory function is dependent on Class I interactions, but neither IL10 nor TGFβ are essential for regulatory cell development or activity.

T-cell suppression mediated by CD8+ T cells has been noted in several animal models of inflammation. They participate in the autoimmune disease model of multiple sclerosis (experimental allergic encephalomyelitis).[76]

Bacterial lipopolysaccharides (LPS) stimulate production of pro-inflammatory molecules through interaction with LPS receptors (TLR4) on various cell types. Intestinal LPMCs normally do not respond to LPS. *H. polygyrus* infection induces mucosal T cells to express TLR4. LPS engagement of these induced TLR4s promotes synthesis of TGF-β rather than release of pro-inflammatory cytokines.[77] Thus, under the influence of helminths, mucosal injury would allow LPS from commensal bacteria to help modulate mucosal inflammation through engagement of TGF-β-producing T cells. This also again suggests that helminths induce regulatory T cells in the mucosa.

Immune-mediated diseases in industrialized countries are increasing in prevalence[1,2] where helminth exposure has become rare.[10] Helminth exposure may bias the immune response and afford protection from these diseases. One such possible biasing mechanism is induction of various immune cells with regulatory functions. Other channels of regulation include induction of regulatory cytokines and functional alterations in pathways of innate immunity. Studying helminths may help us understand the causes of these diseases and assist us in recognizing the immune pathways important for disease prevention and effective treatment.

REFERENCES

1. LOFTUS, E.V. JR. & W.J. SANDBORN. 2002. Epidemiology of inflammatory bowel disease. Gastroenterol. Clin. North Am. **31:** 1–20.
2. BACH, J.F. 2002. The effect of infections on susceptibility to autoimmune and allergic diseases. N. Engl. J. Med. **347:** 911–920.
3. SUMMERS, R.W., D.E. ELLIOTT, J.F. URBAN JR., et al. 2005. *Trichuris suis* therapy in Crohn's disease. Gut **54:** 87–90.
4. SUMMERS, R.W., D.E. ELLIOTT, J.F. URBAN JR., et al. 2005. *Trichuris suis* therapy for active ulcerative colitis: a randomized controlled trial. Gastroenterology **128:** 825–832.
5. SUMMERS, R.W., D.E. ELLIOTT & J.V. WEINSTOCK. 2005. Is there a role for helminths in the therapy of inflammatory bowel disease? Nature Clin. Prac. Gastroenterol. Hepatol. **2:** 62–63.
6. TYSK, C., E. LINDBERG, G. JARNEROT & B. FLODERUS-MYRHED. 1988. Ulcerative colitis and Crohn's disease in an unselected population of monozygotic and dizygotic twins: a study of heritability and the influence of smoking. Gut **29:** 990–996.

7. HALFVARSON, J., L. BODIN, C. TYSK, et al. 2003. Inflammatory bowel disease in a Swedish twin cohort: a long-term follow-up of concordance and clinical characteristics. Gastroenterology 124: 1767–1773.

8. CUTHBERT, A.P., S.A. FISHER, M.M. MIRZA, et al. 2002. The contribution of NOD2 gene mutations to the risk and site of disease in inflammatory bowel disease. Gastroenterology 122: 867–874.

9. ABREU, M.T., K.D. TAYLOR, Y.C. LIN, et al. 2002. Mutations in NOD2 are associated with fibrostenosing disease in patients with Crohn's disease. Gastroenterology 123: 679–688.

10. RADLMAYR, M., H.P. TOROK, K. MARTIN & C. FOLWACZNY. 2002. The c-insertion mutation of the NOD2 gene is associated with fistulizing and fibrostenotic phenotypes in Crohn's disease. Gastroenterology 122: 2091–2092.

11. CALKINS, B.M. 1989. A meta-analysis of the role of smoking in inflammatory bowel disease. Dig. Dis. Sci. 34: 1841–1854.

12. ANDERSSON, R.E., G. OLAISON, C. TYSK & A. EKBOM. 2001. Appendectomy and protection against ulcerative colitis. N. Engl. J. Med. 344: 808–814.

13. DERBY, L.E. & H. JICK. 1998. Appendectomy protects against ulcerative colitis. Epidemiology 9: 205–207.

14. RUSSEL, M.G., E. DORANT, R.J. BRUMMER, et al. 1997. Appendectomy and the risk of developing ulcerative colitis or Crohn's disease: results of a large case-control study. South Limburg Inflammatory Bowel Disease Study Group. Gastroenterology 113: 377–382.

15. SONNENBERG, A., D.J. MCCARTY & S.J. JACOBSEN. 1991. Geographic variation of inflammatory bowel disease within the United States. Gastroenterology 100: 143–149.

16. SHIVANANDA, S., J. LENNARD-JONES, R. LOGAN, et al. 1996. Incidence of inflammatory bowel disease across Europe: is there a difference between north and south? Results of the European Collaborative Study on Inflammatory Bowel Disease (EC-IBD). Gut 39: 690–697.

17. ELLIOTT, D.E., J.F. URBAN JR., C.K. ARGO & J.V. WEINSTOCK. 2000. Does the failure to acquire helminthic parasites predispose to Crohn's disease? FASEB J. 14: 1848–1855.

18. BERNSTEIN, C.N., J.F. BLANCHARD, P. RAWSTHORNE & A. WAJDA. 1999. Epidemiology of Crohn's disease and ulcerative colitis in a central Canadian province: a population-based study. Am. J. Epidemiol. 149: 916–924.

19. LOFTUS, E.V. JR., P. SCHOENFELD & W.J. SANDBORN. 2002. The epidemiology and natural history of Crohn's disease in population-based patient cohorts from North America: a systematic review. Aliment. Pharmacol. Ther. 16: 51–60.

20. ROLON, P.A. 1979. Gastrointestinal pathology in South America. Isr. J. Med. Sci. 15: 318–321.

21. AL SHAMALI, M.A., M. KALAOUI, I. PATTY, et al. 2003. Ulcerative colitis in Kuwait: a review of 90 cases. Digestion 67: 218–224.

22. TEZEL, A., G. DOKMECI, M. ESKIOCAK, et al. 2003. Epidemiological features of ulcerative colitis in Trakya, Turkey. J. Intern. Med. Res. 31: 141–148.

23. HUTT, M.S. 1979. Epidemiology of chronic intestinal disease in middle Africa. Isr. J. Med. Sci. 15: 314–317.

24. SEGAL, I. 1988. Ulcerative colitis in a developing country of Africa: the Baragwanath experience of the first 46 patients. Int. J. Colorectal Dis. 3: 222–225.

25. YANG, S.K., E.V. LOFTUS JR. & W.J. SANDBORN. 2001. Epidemiology of inflammatory bowel disease in Asia. Inflam. Bowel Dis. 7: 260–270.

26. PONGPRASOBCHAI, S., S. MANATSATHIT, S. LEELAKUSOLVONG, et al. 2001. Ulcerative colitis in Thailand: a clinical study and long term follow-up. J. Med. Assoc. Thailand **84:** 1281–1288.
27. CARR, I. & J.F. MAYBERRY. 1999. The effects of migration on ulcerative colitis: a three-year prospective study among Europeans and first- and second- generation South Asians in Leicester (1991–1994). Am. J. Gastroenterol. **94:** 2918–2922.
28. JAYANTHI, V., C.S. PROBERT, D. PINDER, et al. 1992. Epidemiology of Crohn's disease in Indian migrants and the indigenous population in Leicestershire. Q. J. Med. **82:** 125–138.
29. PROBERT, C.S., V. JAYANTHI, A.O. HUGHES, et al. 1993. Prevalence and family risk of ulcerative colitis and Crohn's disease: an epidemiological study among Europeans and south Asians in Leicestershire. Gut **34:** 1547–1551.
30. WRIGHT, J.P., I.N. MARKS, C. JAMESON, et al. 1983. Inflammatory bowel disease in Cape Town, 1975–1980. Part II. Crohn's disease. S. Afr. Med. J. **63:** 226–229.
31. NOVIS, B.H., I.N. MARKS, S. BANK & J.H. LOUW. 1975. Incidence of Crohn's disease at Groote Schuur Hospital during 1970–1974. S. Afr. Med. J. **49:** 693–697.
32. ODES, H.S., D. FRASER & J. KRAWIEC. 1989. Inflammatory bowel disease in migrant and native Jewish populations of southern Israel. Scand. J. Gastroenterol. Suppl. **170:** 36–38.
33. ODES, H.S., D. FRASER, P. KRUGLIAK, et al. 1991. Inflammatory bowel disease in the Bedouin Arabs of southern Israel: rarity of diagnosis and clinical features. Gut **32:** 1024–1026.
34. DUGGAN, A.E., I. USMANI, K.R. NEAL & R.F. LOGAN. 1998. Appendicectomy, childhood hygiene, *Helicobacter pylori* status, and risk of inflammatory bowel disease: a case control study. Gut **43:** 494–498.
35. GENT, A.E., M.D. HELLIER, R.H. GRACE, et al. 1994. Inflammatory bowel disease and domestic hygiene in infancy. Lancet **343:** 766–767.
36. EKBOM, A., C. HELMICK, M. ZACK & H.O. ADAMI. 1991. The epidemiology of inflammatory bowel disease: a large, population-based study in Sweden. Gastroenterology **100:** 350–358.
37. SONNENBERG, A. 1990. Occupational distribution of inflammatory bowel disease among German employees. Gut **31:** 1037–1040.
38. DELCO, F. & A. SONNENBERG. 1998. Military history of patients with inflammatory bowel disease: an epidemiological study among U.S. veterans. Am. J. Gastroenterol. **93:** 1457–1462.
39. HILDEBRAND, H., Y. FINKEL, L. GRAHNQUIST, et al. 2003. Changing pattern of paediatric inflammatory bowel disease in northern Stockholm 1990–2001. Gut **52:** 1432–1434.
40. MOLINIE, F., C. GOWER-ROUSSEAU, T. YZET, et al. 2004. Opposite evolution in incidence of Crohn's disease and ulcerative colitis in Northern France (1988–1999). Gut **53:** 843–848.
41. MOREELS, T.G., R.J. NIEUWENDIJK, J.G. DE MAN, et al. 2004. Concurrent infection with *Schistosoma mansoni* attenuates inflammation induced changes in colonic morphology, cytokine levels, and smooth muscle contractility of trinitrobenzene sulphonic acid induced colitis in rats. Gut **53:** 99–107.
42. ELLIOTT, D.E., J. LI, A. BLUM, et al. 2003. Exposure to schistosome eggs protects mice from TNBS-induced colitis. Am. J. Physiol. **284:** G385–G391.
43. KHAN, W.I., P.A. BLENNERHASSET, A.K. VARGHESE, et al. 2002. Intestinal nematode infection ameliorates experimental colitis in mice. Infect. Immun. **70:** 5931–5937.

44. ELLIOTT, D.E., T. SETIAWAN, A. METWALI, *et al.* 2004. *Heligmosomoides polygyrus* inhibits established colitis in IL-10-deficient mice. Eur. J. Immunol. **34:** 2690–2698.

45. LA FLAMME, A.C., K. RUDDENKLAU & B.T. BACKSTROM. 2003. Schistosomiasis decreases central nervous system inflammation and alters the progression of experimental autoimmune encephalomyelitis. Infect. Immun. **71:** 4996–5004.

46. SEWELL, D., Z. QING, E. REINKE, *et al.* 2003. Immunomodulation of experimental autoimmune encephalomyelitis by helminth ova immunization. Intern. Immunol. **15:** 59–69.

47. ZACCONE, P., Z. FEHERVARI, F.M. JONES, *et al.* 2003. *Schistosoma mansoni* antigens modulate the activity of the innate immune response and prevent onset of type 1 diabetes. Eur. J. Immunol. **33:** 1439–1449.

48. MCINNES, I.B., B.P. LEUNG, M. HARNETT, *et al.* 2003. A novel therapeutic approach targeting articular inflammation using the filarial nematode-derived phosphorylcholine-containing glycoprotein ES-62. J. Immunol. **171:** 2127–2133.

49. NAGAYAMA, Y., K. WATANABE, M. NIWA, *et al.* 2004. *Schistosoma mansoni* and α-galactosylceramide: prophylactic effect of Th1 immune suppression in a mouse model of Graves' hyperthyroidism. J. Immunol. **173:** 2167–2173.

50. BASHIR, M.E., P. ANDERSEN, I.J. FUSS, *et al.* 2002. An enteric helminth infection protects against an allergic response to dietary antigen. J. Immunol. **169:** 3284–3292.

51. MAXWELL, C., R. HUSSAIN, T.B. NUTMAN, *et al.* 1987. The clinical and immunologic responses of normal human volunteers to low dose hookworm (*Necator americanus*) infection. Am. J. Trop. Med. Hyg. **37:** 126–134.

52. LOUKAS, A. & P. PROCIV. 2001. Immune responses in hookworm infections. Clin. Microbiol. Rev. **14:** 689–703.

53. TURNER, J.D., H. FAULKNER, J. KAMGNO, *et al.* 2003. Th2 cytokines are associated with reduced worm burdens in a human intestinal helminth infection. J. Infect. Dis. **188:** 1768–1775.

54. DUNNE, D.W. & E.J. PEARCE. 1999. Immunology of hepatosplenic schistosomiasis mansoni: a human perspective. Microbes Infect. **1:** 553–560.

55. GAUSE, W.C., J.F. URBAN JR. & M.J. STADECKER. 2003. The immune response to parasitic helminths: insights from murine models. Trends Immunol. **24:** 269–277.

56. BANCROFT, A.J., K.J. ELSE, J.P. SYPEK & R.K. GRENCIS. 1997. Interleukin-12 promotes a chronic intestinal nematode infection. Eur. J. Immunol. **27:** 866–870.

57. BORKOW, G., Q. LENG, Z. WEISMAN, *et al.* 2000. Chronic immune activation associated with intestinal helminth infections results in impaired signal transduction and anergy. J. Clin. Invest. **106:** 1053–1060.

58. BENTWICH, Z., Z. WEISMAN, C. MOROZ, *et al.* 1996. Immune dysregulation in Ethiopian immigrants in Israel: relevance to helminth infections? Clin. Exp. Immunol. **103:** 239–243.

59. KULLBERG, M.C., E.J. PEARCE, S.E. HIENY, *et al.* 1992. Infection with *Schistosoma mansoni* alters Th1/Th2 cytokine responses to a non-parasite antigen. J. Immunol. **148:** 3264–3270.

60. PEARLMAN, E., J.W. KAZURA, F.E. HAZLETT JR. & W.H. BOOM. 1993. Modulation of murine cytokine responses to mycobacterial antigens by helminth-induced T helper 2 cell responses. J. Immunol. **151:** 4857–4864.

61. SACCO, R., M. HAGEN, M. SANDOR, *et al.* 2002. Established T(H1) granulomatous responses induced by active *Mycobacterium avium* infection switch to T(H2) following challenge with *Schistosoma mansoni*. Clin. Immunol. **104:** 274–281.

62. SABIN, E.A., M.I. ARAUJO, E.M. CARVALHO & E.J. PEARCE. 1996. Impairment of tetanus toxoid-specific Th1-like immune responses in humans infected with *Schistosoma mansoni*. J. Infect. Dis. **173:** 269–272.

63. MALHOTRA, I., P. MUNGAI, A. WAMACHI, *et al.* 1999. Helminth- and Bacillus Calmette-Guerin-induced immunity in children sensitized in utero to filariasis and schistosomiasis. J. Immunol. **162:** 6843–6848.

64. PARRELLO, T., G. MONTELEONE, S. CUCCHIARA, *et al.* 2000. Up-regulation of the IL-12 receptor beta 2 chain in Crohn's disease. J. Immunol. **165:** 7234–7239.

65. RENNICK, D.M. & M.M. FORT. 2000. Lessons from genetically engineered animal models. XII. IL-10-deficient (IL-10(-/-) mice and intestinal inflammation. Am. J. Physiol. **278:** G829–G833.

66. GORELIK, L. & R.A. FLAVELL. 2000. Abrogation of TGFbeta signaling in T cells leads to spontaneous T cell differentiation and autoimmune disease. Immunity **12:** 171–181.

67. KABASHIMA, K., T. SAJI, T. MURATA, *et al.* 2002. The prostaglandin receptor EP4 suppresses colitis, mucosal damage and CD4 cell activation in the gut. J. Clin. Invest. **109:** 883–893.

68. LYNCH, N.R., I. HAGEL, M. PEREZ, *et al.* 1993. Effect of anthelmintic treatment on the allergic reactivity of children in a tropical slum. J. All. Clin. Immunol. **92:** 404–411.

69. VAN DEN BIGGELAAR, A.H., L.C. RODRIGUES, R. VAN REE, *et al.* 2004. Long-term treatment of intestinal helminths increases mite skin-test reactivity in Gabonese schoolchildren. J. Infect. Dis. **189:** 892–900.

70. JONULEIT, H. & E. SCHMITT. 2003. The regulatory T cell family: distinct subsets and their interrelations. J. Immunol. **171:** 6323–6327.

71. URAUSHIHARA, K., T. KANAI, K. KO, *et al.* 2003. Regulation of murine inflammatory bowel disease by CD25+ and CD25- CD4+ glucocorticoid-induced TNF receptor family-related gene+ regulatory T cells. J. Immunol. **171:** 708–716.

72. LIU, H., B. HU, D. XU & F.Y. LIEW. 2003. CD4+CD25+ regulatory T cells cure murine colitis: the role of IL-10, TGF-β and CTLA4. J. Immunol. **171:** 5012–5017.

73. MOTTET, C., H.H. UHLIG & F. POWRIE. 2003. Cutting edge: cure of colitis by CD4+CD25+ regulatory T cells. J. Immunol. **170:** 3939–3943.

74. FIELD, A.C., L. CACCAVELLI, M.F. BLOCH & B. BELLON. 2003. Regulatory CD8+ T cells control neonatal tolerance to a Th2-mediated autoimmunity. J. Immunol. **170:** 2508–2515.

75. MCGUIRK, P. & K.H. MILLS. 2002. Pathogen-specific regulatory T cells provoke a shift in the Th1/Th2 paradigm in immunity to infectious diseases. Trends Immunol. **23:** 450–455.

76. JIANG, H., S.I. ZHANG & B. PERNIS. 1992. Role of CD8+ T cells in murine experimental allergic encephalomyelitis. Science **256:** 1213–1215.

77. INCE, N.M., T. SETIAWAN, A.M. BLUM, *et al.* 2005. *H. polygyrus* induces TLR4 on murine mucosal T cells that produce TGFβ after LPS stimulation. J. Immunol. **176:** 726–729.

Inflammatory Bowel Disease

Pandora's Box, Present and Future

JÜRGEN SCHÖLMERICH

Klinik und Poliklinik für Innere Medizin I, Klinikum der, Universität Regensburg, D-93042 Regensburg, Germany

ABSTRACT: Current treatment of inflammatory bowel disease is rather effective through it is only working in symptomatic fashion. Most recombinant "biologicals" have not been an overwhelming success. Infliximab has shown clinically relevant efficacy and is used in patients not responding to the standards. Alternatives such as modulating the bacterial-epithelial interaction, tightening of the mucosal barrier and maybe even immunostimulation should be studied since most recent finding on etiology and pathophysiology point to a disturbed barrier with consequent abnormal bacterial epithelial interaction as the main problem in the IBD syndrome. We still need to learn much but we should not focus only on immunosuppressive systems.

KEYWORDS: Inflammatory bowel disease; etiology; pathophysiology; bacteria; biologicals; probiotics

Pandora's box has been said to release a vast number of evils upon mankind. This can definitively not be said for modern inflammatory bowel disease (IBD) research, although we do not know which of the current developments will really lead to progress and benefit for patients. However, due to the fast development of etiological and pathophysiological understanding and of huge investments of industry and researchers into new therapeutic approaches there are in the box, both paths to the future and the possibility of failure.

This review will focus on etiological aspects such as genetics, bacterial-epithelial interactions, and the fact that IBD does not comprise two diseases, but is a whole syndrome. The paper will furthermore discuss the fact that pathophysiology is based on many mediators and cell types, which makes it rather analogous to an orchestra with many instruments. It will then discuss the standard treatment, which is probably better than its image in the view of industry and industry-related researchers. Finally, this paper will discuss the

Address for correspondence: Jürgen Schölmerich, Klinik und Poliklinik für Innere Medizin I, Klinikum der Universität Regensburg, D-93042 Regensburg, Germany. Voice: +49-941-944-7001; fax: +49-941-944-7002.

e-mail: juergen.schoelmerich@klinik.uni-r.de

Ann. N.Y. Acad. Sci. 1072: 365–378 (2006). © 2006 New York Academy of Sciences.
doi: 10.1196/annals.1326.026

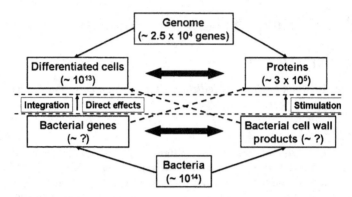

FIGURE 1. Components of the human organism—harmony is needed.

impact of biologicals and "microbiologicals" and in particular the influence of strong paradigms and Wall Street interests.

ETIOLOGY

The human organism has 25,000 genes coding for 300,000 proteins and 10^{13} differentiated cells. The bacteria located in our intestinal tract are at least 10 times greater in number (10^{14}) and have probably many more genes and many bacterial cell-wall products and other components (FIG. 1). Both sides communicate over a vast surface the size of two tennis courts in each of us. Harmony between both sides is required. Without this there will be disease and, in particular, clinical symptoms.

The cotton top tamarin, the only animal spontaneously developing IBD, teaches us two lessons. This animal lives in the forests of Central America without intestinal disease. When taken into captivity it develops IBD and it does so particularly in family clusters. Therefore it is obvious that genetics and environment play a role in this animal as they do in humans. Studies in twins indicating that homozygous twins have a much higher disease concordance compared to heterozygous twins prove a genetic susceptibility, and the fact that the concordance is not 100% indicates the influence of environmental factors. The identification of the first IBD gene— CARD15 coding for the NOD2 protein—brings both sides together.[1-3] The cytoplasmatic protein NOD2 recognizes bacterial cell-wall products, in particular peptidoglycans, and influences the activation of NFκB. We have recently learned that NOD2 signaling interacts with the signaling of toll-like receptors (TLRs) and that this may be one way how deficient action would actually lead to more inflammation.[4] Furthermore, NOD2 seems to be involved in regulation of the production of endogenous antibacterial peptides such as defensins and proapoptotic signaling cascades.[5]

TABLE 1. Influence of NOD2 mutation on survival after stem cell transplantation

	WT	R or D 1 Mutation		R + D heterozygous
GvHD III/IV (%)	19	36	44	58
GvHD intestine (%)	18	36	31	58
Transplantation-associated mortality (%)	20	49	59	83

NOTE: R = recipient; D = donor; WT = wild type.

Both sides of the tennis court influence each other. This is clearly demonstrated by the fact that the bacterial flora of each individual develops in early childhood and remains stable over life and, on the other hand, by the fact that bacterial colonization of the intestinal tract modifies gene expression of intestinal proteins and enzymes.[6]

A very interesting example of influence of NOD2 on epithelial–bacterial interaction in the intestinal tract is the human model of stem cell transplantation. When recipients and donors were analyzed, it turned out that even a heterozygous mutation in either recipient or donor increased graft-versus-host disease in the intestine and transplantation-associated mortality significantly. When both recipient and donor showed a heterozygous mutation, transplantation-associated mortality almost reached 100% (TABLE 1).[7]

Considering that the CARD15 mutations influence the interaction between luminal contents and the mucosal immune system, the question arises of what then leads to the increasing incidence of IBD, because it is not to be expected that the frequency of the genetic alterations has increased over half a century only. Epidemiological studies tell us that there is a rather steep increase in incidence every country, which starts at a different time point in different countries. The earliest rise occurred in Scandinavia, then it went to countries in Central Europe and finally reached Southern Europe. For example, the increase in Greece started in 1980 as far as we know. Meanwhile, the same increses in incidence increase occurs in countries such as Korea, Malaysia, Chile, and Uruguay, among others. This indicates that either "Western" and in particular "Northern European" nutrition or another factor that was earlier broadly present in Northern Europe than in Southern Europe and earlier in Europe than for example in Southeast Asia is responsible for the manifestation of the disease in patients with genetic susceptibility. On the basis of these epidemiological data the "hygiene hypothesis" has been developed. Studies from England demonstrated that the presence of a hot water tub or of a separate toilet for the family in early childhood increased the risk of developing Crohn's disease later on in life by a factor of 3–5.[8] These data have been confirmed in settings outside of Great Britain as well. Interestingly the other mutations thus far demonstrated or at least suggested to play a role in IBD also relate to

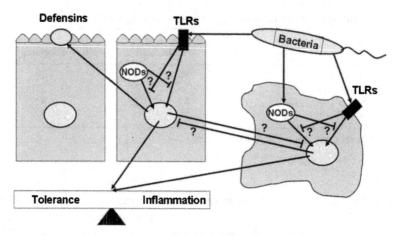

FIGURE 2. Two receptor families recognizing bacteria and modulating epithelial-bacterial interactions determine the balance between tolerance and inflammation.

proteins involved in the transport of bacterial products or the integrity of the intestinal barrier.[9–11]

These genetic and epidemiological data led to the idea that a loss of tolerance against the autologous bacterial flora is indeed the main problem in IBD. Lack of inhibition of TLR signaling, for example, can lead to broken tolerance by induction of costimulatory molecules on dendritic cells and induction of interleukin-6 production, leading to refractoriness of T cells against regulatory cells (FIG. 2).[12] Interestingly the lack of the TLR9, for example, leads to increased severity in experimental models of acute colitis. Furthermore, the transfer of cells from TLR9-deficient donors increases the intestinal inflammation in the severe combined immunodeficiency (SCID) transfer model of chronic colitis (FIG. 3).[13]

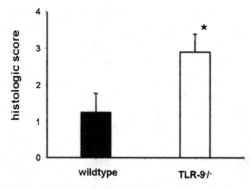

FIGURE 3. Transfer of cells from TLR9-deficient donors leads to increased intestinal inflammation in the SCID-transfer model of colitis.[13]

THE IBD SYNDROME

However, it has to be kept in mind that there is no such thing as one IBD or two IBDs but probably an IBD syndrome comprising many different genotypes and phenotypes. This is obvious for every clinician when looking at the different presentations of Crohn's disease such as, for example, a short stricture at the ileocecal border, an extensive colonic inflammation, upper GI stenosis, or even perianal disease. It will therefore be necessary to finally define all the genotypes and then associate them with the appropriate phenotypes[14] in order to develop understanding and thereby treatment options for this syndrome. It must also be kept in mind that there will be overlap between different genotypes and probably composite genotypes, explaining the wide variety of phenotypes, which have not been defined to a satisfactory extent.

PATHOPHYSIOLOGY

Whereas the understanding of etiology is developing as discussed above, the pathophysiology is much better defined. It actually is not different from the pathophysiology of any other chronic inflammation. An inflammatory stimulus leads to the production of a vast array of cytokines and chemokines, which attract inflammatory cells such as neutrophils and macrophages, which in turn produce another array of mediators such as leukotrienes, platelet-activating factor, reactive oxygen intermediate, and others which finally lead to the destruction of the target cell, in this case the epithelial cell of the gut. Defects in apoptosis of activated immune cells may lead to the chronification of the inflammatory reaction and to a vicious cycle once this system has been started in a susceptible person[15] From this understanding it is obvious that only treatments either eliminating the initial responding cells or the initial signals or interacting with many mediators can be effective in treating the IBD syndrome on the level of the inflammatory reaction. Any other treatment must actually modulate the underlying problem, that is, the disturbed interaction between luminal contents and the intestinal mucosa, most probably the bacterial–epithelial interaction.

STANDARD TREATMENT

What does this imply for our treatment approaches? Fortunately, we are in the lucky situation that our standard treatments are impressively effective.[16] This can be easily seen from current meta-analyses of drugs used in daily practice such as sulfasalazine, mesalazine, and steroids in oral and enema preparations.[17] There is obviously a bias of opinion-leaders regarding severity of IBD and the need for aggressive treatments. Looking at population-based[18–20] data it turns out that fewer than 50% of all patients during their lifetime need

TABLE 2. Assessment of treatment quality in 65 consecutive patients with IBD[25]

	%
5-aminosalicylic acid (ASA) underdosed	64
No rectal treatment with distal colitis	75
Steroids for more than 3 months	77
No prevention of bone loss with steroid treatment	78
No steroid-sparing drugs in patients with long-term steroids	59
Suboptimal dose of azathioprine/6-mercaptopurine	82

steroids. This implies that they can be treated with other drugs less hampered by side effects. This also tells us that the goal of being free of steroids is not a reasonable endpoint for "early aggressive treatment trials." Obviously opinion-leaders mostly working in referral centers are primed by their daily experience to consider the IBD as diseases very difficult to treat. If one takes into account that, for example, cessation of smoking leads to a greater than 50% decrease of the risk of a flare-up during the following 4 years in Crohn's disease,[21] which is a bigger decrease than that achieved with any known drug, it becomes obvious that we have much to learn from epidemiology and from population-based data. Even complications such as fistulae are much less of a problem when looking at population-based data as it appears from referral center studies. Many patients with a fistula, even if they have Crohn's disease, behave like all other non-IBD patients having a fistula. A simple operation may solve the problem.[22]

Furthermore, recent studies make it obvious that we still have not optimized our standard treatment to a reasonable degree. A current analysis tells us that less than 50% of patients were treated according to generally accepted principles (TABLE 2).[23] Furthermore, studies using approaches with combined oral and rectal treatment (TABLE 3)[24,25] or with combinations of drugs provide evidence that there is much to be gained using these mostly pluripotent and well-understood principles. Thus, standard treatment when optimized and used appropriately according to the need of the individual patient is much better than current study results suggest. Well-done epidemiological studies such as in Olmsted County or Copenhagen help a lot in better defining treatment standards.

TABLE 3. Results of combined oral and enema 5-ASA for extensive active UC[24]

8 weeks		Oral 5-ASA, 2 × 2 g/day + Placebo + Enema, 1 g/day (4 weeks)	
Remission	4 weeks (%)	34	44
	8 weeks (%)	43	64[a]
Improvement	4 weeks (%)	62	89[a]
	8 weeks (%)	68	86[a]

[a]Significant.

TABLE 4. Infliximab in patients with ulcerative colitis: results from the ACT I and ACT II trials[28,29]

364/364 patients with active UC: Glucocorticosteroids (GCS) ± Mercartopurine/azathioprine (MP/AZA) in ACT I, 5-ASA, Glucocorticosteroids (GCS) or Mercartopurine/azathioprine (MP/AZA) in ACT II; 0, 2, and 6 weeks results		Dose		
		Placebo	5 mg/kg	10 mg/kg
8 weeks	Response (%)	37.2/29.3	69.4/64.5	61.5/69.2
	Remission (%)	14.9/5.7	38.8/33.9	32.0/27.5
	Mucosal healing (%)	33.9/30.9	62.0/60.3	59.0/61.7
30 weeks	Response (%)	29.8/26.0	52.1/47.1	50.8/60.0
	Remission (%)	15.7/10.6	33.9/25.6	36.9/35.8
	Mucosal healing (%)	24.8/30.1	50.4/46.3	49.2/56.7

NOTE: There were 364 patients in ACT I and 364 patient in ACT II. Treatment was given at 0, 2, and 6 weeks as follows: (GCS) ± MP/AZA in ACT I, and 5-ASA, GCS, or MP/AZA in ACT II.

BIOLOGICALS

However, there still is a group of patients that cannot be sufficiently treated with the standard options. Numerous attempts have been made using pathopysiology-based immunosuppressants or immune modulators to improve the situation. Monoclonal antibodies, soluble receptors, receptor antagonists and many other "biologicals" have been tested. However, only infliximab, a monoclonal antibody against tumor necrosis factor, has been found to be effective to a clinically significant extent without intolerable side effects. This is true for Crohn's disease and ulcerative colitis (UC) (TABLE 4),[26–30] although the results in UC regarding remission induction are probably inferior to those achieved with steroids. Generally it has to be stated that short-term steroid treatment is very effective and helpful, and steroids are vastly underestimated regarding their use in active disease. It is clear that they cannot be used as

TABLE 5. CDP 870 an anti-TNF (tumor necrosis factor) antibody fragment in "active" Crohn's disease [31]

292 patients	Dosing weeks 0, 4, 8			
	Placebo	100 mg	200 mg	400 mg
Clinical response week 12 (%) (CDAI ↓ >100)	35.6	36.5	36.1	44.4
Clinical remission with initial CRP ≥ 10 mg/L	10.7	35.5	32.1	53.1[a]

[a]Significant.
CDAI= Crohn's disease activity index.

long-term treatment in doses needed for this aim, but they should not be disregarded as initial remission-inducing agents.

Many other biologicals have been tested with rather limited success. This may be due in part to the fact that many studies included vast numbers of patients with normal C-reactive protein (CRP), that is at least in Crohn's disease elevated as long as active inflammation is present. When these studies were reanalyzed, stratifying patients according to the CRP levels, it turned out that in most instances patients with increased CRP showed a better response to the anti inflammatory agents compared to placebo, as would be expected in an inflammatory condition, whereas this is not the case in patients included without such signs of inflammation (TABLE 5).[31] This may be due to the fact that many other causes, such as chologenic diarrhea or pain due to fixed stenosis and scar,s lead to an increased "disease activity index," but have nothing to do with active inflammation. Therefore pharmaceutical companies and physicians should reconsider the inclusion criteria. Furthermore, approaches such as epidermal growth factor enemas when given in addition to insufficient oral treatment of distal UC, are certainly better than placebo regarding induction of remission.[32] However, it is rather meaningless to have this "effective" treatment of an insufficiently treated patient with an expensive drug, which also may be considered a procarcinogenic factor in the colon, when alternatives are available. Finally many other approaches that do nor rely on the immunological paradigm, such as granulocyte macrophage-stimulating factor,[33] hormones, and others are available which are certainly not more expensive but probably less prone to causing side effects.[34]

Altogether the list of "biologicals" studied in IBD is impressive but the results are mostly very unimpressive. However, because vast profits are on the horizon, these attempts will continue and need to be considered carefully before implementing them in our daily practice.[34]

Proponents of these new and very expensive approaches, in particular of infliximab, have suggested that early aggressive immunosuppressive treatment in freshly diagnosed patients may be the solution to change the natural history of these disorders. This appears rather unlikely when considering the etiological considerations given above and rests only on the understanding of the more simple general principles of inflammation. However, these proponents have suggested to use this "top-down" strategy in order to change the natural history of the disease. The only trial available[35] studied 130 patients with active, newly diagnosed (less than 4 years) Crohn's disease never treated with glucocorticosteroids or immunosuppressants such as azathioprine or infliximab. The endpoint was "remission without glucocorticosteroids." This again gives glucocorticosteroids too much of an importance because it should better be a comparator and not a target to be eliminated. It turned out that this endpoint was reached more often after 6 but not after 12 months in patients treated initially with infliximab and azathioprine as compared to those treated with budesonide or prednisone in a conventional way. Furthermore, it turned out

TABLE 6. Results of a clinical trial of top-down vs. step-up therapy in Crohn's disease (35)

130 patients with active, newly diagnosed (less than 4 years) CD never treated with GCS, AZA, or Infliximab	Infliximab (5 mg/kg) 0, 2, 6 weeks + AZA 2.5 mg/kg/day (*n* = 65)	BUD (9 mg/day) or PREDNISONE (40 mg/day) tapered (*n* = 65)
Endpoint* reached 6 months (%)	75	48**
12 months (%)	77	64
Still GCS 6 months (%)	0	33**
12 months (%)	0	19**
On AZA 6 months (%)	87	40**
12 months (%)	94	63**
Additional Infliximab (%)	38	15**

*CDAI < 150 GCS **= significant.

NOTE: In a trial reported by hommes et al., 130 patients with newly diagnosed CP and never treated with GCS, AZA, or infliximab were given either infliximab or steroids.

that many more patients were on azathioprine after 6 and 12 months, and in the "top-down" group more patients needed additional or repeated infliximab infusions (TABLE 6).[35] Unfortunately no data on total remission without considering steroid use were given regarding both groups. Thus, it appears that infliximab is somehow equipotent to steroids in induction of remission, but does not really have any clinical or economical advantage as compared to an initial steroid treatment. A total of 19% of patients were still on steroids after 12 months in the "step-up" group. This should be avoided, but otherwise the study does not indicate a need for early aggressive ("top-down") treatment.

MICROBIOLOGICALS

Considering these mostly futile attempts using the pathophysiological understanding for designing treatment approaches (and obtaining Wall Street benefits), the question arises: What are the alternatives? Coming back to the initial considerations of etiology and considering the resulting and broadly accepted hypothesis that there is a disturbed interaction between luminal contents such as bacteria and the mucosa and in particular the epithelial barrier, it is reasonable to act not only on the human immune response, but also on the luminal part of their interaction. This may be possible by modulating the innate immune system, in particular the TLRs, the NOD-systems and readouts such as the defensins. Interestingly the application of bacterial DNA motifs is rather helpful in chronic IBD animal models (FIG. 4).[36] Similarly the application of "probiotics" seems to be effective in such animal models.[37]

As had to be expected probiotic treatments have, been successful also in humans. Initial studies using *Escherichia coli* Nissle, a bacterial "strain" developed almost a century earlier, proved to be equivalent to mesalazine for

TABLE 7. Oral fructo-oligosaccharide for active Crohn's disease [44]

10 Patients 15 g/day for 3 weeks	Initial	3 weeks
Harvey-Bradshaw index	9.8	6.9*
fecal bifidobacteria (log 10 cells/g stool)	8.8	9.4*
IL-10 + dendritic cells (%)expressing TLR 2	1.7	36.8*
TLR 4	3.6	75.4*

*significant

remission maintenance in UC.[38] A number of other studies demonstrated that a mixture of lactobacilli and other bacteria were useful in primary and in secondary prevention of pouchitis in patients after surgery for UC.[39,40] However, lactobacilli strains were not efficient in preventing recurrence of Crohn's disease after surgery.[41,42] More recently it appeared that the strain combination was also effective in inducing remission in UC,[43] but this has to be proven in a controlled randomized trial. Nevertheless, it is generally accepted that probiotics have an effect in IBD. It remains to be defined which strains and which bacterial amounts are useful in which indication.

More recently prebiotics have been tested in very preliminary studies. It has been found that they change the profile of intestinal dendritic cells and the clinical activity in small patient groups (TABLE 7).[44] A controlled trial indicated that substances modulating the barrier such as phosphatidylcholine can be used for treatment of active disease in a successful way.[45] Even more attention was raised by two studies using *Trichuris suis* ova in UC and Crohn's disease, indicating positive effects.[46,47] At least for UC this was even done in a

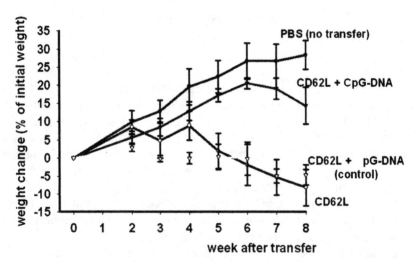

FIGURE 4. Pretreatment with bacterial CpG DNA motifs in the donor prevents weight loss and colitis in the recipient animal in the SCID-transfer model of colitis.[36]

placebo–control study. This vast field of applications of the new paradigm of a disturbed luminal epithelial interaction or, even more focused, bacterial–epithelial interaction, may be the way to the future, although it may well disappoint those who have invested into fancy immunosuppressive drugs.

CONCLUSIONS

In summary, Pandora's box has released many interesting things—good and bad, expected and unexpected. Regarding etiology it has to be considered proven that genetic susceptibility exists—the first genes have been defined. Furthermore, it seems obvious that IBD is a syndrome and that genotypic and phenotypic subgroups with different treatment and prognosis need to be defined. The hygiene hypothesis is the dominant environmental factor and disturbed tolerance to our own enteric flora is broadly accepted. Regarding pathophysiology it is also generally clear that many mediators are involved and that the inhibition of a single mediator does not make much sense. I believe that alternatives to the immunological paradigm have to be examined, in particular the concept of a disturbed barrier, which would render immunosuppressive treatments a concept of the past.

Regarding treatment, it is "comforting" that our standard approaches are rather effective, although they are only working symptomatically and are palliative. Most recombinant, and therefore expensive, principles examined have not been a success. The exception is infliximab, which, has only limited efficacy, however regarding remission and maintenance of remission. Nevertheless, this approach will be continued because the markets are attracting investors and "Wall Street works." In my opinion alternatives should be actively examined that go beyond the immunosuppressive paradigm. Bacterial–epithelial interactions may provide many novel approaches.

It has to be mentioned that the prognosis for IBD with regard to survival has improved to such an extent that survival is almost normal.[20,48] This is a success of the conventional treatment approaches including surgery, glucocorticosteroids, 5-aminosalicylic acid releasing preparations, and conventional immunosuppressants such as azathioprine, 6-mercaptopurine, or methotrexate. A complete healing of the diseases of IBD remains to be achieved, as well as the target of a normal life quality and psychosocial well-being. This has been stated nicely by Lunatscharsky, the first commissar for education and welfare in Russia in 1917: "Complete happiness is nothing else than exceptional harmony in the digestive tract."

REFERENCES

1. OGURA, Y. *et al.* 2001. A frameshift mutation in NOD2 associated with susceptibility to Crohn's disease. Nature **411:** 603–606.

2. HUGOT, J.P. *et al.* 2001. Association of NOD2 leucine-rich repeat variants with susceptibility to Crohn's disease. Nature **411:** 599–603.
3. HAMPE, J. *et al.* 2001. Association between insertion mutation in NOD2 gene and Crohn's disease in German and British populations. Lancet **357:** 1925–1928.
4. WATANABE, T. *et al.* 2004. NOD2 is a negative regulator of Toll-like receptor 2-mediated T helper type 1 responses. Nat. Immunol. **5:** 800–808.
5. WEHKAMP, J. *et al.* 2004. NOD2 (CARD15) mutations in Crohn´s disease are associated with diminished mucosal alpha-defensin expression. Gut **53:** 1658–1664.
6. HOOPER, L.V. *et al.* 2001. Molecular analysis of commensal host-microbial relationships in the intestine. Science **29:** 881–884.
7. HOLLER, E. *et al.* 2004. Both, donor and recipient NOD 2/CARD15 mutations associate with transplant-related mortality and gastrointestinal GvHD following allogeneic stem cell transplantation. Blood **104:** 889–894.
8. GENT, A.E. *et al.* 1994. Inflammatory bowel disease and domestic hygiene in infancy. Lancet **343:** 766–767.
9. PELTEKOVA, V.D. *et al.* 2004. Functional variants of OCTN cation transporter genes are associated with Crohn disease. Nat. Genet. **36:** 471–475.
10. STOLL, M. *et al.* 2004. Genetic variation in DLG5 is associated with inflammatory bowel disease. Nat. Genet. **36:** 476–480.
11. SCHWAB, M. *et al.* 2003. Association between the C3435T MDR1 gene polymorphism and susceptibility for ulcerative colitis. Gastroenterology **124:** 26–33.
12. PASARE, C. & R. MEDZHITOV. 2003. Toll pathway-dependent blockade of CD4+CD25+ T cell-mediated suppression by dendritic cells. Science **299:** 1033–1036.
13. OBERMEIER, F. *et al.* 2005. In vivo CpG DNA/toll like receptor 9 interection induces regulatory properties in CD4+CD62L+ T cells which prevent intestinal inflammation in the SCID transfer model of colitis. GUT **54:** 1428–1436.
14. GASCHÉ, C. *et al.* 2000. A Simple Classification of Crohn's Disease. Inflamm. Bowel. Dis. **6:** 8–15.
15. BEUTLER, B. 2001. Autoimmunity and apoptosis: the Crohn's connection. Immunity **15:** 5–14.
16. SCHÖLMERICH, J. & G. HUBER. 2003. Biological therapies in IBD — anti TNFα and others. Dig. Dis. **21:** 180–191.
17. KORNBLUTH, A.A. *et al.* 1993. Meta-analysis of the effectiveness of current drug therapy of ulcerative colitis. J. Clin. Gastroenterol. **16:** 215–218.
18. SILVERSTEIN, M.D. *et al.* 1999. Clinical course and costs of care for Crohn's disease: Markov model analysis of a population-based cohort. Gastroenterology **117:** 49–57.
19. FAUBION, W.A. Jr. *et al.* 2001. The natural history of corticosteroid therapy for inflammatory bowel disease: a population-based study. Gastroenterology **121:** 255–260.
20. WINTHER, K.V. *et al.* 2003. Survival and cause-specific mortality in ulcerative colitis: follow-up of a population-based cohort in Copenhagen county. Gastroenterology **125:** 1576–1582.
21. COSNES, J. *et al.* 2001. Smoking cessation and the course of Crohn's disease: an intervention study. Gastroenterology **120:** 1093–1099.
22. SCHWARTZ, D.A. *et al.* 2002. The natural history of fistulizing Crohn's disease in Olmsted County, Minnesota. Gastroenterology **122:** 875–880.

23. REDDY, S.I. *et al.* 2005. Are patients with inflammatory bowel disease receiving optimal care? Am. J. Gastroenterol. **100:** 1357–1361.

24. MARTEAU, P. *et al.* 2005. Combined oral and enema treatment with Pentasa (mesalazine) is superior to oral therapy alone in patients with extensive mild/moderate active ulcerative colitis: a randomised, double blind, placebo controlled study. Gut **54:** 960–965.

25. CANDY, S. *et al.* 1995. A controlled double blind study of azathioprine in the management of Crohn's disease. Gut **37:** 674–678.

26. HANAUER, S.B. *et al.* 2002. Maintenance infliximab for Crohn's disease: the ACCENT I randomised trial. Lancet **359:** 1541–1549.

27. SANDS, B.E. *et al.* 2004. Long-term treatment of rectovaginal fistulas in Crohn's disease: response to infliximab in the ACCENT II study. Clin. Gastroenterol. Hepatol. **2:** 912–920.

28. RUTGEERTS, P. *et al.* 2005. A randomized placebo-controlled trial of infliximab therapy for active ulcerative colitis: Act I trial. Gastroenterology **128:** A105.

29. SANDBORN, W.J. *et al.* 2005. Infliximab induction and maintenance therapy for ulcerative colitis: the Act 2 trial. Gastroenterology **128:** A104.

30. JÄRNEROT, G. *et al.* 2005. Infliximab as rescue therapy in severe to moderately severe ulcerative colitis: a randomized, placebo-controlled study. Gastroenterology **128:** 1805–1811.

31. SCHREIBER, S. *et al.* 2003. CDP870, a humanized anti-TNF antibody fragment, induces clinical response with remission in patients with active Crohn's disease. Gastroenterology **125:** 606.

32. SINHA, A. *et al.* 2003. Epidermal growth factor enemas with oral mesalamine for mild-to-moderate left-sided ulcerative colitis or proctitis. N. Engl. J. Med. **349:** 350–357.

33. KORZENIK, J., A. PITTLER & B. DIECKGRAEFE. 2002. Immunostimulation in Crohn's disease: retreatment and maintenance therapy with GM-CSF. Gastroenterology **122:** A432–A433.

34. SCHÖLMERICH, J. 2005. Biological therapies. *In* The Inflammatory Bowel Disease Yearbook. C. N. Bernstein, Ed., pp 111-139.

35. HOMMES, D. *et al.* 2005. Management of recent onset Crohn's disease: a controlled, randomized trial comparing step-up and top-down therapy. Gastroenterology **129:** 371.

36. OBERMEIER, F. *et al.* 2003. Contrasting activity of cytosine-guanosin dinucleotide oligonucleotides in mice with experimental colitis. Clin. Exp. Immunol. **134:** 217–224.

37. SCHULTZ, M., J. SCHÖLMERICH & H.C. RATH. 2003. Rationale for probiotic and antibiotic strategies in inflammatory bowel diseases. Dig. Dis. **21:** 105–128.

38. KRUIS, W. *et al.* 2004. Maintaining remission of ulcerative colitis with the probiotic E. coli Nissle 1917 is as effective as with standard mesalazine. Gut **53:** 1617–1623.

39. GIONCHETTI, P. *et al.* 2000. Oral bacteriotherapy as maintenance treatment in patients with chronic pouchitis. A double-blind, placebo-controlled trial. Gastroenterology **119:** 305–309.

40. GIONCHETTI, P. *et al.* 2003. Prophylaxis of pouchitis onset with probiotic therapy: a double-blind, placebo-controlled trial. Gastroenterology **124:** 1202–1209.

41. PRANTERA, C. *et al.* 2002. Ineffectiveness of probiotics in preventing recurrence after curative resection for Crohn's disease: a randomized controlled trial with Lactobacillus GG. Gut **51:** 405–409.

42. MARTEAU, P. *et al.* 2006. Ineffectiveness of Lactobacillus johnsonii LA1 for prophylaxis of postoperative recurrence in Crohn's disease—a randomized, double-blind, placebo-controlled GETAID trial. Gut **55:** 842–847.
43. BIBILONI, R. *et al.* 2005. VSL#3 probiotic-mixture induces remission in patients with active ulcerative colitis. Am. J. Gastroenterol. **100:** 1539–1546.
44. LINDSAY, J.O. *et al.* 2006. Clinical, microbiological and immunological effects of fructo-oligosaccharide in patients with Crohn's disease. Gut, 348–355.
45. STREMMEL, W. *et al.* 2005. Retarded release phosphatidylcholine benefits patients with chronic active ulcerative colitis. Gut **54:** 966–971.
46. SUMMERS, R.W. *et al.* 2005. Trichuris suis therapy in Crohn's disease. Gut **54:** 87–90.
47. SUMMERS, R.W. *et al.* 2005. Trichuris suis therapy for active ulcerative colitis: a randomized controlled trial. Gastroenterology **128:** 825–832.
48. JESS, T. *et al.* 2006. Survival and cause-specific mortality in patients with inflammatory bowel disease: a long-term outcome study in Olmsted County, Minnesota, 1940–2004. Gut, **doi:** 10.1136/gut.2005.079350.

High Diagnostic Value of ^{18}F–FDG–PET in Pediatric Patients with Chronic Inflammatory Bowel Disease

M. LÖFFLER,[a] M. WECKESSER,[a] C. FRANZIUS,[a] O. SCHOBER,[a] AND K.-P. ZIMMER[b]

[a]Department of Nuclear Medicine, University Hospital of Muenster, Germany, Albert-Schweitzer-Str. 33, 48129 Muenster, Germany

[b]Children's Hospital Muenster, University Hospital Muenster, 48149 Muenster, Germany

ABSTRACT: Diagnosis of chronic inflammatory bowel disease (IBD) in children requires noninvasive, atraumatic diagnostic tools that depict localization and acuity of inflammation and yield only a low radiation dose. This retrospective analysis evaluates the diagnostic potential of FDG-PET. Twenty-six consecutive FDG-PET scans of 23 patients (age: 2–16, years, 14 M, 9 F) with suspected IBD were analyzed in this retrospective study. Results were compared to endoscopic, histologic, and abdominal ultrasound (US) finding. In these examinations, presence of inflammation was evaluated in each patient in 8 bowel segments (score 1–4). Standardized uptake values (SUVs) for FDG–PET were measured for all segments. Sensitivity, specificity, and accuracy were calculated using histology as the standard of reference on a segment-based analysis (pathologic if inflammation score $\geq$ 3 or $SUV_{max}/SUV_{liver} > 1.2$). With histology as the standard of reference, FDG-PET showed a sensitivity/specificity/accuracy of 98%/68%/8%/3 as compared to endoscopy (90%/75%/82%) and US (56%/92%/75%). For the small bowel, FDG-PET was even more reliable (100%/86%/90%). Because of its high sensitivity and accuracy, FDG-PET is an excellent, noninvasive diagnostic tool for IBD. Depicting inflammation in the whole bowel, while being not traumatic, it is attractive for use especially in children. FDG-PET is especially reliable for the small bowel and can inform application of topical therapy.

KEYWORDS: inflammatory bowel disease; FD6-PET; pediatric; Crohn's disease; ulcerative colitis

Address for correspondence: Marcus Loeffler, Department of Nuclear Medicine, University Hospital Muenster, Germany, Albert-Schweitzer-Str. 33, 48129, Muenster, Germany.
e-mail: markus.loeffler@uni-muenster.de

Ann. N.Y. Acad. Sci. 1072: 379–385 (2006). © 2006 New York Academy of Sciences.
doi: 10.1196/annals.1326.014

INTRODUCTION

Children represent 25–50% of patients with chronic inflammatory bowel disease (IBD). Diagnostic latency in Germany is 16–22 month on average[1,2] and the consequent delay in treatment often leads to retardation of growth and development.[3,4] A sensitive examination is still needed to detect early inflammatory changes, showing the site and extension of inflammation as well as its acuity. This is required to initiate topical treatment to avoid side effects of systemic therapy. [18]F fluorodesoxyglucos positron-emission tomography (FDG–PET) is promising in the diagnosis of inflammation[5–8] and its application in children has been established for certain malignant diseases.[9] However, only few published evaluations investigate the use of FDG–PET in IBD[6,10,11] and in the only evaluation with children, histology was not the standard of reference.

PATIENTS AND METHODS

Patients

Twenty-six PET scans were performed in this retrospective study of 23 children (9 F, 14 M; age: 2–16 years, median 12 years). Corresponding examinations (performed less than 10 days before/after PET scan) were endoscopic (colonoscopy with or without gastroduodenoscopy, $n = 18$), histologic ($n = 19$), and ultrasonographic (US) of the bowel/abdomen ($n = 16$). In one patient, the histologic report had no corresponding endoscopy on account of an incompletely written report. Final diagnoses were Crohn's disease ($n = 17$), ulcerative colitis ($n = 2$), infectious colitis ($n = 1$), and juvenile arthritis with concomitant enteritis ($n = 3$) or without enteritis ($n = 2$).

FDG–PET

Written consent from the parents was obtained. The standardized procedure was as follows: minimal fasting period of 4 h; intravenous administration of FDG (3–5 MBq/kg body weight); scanner: ECAT EXACT 921/47 (CTI/Siemens, Knoxville, Tennessee, USA); whole body emission/transmission scans: 6/4 min per bed position (15.9 cm axial FOV). There was no need for sedation. Effective dose was 3–7 mSv for children.[12,13] Evaluation of PET scans was performed blinded to the diagnosis and the clinical symptoms.

Endoscopy with Histology

Examinations were performed with the child under general anesthesia as a standardized procedure. After a written consent from the parents has been

TABLE 1. Evaluation of the diagnostic power of FDG–PET, endoscopy, histology, and ultrasound on a segment-based analysis

	Sens.	Spec.	Ppv.	Npv.	Acc.
Histology as Standard of Reference					
PET	98%	68%	75%	98%	83%
Endoscopy	90%	75%	74%	90%	82%
Ultrasound	56%	92%	87%	69%	75%
Endoscopy as Standard of Reference					
PET	92%	65 %	75%	88%	80%
Histology	74%	90%	90%	75%	82%
Ultrasound	57%	81%	80%	59%	67%

Sensitivity (Sens.), specificity (Spec.), positive predictive value (Ppv.), negative predictive value (Npv.), and accuracy (Acc.) were calculated with histology and endoscopy as the standard of reference. FDG–PET and ultrasound were significantly different to histology and endoscopy ($P <$ 0.05, McNemar). Endoscopy versus histology showed no significant difference ($P = 0.052$).

obtained, upper gastrointestinal tract, colon, and terminal ileum were intubated; biopsy specimens of all segments were taken. The endoscopes used were GIF-V and CF-VI (Olympus). The performing physician was aware of the clinical situation with all examinations and laboratory tests.

Readings and Statistical Analysis

Endoscopy, histology, and ultrasonography were performed in a routine clinical setting and without any blinding, and written reports were analyzed. Inflammation severity was graded (not inflamed to minimally inflamed vs. moderately-to-severely inflamed) for individual bowel segments (duodenum, jejunum, ileum, ascending colon, transverse colon, descending colon, sigmoid colon, rectum). PET scans were analyzed semiquantitatively: standardized uptake values (SUVs) were calculated for all bowel segments and the liver. Diagnostic performance of FDG–PET (pathologic if $SUV_{max}/SUV_{liver} > 1.2$) and of US were calculated (gold standard: histology and endoscopy).

RESULTS

In a segment-based analysis with histology as the standard of reference, FDG–PET showed a sensitivity of 98% (57/58) and a negative predictive value of 98% (40/41). Specificity was 68% (40/59) and positive predictive value 75% (57/76). In the small bowel, FDG–PET showed 9 true-positive results and 18 true-negative results, but only 3 false-positive results and no false-negative result. Two of three false-positive results in the small bowel were similar to the endoscopic readings, indicating the inflammatory activity in those segments was approaching clinical relevance. Further results and clinical examples are shown in TABLE 1 and FIGURES 1 and 2.

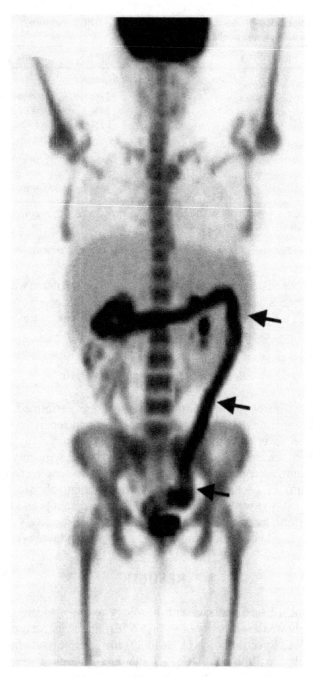

FIGURE 1. Fourteen-year-old female with Crohn's disease; no improvement was seen with systemic treatment. Inflammation in the transverse colon to sigmoid colon is depicted (*arrows*) on FDG–PET, but no small intestine inflammation is seen. Patient became symptom-free with topical therapy (corticoid enema).

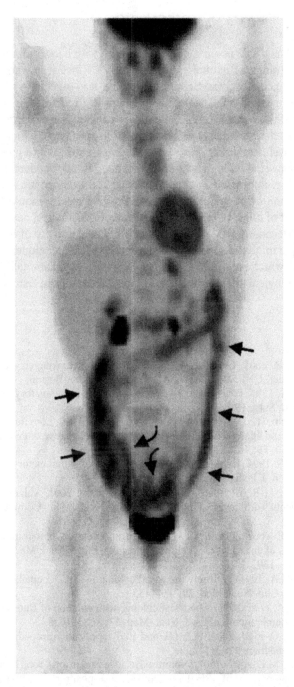

FIGURE 2. Fourteen-year-old female with suspected Crohn's disease. FDG–PET shows inflammation of terminal ileum (*curved arrows*) and colonic frame (*straight arrows*). Therefore, not local, but systemic therapy was applied.

DISCUSSION

FDG–PET is a fast, noninvasive examination with a low radiation exposure of 3–7 mSv (range of natural exposure/year).[13] Since it is well tolerated in contrast to the conventional Sellink procedure, it is especially recommended for the assessment of small bowel involvement in children at an early stage of disease manifestation. FDG–PET identifies affected bowel segments reliably and supplies semiquantitative information of disease activity, including that in the small bowel, furthering differential diagnosis of IBD and guiding topical therapy. Because of its high sensitivity despite its only moderate specificity, FDG–PET is recommended at the beginning of the diagnostic setting as well as for exclusion of bowel inflammation. Positive results should be assessed in the context of clinical, laboratory, endoscopic, histologic, and sonographic evaluation. Because FDG–PET indicates functional activity of inflammation, this technique might be superior to other radiological techniques, such as MR enteroclysis, which are useful to diagnose (advanced) inflammatory processes with morphological alterations, such as bowel stenosis and fistula.

REFERENCES

1. BEHRENS, R. 2001. Chronisch-entzündliche Darmerkrankungen im Kindes- und Jugendalter. UNI-MED. Verlag AG. Bremen-London-Boston.
2. RAINE, P.A. 1984. BAPS collective review: chronic inflammatory bowel disease. J. Pediatr. Surg. **19:** 18–23.
3. HILDEBRAND, H., J. KARLBERG & B. KRISTIANSSON. 1994. Longitudinal growth in children and adolescents with inflammatory bowel disease. J. Pediatr. Gastroenterol. Nutr. **18:** 165–173.
4. HYAMS, J.S. 1994. Extraintestinal manifestations of inflammatory bowel disease in children. J. Pediatr. Gastroenterol. Nutr. **19:** 7–21.
5. LORENZEN, J., R. BUCHERT & K.H. BOHUSLAVIZKI. 2001. Value of FDG PET in patients with fever of unknown origin. Nucl. Med. Commun. **22:** 779–783.
6. KRESNIK, E. et al. 2002. (18)F–FDG positron emission tomography in the early diagnosis of enterocolitis: preliminary results. Eur. J. Nucl. Med. Mol. Imaging **29:** 1389–1392.
7. MEYER, M.A. 1995. Diffusely increased colonic F-18 FDG uptake in acute enterocolitis. Clin. Nucl. Med. **20:** 434–435.
8. HANNAH, A. et al. 1996. Abnormal colonic accumulation of fluorine-18-FDG in pseudomembranous colitis. J. Nucl. Med. **37:** 1683–1685.
9. FRANZIUS, C. et al. 2004. PET/CT and PET: application in pediatric oncology. Nuklearmedizin. **27:** 315–323.
10. NEURATH, M.F. et al. 2002. Noninvasive assessment of Crohn's disease activity: a comparison of 18F-fluorodeoxyglucose positron emission tomography, hydromagnetic resonance imaging, and granulocyte scintigraphy with labeled antibodies. Am. J. Gastroenterol. **97:** 1978–1985.

11. SKEHAN, S.J. *et al.* 1999. 18F-fluorodeoxyglucose positron tomography in diagnosis of paediatric inflammatory bowel disease. Lancet 354: 836–837.
12. HAHN, K. & S. FISCHER. 2002. Radiation dose and radiation protection from paediatric nuclear medicine procedures. Nuklearmedizin. **25:** 90–100.
13. SCHICHA, H. & O. SCHOBER. 2003. Nuklearmedizin. Schattauer. Stuttgart, New York.

Role of Macrophage Metalloelastase in Gut Inflammation

SYLVIA L.F. PENDER,[a] C.K.F. LI,[b] A.D.I. SABATINO,[c]
T.T. MACDONALD,[c] AND M.G. BUCKLEY[a]

[a]Division of Infection, Inflammation and Repair, School of Medicine,
University of Southampton, Southampton SO16 6YD, UK

[b]MRC Human Immunology Unit, The Weatherall Institute of Molecular
Medicine, John Radcliffe Hospital, Headington, Oxford OX3 9DU, UK

[c]Centre for Infectious Disease, ICMS, Barts and the Royal London School of
Medicine and Dentistry, Whitechapel, London E1 2AT, UK

ABSTRACT: Matrix metalloproteinases (MMPs) are involved in a number
of physiological and pathologic processes including the inflammation
found in IBD. We have shown that MMP-3 is upregulated in Crohn's
disease and in ulcerative colitis. This study shows a potential role for
MMP-12 in these idiopathic diseases.

KEYWORDS: immune response; inflammatory bowel diseases; intestine;
macrophages; matrix metalloproteinase; tissue inflammation

Matrix metalloproteinases (MMPs) play a major role in many physiological and
pathological processes such as angiogenesis, wound healing, and inflammation, including that found in inflammatory bowel disease (IBD).[1] Our previous
studies have shown that stromelysin-1 (MMP-3) is upregulated in Crohn's disease and ulcerative colitis (UC).[2] In the present study, we provide evidence of a
potentially important role for MMP-12 in these idiopathic diseases. MMP-12
is a macrophage-specific enzyme, which degrades different substrates, among
which are elastin, laminin, type-IV collagen, fibronectin, and casein. MMP-12
is unable, however, to degrade interstitial collagens or gelatin.[3] It is a 54-kDa
proenzyme that is processed into a 45-kDa and then a 22-kDa active form and is
important for allowing macrophage migration through extracellular matrix.[4]
As macrophages form a significant component in the pathogenesis of IBD,
MMP-12 could play an even more important role in the causation of IBD than
MMP-3.

Address for correspondence: Dr. Sylvia L.F. Pender, Division of Infection, Inflammation, Repair,
Mailpoint 813, Level E, South Academic Block, Southampton General Hospital, Southampton SO16
6YD, UK. Voice: +44-0-23-8079-5081; fax: +44-0-23-8079-5025.
e-mail: s.pender@soton.ac.uk

Ann. N.Y. Acad. Sci. 1072: 386–388 (2006). © 2006 New York Academy of Sciences.
doi: 10.1196/annals.1326.019

In this study, we used gene array analysis and have shown that MMP-12 stands out among the 23 MMPs we screened (including MMP-3) as being most markedly upregulated in a T cell–mediated model of gut injury[5] and in IBD. MMP-12 expression was 11.9- and 7.3-fold higher than in controls in the PWM- and αCD3+IL12-stimulated explant cultures, respectively, whereas MMP-3 expression in the corresponding samples was 8.2 and 5.7, respectively. In IBD tissues we have shown that MMP-12 is increased 7.3-fold in UC and 3.6-fold in Crohn's disease compared to controls. Western blotting has demonstrated that MMP-12 protein is significantly increased in IBD resection samples compared with these of control subjects, and that UC has an even higher expression. Western blotting was also performed on the culture supernatants of *ex vivo* explant cultures[6] and it detected high concentrations of both latent and active forms of MMP-12 in four independent experiments, suggesting that the production of MMP-12 is directly related to T cell or macrophage hypersensitivity as seen in IBD, but without the effect of blood-borne cells such as neutrophils. When purified MMP-12 (3 µg/mL) was used to treat tissue explants,[6] we found that in four independent experiments the epithelium of all the explants was completely destroyed after 4 days of culture. At 0.3µg/mL, the epithelium of the explant was partially abolished. Immunostaining confirmed the disappearance of the epithelium after MMP-12 treatment. The basement membrane and smooth muscle actin of the explant were still intact at low doses of MMP-12; however, they were completely destroyed by high doses. When trinitrobenzene sulphonic acid (TNBS) was administered to the colons of MMP-12 knockout mice ($n = 14$) for 7 days, no mucosal damage was seen histologically on H&E stain. However, severe colitis was observed in wild-type control mice (C57BL/6, $n = 29$). Colons of wild-type mice but not knockout mice were significantly thickened after TNBS treatment.

These data indicate that local immune responses can increase MMP-12 expression in resident lamina propria macrophages, and that MMP-12 might play a significant part in tissue inflammation in IBD.

ACKNOWLEDGMENT

This study is supported by the Board Medical Research Programme, Los Angeles, USA.

REFERENCES

1. PENDER, S.L. & T.T. MACDONALD. 2004. Matrix metalloproteinases and the gut— new roles for old enzymes. Curr. Opin. Pharmacol. **4:** 546–550.
2. HEUSCHKEL, R.B., T.T. MACDONALD, G. MONTELEONE, *et al.* 2000. Imbalance of stromelysin-1 and TIMP-1 in the mucosal lesions of children with inflammatory bowel disease. Gut **47:** 57–62.

3. GRONSKI, T.J. JR., R.L. MARTIN, D.K. KOBAYASHI, *et al.* 1997. Hydrolysis of a broad spectrum of extracellular matrix proteins by human macrophage elastase. J. Biol. Chem. **272:** 12189–12194.
4. SHIPLEY, J.M., R.L. WESSELSCHMIDT, D.K. KOBAYASHI, *et al.* 1996. Metalloelastase is required for macrophage-mediated proteolysis and matrix invasion in mice. Proc. Natl. Acad. Sci. USA **93:** 3942–3946.
5. SALMELA, M.T., T.T. MACDONALD, D. BLACK, *et al.* 2002. Upregulation of matrix metalloproteinases in a model of T cell mediated tissue injury in the gut: analysis by gene array and in situ hybridisation. Gut **51:** 540–547.
6. PENDER, S.L., S.P. TICKLE, A.J. DOCHERTY, *et al.* 1997. A major role for matrix metalloproteinases in T cell injury in the gut. J. Immunol. **158:** 1582–1590.

IL-10 Gene-Deficient Mice Lack TGF-Beta/Smad-Mediated TLR2 Degradation and Fail to Inhibit Proinflammatory Gene Expression in Intestinal Epithelial Cells under Conditions of Chronic Inflammation

PEDRO A. RUIZ,[a] ANNA SHKODA,[a] SANDRA C. KIM,[b]
R. BALFOUR SARTOR,[b] AND DIRK HALLER[a]

[a]*Else-Kroener-Fresenius Centre for Experimental Nutritional Medicine,*
Technical University of Munich, 85350 Freising-Weihenstephan, Germany

[b]*Department of Medicine, University of North Carolina, Chapel Hill,*
North Carolina, USA

ABSTRACT: Nonpathogenic enteric bacterial species initiate and perpetuate experimental colitis in interleukin-10 geneeficient mice (IL-10$^{-/-}$). Bacteria-specific effects on the epithelium are difficult to distinguish because of the complex nature of the gut microflora. We showed that IL-10$^{-/-}$ mice compared to wild-type mice fail to inhibit pro-inflammatory gene expression in native intestinal epithelial cells after the colonization with colitogenic Gram-positive *Enterococcus faecalis*. Of interest, pro-inflammatory gene expression was transient after 1 week of *E. faecalis* monoassociation in IECs from wild-type mice but persisted after 14 weeks of bacterial colonization in IL-10$^{-/-}$ mice. Accordingly, wild-type IECs expressed phosphorylated NF-kappaB subunit RelA (p65) and phosphorylated Smad2 only at day 7 after bacterial colonization, whereas *E. faecalis*-monoassociated IL-10$^{-/-}$ mice triggered persistent RelA but no Smad2 phosphorylation in IECs at days 3, 7, 14, and 28. Consistent with the induction of TLR2-mediated RelA phosphorylation and pro-inflammatory gene expression in *E. faecalis*-stimulated cell lines, TLR2 protein expression was absent after day 7 from *E. faecalis*-monoassociated wild-type mice but persisted in IL-10$^{-/-}$ IECs. Of note, TGF-beta-activated Smad signaling was associated with the loss of TLR2 protein expression and the inhibition of

Address for correspondence: Dr. Dirk Haller, Else-Kroener-Fresenius Centre for Experimental Nutritional Medicine, Technical University of Munich, 85350 Freising-Weihenstephan, Germany. Voice: +49-8161-71-2026; fax: +49-8161-71-2097.
e-mail: haller@wzw.tum.de

Ann. N.Y. Acad. Sci. 1072: 389–394 (2006). © 2006 New York Academy of Sciences.
doi: 10.1196/annals.1326.023

NF-kappa Bependent gene expression in *E. faecalis*-stimulated IEC lines. In conclusion, *E. faecalis*-monoassociated IL-10$^{-/-}$ but not wild-type mice lack protective TGF-beta/Smad signaling and fail to inhibit TLR2-mediated pro-inflammatory gene expression in the intestinal epithelium, suggesting a critical role for IL-10 and TGF-beta in maintaining normal epithelial cell homeostasis in the interplay with commensal enteric bacteria.

KEYWORDS: chronic intestinal inflammation; intestinal epithelial cells; *Enterococus faecalis;* nuclear factor (NF)-κB; toll-like receptor (TLR) 2; TGF-β/Smad signal transduction

INTRODUCTION

Gastrointestinal infections, the genetic predisposition to dysregulated mucosal immune responses, and the concurrent prevalence of certain environmental triggers in developed countries are strong etiologic factors for the development of chronic intestinal inflammation including ulcerative colitis and Crohn's disease.[1,2] Microbial agents of the normal enteric microflora are involved in each of the current etiologic theories of these immunologically mediated idiopathic disorders.[3] Commensal bacterial strains from the species *Enterococcus faecalis (E. faecalis)* have been shown to be particularly important to the induction of colitis in gnotobiotic IL-10 gene-deficient (IL-10$^{-/-}$) mice.[4] The intestinal epithelium must interact with and adapt to a constantly changing environment by processing the combined biological information of luminal enteric bacteria as well as host-derived immune signals in order to maintain gut homeostasis. Intestinal epithelial cells (IECs) constitutively express or can be induced to express toll-like receptors (TLRs) and a wide range of inflammatory cytokines.[5] Most of these molecules are transcriptionally regulated by the transcription factor NF-κB.[6] We hypothesize that changes in the homeostasis of bacteria- and host-derived signal transduction at the epithelial cell level may lead to functional disturbances of the intestinal epithelium and to the development of chronic inflammation in the susceptible host.[7-10]

RESULTS AND DISCUSSION

In this study, we demonstrate that *E. faecalis*-monoassociated wild-type (WT) and IL-10$^{-/-}$ mice differentially induce TLR2-mediated NF-κB and TGF-β/Smad signaling in the intestinal epithelium. Real-time PCR analysis (FIG. 1 A) showed that *E. faecalis* monoassociation triggered IP-10 gene expression in WT and IL-10$^{-/-}$ IECs after the first week of bacterial colonization, well before the onset of histopathologic changes. In contrast to the

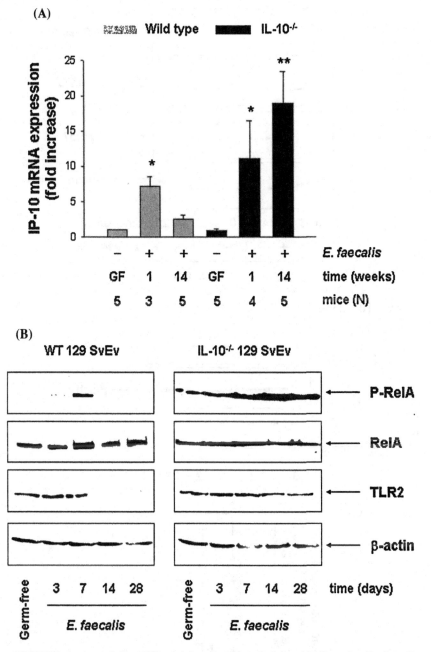

FIGURE 1. A and **B**: Differential activation of the epithelium in *E. faecalis*-mon-oassociated wild-type and IL-10$^{-/-}$ mice. Germ-free WT and IL-10$^{-/-}$ mice were colonized with *E. faecalis* and were killed at day 3, 7, 14, and 28 as well as 14 weeks. IP-10 gene expression (**A**, Light Cycler PCR), phospho-RelA, and TLR2 protein expression (**B**, Western blot analysis) were measured in isolated primary IECs.

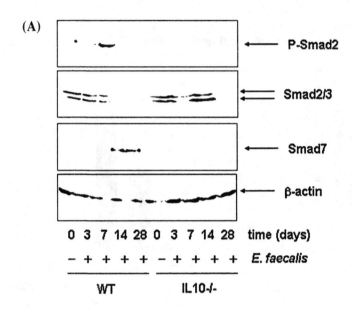

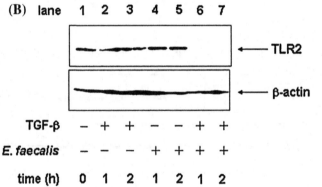

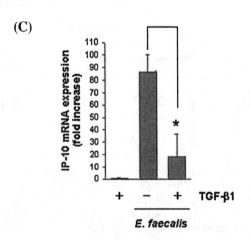

transient IEC activation in WT mice, IP-10 expression persisted in IL-10$^{-/-}$ IEC at late stages of bacterial colonization (14 weeks) and was associated with the development of severe colitis. In addition, *E. faecalis* triggers transient RelA (p65) phosphorylation in WT mice, but persistent RelA phosphorylation in IL-10$^{-/-}$ mice (FIG. 1 B), suggesting an intrinsic defect of IL-10$^{-/-}$ mice to control transient induction of NF-κB activity and proinflammatory gene expression in the intestinal epithelium following bacterial colonization. Consistent with the finding that *E. faecalis* induces TLR2-mediated RelA phosphorylation and NF-κB-dependent IP-10 gene expression in epithelial cell lines (data not shown), TLR2 protein expression was absent in native IEC after the first week from *E. faecalis*-monoassociated WT mice but persisted in IL-10$^{-/-}$ mice (FIG. 1 B). Although the purpose of TLR signaling is to alert and protect the host,[11,12] the unbalanced activation of these innate signaling pathways due to host genetic predispositions may turn a physiological response into a pathological situation of chronic inflammation. The second key feature of our present study is the observation that the lack of Smad2 phosphorylation in IECs from *E. faecalis*-monoassociated IL-10$^{-/-}$ mice is associated with persistent TLR2 protein expression under conditions of chronic inflammation (FIG. 2 A). Interestingly, TGF-β-activated Smad2 signaling triggers TLR2 protein degradation in *E. faecalis*-stimulated MODE-K cells (FIG. 2 B) and inhibits IP-10 gene expression (FIG. 2 C). These results are consistent with previous observations in TGF-β receptor transgenic mice, demonstrating that the blockade of TGF-β signaling at the epithelial cell level resulted in the development of colitis in these mice.[13] It seems an attractive hypothesis that host-derived feedback mechanisms control the status of "physiological inflammation" in the epithelium by maintaining low levels of TLR expression through the induction of IL-10–mediated TGF-β responses under normal conditions.[14,15] However, the unbalanced activation of innate immune responses toward luminal enteric bacteria in the absence of host-derived negative regulators may lead to persistent epithelial cell activation and the development of chronic intestinal inflammation.[16]

FIGURE 2. A–C: Differential induction of protective TGF-β-mediated Smad signaling in the epithelium in *E. faecalis*-monoassociated wild-type and IL-10$^{-/-}$ mice. Germ-free WT and IL-10$^{-/-}$ mice were colonized with *E. faecalis* and were killed at day 3, 7, 14, and 28. Phospho-Smad2, Smad2, and Smad7 were measured in primary isolated IECs (**A**, Western blot analysis). TGF-β triggers TLR2 protein degradation in *E. faecalis*-stimulated MODE-K cells (**B**, Western blot analysis). TGF-β inhibits *E. faecalis*-induced IP-10 gene expression in MODE-K cells (**C**, Light Cycler PCR).

REFERENCES

1. LOFTUS, E.V., JR. 2004. Clinical epidemiology of inflammatory bowel disease: incidence, prevalence, and environmental influences. Gastroenterology **126**: 1504–1517.
2. AHMAD, T. *et al.* 2004. Clinical relevance of advances in genetics and pharmacogenetics of IBD. Gastroenterology **126**: 1533–1549.
3. SARTOR, R.B. 2004. Therapeutic manipulation of the enteric microflora in inflammatory bowel diseases: antibiotics, probiotics, and prebiotics. Gastroenterology **126**: 1620–1633.
4. KIM, S.C. *et al.* 2005. Variable phenotypes of enterocolitis in interleukin 10-deficient mice monoassociated with two different commensal bacteria. Gastroenterology **128**: 891–906.
5. CARIO, E. 2005. Bacterial interactions with cells of the intestinal mucosa: toll-like receptors and NOD2. Gut **54**: 1182–1193 Epub 2005 Apr 19.
6. HALLER, D. & C. JOBIN. 2004. Interaction between resident luminal bacteria and the host: can a healthy relationship turn sour? J. Pediatr. Gastroenterol. Nutr. **38**: 123–136.
7. HALLER, D. *et al.* 2002. IKK beta and phosphatidylinositol 3-kinase/Akt participate in non-pathogenic gram-negative enteric bacteria-induced RelA phosphorylation and NF-kappa B activation in both primary and intestinal epithelial cell lines. J. Biol. Chem. **277**: 38168–38178.
8. HALLER, D. *et al.* 2003. Transforming growth factor-{beta}1 inhibits non-pathogenic gram negative bacteria-induced NF-{kappa}B recruitment to the interleukin-6 gene promoter in intestinal epithelial cells through modulation of histone acetylation. J. Biol. Chem. **278**: 23851–23860.
9. HALLER, D. *et al.* 2004. Differential effect of immune cells on non-pathogenic gram-negative bacteria-induced nuclear factor-kappaB activation and pro-inflammatory gene expression in intestinal epithelial cells. Immunology **112**: 310–320.
10. RUIZ, P.A. *et al.* 2004. 15-deoxy-delta12,14-prostaglandin J2-mediated ERK signaling inhibits gram-negative bacteria-induced RelA phosphorylation and interleukin-6 gene expression in intestinal epithelial cells through modulation of protein phosphatase 2A activity. J. Biol. Chem. **279**: 36103–36111 Epub 2004 Jun 15.
11. MEDZHITOV, R. & C.A. JANEWAY, JR. 2002. Decoding the patterns of self and nonself by the innate immune system. Science **296**: 298–300.
12. RAKOFF-NAHOUM, S. *et al.* 2004. Recognition of commensal microflora by toll-like receptors is required for intestinal homeostasis. Cell **118**: 229–241.
13. HAHM, K.B. *et al.* 2001. Loss of transforming growth factor beta signalling in the intestine contributes to tissue injury in inflammatory bowel disease. Gut **49**: 190–198.
14. FUSS, I.J. *et al.* 2002. The interrelated roles of TGF-beta and IL-10 in the regulation of experimental colitis. J. Immunol. **168**: 900–908.
15. DI GIACINTO, C. *et al.* 2005. Probiotics ameliorate recurrent Th1-mediated murine colitis by inducing IL-10 and IL-10-dependent TGF-beta-bearing regulatory cells. J. Immunol. **174**: 3237–3246.
16. RUIZ, P.A. *et al.* 2005. IL-10 gene-deficient mice lack TGF-beta/Smad signaling and fail to inhibit proinflammatory gene expression in intestinal epithelial cells after the colonization with colitogenic *Enterococcus faecalis*. J. Immunol. **174**: 2990–2999.

Perinodal Adipose Tissue and Fatty Acid Composition of Lymphoid Tissues in Patients with and without Crohn's Disease and Their Implications for the Etiology and Treatment of CD

EDWARD D.A. WESTCOTT,[a,b,c] CHRISTINE A. MATTACKS,[c]
ALASTAIR C.J. WINDSOR,[b] STELLA C. KNIGHT,[a]
AND CAROLINE M. POND[c]

[a]Antigen Presentation Research Group, Imperial College, London,
Northwick Park and St. Mark's Campus, Harrow, HA1 3UJ, UK

[b]Department of Surgery, St. Mark's Hospital, Harrow, HA1 3UJ, UK

[c]Department of Biological Sciences, The Open University, Milton Keynes,
MK7 6AA, UK

ABSTRACT: The physiological bases for roles of adipose tissue and fatty acids in the symptoms and dietary treatments of Crohn's disease are poorly understood. The hypothesis developed from experiments on rodents that perinodal adipocytes are specialized to provision adjacent lymphoid tissues was tested by comparing the composition of triacylglycerol fatty acids in homologous samples of mesenteric adipose tissue and lymph nodes from patients with or without Crohn's disease. Mesenteric perinodal and other adipose tissue, and lymph nodes, were collected during elective surgery for Crohn's disease and other conditions. Fatty acids were extracted, identified, and quantified by thin-layer and gas-liquid chromatography. Perinodal adipose tissue contained more unsaturated fatty acids than other adipose tissue in controls, as reported for other mammals, but site-specific differences were absent in Crohn's disease. Lipids from adipose and lymphoid tissues had more saturated fatty acids, but fewer polyunsaturates in Crohn's disease patients than controls. In adipose tissue samples, depletion of n-3 polyunsaturates was greatest, but n-6 polyunsaturates, particularly arachidonic acid, were preferentially reduced in lymphoid cells. Ratios of n-6/n-3 polyunsaturates were higher in adipose tissue but lower in lymphoid cells in Crohn's disease patients than in controls. Site-specific differences in fatty acid composition in normal human mesentery are consistent with local interactions between lymph node lymphoid cells and adjacent adipose tissue. But these

Address for correspondence: Prof. Caroline M. Pond, Department of Biological Sciences, The Open University, Milton Keynes, MK7 6AA, UK. Voice: +44-1908-655077; fax: +44-1908-654167.
e-mail: c.m.pond@open.ac.uk

Ann. N.Y. Acad. Sci. 1072: 395–400 (2006). © 2006 New York Academy of Sciences.
doi: 10.1196/annals.1326.034

site-specific properties are absent in Crohn's disease, causing anoma-
lies in composition of lymphoid cell fatty acids, which may explain the
efficacy of elemental diets containing oils rich in *n*-6 polyunsaturates.

KEYWORDS: triacylglycerols; phospholipids; arachidonic acid; lymph
nodes; site-specific properties

INTRODUCTION

Comparative and experimental studies show that perinodal adipose tissue
surrounding mammalian lymph nodes is physiologically specialized for local
interactions with lymphoid cells.[1,2] The composition of fatty acids in lipids
of lymph node and tissue-derived lymphoid cells is similar to that of adjacent adipocytes, indicating that they supply nutrients that support immune
responses.[3,4]

Triacylglycerols and phospholipids of perinodal adipose tissue contain pro-
portionately more polyunsaturated fatty acids (PUFAs).[5] This property can be
measured accurately in samples that have been stored frozen and thus used to
identify perinodal adipose tissue. The roles of dietary lipids in Crohn's disease (CD) are paradoxical. Fish-oil diets rich in *n*-3 PUFAs relieve CD and
other chronic inflammatory conditions.[6,7] Fatty acid compositions of blood
cell phospholipids and adipose tissue triacylglycerols are anomalous in CD.[8]
Blood-borne mononuclear cells contain more, not less, *n*-3 PUFAs in CD than
controls.[9] Arachidonic acid (20:4*n*-6) in blood mononucleocytes from CD patients is very low.[9] Elemental diets containing arachis oil (high in linoleic acid,
18:2*n*-6) were as effective for acute CD as high-dose oral steroids,[10] and better than diets high in anti-inflammatory *n*-3 fatty acids.[11,12] Supplying more
dietary *n*-6 PUFAs relieves inflammatory symptoms most efficiently.[11]

Crohn *et al.*[13] described abnormally thickened mesenteries and fat-wrapping
in 1932. Such selective hypertrophy suggests that the adipose tissue is abnormal
but the nature of the defect, and its relationship to CD symptoms and clinical
outcomes, remain unknown.[14]

METHODS AND RESULTS

As described elsewhere,[15] perinodal adipose tissue and the enclosed mesenteric lymph node and remote-from-node mesenteric and abdominal subcutaneous adipose tissue, were obtained from 10 patients undergoing ileal resection
for CD, and from 7 controls (familial adenomatous polyposis, enterocutaneous
fistulas following surgical misadventure, or benign right-sided colonic polyp).
Samples were frozen within 2 h and stored and transported at –20°C. Triacylglycerol and phospholipids were extracted from each sample and their

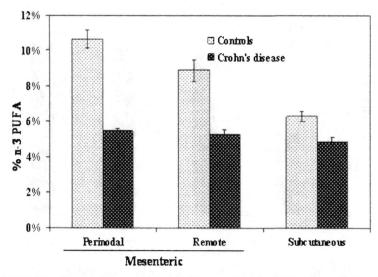

FIGURE 1. The relative abundance of all detectable *n*-3 PUFAs (mostly C18: $3n = 3$) in mesenteric and subcutaneous adipose tissue from control (pale bars; N = 7) and CD (dark bars; N = 10) patients.

fatty acids converted to methyl esters that were separated and identified using gas-liquid chromatography.

In the controls, but not in CD patients, mesenteric adipose tissue has more PUFAs than subcutaneous adipose tissue and the perinodal adipose tissue has more than remote-from-lymph nodes (FIG. 1). The perinodal adipose tissue of normal humans has the site-specific fatty acid composition expected from previous studies of rodents[5] and other monogastric mammals,[16] but this property is absent in CD. In controls, *n*-6/*n*-3 PUFAs are similar in lymphoid cells and their perinodal adipocytes (FIG. 2), but mesenteric lymph node lymphoid cells from CD patients contain fewer *n*-6 PUFAs, even though CD adipose tissue has more *n*-6 PUFAs than controls. More detailed analysis of the phospholipid fatty acids in lymphoid cells released from the mesenteric lymph node (TABLE 1) shows that arachidonic acid, docosahexaenoic acid, and the corresponding C18 PUFAs are much lower in the lymphoid cells of CD patients than in controls. These data are consistent with the conclusion that, as in rodents,[3] the phospholipid fatty acids that comprise the membranes of lymph node lymphoid cells in normal people are derived mainly from triacylglycerol fatty acids in the adjacent perinodal adipose tissue, but the adipocytes surrounding lymph nodes of CD patients fail to supply structurally and metabolically important fatty acids to adjacent lymphoid cells. Lack of the dietary essential arachidonic acid and docosahexaenoic acid may seriously disrupt production of eicosanoid or docosanoid messenger molecules that are important in cell signaling.

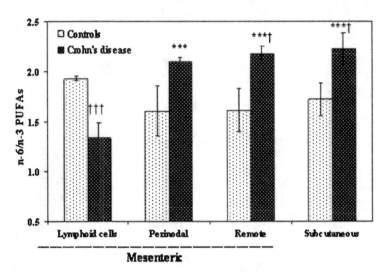

FIGURE 2. The ratio of n-6/n-3 PUFAs in mesenteric lymph node lymphoid cells and in mesenteric and subcutaneous adipose tissue from control (pale bars; N = 6 lymphoid cells, N = 7 adipose tissue) and CD (dark bars; N = 9 lymphoid cells, N = 10 adipose tissue) patients. n-6/n-3: adipose tissue = (C18:2n-6/C18:3n-3); lymphoid cells: n-6/n-3 = ([C18:2n-6 + C18:3n-6 + C20:3n-6 + C20:4n-6)/(C18:3n-3 + C20:5n-3 + C22:6n-3]). Student's t-test: ratios from lymphoid cells compared with those from perinodal adipose tissue: ***$P < 0.001$; control and CD perinodal adipose tissue: [†]$P < 0.05$; [†††]$P < 0.001$. (From Westcott et al.[15])

TABLE 1. The fatty acid composition of lipids extracted from lymphoid cells from mesenteric lymph nodes (Data simplified from Westcott et al.[15])

Fatty Acid		Controls (N = 6)	Crohn's Disease (N = 9)
Palmitic	C16:0	18.8 ± 2.0	25.4 ± 0.08**
Linoleic	C18:2n-6	6.6 ± 0.9	2.4 ± 0.05***
α-Linolenic	C18:3n-3	3.3 ± 0.7	1.9 ± 0.2*
Arachidonic[a]	C20:4n-6	2.6 ± 0.4	0.64 ± 0.02***
Docosahexaenoic[b]	C22:6n-3	1.8 ± 0.3	1.3 ± 0.02*

[a]Immediate precursors of eicosanoid cell signals.
[b]Immediate precursors of docosanoid cell signals.
[b]Student's t-test differences between control and CD values significant at: *$P < 0.0$; **$P < 0.01$; ***$P < 0.000$.

CONCLUSIONS

1. Perinodal adipose tissue identified by site-specific fatty acid composition is present, as expected, in normal human mesentery but not in CD.

2. The fatty acid composition of perinodal, but NOT subcutaneous, adipose tissue correlates with that of lymphoid cells. So, analysis of superficial

adipose tissue biopsies would not adequately reveal the lipids available to lymphoid cells *in vivo*.

3. Although adequate in the adipose tissue, fatty acid precursors of eicosanoid and docosanoid signal molecules are low in mesenteric lymphoid cells in CD, possibly because perinodal adipocytes do not supply fatty acids to adjacent lymphoid cells.

4. Defective perinodal adipose tissue may underlie the adipose and immunological abnormalities in CD and may explain the paradoxical clinical finding that elemental diets high in *n*-6 PUFAs work better than those high in anti-inflammatory *n*-3 PUFAs.[9,10]

ACKNOWLEDGMENTS

E.D.A.W. was supported by S.L.A. Pharma (UK) Ltd. Watford WD25 7SA. S.C.K.'s research is supported by the MRC.

REFERENCES

1. POND, C.M. 2003. Paracrine relationships between adipose and lymphoid tissues: implications for the mechanism of HIV-associated adipose redistribution syndrome. Trends Immunol. **24:** 13–18.
2. POND, C.M. 2005. Adipose tissue and the immune system. Prostaglandins Leukot. Essent. Fatty Acids **73:** 17–30.
3. POND, C.M. & C.A. MATTACKS. 2003. The source of fatty acids incorporated into proliferating lymphoid cells in immune-stimulated lymph nodes. Brit. J. Nutr. **89:** 375–382.
4. MATTACKS, C.A. *et al.* 2004. Site-specific differences in the fatty acid compositions of dendritic cells and associated adipose tissue in popliteal depot, mesentery and omentum, and their modulation by chronic inflammation and dietary lipids. Lymph. Res. Biol. **2:** 107–129.
5. MATTACKS, C.A. & C.M. POND. 1997. The effects of feeding suet-enriched chow on site-specific differences in the composition of triacylglycerol fatty acids in adipose tissue and its interactions in vitro with lymphoid cells. Brit. J. Nutr. **77:** 621–643.
6. MIURA, S. *et al.* 1998. Modulation of intestinal immune system by dietary fat intake: relevance to Crohn's disease. J. Gastroenterol. Hepatol. **13:** 1183–1190.
7. CALDER, P.C. 2003. *n*-3 polyunsaturated fatty acids and inflammation: from molecular biology to the clinic. Lipids **38:** 343–352.
8. GEERLING, B.J. *et al.* 1999. Fat intake and fatty acid profile in plasma phospholipids and adipose tissue in patients with Crohn's disease, compared with controls. Am. J. Gastroenterol. **94:** 410–417.
9. TREBBLE, T.M. *et al.* 2004. Peripheral blood mononuclear cell fatty acid composition and inflammatory mediator production in adult Crohn's disease. Clin. Nutr. **23:** 647–655.
10. O'MORAIN, C. *et al.* 1984. Elemental diet as primary treatment of acute Crohn's disease: a controlled trial. Br. Med. J. **288:** 1859–1862.

11. GASSULL, M.A. *et al.* 2002. Fat composition may be a clue to explain the primary therapeutic effect of enteral nutrition in Crohn's disease: results of a double blind randomised multicentre European trial. Gut **51:** 164–168.
12. BELLUZZI, A. 2002. n-3 Fatty acids for the treatment of inflammatory bowel diseases. Proc. Nutr. Soc. **61:** 391–395.
13. CROHN, B.B. *et al.* 1932. Regional ileitis, a pathologic and clinical entity. J. Am. Med. Assoc. **99:** 1323–1329.
14. SCHÄFFLER, A. *et al.* 2005. Mechanisms of disease: adipocytokines and visceral adipose tissue-emerging role in intestinal and mesenteric diseases. Nat. Clin. Pract. Gastroenterol. Hepatol. **2:** 103–111.
15. WESTCOTT, E.D.A. *et al.* 2005. The fatty acid compositions of lipids in mesenteric adipose tissue and lymphoid cells in patients with and without Crohn's disease and their therapeutic implications. Inflamm. Bowel Dis. **11:** 820–827.
16. POND, C.M. 2003. The contribution of wild animal biology to human physiology and medicine. Écoscience **10:** 1–9.

Intestinal Epithelial Antigen Induces CD4$^+$ T Cells with Regulatory Phenotype in a Transgenic Autoimmune Mouse Model

ASTRID M. WESTENDORF,[a] DUNJA BRUDER,[a] WIEBKE HANSEN,[a] AND JAN BUER[a,b]

[a]*Department of Mucosal Immunity, German Research Centre for Biotechnology, Braunschweig, Germany*

[b]*Institute of Medical Microbiology, Hannover Medical School, Hannover, Germany*

ABSTRACT: Regulatory T cells play a crucial role in the control of immune responses in the intestinal mucosa and their absence may predispose to inflammatory bowel disease (IBD). However, the induction of regulatory T cells at sites of mucosal inflammation is not yet fully understood and may involve antigen presentation by local immature dendritic cells and/or intestinal epithelial cells (IECs). VILLIN-HA mice, which express the hemagglutinin (HA) from influenza virus A exclusively in enterocytes of the intestinal epithelium, were matched with T cell receptor (TCR)-HA mice expressing an $\alpha\beta$-TCR which recognizes a major histocompatibility complex (MHC) class II-restricted epitope of HA in order to determine the impact of antigen presentation by IECs on CD4$^+$ T cell immunity. In VILLIN-HA × TCR-HA mice, peripheral HA-specific lymphocytes showed an activated phenotype and increased infiltration into the intestinal mucosa without destruction of the intestinal epithelium. Mucosal lymphocytes from VILLIN-HA × TCR-HA mice secreted lower amounts of interferon-γ (IFN-γ) and interleukin-2 (IL-2) and exhibited an increased expression of interleukin-10 (IL-10), Nrp-1, and Foxp3, molecules published as markers for regulatory T cells. IECs can take up and process antigen but the antigen presentation capacity of these cells is often inefficient. Functional and molecular characterization of IECs from VILLIN-HA and VILLIN-HA × TCR-HA transgenic mice revealed a direct role in the induction of CD4$^+$ T cells with a regulatory phenotype that maintain intestinal homeostasis.

KEYWORDS: intestinal immunity; transgenic mouse model; regulatory T cells; intestinal epithelial cells

Address for correspondence: Astrid M. Westendorf, Ph.D., Department of Mucosal Immunity, German Research Centre for Biotechnology, Mascheroder Weg 1, D-38124 Braunschweig, Germany. Voice: +49-531-6181942; fax: +49-531-6181748.
e-mail: awe@gbf.de

Ann. N.Y. Acad. Sci. 1072: 401–406 (2006). © 2006 New York Academy of Sciences.
doi: 10.1196/annals.1326.035

INTRODUCTION

The intestinal immune system is constantly undergoing low-grade inflammation that appears to be related to the presence of luminal bacteria.[1] This inflammation is also called physiologic inflammation, in which the gut is poised for, but actively restrained from, full immunologic responses. The mechanisms responsible for controlled inflammation remain poorly defined and probably involve multiple cell types and pathways. Different populations of regulatory T cells, T helper (T_H)3 cells, $CD4^+CD25^+$ or $CD4^+CD45RB^{low}$ T cells or $CD8^+$ suppressor T cells[2-4] have been described as being involved in controlling intestinal inflammation. These regulatory cells mediate suppression in surrounding T cells most likely by secretion of regulatory cytokines, such as interleukin-10 (IL-10) or TGF-β and inhibit inappropriate immune responses toward harmless mucosal antigens.[5,6] Although it is known that intestinal epithelial cells (IECs) are involved in the induction of innate immune responses, particularly in the regulation of uncontrolled T cell responses[7,8] (e.g., by secreting cytokines),[9,10] their role in inducing $CD4^+$ T cell immunity is not yet fully understood. Thus, the purpose of this investigation was to determine the potential of IECs for expression and presentation of a specific self-(auto-) antigen and to induce $CD4^+$ T cell immunity *in vivo*.

RESULTS AND DISCUSSION

In order to investigate the consequences of antigen expression by IECs on the outcome of mucosal homeostasis, we generated transgenic mice expressing the hemagglutinin (HA) from influenza virus A as model antigen under control of the enterocyte-specific VILLIN promoter.[11] This promoter directs protein expression to undifferentiated and mature epithelial cells in the small intestine and colon.[12] Crossing these mice with transgenic animals that express $\alpha\beta$-T cells specific for HA resulted in an animal with autoreactive T cells that recognized HA as a "self" antigen restricted to the IECs. We demonstrate here that in these animals the expression of a self-antigen by IECs is sufficient to trigger the development of autoimmune intestinal inflammation (FIG. 1A). However, the inflammation we found was far less severe than in other models of inflammatory bowel disease (IBD), suggesting that inflammation is partially controlled by regulatory mechanisms. Furthermore, we studied the proliferative capacity and cytokine profiles secreted by mucosal lymphocytes from the transgenic animals in response to antigen stimulation. Whereas intraepithelial lymphocytes (IELs) and lamina propria lymphocytes (LPLs) from TCR (TCR)-HA mice, as well as LPL from VILLIN-HA × TCR-HA transgenic mice, proliferated in a dose-dependent manner, the proliferative capacity was drastically reduced and even abrogated in IELs from VILLIN-HA × TCR-HA mice. The secretion of the classical T_H1 effector cytokines (IFN-γ) and IL-2

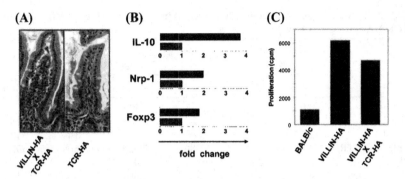

FIGURE 1. (A) VILLIN-HA × TCR-HA transgenic mice are characterized by infiltration of lymphocytes in the lamina propria and intestinal epithelium. Intestinal villi are distended by increased numbers of lymphocytes (*right panel*) when compared to intestinal villi of TCR-HA transgenic mice (*left panel*). **(B)** IL-10, Nrp-1, and Foxp3 expression levels of HA-specific LPL. HA-specific CD4+ LPL were sorted from TCR-HA (*grey bars*) and VILLIN-HA × TCR-HA (*black bars*) transgenic mice. Total RNA was prepared, reverse-transcribed, and mRNA expression levels determined in real-time RT-PCR assays. Mean relative regulation is indicated. Results are from pooled individual mice (*n* > 3) and obtained in duplicate real-time RT-PCR assays. RPS9 mRNA expression served as housekeeping gene control. **(C)** Antigen-presenting capacity of IECs from VILLIN-HA transgenic mice. IECs were isolated from VILLIN-HA, VILLIN-HA × TCR-HA transgenic and BALB/c mice and incubated for at least 72 h with HA-specific CD4+ T cells. Proliferation was measured by ³[H]thymidine incorporation.

was decreased, whereas secretion of the pro-inflammatory cytokines tumor necrosis factor-α (TNF-α), monocyte chemoattractant protein-1 (MCP-1), and interleukin-6 (IL-6) was increased, indicating that while T cells were capable of responding to antigen, the nature of the response was markedly altered. This raises the possibility that a steady-state was reached between regulatory and inflammatory mechanisms, maintaining chronic persistent inflammation. To pursue this hypothesis further, we did comprehensive gene expression profiling of mucosal lymphocytes from VILLIN-HA and VILLIN-HA × TCR-HA transgenic mice and found that autoreactive LPLs and IELs expressed increased levels of the cytokine IL-10 and several genes associated with regulatory T cells (TABLE 1). While some of these genes might simply reflect T cell activation (e.g., OX40, GITR), others such as Nrp-1[13] and especially Foxp3[14] are currently accepted as the best markers for regulatory T cells. Nrp-1, Foxp3, and IL-10 mRNA expression in HA-specific LPLs was therefore confirmed by real-time RT-PCR (FIG. 1B).

Our study suggests that the chronicity of the inflammation, which is the result of a balance between pro- and anti-inflammatory pathways, involves the induction of regulatory T cells. Factors underlying this regulatory network are at present unknown. With the emerging evidence for the existence of different lines of regulatory T cells, the issue of the origin of prospective regulatory

TABLE 1. Selected genes differentially expressed in LPL and IEL from VILLIN-HA × TCR-HA and TCR-HA mice

| Name | Regulation Fold Increase | | Signal Intensity | | | |
	LPL	IEL	LPL stg	LPL dtg	IEL stg	IEL dtg
$\alpha_E\beta_7$	3.0	1.7	135	399	1,206	2,075
Nrp-1	3.5	3.9	25(a)	87	69(a)	269
IL-10	2.6	5.0	288	745	144	713
Tnfrsf18/GITR	3.1	1.2	2,384	7,324	669	772
PD1	4.1	2.8	349	1,446	87(a)	247
Tnfrsf4/OX40	4.2	3.8	1,386	5,804	398	1,494

Total RNA from sorted HA-specific CD4$^+$ T cells was isolated using the RNAeasy kit (Qiagen). Quality and integrity of total RNA isolated from 10^5 sorted T cells was assessed by running all samples on an Agilent Technologies 2100 Bioanalyser. Expression analysis was performed according to the Affymetrix small sample target protocol.

stg: TCR-HA; dtg: VILLIN-HA × TCR-HA; (a): absent, defined by the Affymetrix software algorithm. Results are from pooled individual mice ($n > 3$).

T cells in the intestine becomes more important. IECs are involved in the induction of innate immune responses, particularly in the regulation of uncontrolled T cell responses[7,8] (e.g., by secreting cytokines).[9,10] The ability of IECs to constitutively express molecules involved in antigen presentation including MHC class I and II, and to take up and process soluble antigens, suggests they can also act as antigen presenting cells.[15–17] Lack of costimulatory molecules on the surface of IECs might result in anergy of T cells or the induction of regulatory cells and may be important for maintaining immune homeostasis by suppression of T cell immune responses (FIG. 2). In our model, we clearly found that IECs of VILLIN-HA and VILLIN-HA × TCR-HA transgenic mice,

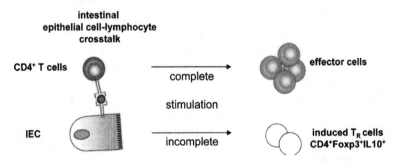

FIGURE 2. Model for the generation of effector and regulatory CD4$^+$ T cell responses in the intestine. Naive lymphocytes are able to enter the intestine. There, they can interact with IECs that have assimilated antigens. Interactions with IECs can subsequently stimulate the naive lymphocytes completely and induce their differentiation into effector lymphocytes. However, incomplete stimulation of naive CD4$^+$ T lymphocytes in the intestine via IECs might result in T cells with a regulatory phenotype.

but not of BALB/c mice, induce proliferation of TCR-HA transgenic T cells (FIG. 1C). Furthermore, co-culture of IECs from VILLIN-HA and VILLIN-HA × TCR-HA mice with naive HA-specific T cells resulted in Foxp3$^+$ CD4$^+$ T cells, highly suggestive of induced regulatory T cells. These studies suggest that IECs are able to directly present self-(auto-) antigens leading to the induction of local regulatory T cells. In the context of chronic mucosal inflammation, this might prevent progression toward overt autoimmunity.

REFERENCES

1. BRANDTZAEG, P., K. VALNES, H. SCOTT, et al. 1985. The human gastrointestinal secretory immune system in health and disease. Scand. J. Gastroenterol. **114**(Suppl.): 17–38.

2. MILLER, A., O. LIDER, A.B. ROBERTS, et al. 1992. Suppressor T cells generated by oral tolerization to myelin basic protein suppress both in vitro and in vivo immune responses by the release of transforming growth factor beta after antigen-specific triggering. Proc. Natl. Acad. Sci. USA **89**: 421–425.

3. MOWAT, A.M., A.G. LAMONT, S. STROBEL & S. MACKENZIE. 1987. The role of antigen processing and suppressor T cells in immune responses to dietary proteins in mice. Adv. Exp. Med. Biol. **216A**: 709–720.

4. SAKAGUCHI, S. 2000. Regulatory T cells: key controllers of immunologic self-tolerance. Cell **101**: 455–458.

5. LUDVIKSSON, B.R., D. SEEGERS, A.S. RESNICK & W. STROBER. 2000. The effect of TGF-beta1 on immune responses of naive versus memory CD4+ Th1/Th2 T cells. Eur. J. Immunol. **30**: 2101–2111.

6. STROBER, W., B. KELSALL & T. MARTH. 1998. Oral tolerance. J. Clin. Immunol. **18**: 1–30.

7. SHAO, L., D. SERRANO & L. MAYER. 2001. The role of epithelial cells in immune regulation in the gut. Semin. Immunol. **13**: 163–176.

8. ALLEZ, M., J. BRIMNES, I. DOTAN & L. MAYER. 2002. Expansion of CD8+ T cells with regulatory function after interaction with intestinal epithelial cells. Gastroenterology **123**: 1516–1526.

9. NEISH, A.S., A.T. GEWIRTZ, H. ZENG, et al. 2000. Prokaryotic regulation of epithelial responses by inhibition of IkappaB-alpha ubiquitination. Science **289**: 1560–1563.

10. KAGNOFF, M.F. & L. ECKMANN. 1997. Epithelial cells as sensors for microbial infection. J. Clin. Invest. **100**: 6–10.

11. WESTENDORF, A.M., M. TEMPLIN, R. GEFFERS, et al. 2005. CD4+ T cell mediated intestinal immunity: chronic inflammation versus immune regulation. Gut **54**: 60–69.

12. PINTO, D., S. ROBINE, F. JAISSER, et al. 1999. Regulatory sequences of the mouse villin gene that efficiently drive transgenic expression in immature and differentiated epithelial cells of small and large intestines. J. Biol. Chem. **274**: 6476–6482.

13. BRUDER, D., M. PROBST-KEPPER, A.M. WESTENDORF, et al. 2004. Neuropilin-1: a surface marker of regulatory T cells. Eur. J. Immunol. **34**: 623–630.

14. BLAIR, P.J., S.J. BULTMAN, J.C. HAAS, et al. 1994. CD4+CD8- T cells are the effector cells in disease pathogenesis in the scurfy (sf) mouse. J. Immunol. **153**: 3764–3774.

15. CAMPBELL, N., X.Y. YIO, L.P. SO, *et al.* 1999. The intestinal epithelial cell: processing and presentation of antigen to the mucosal immune system. Immunol. Rev. **172:** 315–324.
16. HERSHBERG, R.M., D.H. CHO, A. YOUAKIM, *et al.* 1998. Highly polarized HLA class II antigen processing and presentation by human intestinal epithelial cells. J. Clin. Invest. **102:** 792–803.
17. BLUMBERG, R.S., W.I. LENCER, X. ZHU, *et al.* 1999. Antigen presentation by intestinal epithelial cells. Immunol. Lett. **69:** 7–11.

Toll-Like Receptor Expression and Response to Specific Stimulation in Adipocytes and Preadipocytes

On the Role of Fat in Inflammation

J. PIETSCH, A. BATRA, T. STROH, I. FEDKE, R. GLAUBEN, B. OKUR, M. ZEITZ, AND B. SIEGMUND

Charité–Universitätsmedizin Berlin, CBF, Medizinische Klinik I, Hindenburgdamm 30, 12200 Berlin, Germany

ABSTRACT: Data in this study indicate that both adipocytes and preadipocytes express abroad set of TLRs and they also respond to specific stimulation by cytokine production. The may be of relevance to Crohn's disease and a suggests a closer link between adipose tissue and innate immunity.

KEYWORDS: adipocytes; innate immunity; toll-like receptors

So far adipose tissue has mainly been recognized for its role in energy homeostasis. However, data from the last years suggest a close link between adipose tissue and the immune system. For example, adipose tissue is a potent producer of proinflammatory cytokines including IL-6 and TNF-α.[1] Furthermore, adipocytes are the main source of leptin, an adipocytokine that exerts stimulatory effects on various cells from innate and adaptive immunity.[2] A more recent study by Charrire et al. provided evidence that preadipocytes, the precursors of adipocytes, can convert into macrophage-like cells, therefore further linking adipose tissue to innate immunity.[3]

To gain additional information about the interplay between adipose tissue and innate immunity we evaluated whether preadipocytes and adipocytes express functional toll-like receptors (TLRs), a group of pattern-recognition receptors expressed on various cells from innate immunity. Furthermore, we were interested in the possible influence of leptin on TLR expression as well as responsiveness.

Address for correspondence: J. Pietsch, Charité–Universitätsmedizin Berlin, CBF, Medizinische Klinik I, Hindenburgdamm 30, 12200 Berlin, Germany.
e-mail: jeannette.pietsch@freenet.de

Ann. N.Y. Acad. Sci. 1072: 407–409 (2006). © 2006 New York Academy of Sciences.
doi: 10.1196/annals.1326.021

Preadipocyte cell lines were established from the mesenteric fat of wild-type C57BL/6 (BL6) as well as leptin receptor C57BL/KSlep$^{db/db}$ (db/db) and leptin-deficient C57BL/6lep$^{ob/ob}$ (ob/ob) mice, and commitment to the adipocyte lineage was verified in these cells as well as in the similarly studied 3T3L1 cells by induction of differentiation to adipocytes according to standard protocols.[4] Expression of TLR1 to 9 mRNA was tested by PCR and the presence of TLR protein was evaluated by Western blot analysis. Functionality of receptors was tested by TLR-specific stimulation and subsequent evaluation of cytokine production.

Using PCR, expression of various TLR-specific mRNAs was detected in preadipocytes from all cell lines. However, TLR mRNA panels showed leptin dependency and were broadest in the absence of leptin signaling (db/db and ob/ob: TLR 1–9; BL6: TLR 1–7; 3T3L1: TLR 1–4, 6). Interestingly, maturation to adipocytes affected TLR mRNA panels only slightly, but differed between the cell lines studied. Whereas ob/ob and BL6 cells lost TLR7 mRNA, 3T3L1 adipocytes gained expression of TLR9 mRNA.

To confirm expression of the various TLRs on the protein level, Western blot analysis was performed. All TLRs tested (TLR2, TLR3, TLR5, TLR7, and TLR9) were detectable in lysates of preadipocytes and adipocytes from the various cell lines.

To verify the functionality of the TLRs, cells were cultured in the presence of TLR-specific ligands, namely: zymosan (TLR2), poly I:C (TLR3), LPS (TLR4), flagellin (TLR5), loxoribine (TLR7), and ODN 1668 (TLR9). Following 3 days of culture, supernatants were harvested and tested by enzyme-linked immunosorbent assay (ELISA) for the presence of IL-6, TNF-α, and IL-10, all cytokines known to be produced by adipose tissue. However, IL-10 was below detection limit in all samples studied and significant production of TNF-α was restricted to db/db cells. Remarkably, all cell lines were potent producers of IL-6, with cytokine production being significantly higher (10–40-fold increased) in db/db and ob/ob cells than in WT cells. Furthermore, as our prior results intimated, ob/ob and db/db cells were responsive to a broader set of TLR ligands than were WT cells, with LPS being the sole TLR ligand that induced IL-6 production in preadipocytes and adipocytes from each cell line.

In summary, our data indicate that both adipocytes and preadipocytes not only express a broad set of TLRs, but also respond to specific stimulation by cytokine production. Interestingly, both, TLR mRNA panels as well as TLR responsiveness show leptin dependency, indicating a yet unknown effect of leptin. This TLR responsiveness of cells from adipose tissue might not only be of relevance in regard to the hypertrophy of mesenterial fat and bacterial translocation seen in Crohn's disease but suggests an even closer link between adipose tissue and innate immunity than described so far. Thus, adipocytes as well as preadipocytes should be considered as new members of the innate immune system.

REFERENCES

1. COPPACK, S.W. 2001. Pro-inflammatory cytokines and adipose tissue. Proc. Nutr. Soc. **60:** 349–356.
2. RAJALA, M.W. & P.E. SCHERER. 2003. Minireview: the adipocyte—At the crossroads of energy homeostasis, inflammation and atherosclerosis. Endocrinology **144:** 3765–3773.
3. CHARRIÈRE, G. *et al.* 2003. Preadipocyte conversion to macrophage. J. Biol. Chem. **278:** 9850–9855.
4. STUDENT, A.K. *et al.* 1980. Induction of fatty acid synthetase in differentiating 3T3-L1 preadipocytes. J. Biol. Chem. **255:** 4745–5.

Index of Contributors